ECONOMICS
IN
HEALTH CARE

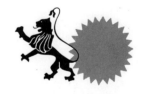

ASPEN SYSTEMS CORPORATION

GERMANTOWN, MARYLAND

1977

Library of Congress Cataloging in Publication Data

Main entry under title:

Economics in health care.

A selection of papers presented in Inquiry from
1966-1977.
Includes bibliographical references.
1. Medical economics—Addresses, essays, lectures.
I. Berman, Howard J. II. Weeks, Lewis E.
[DNLM: 1. Economics, medical. W74 B516e]
RA 410.E35   338.4'7'36210973   77-10860
ISBN 0-89443-026-2

Library of Congress Catalog Card Number: 77-10860
ISBN: 0-89443-026-2

Printed in the United States of America
1 2 3 4 5

To
James E. Veney and Valeda Slade
For all they did to make this possible

Contents

vii **Preface**

1 **Part I—Introduction**

1 Health Care Economics: An Overview
Kong-Kyun Ro

11 **Part II—Framework of Analysis**

13 Health and Public Policy
Herman M. Somers

23 An Economist's View of the Health
Services Industry
Richard M. Bailey

39 Toward the Political Economy
of Medical Care
Sander Kelman

49 A Survey of Economic Models
of Hospitals
Philip Jacobs

63 **Part III—Demand and Supply Analysis**

65 Empirical Research on the Demand
for Health Care
Hyman Joseph

77 Medical Manpower Models: Need,
Demand and Supply
*Judith R. Lave, Lester B. Lave and
Samuel Leinhardt*

107 A Comparison of Hospital Utilization
and Costs by Types of Coverage
Robert Williams

121 The Relationship of Multiple Health
Insurance Coverage and
Hospital Utilization
Bernard Ferber

133 Income and the Use of Outpatient
Medical Care by the Insured
*Joel W. Kovner, L. Brian Browne and
Arnold I. Kisch, M.D.*

141 Trends in Physicians' Patient Volume
Glenn Wilson and James W. Begun

147 The Relationship of Cost
to Hospital Size
W. John Carr and Paul J. Feldstein

167 Case Mix and Resource Use
*John D. Thompson, Robert B. Fetter
and Charles D. Mross*

181 On Grouping Hospitals for Economic
Analysis
Ralph E. Berry, Jr.

189 **Part IV—Pricing and Efficiency**

191 Incremental Pricing Would Increase
Efficiency in Hospitals
Kong-Kyun Ro

201 Efficiency, Incentives and
Reimbursement for Health Care
Mark V. Pauly

219 Prospective Reimbursement of Hospitals
William L. Dowling

237 Incentive Reimbursement as an Impetus
to Cost Containment
Carol McCarthy

247 Consumer Response to Incentives Under
Alternative Health Insurance Programs
Bernard Friedman

251 **Part V—National Health Insurance and Alternate Modes of Delivery**

253 Economic Effects of National Health Insurance
Sylvester E. Berki

273 A Design for a Health Insurance Experiment
Joseph P. Newhouse

297 Estimating the Cost of Health Insurance Programs
David M. Barton and Robert H. Smiley

309 An Evaluation of Prepaid Group Practice
Avedis Donabedian

335 A Financial Planning Model for Evaluating the Economic Viability of Health Maintenance Organizations
John R. Coleman and Frank C. Kaminsky

349 Poverty and Health: A Re-Examination
Myron J. Lefcowitz

361 **Part VI—Applications**

363 Cost Benefit and Cost Effectiveness Analyses in the Health Field: An Introduction
Royal A. Crystal and Agnes W. Brewster

373 Application of Cost-Benefit Analysis to a PKU Screening Program
Kenneth C. Steiner and Harry A. Smith

381 The Application of Economic Analysis to Evaluation of Alcoholism Rehabilitation Programs
J. Michael Swint and William B. Nelson

391 Economics of Disease Prevention: Infectious Kidney Disease
Fredric C. Menz

407 Hospital Costs in Massachusetts: A Methodological Study
Martin S. Feldstein and James Schuttinga

Preface

In its 14 years, *Inquiry* has published a number of landmark papers. Many of these works have been concerned with what was, at the outset of *Inquiry*, the emerging discipline of health economics. As health economics has matured, gaining status as an important area of economic thought and study, the need for teaching references and resource literature has increased. Recognizing both the growing necessity for a comprehensive selection of major health economics writings and the high quality of the contributions published in *Inquiry*, a decision was made to develop this anthology.

The papers selected for presentation span an 11-year period, from 1966 to 1977. Some of the writings have been designated as required reading in graduate programs for health services administration. Some also have become permanent references for practitioners, health planners, policy-makers, and legislators. Other papers within this anthology have been circulated less widely. Nonetheless, they contain findings and conclusions that are valid and provocative. Hence, the editors included them.

In all, each of the papers presented in this collection constitutes an important contribution to the literature. Each deserves the enduring reference qualities that only the medium of a book can provide.

This preface would not be complete without a word of appreciation to those most closely involved with the development of this anthology. The editors therefore wish to express their gratitude to the authors for submitting their research for publication in past issues of *Inquiry*. Without them, of course, this volume would not exist. In addition, acknowledgements are due Marilyn H. Cutler, managing editor of *Inquiry*, who guided the anthology through copy editing and production, and Annie Marie Chevalier, editorial assistant of *Inquiry*, who carefully assembled its contents for the editors.

Lewis E. Weeks
Howard J. Berman

Ann Arbor, Michigan
Chicago, Illinois
June 1977

Part I

Kong-Kyun Ro

Health Care Economics: An Overview

Professor Herbert Klarman, a pioneer in health economics, wrote the first book which has the title of *The Economics of Health* in 1965.[13] The object of this book was "to engage the interest of economists in the problems of (the) health field (13, p. 1.)" Since then, numerous books bearing similar titles have been written and research findings in health economics have appeared in numerous articles. It is interesting to note that Professor Klarman's book, which contained an extensive bibliography, listed 230 references. Seven years later, in another book, *Hospital Economics*,[6] the main contribution of which was an extensive bibliography, Professor Sylvester Berki listed 446 references.

The nearly doubling of references between 1965 and 1972 is a good indication of the rate of growth of research output in health economics. If one were to compile an extensive bibliography in this field today, 800 important references could easily be listed reflecting the shortening of the time during which research output has doubled from seven to five years. The pace of growth of doctoral dissertations in health economics is similar to that of published references. The December 1976 issue of the *American Economic Review* listed 19 doctoral dissertations in the health

field. In 1970, (A.E.R., December, 1970) the number was 8.

Why does one single out the health sector and come up with the name health economics? Agricultural economics, transportation economics and more recently urban economics are forerunners. The reasons for naming the above have been: 1) the importance and public concern focused on these areas of economic inquiry, and 2) the belief that these areas have unique characteristics which distinguish themselves from other areas of economic inquiry.

Factors Contributing to the Growth of Interest and Research Output in Health Economics

Although numerous factors have contributed to the rapid growth of interest and research output in health economics in recent years, three are important. First, expenditures for health services have increased rapidly since the end of World War II, accounting for a steadily increasing proportion of personal consumption expenditures and the Gross National Product. Second, a consensus is held by all groups within the political spectrum that everyone should have access to health services regardless of financial status. Third, the health industry is largely insulated from the market system of rewards and admonitions, thus efficient operation is not a necessity for the survival of its individual members. If an increasing portion of

Kong-Kyun Ro, Ph.D., is Director of Economic Analysis for the Blue Cross Association and Visiting Lecturer of Economics at the University of Illinois, Chicago Circle Campus.

1

a nation's resources were allocated to the products of a competitive industry, it would be of no particular concern to the general public nor to policy-makers. It simply would be a phenomenon of the dynamic process of the economy. The rising costs of health services are a public concern because the health industry is not subject to rigorous processes of competition, yet its product is considered to be one of the necessities of life.

The crux of the problem is that health service is one among a handful of industries in which there is an emerging consensus to eliminate financial barriers to access; at the same time, it is one of the few industries that has no built-in mechanism to promote efficiency. Every means available to guarantee access to health services invariably reduces consumer concern about efficiency; similarly, the prevailing methods of reimbursement tend to reduce provider efficiency. Hence, a unique matching of sociopolitical reality occurs in which the demand for health services becomes highly inelastic in comparison with the structure and pricing system of the health industry. This results in an ever-increasing portion of the nation's resources being allocated to health services without any assurance that these resources are being spent efficiently.

In the early Sixties, the response of economists to the increasing demand for research in the health field was unenthusiastic, if not totally negative. Analyses of economic problems of health services were relegated to a virtual no-man's-land. As recently as 1969, for example, the index of economic articles prepared by the American Economic Association listed for the first time "Economics of Health" as a subject under Welfare, Health, and Education. Prior to that, "Medical Economics" was listed under Health, Education, Welfare, and Poverty.

Of late, an increasing number of economists have directed their attention to the health field because demand for their contribution increased and because new theories have developed that dovetail more closely with analysis of problems of health than did traditional theories. The stepped-up demand for economists in the health field parallels directly the steadily increasing support for economic research, the burgeoning opportunities for economists in teaching and nonacademic positions within the health field and, finally, the increasing use of economists at policy levels.

There are five areas in which development of new theories have been particularly helpful for economists in analyses of the health services industry: 1) human capital; 2) transaction costs and uncertainty; 3) household production and the value of time; 4) technological change and diffusion; 5) interdependent utilities.[24]

With the upsurge in published articles on health economics by prominent economists, health economics has moved into the mainstream of economic thought. Following is a list of several landmark publications. Kenneth Arrow, Nobel Laureate, wrote an article, "Uncertainty and the Welfare Economics of Medical Care," published in the *American Economic Review* in 1963.[2] This touched off the debate on the moral hazard of health insurance. Martin Feldstein's book, *Economic Analysis for Health Service Efficiency*, was published in 1967.[8] Under the initiative of Victor R. Fuchs, the prestigious National Bureau of Economic Research (NBER) began research on health economics in 1966. The first book resulting from NBER research, *Essays in the Economics of Health and Medical Care*, was published in 1972.[10]

Special Characteristics of Health Services as an Economic Commodity

As mentioned earlier, one reason for singling out health services as a special subject of economic inquiry is because they differ significantly from other commodities. Some individuals argue that health services are markedly different from the generality of goods and services and possess certain characteristics that make the market sector unsuited for their production and distribution. Health services, therefore, should be treated as public goods. At issue is whether health care is sufficiently apart from the generality of commodities so that if it were left to make its way in the market system, a substantial malallocation of resources would result.

Next, let us consider the distinctive economic features of health care. The following characteristics are cited most frequently: 1) health care as a mixture of consumption and investment elements; 2) departure of the health industry from the norm of competition; 3) external effects and indivisibility; 4) consumer ignorance of the content of health care; 5) health care as a right.[13]

Health and Health Care as an Investment

Recognition of health as an investment traces back to the 1960s when Theodore W. Schultz wrote a series of articles on the subject of human capital. The first of these articles was published in 1960 and titled "Capital Formation by Education" (December 1960)[20]; the next, "Investment in Human Capital," appeared in March 1961.[21] Later on, Selma J. Mushkin included health, in addition to education, as an investment in her article titled "Health as an Investment," published in October 1962.[16] Eleven years after that, Michael Grossman formulated and defined rigorously the concept and implications of health as human capital.[11]

The recent recognition of health as an investment, together with the increasing interest in research on health as capital, is a result of a shift of emphasis from investment in physical to investment in human capital in the methodology of economic planning; it also represents a movement toward "generalized capital accumulation theory."[12] Discussions, however, of the investment in human capital have been confined for the most part to educational capital and knowledge embodied in the human population.[7] Schultz warned that "by concentrating on education we are in danger of losing sight of other sources of human capital, and, not seeing their contributions, crediting some of them to education."[22] Meanwhile, the increasing public interest in health economics is forcing economists to take a more balanced view of health versus education as sources of investment in human capital.

Flaws in the Market System for Production and Distribution of Health Services

Market imperfections in industries characterized by the presence of monopoly or oligopoly behavior have led to higher prices and lower utilization of resources than those in competitive industries. But market imperfections in health care—particularly in the medical industry—appear to have resulted in higher prices and overutilization of resources by this industry in the United States. This has occurred because market imperfections in the health industry have created a situation wherein providers are placed in a position to generate and manipulate the demand for their product at prices that guarantee the targeted amount of income. In this setting, overutilization of resources may occur because any creation of demand by suppliers is supported by the third-party payment of bills.

The market structure of the medical care industry is a neglected area of research, ergo the need to study further the underlying causes of market imperfections of the industry. In particular, physicians' behavior under the present market and institutional conditions should be examined. Physicians play a central role in the health care that individuals receive. It is this anomaly in the medical market that is the cause of malallocation of resources in the health sector versus the rest of the economy.

Uwe Reinhardt has made a significant contribution through his formulation of a physicians' behavior model.[18] The model is similar to the behavior model of firms in monopolistic and oligopoly markets. According to Reinhardt, an increase in the supply of physicians is likely to lead to physician-induced increases in demand per patient. If such demand increases fail to offset a decline in revenues caused by the decline in the number of patients coming to individual physicians, it likely will lead to increases in physicians' fees. Thus, this macropolicy of increasing aggregate supply of physicians is destined to failure unless the medical market structure is overhauled.

External Effects

Included in the measurement of economic impact of diseases is the study of external effects of disease prevention and treatment. Burton A. Weisbrod formulated a model to study external effects of disease in 1961.[23] Since then, numerous studies have included external effects of disease in their research.[3] But as an important source of external effects, health care has lost its importance owing to the virtual disappearance of communicable diseases in recent years. The potential of external economies in production exists in the drug industry, but patent laws and the lack of competition preclude its realization under the circumstances.

Consumer Ignorance of the Content of Health Care

Some recent progress has been made toward demystifying medicine. The reason: a rise in consumer awareness. But ignorance of what the consumer is buying in the health industry remains more prevalent than in other industries. Moreover, research examining the implications of consumer ignorance in the health industry has been totally lacking. The economics of information and uncertainty should provide a useful starting point for future research in this area.

Health Care as a Right

Based on the proposition that health care is a necessity of life, consensus has been emerging that everyone ought to have access to health care regardless of financial status. It has been argued that the amount of resources allocated to health care throughout the market place (defined as the optimum amount in welfare economics) is less than the "social optimum" in the case of health services. The validity of such political or ethical postulates cannot be resolved on the basis of economics.

Economists nonetheless can point to the fact that when more resources are allocated to one necessity of life, fewer resources are allocated to other real or imagined necessities of life. The problem of economic overutilization of resources in the health industry becomes all the more serious when it is realized that such political belief entails an increase in demand for products which are provided by noncompetitive suppliers in a market that contains imperfections. The assumption underlies the historical fact that a discrepancy exists between the social optimum and the economic optimum of resources allocated to health care as far as government participation in various health care programs is concerned. In his book published in 1968, Odin W. Anderson set forth the issues involved and documented the history of involvement of the public sector in the health field in the United States.[1]

Health Services as an Input for the Production of Health

Most of the basic textbooks define economics as the study of how scarce resources are allocated among competing ends. Following this tradition, health economics can be defined as the study of how scarce resources are allocated between the health sector and other sectors of the economy, as well as how resources are allocated within the health sector among different components that contribute to or produce health.

Figure I provides a schematic view of health economics according to the following definition: Maximization of "utility" is the objective of the economic system depicted by Figure I. If all output is divided into two components—health and others—the first task of health economics is the study of what the optimum allocation of resources is between the two components. If shifting any resources from one to the other results in an increase in utility, the existing allocation is suboptimum. Given the practical application of this definition, the study of health economics should enlighten the national debate on priority between health and other objectives for given relative real costs.

Next, health economics studies of allocation of resources among the components, or inputs, of health. The optimum allocation of resources calls for equating the ratio of the marginal physical product (MPP) of health services to their prices with that of the MPP of environmental factors to their prices. Departure from optimum allocation under the present market structure is likely to occur, because the effective price of health services to consumers is less than the total price charged and because providers do not practice marginal cost pricing. Thus, both the third-party payment of health care and the market imperfection of the health care industry tend to lead to more than optimum allocation of resources to health services and to less than optimum allocation of resources to other inputs of health.

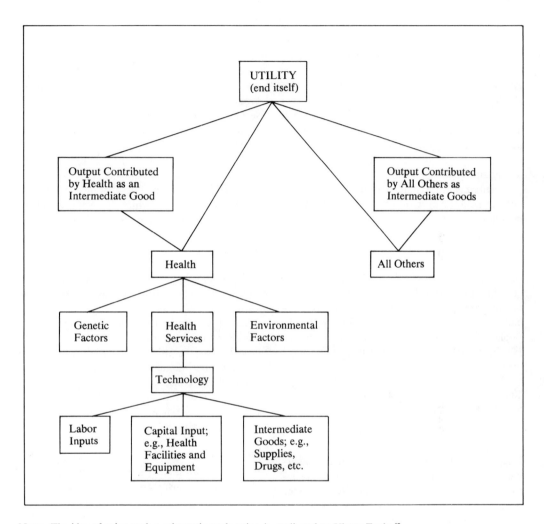

Note: The idea of using such a schematic exploration is attributed to Victor Fuchs.[25]

Figure I. Schematic view of resource allocation into and within the health sector

Viewed this way, spending less for health care is not a question of sacrificing the nation's health for the sake of economy. Rather, it is a question of improving health at the same cost or lower cost while maintaining the same level of health by shifting resources between different inputs for health.

The third level at which health economics studies resource allocation is that of allocation among three broad categories of inputs for the production of health services. As long as technology does not dictate a fixed input-mix, the optimum allocation of resources calls for the same condition; that is, the equation of the ratio of the MPP of an input to its price to that of any other input to its price. The current debate concerning use of sophisticated and complex equipment can be analyzed in terms of the ratio of its contribution to output (health care) relative to its price, compared with the same ratio for other inputs such as labor or drugs.

When examined within the context of health economics, the argument for substituting input of allied health personnel for that of physicians is based on the assumption that the ratio of the MPP of support personnel to its price is higher than the same ratio for physicians. Recognition of such an assumption and examination of its validity belong to health economics studying resource allocation at its fifth level (see Figure I). To be sure, the quest does not stop here. At the sixth level, for example, health economics studies resource allocation among different specialties of given categories of labor, such as physicians and nurses. The study of resource allocation among the increasing subdivisions of inputs can be applied to capital inputs and intermediate goods as well.

Awareness of the nature of health economics enables us to analyze all economic problems of health in terms of resource allocation. Promoting this awareness and the systematic analysis of resource allocation in the health sector is the most valuable contribution made by health economics. Victor R. Fuchs made a major contribution toward the understanding of health economics as the study of resource allocation (as it pertains to the health sector) with publication of his article "Contribution of Health Services to the American Economy" in 1966.[9]

Empirical Analyses of Demand for and Supply of Health Services

What is the cause of rapid inflation in the health sector? Is there a shortage of physicians? What will be the cost of national health insurance? How much savings can be made by introducing a deductible and/or coinsurance feature into health insurance? What is the health manpower requirement of the 1980s?

These are among the important questions asked by policy-makers and by the public. For general economic commodities, the invisible hand of the market system is expected to solve these questions automatically, as buyers and sellers interact at the market place. In the health sector, market imperfection and increasing financial involvement of governments at all levels and the third-party payment methods preclude entrusting the invisible hand to the task. Hence, empirical analyses of demand for and supply of health services are essential in health economics.

Traditionally, demand studies have grouped all factors affecting demand into three categories: price (relative); income (buyer's); taste (H. Joseph). An accurate estimate of

price elasticity of demand for health services is essential in projecting effects of various kinds of (national) insurance, deductible, and co-insurance features. Before Medicare and the spread of health insurance of service benefit-type payment, the price elasticity for health services tended to be underestimated. The dramatic increase in demand for health care since Medicare and other demand increasing programs have forced economists to re-estimate the price elasticity of demand.

It is important to note that health services include components which have many substitutes. To illustrate, inpatient hospital care includes hotel-type and other general nursing services that can be provided through suitable care in the home. This point is supported by a study showing that those living alone tend to stay hospitalized longer than those living with relatives.[19]

Another important factor to recognize in studies of price elasticity of demand for health care is that the price of health care has two components: nominal price charged and the value of the consumer's time.[25] If a person is self-employed, the cost of his foregone income—in other words, the cost of his time while hospitalized—may be a more important factor in deciding how long to stay in the hospital than is the total hospital charge paid mostly by a third party. Waiting and travel time also are costs consumers take into account when seeking health care.

In many instances, studies of price elasticity of demand have taken the form of studies of effects of various types of insurance on utilization (R. Williams, B. Ferber, and J. Kovner, et al.). In these studies, price can be measured by the amount of out-of-pocket expenses as determined by various insurance coverages. Some studies include proxy variables for the cost of time as another component of price.

Depending on measurements used and methods of controlling the effects of other variables on demand, past estimates of price elasticity of demand for various components differ significantly. According to a Rand study, when price is measured by price multiplied by co-insurance, price elasticity for length of hospital stay is estimated at –0.07 with a standard error of 0.035; for admissions, it is –0.22 with a standard error of 1.11; for hospital expenditure the figure is −0.34. For physician services, the price elasticity is −0.06 for office visits with a standard error of 0.03, and −0.2 for physician expenditure with a confidence interval from −0.05 to −0.35.[17]

Studies of income elasticities of demand for health services face more problems than do those of price elasticity of demand. Here is a typical situation: A serious source of bias exists owing to the correlation between one's income and the kind of diseases for which one seeks medical or hospital care. A second source of bias exists owing to the correlation between one's income and cost of one's time. Some studies attempt to avoid the first kind of bias by measuring the quantity demanded as services provided per given episode of disease and also by using a measure of permanent income for the income variable, rather than current income. The second type of bias could be reduced by differentiating between earnings and income and also between self-employed people and those who have fully paid sick leaves.

The first type of bias may arise when the quantity demanded is measured by the number of various categories of services received. Simple correlation of such measures of quantity demanded and income would show that some categories of services are correlated negatively and others positively with income (Kovner, et al.). This does not mean that some categories of services are inferior goods and others normal goods. Instead, it suggests taking the perspective that when seeking care for a given disease, one's choice of input-mix depends on his income. An example of the second kind of bias may arise in the instance when the length of the hospital stay is correlated negatively with the patient's income.[15] This may not be a case of negative income effect, but rather a case of a price effect in which high income reflects a higher cost of time of hospitalization because of a higher foregone income while hospitalized.

Efficiency in the Health Services Sector

As I see it, the central concern of health economics is efficiency: X-efficiency and allocative efficiency.[26] X-efficiency is achieved when an industry, a company, or a nation is producing on the frontier of the production possibility curve for given resources and technology. Allocative efficiency is achieved when a resource is allocated optimally, given scarcity of resources and consumer preferences. In a purely competitive economy, both kinds of efficiency are achieved automatically through the market system. Mounting concern is shared among economists about efficiency in health services, owing to increasing awareness that there is considerable departure from the norm of competition.

There are other industries in which market imperfection tolerates provider inefficiency and leads to income redistribution from consumers to providers. As mentioned before, the exceptional thing about the health care industry is the matching of an imperfect market condition, in which there is no mechanism to ensure provider efficiency, with the condition of discrepancies between the price received by suppliers and that paid by consumers out-of-pocket. This coexistence of two anomalies creates further allocative problems since the health care sector is the type of service industry whose productivity lags behind that of the manufacturing industry under even the best of conditions.

The nature of the technological problem of industry can be appreciated when it is observed within the framework of William Baumol's macroeconomic model of unbalanced growth.[4] Baumol developed a two-sector model according to the technological structure of industry. In the "progressive sector," labor productivity increases at a continuously compounded rate while it remains constant in the "non-progressive sector." The role played by labor differentiates the two sectors. Labor is primarily an instrument, "an incidental requisite for the attainment of the final product" in the progressive sector, whereas in the nonprogressive sector, "labor is itself the end product."

According to this model, if one assumes wage diffusion where money wages in the nonprogressive sector rise in pace with money wages in the progressive sector (with or without a lag), industries in the nonprogressive sector have two alternatives. Either outputs of this sector vanish ultimately or their cost increases without limit. The former alternative is likely to occur when the demand for output is elastic. The latter alternative is likely to occur if government or other sources sustain the demand for output and/or demand is highly inelastic. The demand for health care is sustained by a third-party payment system and government subsidies, and furthermore, it is produced in a non-competitive industry. As a result, its output has not declined but its cost has been rising rapidly and the continuation of rapid increase in the near future appears certain.

There is a tendency among suppliers to point to the technological structure of the industry as the cause of rapid cost inflation of its output in recent years. The economists' concern is whether health care is produced at the frontier of the production possibility, given the technological nature of the industry. Their concern appears to be justified, owing to the fact that there is a considerable distance to go before achieving X-efficiency in the industry. Consequently, various proposals are made to rectify some of the undesirable consequences of anomalies within the health care industry. An example is the growing number of proposals to improve producer efficiency by introducing incentive features into the reimbursement system.

Alternative modes of service delivery also have been proposed. Prepaid group practices and HMOs are evaluated here as a possible solution (Donabedian and Coleman, et al.). To rectify the undesirable consequences of anomalies stemming from triple roles assumed by physicians in the United States, legal and other institutional changes are suggested. Illustrations of these proposed changes include guaranteed free entry to the medical profession to all "qualified" applicants, enabling allied health personnel to compete with physicians at the point of entry,[18] and requiring all physicians to work on a salary basis.

To improve consumer efficiency, various proposals have been made to establish a direct link between the price received by the provider and the price paid by consumers out-of-pocket (Friedman). Incremental pricing of hospital care also is suggested as a way to improve both consumer and producer efficiency (Ro).

If marginal pricing is practiced in such a way that a consumer's out-of-pocket payment reflects the marginal cost of the services he receives, then consumer and provider efficiency is improved. At the same time, hospitals can reduce overhead costs by stabilizing demand fluctuation through a system of giving consumers an incentive to come at off-peak days for nonemergency treatment.

Even if adopted, some proposals lack effectiveness in introducing incentives for efficiency, while others do not possess the political feasibility of being adopted in the first place. The best hope of achieving efficiency in the health sector lies in the change of the sociopolitical climate. This would enable the nation to adopt some drastic changes in the modus operandi of production and distribution in the health services industry.

Summary and Concluding Remarks

Consensus continues to grow that everyone ought to have access to health services. This consensus has prompted private and government responses in the form of spreading health insurance, Medicare and Medicaid. The public, in turn, has become increasingly aware of the results of these responses as is reflected in the rapid growth of health care prices and greater portions of the nation's resources being allocated to the health care industry.

If rising health care prices were the necessary and inevitable result of the interplay of supply and demand in a competitive market, the increasing portion of the nation's resources allocated to the health care industry would be of no alarming concern to the general public nor to policy-makers. It simply would be a phenomenon of the dynamic process of the economy. As things stand, however, the rising costs of health services *are* a public concern, because the health services industry is insulated largely from the market system of rewards and admonitions and because the consumer demand for health services is expressed through the third-party payment system. The market structure of the health industry, plus the discrepancy between the price paid to suppliers and that paid by consumers out-of-pocket, creates a situation in which there is no mechanism to ensure provider or consumer efficiency.

Heightened awareness of problems created by this unique situation have contributed to the rapid growth of interest and research output in health economics. Economists have been called upon increasingly to participate in formulating policies. At the same time, new economic theories have been developed which are more useful in analyzing economic problems of health care and health than were the traditional ones. The effect has been mutually reinforcing wherein more economists have been encouraged and enticed to study the health field and this, in turn, has led to the development of more new economic theories to deal with its problems. The result has been an expanded output of high quality research in health economics during recent years.

Numerous proposals have been made for improving efficiencies. Among them: To approximate the market system of pricing, various incentive reimbursement formulae and marginal cost pricing have been suggested (Ro, Pauly, Dowling, and McCarthy); to improve the operational aspects of the health care industry, application of the latest techniques of management science have been proposed (Coleman and Kaminsky); to modify and improve behavior patterns of the health care industry, alternative modes of delivery, various forms of government regulation, institutional, and peer overseeing mechanisms have been proposed (Donabedian and Newhouse). To date, though, all of these proposals have had only limited success.

At the same time that policy-makers and health economists continue to seek politically acceptable methods of improving efficiency in the health industry, what is politically acceptable has been changing—slowly yet unmistakably. With these two forces at work, eventual changes surely will emerge to place health care efficiency on a level that everyone can live with.

References and Notes

1 Anderson, Odin W. *The Uneasy Equilibrium*. New Haven: College and University, 1968.

2 Arrow, Kenneth. "Uncertainty and the Welfare Economics of Medical Care," *The American Economic Review*, *53* (December 1963), 941–973.

3 Barlow, Robin. "The Economic Effects of Malaria Eradication," *The American Economic Review*, *57* (May 1967), 130–148.

4 Baumol, William J. "Macroeconomics of Unbalanced Growth: The Anatomy of Urban Crisis," *The American Economic Review*, *56* (June 1966), 415–426.

5 Becker, Gary S. "A Theory of the Allocation of Time," *The Economic Journal, 75* (September 1965), 493–517.

6 Berki, Sylvester. *Hospital Economics*. Lexington: Heath, 1972.

7 Blaug, Mark. *Economics of Education: A Selected Annotated Bibliography*. Oxford and New York: Oxford University Press, 1966.

8 Feldstein, Martin. *Economic Analysis for Health Service Efficiency*. Amsterdam: North Holland Publishing Company, 1967.

9 Fuchs, Victor R. "Contribution of Health Services to the American Economy," *Milbank Memorial Fund Quarterly, 44, part 2* (October 1966), 65–101.

10 Fuchs, Victor R., ed. *Essays in the Economics of Health and Medical Care*. New York: National Bureau of Economic Research, 1972.

11 Grossman, Michael. "On the Concept of Health Capital and the Demand for Health." *Journal of Political Economy 80*, No. 2 (March–April 1972), 223–56.

12 Johnson, Harry G. "Toward a Generalized Capital Accumulation Approach to Economic Development," in *Residual Factors and Economic Growth*. Paris: Organization for Economic Cooperation and Development, 1961, pp. 219–225.

13 Klarman, Herbert. *The Economics of Health*. New York and London: Columbia University Press, 1965.

14 Klarman, Herbert. "Syphilis Control Programs," in Robert Dorfman, ed. *Measuring Benefits of Government Investments*. Washington, D.C.: The Brookings Institution, 1965.

15 Leibenstein, Harvey. "Allocative Efficiency vs. 'X-efficiency'," *The American Economic Review, 56* (June 1966), 392–415.

16 Mushkin, Selma J. "Health as an Investment," *Journal of Political Economy, 70, no. 5, part 2* (October 1962), 129–157.

17 Newhouse, Joseph P. and Phelps, Charles E. "New Estimates of Price and Income Elasticities of Medical Care Services," in Richard N. Rossett, ed. *The Role of Health Insurance in the Health Sector*. New York: National Bureau of Economic Research, 1976.

18 Reinhardt, Uwe E. *Physician Productivity and the Demand for Health Manpower*. Cambridge: Ballinger, 1975.

19 Ro, Kong-Kyun. "Patient Characteristics, Hospital Characteristics and Hospital Use," in Victor R. Fuchs,

ed., *Essays in the Economics of Health and Medical Care*. New York: National Bureau of Economic Research, 1972.

20 Schultz, Theodore W. "Capital Formation by Education," *Journal of Political Economy, 68* (December 1960), 571–583.

21 Schultz, Theodore W. "Investment in Human Capital," *The American Economic Review, 51* (March 1961), 1–14.

22 Schultz, Theodore W. "The Reckoning of Education as Human Capital," in W. Lee Hansen, ed. *Education, Income and Human Capital*. New York: National Bureau of Economic Research, 1970.

23 Weisbrod, Burton A. *Economics of Public Health*. Philadelphia: University of Pennsylvania Press, 1968.

24 This list is based upon a reference prepared by Victor Fuchs.

25 The role of the cost of time in influencing consumer behavior has been formulated systematically by Gary S. Becker.[5]

26 These terms are coined by Harvey Leibenstein in his article.[15]

Part II

Framework Of Analysis

This opening section provides perspective on the role that economics can play in analyzing and financing solutions to health and medical care problems. It also supplies some background on the economic and political nature of these problems.

In the first paper, Herman Somers presents the sociopolitical and economic background of problems of health and medical care. He contends that the factors which complicate the health care system are not so much those elements that contribute to the failure of the market system to solve its problems. Rather, says Somers, it is the fact that, in spite of the extensive amount of public financing, health care remains predominantly a private industry.

Somers provides insight into the political process by explaining why there is no cohesive national policy on health. He points out that in a case such as national health policy, the controversy is many-faceted and deeply felt. In a democratic society such as ours, therefore, one must learn to live with inconsistencies and compromises. Somers endorses marginalism in politics; by this he means that when the bargaining process gets messy, progress should be made and measured incrementally.

As for allocative efficiency, Somers—like many other economists—thinks that the shifting of resources from health and medical care to other factors that contribute to health will promote allocative efficiency in the production of health.

The second paper, by Richard Bailey, demonstrates how basic concepts in economics can be applied to health care issues. Useful analyses of the medical care market in terms of competitive and monopoly models are presented.

In the third paper, Sander Kelman offers a contrast to Bailey in that Kelman uses a "dialectical" model to analyze health issues. Whereas Bailey relies on microtheory to give a background, Kelman's analyses are based on what appear to be the Marxian theory of history.

Finally, the paper by Philip Jacobs deals with the important issue of the behavior model of hospitals. An incisive survey of economic models of hospitals is set forth. Various models presented here attest to the fact that hospitals are an anomaly as a firm in microtheory.

11

Robert D. Eilers
Memorial Lecture

Leonard Davis Institute
of Health Economics
University of Pennsylvania
February 26, 1975

Health and Public Policy
Originally Published in June 1975

Herman M. Somers

Reprinted with permission of the Blue Cross Association, from *Inquiry:* Vol.XII, No.2, pp.87-96. Copyright © 1975 by the Blue Cross Association.

Complaints are frequent that the United States lacks a national health policy. What that allegation means is rarely made clear. Policy means different things to different people. But, if by policy one means legislative and governmental administrative actions, it is conspicuous that this nation has been spawning health policies at a proliferating and bewildering rate ever since World War II. Keeping up with the multiplicity of policies has become a formidable challenge, and few succeed.

In this fiscal year the nation is spending for health and medical care about $116-billion;[1] in 1950, we spent $12-billion. That is almost a 10-fold increase. On a per capita basis we have moved from about $78 to an estimated $530 per person. Even in constant dollars—removing the influence of inflation—the increases are almost as impressive. The public portion of these expenditures has accelerated at a far more rapid pace than the total. Government, at all levels, spent well over $41-billion for health care in 1974, compared to $3-billion in 1950. During the 10-year period, 1965 to 1974, government increased its payments by 333 percent. Public expenditures moved from 25 percent of the total in 1950 to 40 percent in 1974.[2]

Herman M. Somers Ph.D. is Professor of Politics and Public Affairs, Woodrow Wilson School of Public and International Affairs, Princeton University (Princeton, NJ 08540).

This is the first in a series of annual lectures on health care topics presented by the Leonard Davis Institute in memory of Dr. Robert D. Eilers, who was founder and director of the Institute until his untimely death on March 1, 1974. For the five years prior to his death, Dr. Eilers was a valued member of the Editorial Board of Inquiry. *We are pleased to have the honor of publishing this first lecture in the memorial series.*

This, I submit, in itself represents a policy—and an important one. Government has now committed itself to massive expenditures for health care. It has allotted progressively larger portions of the government budget and induced steadily higher proportions of our total wealth —gross national product—to this field. This has been accompanied by governmental involvement in the full spectrum of health activities.

Access

The largest and most obvious outlet for these expenditures has been the attempt to enlarge access to health care through such programs as Medicare and Medicaid. Precise data are not available, but the indications are that utilization of health services has been substantially increased, probably more than doubled per capita since 1950. In recent years the poor on average have become as active utilizers of services as the rest of the population, although, of course, they need much more—and other serious historical inequities remain. In fact, to a large extent it has been the improvement in the circumstances of the relatively deprived that has helped sensitize us to the many gross inequities that remain.

There have been unhappy and unplanned "side effects" of these new expenditures such as an acceleration of an already serious inflation of prices and costs, and various abuses and corruption, particularly in nursing homes.

Research and Construction

For some time now, government has been paying for more than 90 percent of all serious biomedical research in this country. This is an important policy. There are many who are convinced that by far the most important improvements we can look forward to in health care are likely to result from the products of the research centers rather than direct expenditures for health services.

But, here too, there are many protests about undesirable "side effects." It is alleged that an unduly large proportion of physicians have been diverted from delivery of health care to research, and that the large research grants flowing from government to medical schools have distorted the teaching functions of the schools.

Government has also steadily increased its financial support for construction of medical facilities: hospitals, clinics, etc. Last year more than a third of all construction costs for both private and public facilities was paid for by government.

Medical Manpower

A few years ago the nation decided on an all-out drive to increase the supply of medical manpower, in all categories. Federal support for health professions education reached its legislative apogée with the passage of the Comprehensive Health Manpower Training Act of 1971. Massive support has been furnished to encourage increased enrollments and development of new schools.

Between 1968 and 1974, 20 new medical schools were created, bringing the total to 114, which was 25 percent more schools than in 1951. The number of students increased even more rapidly. In 1974 we graduated 84 percent more M.D.s than in 1951, and 42 percent more than in 1968. The accelerating trend is perhaps best indicated by pointing out that the first-year class in medical schools in 1973–1974 was 14,124, and this was 25 percent more than that year's graduating class.[3] As a result of such movement, the physician/population ratio rose to a record high in 1974, and now compares favorably with any other Western society.

This policy also is subject to mounting attacks. There are increasing fears that we may have gone too far and that we are moving toward a costly surplus of physicians. (The province of Ontario has recently undertaken to limit the admission of additional physicians in order to contain costs; the government calculates that every additional physician generates at least $150,000 of additional medical costs annually.) It is also questioned whether medical schools have been encouraged to operate on too extravagant a scale. There are increasing allegations that the training the schools are offering with the new money is, in fact, not being directed toward meeting the health needs that were the justification for the additional financial support. The schools are being blamed for an excessive movement to specialization, so that even though we increase the supply of physicians there is a decline in the number available for primary care.

There are increasing protests that at the same time that we have been rapidly expanding our own supply of physicians we have been encouraging an even more rapid entry of foreign medical graduates, whose training for delivery of health services is widely questioned. In 1972, 46 percent of all new licentiates were FMGs.[4] In each of the last four years for which data are available (1970–1973), the number of FMGs admitted to the United States exceeded the total number graduated that year from U.S. medical schools. The wide use of undereducated physicians, often unlicensed, who have either not taken or have failed a licensing examination, and who have never passed a proficiency examination, was recently labeled a "medical underground" in one of our leading medical journals.[5]

The federal government has tried to cope with the problem of geographic imbalance by subsidizing clinical facilities in rural and underserved areas and by creation of the National Health Service Corps, which subsidizes young physicians who agree to serve for a limited period in underserved areas. Its history is yet too brief to evaluate results.

Structure and Organization

Government has even undertaken to reform the organization and structure of the delivery system. Almost 30 years ago, the Congress passed the Hospital Survey and Construction Act, commonly known as Hill-Burton. The preamble of that Act has often been described as one of the most advanced statements of public policy ever made in this country for the development of regionalized medical care. The legislation, many times renewed over the following years, did stimulate and help finance thousands of new and modernized hospital beds, particularly in rural areas.

Now the complaint is that the country is substantially over-bedded and that this is a major factor in the inflation of costs. Many people are calling for an absolute moratorium on all construction and expansion of hospital capacity. Moreover, no visible progress has been made toward regionalization or rationalization of services or health care institutions. Clearly, a public policy pronouncement, however earnest its intent, is not to be confused with a pragmatic achievement.

With a similar goal, the Congress passed the Regional Medical Program legislation in 1965 (P.L.89-239). Some very useful individual and special projects mark the history of RMP, but its underlying goal of regionalization completely eluded the program, which is now entering its final days.

In 1966, Congress passed the Comprehensive Health Planning Act (P.L. 89-749), subsidizing the operation of health planning agencies in every state and in smaller geographic areas throughout the country. The functions of such agencies were only vaguely defined, but systemization of health care delivery was a primary policy intent. CHP is now being phased out in favor of a new legislative effort, the National Health Planning and Resources Development Act of 1974 (P.L.93-641). But we are no closer to systemization now than we were in 1966, and fragmentation remains the most conspicuous hallmark of the delivery structure.

Both the legislation of 1966 and the new 1974 law contain ringing declarations of public policy in their preambles. The 1966 Act declared that access to adequate health care was a right of every citizen; and the 1974 Act opens with the statement, "The achievement of equal access to quality health care at a reasonable cost is a priority of the Federal Government." A priority is, I presume, intended to be a policy, but it would not be fair to expect the 1974 law alone to bring us very much closer to the goal than did the 1966 legislation.

HMOs

Five years ago, in 1970, the Department of Health, Education and Welfare, then under Elliot Richardson, proclaimed with considerable fanfare that the promotion and support of health maintenance organizations was to be the "centerpiece" of the Administration's health care strategy, because HMOs represented a more efficient way of organizing and delivering health services. HEW announced its intention of spotting the country with enough HMOs to be available to 90 percent of the population by 1980.[6]

HEW promptly undertook to furnish financial support for the policy, even in advance of congressional action. In 1973, Congress finally enacted the Health Maintenance Organization Act, authorizing $375-million to assist in the financing of HMOs. It also undertook to stimulate HMOs by passing a mandatory requirement that all employers of 25 or more employees covered by the Fair Labor Standards Act must, in their employee health insurance plan, offer an HMO option to each employee, wherever one exists. It also authorized the bypassing of any restrictive state laws against HMOs.

Despite all this, the movement toward HMOs has been disappointingly slow. Best estimates are that HMOs are now serving about six to seven million people, less than 4 percent of the population.[7] It has again been made clear that even laws, public policy, and public monies do not rapidly alter patterns of behavior of consumers or providers, and that human institutions have a stubborn tenacity for survival.

Experience and Perspective

This list is, of course, only a sampling of some of the better known federal activities of recent years and omits mention of a significant multitude of state actions. Yet I have found that in our impatience for more progress and new action, we often tend to overlook or understate the extraordinary volume and variety of past and present governmental efforts—currently costing about $43-billion a year and sweeping upward. The amount of experience we have accumulated with governmental activity in health care is now prodigious; it should be instructive. Yet the historical experience seems in the main to go unappraised, almost unnoticed, as I believe examination of current literature and contemporary policy debate will confirm. It is commendable and necessary to look ahead, but it is also prudent to look back periodically. It may add enlightenment to our vision of the future.

The lessons of our experience are numerous and widely suggestive. However, I will confine myself to two areas: the first concerns the politics of health, and the second has to do with the effect of medical care on health, a matter that has become of profound concern to me.

Politics and Policy

When people complain about a lack of national policy, they obviously cannot mean quite that, as it is too apparent that policies are legion. They are really saying that they are displeased with the policies; or, more frequently, they complain that the various policies lack coherence, that they are frequently contradictory, often fragmentary, tentative and halting.

This is, of course, very true. I do find puzzling, however, the apparent notion that this in some way differentiates the health field from other areas of public concern. That phenomenon characterizes foreign policy, economic policy, labor policy, welfare policy, and all others of importance. With some variations in particulars, related to each field, the reasons are essentially the same. The policies emerge from essentially the same political process.

In a country of continental dimensions, large issues cut across a multitude of diverse and conflicting interests, and the stakes are often high. We are sometimes told government is not responsive. Yet the problems people point at usually are direct consequences of the fact that governmental machinery, both legislative and administrative, dances to many tunes because it *is* responsive. It is, as it must be, responsive to diverse constituencies pursuing different goals. It marches to discordant beats of varied drummers, each of whom has a large enough drum to be heard and respected—each of whom has some power base among the multitude of power centers in our society, rarely powerful enough to get its own way but influential enough

to be able to stop the opposition from getting its way.

The normal pattern is either to accept stalemate or to get some kind of action through a process of bargaining, compromise, and accommodation. This may come about in a settlement that gives two or three proponents of divergent policies their own partial victories on condition they permit the others to have their victories simultaneously. Or, the bargaining may lead to elimination or softening of particular provisions that are completely offensive to one or more large interests too strong to be overcome, resulting in a program that is acceptable to the majority of interests, although not fully satisfactory to any of them. Not surprisingly, such legislation will tend to be general, ambiguous, even conflicting, and subject to many different interpretations and actions at the administrative level.

Similar pressures impinge upon and influence the administrative policy process. As a result we frequently hear demands for reorganization or "coordination" of the administrative structure. There is almost always a good case to be made for reorganization—if only to avoid bureaucratic arteriosclerosis—but no amount of reorganization is likely to produce full agreement on goals, or how best to achieve them, or end the fragmentation among health interests. Policies, administrative and legislative, will reflect these realities.

This, of course, tends to sound messy and unsatisfactory, especially if, in our mind's eye, we envision the alternative as being a clear and coherent expression of policy that we support. It may not seem quite so unsatisfactory, and the messiness more tolerable, if we consider the possibility that the clear and coherent policy could be one that we would utterly deplore. A winner-take-all game is only attractive to the winner.

In any case, where controversy is many-faceted and deeply felt, the only way to a unified and consistent national policy is through authoritarianism. Those who would function effectively in a democratic society learn to live with inconsistencies and compromises and try to make progress incrementally within a bargaining process. It may rankle, but as Woodrow

Wilson wrote a long time ago, "It is a strenuous thing this living the life of a free people." I often think of the appropriateness of George Shultz's observation when be became the first director of the Office of Management and Budget a few years ago, "Those who can't stand ambiguity can't be creative here."

Some Special Factors

There are, additionally, some special complicating factors in the case of health care. Among these are, first, that despite the great degree of public financing, health care remains predominantly a private sector industry. The creation and administration of public policy for a widely dispersed and varied set of enterprises dominated by the private sector involves numerous delicate legal and bureaucratic complexities. Things often have to be done by indirection and devising of roundabout procedures.

Second, there are historical and practical problems of intergovernmental relations. Historically and, many believe, constitutionally the states are the regulators of health care. They alone, for example, license practitioners and institutions and set standards. By its inherent character as a personal and individualized service, health care is provided at the local level. The problems of reconciling into a national policy the interests and functions of all levels of government that must be involved are both sensitive and formidable.

Third, health care is full of unresolved issues about which our factual knowledge is sparse and uncertain. For example, we have been debating the question of quality of care for a long time and most people accept the idea that some sort of policy is needed to assure a reasonable standard of quality. But the concept of quality is as elusive as it is important. There is little agreement on its definition, or on criteria, or upon how one goes about effectuating quality controls.

The problem is illustrated by the Professional Standards Review Organizations (PSRO) legislation passed by Congress two years ago (P.L.92-603). The purpose was the monitoring and promotion of quality of care as well as cost containment. Necessarily, the law states mainly high level objectives; it could not and does not

attempt to spell out what quality is. It leaves that to the administrators and the hundreds of local PSRO organizations, most yet to be established, to determine. We are all aware of the struggles, the compromises, and the evasions now in progress in the attempt to find acceptable standards and procedures. The American Medical Association has, in another context, taken court action against the government, claiming that it does not have the power to mandate peer review. And a great many physicians honestly fear that the process could actually prove a set-back to quality. Yet, it is clear that protection of quality does require professional peer review, within a context of public accountability, and all one can do is to explore within such parameters.

Another example is the delivery system. For a great many years we have been hearing eloquent demands that the delivery system needs to be reformed. By now most people appear to agree that reform is desirable, if not necessary. But what kind of reform? What specifically are the next steps? Here the consensus collapses. There appear to be as many different notions of how best to reorder delivery as there are advocates of reform. And, as in the case of quality, none can definitively demonstrate that he is right or that his reform would really be an improvement. The policy process becomes ensnared in situations where no witnesses can offer persuasive positive facts.

There is thus a certain inevitability about the vagueness, the complexity, and the unresolved issues that characterize our most recent assault on the problem of systemization, the National Health Planning and Resources Development Act of 1974, which was signed into law on January 4, 1975. This law is also facing a court test by the AMA. The Act, among other things, replaces Hill-Burton, Comprehensive Health Planning, and the Regional Medical Program, and moves on to a somewhat different track. The mood is frankly experimental and exploratory. It is hoped that the uncertainties and conflicts will be worked out in the process of administrative action, and that at least some framework for regulation may be available by the time national health insurance arrives on the scene.

There is little doubt that we will be in for

more frustrations and aggravation. But I would plead for tolerance and restraint. When we cannot be sure of the right road, cautious probing may be the only sensible behavior. Certainly it is better than endless debate and no action.

A final point is perhaps only a corollary—it is a reminder of the limits of human and institutional capacities. Not everything we would like to see done can be done. Not everything that can be done lies within the competence of the federal government. Whenever we discover an inefficiency or an inequity or a malfunctioning that seems to need correcting, we almost instinctively say, why does not the federal government change all that?

If there is anything that should have become visible in the last decade or more it is that there are severe limits on what large bureaucracies can do well, or do at all. Our politicians are responsive—perhaps too much so. If strong enough demands are made they will respond, even when they know the proposed solution may not work. So, if we are tired of failures, we need to be more selective in what we demand of government. We have to develop a greater consciousness of the technical and administrative problems that accompany grand scale proposals. We have to ask: desirable or not, can this program be carried out by government? And, are governmental monopolies any healthier for society than private monopolies? It is one thing to enunciate lofty goals, but quite another to know how to implement them.

National Health Insurance

These political observations seem to have immediate pertinence to at least one major current issue of concern to everybody interested in health care—the debate over national health insurance. For several years now, people have been led to expect that a comprehensive national plan would be passed in that year, and many are still saying, "this year for sure." The fact is that no bill of any description has even been reported out by any committee in either House. People have apparently been misled by the fact that every important interest group —from the AMA to the AFL-CIO to the Health Insurance Association of America and the Administration—has sponsored some sort of NHI proposal, and a majority of congressmen, as well as the public, appear to be in favor of a national plan.

This is misleading because the proposals of the various groups differ sharply on the essentials: how the program will be financed; who will administer it; the scope of the program; and the like. Thus far, most of the leading contestants have not been willing to participate in the normal political process; they have refused to bend or bargain. The result has been a drawn-out stalemate. If postures do not change this will continue because no proposed plan can now, or in the foreseeable future, command anything resembling a majority. Some of the purists allege with pride that they are "standing on principle" when they refuse to compromise. But the nation has been paying a heavy price for their "purity." If the parties had been amenable to compromise, the country could already have been started on the road to comprehensive national health insurance. It would have been a modest and incomplete start, but one that could be added to and adjusted incrementally over the ensuing years. This continues to be true. If the chief contending forces are willing to accept something much smaller than their proposals contemplate, we could have legislation in this session of the Congress. Otherwise, stalemate is sure to continue.

Health Care and Jobs

One last point about the politics of health. The enormous growth of the health care economy has made it a leading source of employment and an important economic prop for many communities. There are now 4.5 million persons employed in the industry, not counting the large number engaged in the manufacture of pharmaceuticals and in the health insurance business. It is one of the largest employers in the nation. Thus, debates over proposals for particular health care expenditures or programs often, in reality, relate more to economic protectionism for providers of all stripes, employees, industries, and communities than they do to health —although the public rhetoric is of course aimed at health. An increasing number of strong vested interests have developed, as is inevitable in a $100-billion industry with so much at stake—and this means more pockets of resistance to change irrespective of basic ideological orientation.

When it was proposed to close some public health hospitals, the real issue became not whether those hospitals were still serving a useful purpose, but the economic blow it would represent to the communities in which they were located. When a new neighborhood health center is under discussion, the central issue is often the employment opportunities it will offer to local people. When a hospital reorganization or merger is contemplated, the position of employee unions will be determined by its effect upon jobs, and the position of the medical staffs by the effects on their practices.

I am not one to take the problem of employment and unemployment lightly, especially in times like the present. But it is always useful to recognize what the real issue is and to understand that many alleged health care decisions are being taken on grounds that have little or nothing to do with health as such, and that most of the pressures influencing health care policy are actually generated from within the health care industry itself.

Health Services and Health

I now turn to a second broad lesson of recent history. In the waves of enthusiasm for opening up previously barricaded access to medical care, we may have lost our sense of proportion. When people speak of national health policy it usually turns out that they are really talking about health care policy—or, more specifically, medical care. This can be dangerously misleading, for the two are not the same. Our goal presumably is, or should be, health. Medical care is not an end in itself, but one of the instrumentalities toward achievement of health. The utility of medical care as a purveyor of better health can easily become overvalued in relation to the many other factors determining health, and extreme overemphasis on medical care can threaten both the quality of medical services themselves as well as the public health.

The spectacular increases in health care expenditures and in utilization of medical services in recent years has not been accompanied by improvement in the health of Americans, as measured by any available indices of health status. After half a century of steady and marked improvement, the crude death rate for the United States ceased to improve during the 1960s and into the 1970s. It has remained virtually stable for well over a decade, fluctuating between 9.3 and 9.7 per thousand. The age-adjusted death rate was 7.6 in 1960, 7.3 in 1969, 9.5 for males both years.[8]

When the data are broken down by age and sex it appears that the overall stability obscures particulars that are far more disturbing. The general stability resulted primarily from the changing age composition of the population. During the 1960s, there was a decline in the infant population (under one year), which has a death rate far above the general or crude rate. On the other hand, the population in the low-risk age groups, between five and 44, increased.[9] This tends to give the overall rate a more favorable skewing.

There has been improvement in infant mortality and length of life for females, and in the control of some remaining infectious diseases such as measles. But these gains have been offset by increases in lung cancer, emphysema, cirrhosis of the liver, motor vehicle accidents, suicide, homicide, and diabetes mellitus.

During the 1960s, death rates rose in every five-year age group from 15 years through 44 years. Significant improvement was registered only for the very young (under five years of age) and the old, particularly those 75 and over.[10]

Death rates of young and middle-aged American males are rising sharply. Mortality for white men, aged 15–24, rose 22 percent. For nonwhites, the rise was a shocking 42 percent. Mortality increases, smaller but still significant, apply to all white males under 45 and to all nonwhites under 75. The leading factors in the upturn for young men, 15–24 years, were motor vehicle accidents, suicide, and homicide.

For those between the ages of 25 and 44, the leading culprits were the automobile, homicide, lung cancer, suicide, and cirrhosis of the liver. For men between 45 and 64, there were substantial increases in the death rate due to lung cancer, emphysema, diseases of the heart and circulatory system, bronchitis, and cirrhosis. There were also substantial increases in the death rates for white women at ages 15–24 and 35–44 years, and for women of other races at ages 15–24 years.

While the overall death rates remain stable, it appears that the most productive years of life for American men are being foreshortened. Disablement and morbidity are not as well reported as deaths. But it can be readily inferred that increased death rates are accompanied by similar or larger morbidity and disability changes from the same causes.

Mortality Rates and Medical Care

It should be noted that the mortality data show a preponderant incidence of preventable causes, but generally not of the kind that lend themselves to medical "cure." They reflect primarily the consequences of life-style and personal behavior and portray circumstances wherein conventional medical intervention is usually too late. The availability of medical care is clearly not the major problem.

The rapidly increasing differential in male-female life expectancy is also revealing. In 1920, the average female baby could expect to live only one year longer than the average male baby; in 1972 the differential was 7.7 years and growing,[11] which explains the rapid increase of widows in our population. In 1910, there were 106 males for every 100 females in the United States; in 1972, only 95. Especially interesting is the fact that sex differentials have become more important than racial differentials in life expectancy. The average black female baby can now expect to live about a year longer than the average white male baby; three years longer in California. Certainly the genetic make up of males and females has not been altered in recent years. Nor is there a difference in access to health care among males and females. The explanation appears to lie primarily in different life-styles, not in the amount of medical care.

Another revealing statistical phenomenon is that the traditional relationship between life expectancy and per capita income has vanished, except among the very poor.[12] Although high income groups have better access to modern medical care, their health is no better than among middle and lower-middle classes. In fact, evidence indicates that higher incomes often seem to do more harm than good for health. Again, the explanation appears to lie in life-style of the affluent rather than medical care.

Diminishing and Disappearing Returns

Nobody questions that availability of a certain amount of medical care is of great importance and that therapeutic medicine has made significant contributions to improvement in health status. But scholars are increasingly recognizing that additional increments of medical services can eventually lead to diminishing returns. The marginal value of added care is eventually reduced to a point where it does not repay the investment. More important, it is possible for the marginal value to reach zero or even become negative. Duncan Neuhauser, of the Harvard School of Public Health, has suggested the possibility that we may have reached or passed that point in the United States.[13]

There is increasing evidence of the diminishing relative importance of traditional therapy in all advanced societies, and the problem is receiving increased attention of scholars in many countries. Among the growing number of authorities who have been calling into doubt the value of proliferating service expenditures or the burgeoning of increasingly elaborate techniques are A. L. Cochrane, Thomas McKeown, and Brian Abel-Smith in England; A. D. Frazier in Canada; Anne R. Somers and Victor Fuchs in the United States.

The available evidence suggests to me that we have reached a stage where we must examine with care, and some skepticism, any proposal to throw more money and resources into the health care machine, although there is no question that the machine could absorb infinite amounts. As Enoch Powell, the former Minister of Health in Great Britain, reported about a decade ago, "There is virtually no limit to the amount of medical care an individual is capable of absorbing."[14] The caution I urge is not primarily for purposes of trying to save money but because of a concern for health.

First, we must keep in mind that we live in a world of limited resources, and thus every expenditure represents a choice among alternatives. If we feed the health care machine additional resources that do not add to positive health, we are depriving ourselves of the opportunity to use such resources in other pursuits where we know the marginal gains can be great: better food, improved housing, a cleaner environment, etc. Second, we may be nurturing a comfortable illusion that better health is simply for sale, and deflecting people from behavior that can prove more fruitful to health.

Dr. René Dubos, one of the world's most respected health authorities, told us several years ago that "Therapeutic medicine is probably now entering a phase of medically diminishing returns."[15] It now seems that the greatest potential for improving the health of the American people is probably not to be found in increasing the number of physicians or hospital beds, but rather in what people can be taught and motivated to do for themselves, in influencing personal behavior and attitudes.

This is hardly a new thought. Writing almost 35 years ago, Dr. Henry Sigerist, the great medical historian, said, "The state can protect society very effectively against a great many dangers, but the cultivation of health, which requires a definite mode of living, remains, to a large extent, an individual matter."[16] But individual activity and behavior can be promoted, aided, and encouraged by the state in many ways. We have not acted on such knowledge.

Discipline is more demanding than shopping for health. Moreover, there is no significant interest group, no professional constituency, no lobby, for health itself—only for health services that can be purchased. Thus, we may be in danger of inflating ourselves into an over-medicated society and increasingly exposing ourselves to iatrogenic illness.

Make no mistake, I am not advocating a retreat into the past or an abandonment of medical services. There is much to be done in health care itself. I strongly favor and advocate comprehensive national health insurance, I was pressing for prepaid group practice many years before it became a popular cause, and I feel it essential that we have a more equitable deployment and distribution of the resources we devote to health care. What I am pleading for here is some sense of balance in resource allocation, that we invest a reasonable proportion of future dollars, and a larger part of present dollars, in positive health promotion, including prevention (by which I do *not* mean primarily more and earlier visits to the doctor), health education, and health motivation. Nobody can guarantee results in health, whatever road we take. But it does seem reasonably clear that the prospective pay-off for investment in health promotion represents a far better bet for society than still more investment in an already prodigious health care economy. "In order to build its own future, each generation must learn both to utilize its past and to escape it."[17]

References and Notes

1 Department of Health, Education and Welfare. *Estimated Health Expenditures Under Selected National Health Insurance Bills—A Report to Congress*, July 1974 (processed), p. 3.
2 Worthington, N. L. "National Health Expenditures, 1929–74," *Social Security Bulletin*, February 1975, p. 5.
3 *Journal of the American Medical Association*, November 19, 1973, pp. 910, 918. Estimates, 1973–74, from Association of American Medical Colleges.
4 Association of American Medical Colleges, Task Force on Foreign Medical Graduates. *Graduates of Foreign Medical Schools in the United States: A Challenge to Medical Education* (Washington, D.C.:

AAMC, March 22, 1974) Table 1. Also, Department of Health, Education and Welfare. *The Foreign Medical Graduate and Physician Manpower in the U.S.* DHEW Publication No. (HRA) 74-30; (Washington, D.C.: DHEW, 1974).
5 Weiss, R. J., *et al.* "The Effect of Importing Physicians—Return to a Pre-Flexnerian Standard," *New England Journal of Medicine* 290:1453–1457 (June 27, 1974); and Weiss, *et al.*, "Foreign Medical Graduates and the Underground," *New England Journal of Medicine* 290:1408–1413 (June 20, 1974). Also see: Dublin, T. D. "Foreign Physicians: Their Impact on U.S. Health Care," *Science* 187:407–414 (August 2, 1974).

6 Department of Health, Education and Welfare, Office of the Secretary. *Towards a Comprehensive Health Policy for the 1970s—A White Paper* (Washington, D.C.: DHEW, May 1971) p. 37.

7 Department of Health, Education and Welfare, Health Services Administration, Bureau of Community Health Services. *Community Health Service* (Washington, D.C.: DHEW, April 1974).

8 *Statistical Abstract of the United States, 1974*, p. 60; Department of Health, Education and Welfare, National Center for Health Statistics. *Mortality Trends: Age, Color, and Sex, United States, 1950–69*, Series 20, No. 15 (1973) p. 14.

9 *Ibid.*, p. 3 ff.

10 These and data in the next three paragraphs are from *ibid*; Department of Health, Education and Welfare, National Center for Health Statistics. *Mortality Trends for Leading Causes of Death: U. S., 1950–69* Series 20, No. 16 (1974); and *Leading Components of Upturn in Mortality of Men: U.S. 1952–67* (1971).

11 Department of Health, Education and Welfare, National Center for Health Statistics. *Vital Statistics of the United States, 1972: Vol. 11* Section 5, Life Tables, DHEW Publication No. (HRA) 75-1147, p. 5–15.

12 Fuchs, Victor R. *Who Shall Live?* (New York: Basic Books, Inc., 1975) p. 31 ff.

13 Neuhauser, Duncan. "The Future of Proprietaries in American Health Services," in: Havighurst, C. C. (ed.) *Regulating Health Facilities Construction* (Washington, D. C.: American Enterprise Institute for Public Policy Research, 1974) pp. 233–237.

14 Powell, J. Enoch. *Medicine and Politics* (London: Pitman Medical Publishing Co., 1966) ch. 4.

15 Dubos, René. *Man, Medicine, and Environment* (New York: New American Library, 1968) p. 119.

16 Sigerist, Henry. *Medicine and Human Welfare* (New Haven: Yale University Press, 1941) p. 103.

17 Davis, Michael M. *Medical Care for Tommorrow* (New York: Harper and Brothers, 1955) p. 434.

Richard M. Bailey

An Economist's View of the Health Services Industry

Originally Published in March 1969

An economist's perspective on developments in the field of health may be compared with analyses that economists make of business organizations and other industries in our society. The rationale of the economist for viewing the production of health services as an industry is based largely on the observation that medical services are produced and sold in our society in a manner not very different from the way in which other goods and services are sold. Specifically, though health professionals like to talk about the "need" for medical care, by and large our health organizations and institutions are structured to respond only to an expressed demand. "Need" is a nice professional concept, but the kinds of health services traditionally produced are those which can be sold in the marketplace. They are medical services which meet the test of the marketplace: services which the public is willing to pay for because of a reasonable expectation that these will be visibly beneficial to them.[1]

Richard M. Bailey, D.B.A., is Assistant Professor of Business Administration and Public Health, University of California at Berkeley. This paper is based upon a speech delivered at a conference on "The Planning Process: Physician-Consumer Involvement," sponsored by the California Medical Education and Research Foundation, in San Francisco, July 18-20, 1968.

The Production of Medical Services

Historically, medical services have generally been produced by relatively small scale medical practices or, to make the business analogy even stronger, medical firms, where the physician has been the key factor in the production of all health services. Traditionally, these services have been highly personalized and have led to many discussions about the sacred and close physician-patient relationship. These physician services have been tailored to what the physician interprets as the patient's requirements, that is, what kind of care he may require. To put a little more perspective on this analysis by backtracking 40 or 50 years to a time when medical knowledge was much more limited than it is today, we would probably have to admit that much of the physician's service contained a large component of tender, loving care and human concern, and a relatively small amount of scientific information. Usually the physician saw the patient only when the patient was quite ill and suffering from obvious physical discomfort. This pattern of seeking medical care remains prevalent today. Most patients do not buy services from the physician unless they feel some real discomfort or otherwise sense a problem. Problems defined as minor by the patient are cared for in a multitude of ways: with home remedies, neglect, or what have you. The important point is that the patient comes to the physician only when he is concerned or ill.

Role of the Physician

How, then, has the physician responded to the patient? It should be recognized that the physician is cast in a role somewhat different from that of most producers: the physician-patient relationship may be more properly conceived of as agent-principal rather than producer-consumer. The patient is analogous to the principal in law. He employs an agent, the physician, to act in his best interest. So, the transaction between patient and physician can hardly be regarded as a straight across-the-table bargaining activity in which the patient asks about which services will be produced and what price will be charged. Rather, the patient asks the physician to provide services that the physician believes will contribute to the patient's well-being. Because the physician has taken on this kind of agent or trustee responsibility, the medical profession has, over time, conceived of the process of medical services production as unique. It has opposed the idea that the delivery of medical services can involve a common production process. Much emphasis has been placed upon the "tailor-made" aspects of the transaction. To use commercial terms, we might say that the services typically produced by the physician have been of a job-order type. They have been specially packaged to meet a particular patient requirement for services; they are not mass-produced. Medical services are simply not discussed in terms that refer to a high volume, standardized way of production as is done in most goods and service industries.

Another interesting observation is that those medical services typically produced are primarily only those deliberately sought by the patient. There has been no great promotional effort by the medical profession to sell *more* or *different*

kinds of medical services. In fact, a whole body of medical ethics has prevented advertising to create a demand and encourage people to seek more medical services. Indeed, the emphasis has often been placed on discouraging more demand.[2] It is also apparent that the services made available by physicians have been largely curative. Curative services can be sold.[3] Curative services derive from a felt need on the part of the patient. When the patient is ill, the encounter with the physician holds forth some real prospect of being beneficial to him. In this instance, it becomes rational for the patient to go to the physician and buy medical services. This is the way our health service system is largely organized today—on the basis of providing those services that can be sold in a free market setting. But note that this is a limited bundle of services. It may not begin to cover the spectrum of services that should be made available.

Distribution of Medical Services

Concern is expressed today about the distribution of medical services. This problem is closely related to the traditional way of selling medical care. In areas where demand is strong, incomes are high, and people are educated sufficiently to have high expectations from medical services, there we find most of the physicians. Of course, an adequate population base is necessary, but even within a community such as San Francisco, or New York, or Atlanta, the density of physicians and the quantity of services provided are definitely centered in a few geographic areas. Physicians are located where the demand for their services is strong. We likewise find other medical facilities grouping around these sources of strong demand—hospitals, convalescent homes, and related establishments.

Consumer Demand for Health Services[4]

Given that the purchase of most medical services has been in a market setting wherein the consumer has selected and paid for these services as he has when buying other goods, attention now turns to the way in which this market has functioned. A fundamental point to be made in this context is that the consumer has demanded only those medical services which have appeared to be rational for him to buy—services from which he might reasonably expect to receive a visible payoff. We might classify these demands for medical services by order of urgency and, hence, the priority in which medical care has been sought. They are:

1 Demand arising from an emergency/ serious situation, where life or death are the alternatives.

2 Demand for treatment of not-so-serious conditions, such as an acute illness where life is not threatened, or a chronic illness where management of the problem is needed. In these cases, it is likely that physical and/or mental discomfort are present.

3 Demand for medical services to detect developing medical problems early, which may make proper management of the condition more efficacious.

Consumer Demand for Life-Sustaining Health Services

Economists refer to the concept of utility as meaning the value that the consumer expects he will receive from his purchase of this or that good or service. Applying this concept to the three types of demand for medical care, one might say that the consumer could expect the greatest utility to be derived from a medical service that is life-saving in nature; less utility from the alleviation of an acute or chronic condition; and, perhaps, to exhibit an ambivalent attitude of either very small or even negative utility regarding the purchase of preventive medical services.

As concerns the prevention of death or serious disabilities, is there any doubt why consumer demand has been strongest (and

public expression of urgency greatest) for services that prevent quick death or serious disabling consequences? The great majority of people have a strong desire for services of this type; few have a fervent death wish or like to see others die or be in great pain. We see evidence of this demand expressed in the supply of the many acute-care hospitals which dot the countryside and in the large number of hospital-oriented medical and surgical specialists who are concerned with repairing bodies broken either physically or by damaging disease. Moreover, we even see this expression of demand in the predominant types of health insurance policies that are marketed in this country; these place principal emphasis upon hospital care for acute conditions, with payment being for quite limited duration and the illnesses or accidents covered being those requiring surgery or intensive medical treatment to avoid death or permanent disability.

Consumer Demand for Health Services to Alleviate Acute or Chronic Conditions

The demand for medical services intended to alleviate acute problems that are not life-threatening has been growing rapidly in recent years as the result of numerous factors. Among these are increased patient awareness of the physician's ability to treat such problems (largely related to better drugs and medicines), higher incomes, availability of services, and so on. Patients visiting physicians for such complaints often make up what is known in the trade as the "bread and butter" work of medical practice. These are medical services with which the physician has become quite familiar, and though he personally may not receive as much psychic satisfaction from producing such services as he would from participating in the more dramatic act of saving lives, he is comfortable within this productive role. Thus, as demand for medical care has grown in the aggregate, and many of the earlier killer diseases such as smallpox and polio have been brought under control by vaccination, most physicians have found demand for this type of service growing more markedly than any other.

Economists frequently engage in sharp debates over the nature of certain goods and services in their attempts to classify them as investment or consumption goods. Investment goods are often regarded as those which generate a payoff to the individual or society over a comparatively long period of time and may, in fact, be necessary prerequisites to further productive work. Consumption goods are assumed to yield short-run benefits to the purchaser and, in one way or another, produce some pleasure for the user while being consumed. Applying these investment/consumption criteria to medical services is fraught with problems, but a gross example might be to say that the purchase of an appendectomy for a 14-year-old boy could be called an investment expenditure, while the purchase of an office visit to a dermatologist for removal of a wart on his hand could be called a consumption expenditure. The former may be essential to the preservation of life; the latter to make one's hands more beautiful. It is quite probable that the utility of the first operation exceeds by a wide margin that of the second. Yet, it is this latter type of demand for medical services that is growing rapidly in our generally affluent economy, a type of demand that seems to be more influenced by the income level of the patient than anything else.

As noted above, insurance companies have found the demand for health insurance coverage greatest in those instances where life is at stake. Barring a major catastrophe, demands for medical services of this type are reasonably predictable; they are not services that are willingly sought and thus subject to the personal fancy of the patient. The demand for medical services to alleviate relatively minor problems or self-limiting conditions, however, is subject to widely different and highly unpredictable influences. It is for this reason that insurance companies are reluctant to write policies covering such services unless there is a substantial self-insurance clause in the contract requiring the patient to pay the first $100 or $200 of claims each year. (Both Title XVIII and Title XIX of the Social Security Amendments of 1965 recognize this problem and require that initial costs be borne by the patient each year, normally the first $50.) Since demand by consumers for these services is high and growing, we find physicians and medical institutions organized to produce these services in large quantity. However, just as we find individual patients according lesser priority to these services than to those of a life-threatening type, so also we find hospitals and physicians ranking these services similarly. They are, in a sense, less important. They are more likely to be consumption goods than investment goods.

Consumer Demand for Preventive Health Services

Turning finally to the demand for medical services which emphasize early detection or the prevention of illness, we confront a situation which illustrates most clearly the problems created by consumer ignorance. Economic theory grants that the consumer is rational in making purchases. He considers the various products and services that his tastes dictate; he weighs the expected utility of possessing one or another of the goods or services, taking into account his income and the relative prices of each alternative; and then he makes his decision with the view of maximizing total utility. All of these decision-making activities presuppose that the consumer is well-informed about the choices at hand. Now we find him presented with a new medical service—a service which may detect a disease in its incipient stages or prevent future illness. How is he to evaluate its utility? How can he express a level of effective demand that will lead to the production of the service?

If the consumer is rational, he will not buy preventive health services unless he can be convinced that the marginal utility of the service will exceed the marginal utility derived from purchasing some other goods or services. But who can be so convinced? Perhaps a person who is aware that he is in a high risk group. Perhaps a preventive service can be urged upon a patient who is already in the physician's office or hospital for some other reason. In such a case, the marginal cost of the preventive service may appear to be low (or even zero if the service can be disguised as part of the total bill which is covered by insurance). But how can the demand for preventive services be self-generated when the consumer is so often unaware of their existence or, if aware, finds it literally impossible to evaluate how beneficial they may be to him personally? In decision-theory terms, the potential consumer is being asked to evaluate a purchase decision problem which is filled with uncertainty. There is little opportunity to measure the size of the risk that is undertaken by failure to purchase the service. The data do not exist in most instances. Thus, the purchase of preventive services presents a case of consumption under a high degree of uncertainty leading to what appears to be a rational decision on the part of most consumers: a decision *not* to purchase such services.[5]

Effect of Income on Demand for Health Services

Since our focus is upon consumption theory, let us now discuss the influence that purely economic factors—income and prices—may have upon the decision to purchase various kinds of medical services. Since hard data are not available, we will use graphs to present such relationships. In a sense, these are the author's hypotheses about the effect of income and price upon aggregate medical demand—the way that the population as a whole may behave in its demand for health services.

Income and Demand for Life-Sustaining Services

The effect of income on the demand for medical services to treat serious illnesses falls along a spectrum ranging from high to low. We say that the income effect is high if an aggregate increase in income leads to a more than proportional increase in the demand for these services. Conversely, if there is only a slight increase in demand with an increase in income, the income effect is low. Using a chart whose vertical axis measures income (Y) and whose horizontal axis measures the quantity of these services demanded (Q), the demand curve for life-sustaining health services probably looks like this:

Figure I. Consumer demand for life-sustaining health services as a function of income

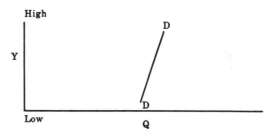

The demand curve DD reflects a relatively slight effect of income on the demand for services to treat emergency/serious illnesses. That is, level of income may not play a major role in the quantity of such services demanded, except in the sense that the higher one's income the greater may be one's access to the institutions and personnel producing such services. However, heart attacks, cancer, automobile accidents, strokes, and appendicitis strike the rich as well as the poor with approximately equal frequency. Moreover, the health care delivery system rarely closes its doors to people who need such services even though they may not have the income with which to pay for the services. People with emergency or life-threatening medical problems are usually able to enter the medical care delivery system in one way or another without first considering if they have the means to pay. They have a vital and immediate need; they are accepted for treatment; their income is considered later. This opportunity to receive some care coincides with the section of medical ethics which says that no patient will be denied access to medical care if he is in real need. Surely, the care that the poor receive may not be of equal quality with that received by the more affluent patient, but generally some care is available. Of course, as time passes and the population grows, we may see an increase in demand for treatment of emergencies or serious illnesses. But such demand is not usually a direct function of individual income at any particular point in time. Demand for these services, then, is not seen as being particularly sensitive to income of the patient.

*Income and Demand for Other
Curative Services*

Turning to the effect of income level upon the demand for curative services to treat problems that are not life-threatening, we might see a set of relationships as follows:

Figure II. Consumer demand for health services to alleviate minor health problems as a function of income

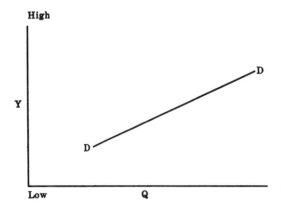

The demand curve DD reflects a strong income effect on the demand for these services. The explanation advanced for this relationship is based on two points: 1) the superior nature of medical services vis-à-vis most other goods and services and, 2) the fact that, with higher incomes, the marginal utility of other goods or services which might have been very high when incomes were low now diminishes rapidly, and medical services yield relatively higher utility. Of course, we also find the linkage between education and income level to be very strong. Hence, other factors explaining the increased demand for services to alleviate these acute but not death-inducing illnesses may be related to a different set of values, or to the possession of more information which leads to greater rationality in the allocation of one's income.[6]

It bears note that coverage of these services under either public programs or private insurance contracts results in a subtle increase in the individual's income, an increase, however, that can be spent in only one manner, for the purchase of medical services. Small wonder why third party payment for such services is viewed as a "bottomless pit" into which a very substantial amount of expenditures may rapidly be absorbed.

*Income and Demand for Preventive
Services*

Our final concern is with the effect of income level on the demand for preventive health services. Conceptually, this demand might be pictured thusly:

Figure III. Consumer demand for preventive health services as a function of income

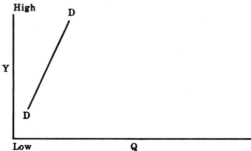

In this case, we find the total quantity of such services demanded to be low at all income levels (the curve is close to the vertical axis), with perhaps some slight increased propensity to consume these services at the highest income levels. Here, we return to the issue of consumer rationality: Why does the demand for these services appear to be so small? The apparent answer is found in the very uncertain knowledge that the consumer possesses about the value of such services from a medical viewpoint and, accordingly, their dollar value. Spending $100 for a series of tests that are interpreted by the physician as indicating that the patient is in good health may merely confirm what the person already believed to be true. With higher incomes, $100 may seem to be a small price to pay for such assurances; however, greater utility may be attached to the purchase of other goods or services that provide more immediate gratification.

Effect of Price on the Demand for Health Services

In the three diagrams that follow, we picture the effect of price (P) upon the aggregate quantity demanded (Q) of certain health services. These diagrams are shaped like the more traditional demand curves found in economics textbooks, whereas the prior diagrams relating income to demand are seldom used quite this way. Again, remember that these are hypotheses of the authors.

Price and Demand for Life-Sustaining Services

Applying this concept to the demand for emergency/serious services results in the graph shown in Figure IV.

Here, we find the quantity demanded relatively insensitive to price of the service. The reason, again, is that these services are generally not consumed under what might be called "pleasant circumstances." Hence, price may neither act much as a

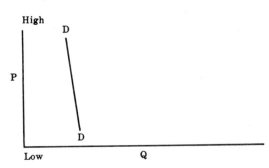

Figure IV. Consumer demand for life-sustaining health services as a function of price

deterrent nor incentive to use. It would be wrong, of course, to assume that there is no effect of price on the demand for these services: witness the effect of hospitalization insurance coverage on the use of hospitals. Insurance, in this case, acts to reduce the out-of-pocket cost of the medical and hospital services to the patient below the going market price. A lower price may then result in a shifting of marginal utilities among various alternative goods or services. But confusion abounds here too. If the medical problem is truly serious, the possession of hospital insurance may merely accelerate the use of the service—the transaction may not be delayed until there is no alternative but hospitalization. It may also be true that many of the medical reasons for hospitalization are not for the treatment of emergency/serious conditions. Some misclassification of the medical problem may arise so that the cost of care can be shifted from the patient to the insurance company. In summary, casual observation of the effect of price on the demand for emergency medical services may indicate a rather close relationship, but if one examines more closely the nature of these services and what they are for, it becomes doubtful if price is as important a factor as assumed.

Price and Demand for Other Curative Services

The effect of price upon the demand for nonserious, curative medical services probably is quite strong, as shown in Figure V.

In this case, we find the total quantity of such services demanded to be low at all income levels (the curve is close to the vertical axis), with perhaps some slight increased propensity to consume these services at the highest income levels. Here, we return to the issue of consumer rationality: Why does the demand for these services appear to be so small? The apparent answer is found in the very uncertain knowledge that the consumer possesses about the value of such services from a medical viewpoint and, accordingly, their dollar value. Spending $100 for a series of tests that are interpreted by the physician as indicating that the patient is in good health may merely confirm what the person already believed to be true. With higher incomes, $100 may seem to be a small price to pay for such assurances; however, greater utility may be attached to the purchase of other goods or services that provide more immediate gratification.

Effect of Price on the Demand for Health Services

In the three diagrams that follow, we picture the effect of price (P) upon the aggregate quantity demanded (Q) of certain health services. These diagrams are shaped like the more traditional demand curves found in economics textbooks, whereas the prior diagrams relating income to demand are seldom used quite this way. Again, remember that these are hypotheses of the authors.

Price and Demand for Life-Sustaining Services

Applying this concept to the demand for emergency/serious services results in the graph shown in Figure IV.

Here, we find the quantity demanded relatively insensitive to price of the service. The reason, again, is that these services are generally not consumed under what might be called "pleasant circumstances." Hence, price may neither act much as a

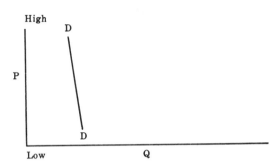

Figure IV. Consumer demand for life-sustaining health services as a function of price

deterrent nor incentive to use. It would be wrong, of course, to assume that there is no effect of price on the demand for these services: witness the effect of hospitalization insurance coverage on the use of hospitals. Insurance, in this case, acts to reduce the out-of-pocket cost of the medical and hospital services to the patient below the going market price. A lower price may then result in a shifting of marginal utilities among various alternative goods or services. But confusion abounds here too. If the medical problem is truly serious, the possession of hospital insurance may merely accelerate the use of the service—the transaction may not be delayed until there is no alternative but hospitalization. It may also be true that many of the medical reasons for hospitalization are not for the treatment of emergency / serious conditions. Some misclassification of the medical problem may arise so that the cost of care can be shifted from the patient to the insurance company. In summary, casual observation of the effect of price on the demand for emergency medical services may indicate a rather close relationship, but if one examines more closely the nature of these services and what they are for, it becomes doubtful if price is as important a factor as assumed.

Price and Demand for Other Curative Services

The effect of price upon the demand for nonserious, curative medical services probably is quite strong, as shown in Figure V.

uncertainty attached to the value of such services. Reducing prices substantially (moving down the DD curve) might bring a one-shot increase in demand by people whose tastes incline in this direction. Beyond that, special efforts to increase consumption would probably be needed (DD[1] curve)—but, of course, any efforts that could be made to lower the price of such services closer to zero should prove a great inducement to additional consumption.

Demand Responsive to Economic Factors

To summarize this section on consumer demand for medical services, it should be emphasized that with the exception of demand for emergency, life-saving care— which is not very responsive to either price or income—the demand for other curative services is quite responsive to purely economic factors. Demand for preventive services shows some relationship to income and price levels but to generate any substantial increases in demand, educational efforts coupled with price changes would be required. Accepting the thesis that consumers are basically rational in their decision-making about prospective expenditures (limited primarily by their knowledge of benefits to be derived from various medical services), we may better understand why some services are widely sought even though they may not be highly regarded by physicians, and other services are not purchased although health professionals might give high priority to such consumption. Uncertainty is a very important element in consumer decision-making and when it is present, individual calculations of utility to be derived from a given expenditure may result in purchases that do not optimize the person's best interests. But can the consumer be blamed for such lack of knowledge? It may be that many health services are not like other goods and services. Hence, reliance upon market processes to generate an optimal level and mix of demand can lead to some undesirable resource allocations.

The Medical Market Place

The prior discussions of the traditional market for medical services and what seem to be the major economic factors influencing the demand for various kinds of services leads us now to focus upon some private market strengths and weaknesses. Specifically, where does the private market do a good job of allocating resources and where may it be inadequate? In our country, the underlying concept of the value of producing goods and services in a free market setting is based upon the belief that the market is an efficient allocator of resources. By this it is meant that if one accepts as given the income distribution existing among various groups in society —or within any given group, for that matter—then if a good or a service is demanded by an individual who is willing and able to pay for it, producers will respond to provide these services. In this context, we believe that the market is an efficient allocator for it provides the individual with the opportunity to spend his income to attain maximum satisfaction. But this opportunity to spend is always subject to his ability to spend *his* income. If one person has an income of $20,000 a year, he may spend that income differently from the way I might spend $20,000 a year—and that is well and good. We further believe that having this freedom to spend and to select from a wide variety of goods and services in the market is very important to maintaining other individual freedoms. A quite different pattern of expenditures may also be expected when consumers have vastly different levels of income, say, $20,000 per year and $2,000 per year. Even here, economic theory posits that each consumer will have the greatest opportunity to satisfy his desires if markets are free and consumer choice is broad.

The point that needs to be stressed is that for this market to work effectively and to distribute goods and services to various consumers at low prices, it is important that the producers be highly competitive. It is important that the consumer have many options to buy various kinds of goods or services at various prices, at various levels of quality, and in a variety of combinations. If the market is to work effectively, the consumer also must be sufficiently knowledgeable to discriminate in his choices, to know what he is buying, and to be able to discern the relative value of particular goods or services. If we find that producers are competing, and if the consumer is informed, then we can take another step. We can say that in this kind of market setting, consumer well-being will be maximized by encouraging producers to organize their activities to maximize their own best interests.[7] Consumer and producer interests harmonize in a competitive marketplace because strong competition among producers leads to providing a variety of services at low prices. Another way to say this is that the self-interest both of consumers and of producers is served when producers are highly competitive. This leads to the rationalization of profit maximization among producers because, in a competitive market, the producer is able to maximize his profits only by offering services at low prices. If consumers are not satisfied with the producer's prices or services, they will refuse to buy his output and will soon put him out of business. Someone else who responds to the consumers' demands will get the business.

Competition in Medicine

The purpose of this discussion about the marketplace is to lead to a focus on the health services industry. In the field of health, many physicians have traditionally held somewhat fallacious beliefs about the degree of competition existing in medicine. One of these beliefs is that medicine is highly competitive. Economists, on the other hand, are quite inclined to downgrade the free competition explanation of medical practice and to describe the industry as a distinct form of monopoly. The reasons given by economists are:

1 In a highly competitive industry, prices are set by the forces of supply and demand as they interact in the marketplace. In the case of medical practice, prices are set by individual producers who have a high degree of discretion to discriminate in pricing as they see fit.

2 In a competitive industry, price competition is used between producers as a means of attracting a greater number of consumers. In medical practice, the use of price as a competitive instrument is frowned upon and declared to be unethical.

3 In a competitive industry, the product or service that is offered for sale generally is homogeneous. In medical practice, the service offered is conventionally treated as heterogeneous ("individual health care"), with considerable differentiation occurring both in the mix and number and quality of services produced.

4 In a competitive industry, the consumer has the opportunity to be well informed and is able to bargain among the producers to obtain the best terms of sale. In the market for medical services, the consumer is not well informed. He selects his physician on the basis of highly subjective criteria and, after the selection is made, is in a relatively weak position to bargain on price, other services to be purchased, or to whom referral for additional attention will be made, since advertising is unethical.

5 In a competitive industry, there is ready ease of entry into the industry. In medical practice, there are numerous barriers to entry. Nationally, these barriers are erected through the educational process. At the state level, the barriers are maintained by the licensing of physicians. At the local level, medical societies and hospital staffs act as barriers to entry into practice.[8]

By the very way in which medical services are provided, we are saying implicitly that these services are no different from other goods and services. Those who want to buy medical services and have the income to purchase them can do so (subject to being informed as to what is purchased). We have assumed that there is competition and, therefore, as the consumer enters this marketplace to buy medical services, he does so in a setting where the resources supposedly are allocated effectively. Many statements in medical publications are based upon these ideas. Accordingly, physicians are encouraged to act in their own best economic interest, feeling that consumer well-being also will be served well.

I do not believe we can say that if the physician acts in his own economic interest this will benefit the consumer. Of course, there is much conflict in the language here, even within the medical profession. What needs to be recognized, though, is that if one accepts the statements about problems of competition in medicine and about the lack of consumer information or education concerning medical services, it becomes almost impossible to say that the typical market setting for the provision of medical services can solve all the problems in this field today. Some services are not bought because of lack of income; some services are not purchased because the price is too high; some services are not even produced because physicians do not see much of a market for them. Overriding all these matters is the lack of competition in the industry.

Physician-Producers in Strong Position

In summary, an overview of the medical practice industry reveals that the producers are in a very strong bargaining position relative to the consumers. Over the last 20 to 25 years, as demand for medical care has grown for a variety of reasons, the power of the physician-producers in the marketplace has been strongly evident. Because consumers have not been in a good bargaining position, the physician-producers have not been subjected to pressures to be more efficient in their productive activities. The strong demand, moreover, has made it easier for physicians to raise their prices rather than to increase efficiency. If the industry were more competitive, such price increases would not be possible because the competitive incentives to increase efficiency and to reorganize the production process would work to the consumers' advantage, not to the advantage of the producer.

Government's Role in the Medical Marketplace

Recently, the medical profession has felt itself besieged by all sorts of pressures from the federal government. Why does government intervene in the marketplace to change certain ground rules? Economists hold that there are three justifiable reasons.[9] One reason is to supply services—often called pure public goods—that simply cannot be provided in the normal market setting. We could not maintain a very good army if different persons decided to buy one day per month of a soldier's time, or one tread for a tank, or one life preserver for some ship, and so on. Market transactions are also inadequate for the purchase of police and fire protection and a number of other goods or services where we know that production would not occur if they were sold only in a market setting. Economists say that these goods possess externalities—benefits that accrue to many individuals without their paying directly. As an example, if I hired my own army to help protect the city in which I live, all other people would get a free ride on my army, they would receive benefits without sharing the costs. Moreover, there probably would be an under-purchase of defense services. To provide adequate "essential" services we recognize that they must be purchased by the public so that everyone shares in the cost who benefits from the externalities.

A second reason why government intervenes in economic affairs is to affect the income distribution. Typically, in this country, such intervention is designed to benefit only those persons who suffer the grossest inequalities of income. Hence, we have social security and welfare programs which tax the more affluent and redistribute resources to the poor.

The third area of government intervention is in purchasing goods and services where the market operates less than full time. Examples of some quasi-public goods are such things as highways and research. Certainly, highways and bridges could be private ventures and we could pay each time we drive over them. Research also could be purchased privately. There is the general feeling, however, because of externalities, that not enough research or highways or bridges would be produced to meet the public need. Therefore, government intervenes and produces, or pays to have produced, some of these goods and services.

Market Setting Inadequate for Health Services

I submit that many of the activities of the health services industry fall into the category of quasi-public goods. There is a belief in the public sphere that the market does not work part of the time and does not provide an adequate quantity of medical services. For various reasons, medical services are considered important —more important than certain other kinds of services and goods whose production is left purely in the private market. There is the feeling that these services should be made available to more people—that medical care is a right, not a privilege. The statement implies that medical services should not be denied because of income considerations. Moreover, we are recognizing that the many externalities of medical care make this a unique service. We have witnessed actions by government to stamp out communicable diseases. Here

the idea of externalities comes across very strongly. That is, if in trying to eliminate a highly communicable disease we left it solely up to each individual to purchase a vaccine, we would soon have some difficult medical problems on our hands. This could occur because some people would purchase the services and get some benefits, and others would not. Those not able to purchase the services for a variety of reasons (poverty, ignorance, because they are children, and so forth) would be exposed to the disease, and the problem of externalities would be evident. Thus, public policy indicates that problems of communicable disease and sanitation are so important to large numbers of people that they must be dealt with outside of the market setting.

Health Services Rationale Changing

Another point needs brief mention: The rationale regarding health services has changed over time. Part of today's basis is the new concept of the significance of human beings in matters of economic growth. In the past, most growth in the economy was attributed to an increasing abundance of material capital. Now we find the balance has shifted and human capital turns out to be relatively more important—and more scarce.[10] Increasingly, we look at health expenditures in part as investment and in part as consumption. From a national economic policy point of view, it is a wise investment to pay today to obviate some medical problems tomorrow. Prevention now may keep the recipient from becoming totally dependent on society in 10, 20, or 30 years. These public expenditures for specific kinds of personal health services may be viewed as part of a national investment policy.[11] Justification for public investment in personal health is that healthy people are more productive in the long run.

The concept that considers health services to be consumption goods fits in nicely with the various demands for health services mentioned earlier. We usually fail to consider that if a youngster does not get adequate medical care (either because his family neglects his physical needs or has inadequate income to pay for medical services) this neglect may impose a burden on society at some later date if he suffers a serious disabling illness. For all of these reasons—problems of the market setting and of the nonavailability of certain services—government has found a rationale to enter the marketplace and to say that medical care is a right, not a privilege.

Defining medical care as a right and not as a privil ge implies a number of long-term and serious changes in the organization of our delivery system for health services. Assuming government is serious in its purpose, there are several options opened for action. The first is for government to set itself up a a major producer of medical services. The rationale to be employed is that there is something wrong with the way these services are provided today: there are not enough of them; they are not adequately distributed; or there is not enough variety. The government could then move in and become a new, large producer of these services.

As a second option, government might shun the production route and become a large consumer, acting in the consumer interest both for services purchased directly and for production of medical services in general. Government seems to have selected this option and is now moving rapidly and forcefully to enlarge its role as a consumer of health services. In fact, government seems to be anxious to be rid of the producer role that it has had, in part, in the past. Public production of health services traditionally has occurred in city health departments, county hospitals, city clinics and VA hospitals. The passage of various pieces of legislation in the last few years has literally worked to destroy many of these governmental health services producing institutions, and government now is oriented to creating incen-

tives for private producers to replace some of these public organizations.

Incentives for Private Production

Let us consider some of these incentives for private production. First, we have the establishment of the Regional Medical Programs. This is a direct governmental attempt to affect the production of medical services at the regional level. Three years ago the Group Practice Facilities Act was passed, based upon public reasoning that there should be more large, comprehensive group medical practices. Incentives—subsidies, if you will—are provided to private physicians to encourage them to form new kinds of organizations for the production of medical services. In 1966, Comprehensive Health Planning legislation was passed by Congress. The focus of this legislation is very broad, but its intent is clear: to place the responsibility for careful planning and organization of the health care delivery system at the local level. All parts of the community are encouraged to consider what is desirable and necessary to make health services broadly available. The Federal government views its role largely as offering seed money to assist the planning process.

Government as a Collective Consumer

Government acts as a major consumer in the sense that it specifically purchases services for some population groups under both Medicare and Medicaid legislation. The major point here is that government is concerned with the market setting, the distribution, and the availability of various kinds of medical services. Government is concerned that the market cannot resolve these problems by itself, especially if we define access to health services as a right. In this way, government behaves like a collective consumer—either creating incentives for production of new services or providing funds for people to buy services where and as they will.

Not only is government thus defined as a collective consumer, it is a considerably better-informed consumer than the average person, in part because it employs many professionals. And, as an informed consumer, government is now asking many new questions about the whole organization of the health care industry: questions about the kinds of services being produced; whether they really accomplish anything; whether they improve health.

These questions have a great bearing on the mix of medical demands. As an economist, I see an interesting situation developing. Within the medical profession specifically, and within the whole industry generally, there are many monopoly powers; monopoly powers with which the individual consumer has been unable to cope in the past. But now, government is entering the scene in its new role of collective consumer and, in the process, is starting to behave like a monopsonist—a very powerful purchaser. Some conflict is inevitable. It is a natural result when any powerful producer meets any powerful consumer head-on. The situation developing in the health field today is analogous to Sears, Roebuck's treatment of its suppliers: "Meet certain standards, or we will buy elsewhere." Government, as an informed consumer with many dollars to spend, is beginning to ask questions not only about the availability of services but about their application at a point in time in the development of a disease when the services will be most effective. In so doing, government's attitude is to create positive financial incentives to encourage private producers to make these services available.

As an example, let us take a given disease—measles. For many years, the treatment of measles was largely in the private sector. People who had the disease, or who sought to purchase an effective vaccine when it became available, were the ones who received care. Parents subconsciously or consciously made decisions for their children—either to let them catch measles and then seek treatment, or to take the child for a vaccination and effectively eliminate the problem. In this setting, measles continued to be a large problem nationally, even after the vaccines were developed because many people did not have their children vaccinated. Now, government as a collective consumer is looking not only at measles but at many other kinds of diseases with one question in mind: What is the best point in time to confront this disease? And, it may well be, as with the measles example, best to say: Eliminate it at its source. Make sure that vaccines are provided for everyone, and back up the availability with strong efforts to get everyone vaccinated.

Government Questions Past Approach

The focus and organization of our medical system in the past has been to deal with problems after the patient has contracted an illness, to deal with problems when the individual sees it directly beneficial for him or his child to see the doctor; or to repair damage that has already occurred. As an informed consumer, government has questioned this approach and accordingly has conducted a number of studies in recent years on cancer, heart, kidney disease, automobile accidents, and so on.[12] The answers that keep coming to the fore would warm an epidemiologist's heart: to be effective in caring for most of these problems, intervention must come early.

If government continues with these analyses and concludes—as an effective, informed consumer—that the best way to obtain these services, or to have these illnesses or diseases treated properly, is to tackle them early, then several actions are likely to follow. One, government may begin to create financial incentives to encourage the private production of these medical services—many of which are barely produced today and many of which are not produced at all because they have not been salable in the private market. This may mean simply that we are going to see an increasing emphasis placed upon the producton of preventive services, not only preventive services in the form of annual examinations, but preventive services which carry many implications in terms of changing the whole nature of the medical services production process. Physicians have been reluctant to talk about mass production. All medical services are seen as job-ordered, tailored to the individual patient. In looking after the individual patient, though, physicians too often neglect society. But if instead of the individual buying services at the moment he feels a "real" need, you start asking questions about buying services at the time when they will be most effective for large groups of people, it may mean that physician involvement ultimately will be minimal, or that the production process will be markedly different from that which we now experience.

Summary

The economist's approach is to ask the direct question: How does one get goods or services produced that are in line with society's needs? Generally, the economist does *not* say, "Go start a new governmental firm to produce these services." Rather, he encourages the private production of these services by making it profitable. The analyses that we have covered, which deal with atttacking diseases early in their development, can be transferred into specific goals. If government wants to achieve these goals, it may do so by rewarding those producers who respond to these goals. Conversely, the public attitude may make it financially difficult for those who do not respond to meet this kind of demand.

The implications of these changes—for the medical profession, for all the health professions, and for the traditional production process—are great. It means taking a new look at what needs to be done; what services need to be produced in the future. We are saying that individual market demand criteria are not the *only* existing criteria. Increasingly, government seems ready to funnel funds into areas where the payoff to society seems higher. This may be in producing services in ways quite different from those we are accustomed to today. It may mean the complete reorganization of many of the institutions of health. But I do not see government anxious to use force to bring change. Rather, I see government using financial (economic) incentives to effect changes that have seemed only idealistic before. As a society, we are searching for objectives; then exploring ways to make them financially attractive for producers to respond accordingly. The changes that are occurring in the health field need to be viewed in this overall context. The simple phrase that medical care is a right and not a privilege implies tremendous changes in the kinds of medical services that need to be produced, how they will be distributed, how the professions will interact with one another, and how various organizations will respond to meet the needs.

If the marketplace were really adequate, if consumers were really informed, and if there were not powerful professional interests, then we could say, let the market solve the problem. But, I think we must admit that none of these conditions holds today. As we focus more on the problem of the provision of health services, where they are most effective, and how they can be produced, it is to be expected that government will increasingly create incentives for physicians to change, to respond to these new markets. And they will be *new* markets. This must be kept in mind. By so doing, we may be able to surmount any philosophical bugaboos that are carryovers from the days of pure laissez-faire medicine and realize that both health personnel and institutions now need to respond to a new set of market demands in our society.

Sander Kelman

Reprinted with permission of the Blue Cross Association, from *Inquiry:* Vol.VIII, No.3, pp.30-38. Copyright © 1971 by the Blue Cross Association.

Toward the Political Economy of Medical Care

Originally Published in September 1971

Medical care—like poverty, urban problems, and economic development—is one of those areas of social concern in which all disciplines of social science are generally considered to have a legitimate research function. Hence, we find sociologists, social psychologists, economists, political scientists, regional planners, and operations researchers bringing their own particular disciplinary biases to bear on problems in the medical care system,[1] and forcing the institutions and data of that system into the paradigms of their respective disciplines.

Yet, Western functionalist[2]-oriented social science (and its roots in German Idealism and August Comte) has been often criticized for 1) being ahistorical, 2) lacking in critical analysis, and 3) emphasizing technique at the expense of content.[3] Still, this type of analysis and its applications continue to thrive in the universities.

Rather than restating these criticisms and trying to explain why they have not been heeded, this article will simply attempt *to make the case* for a political economic analysis of the American medical care system that is at once historical in approach and critical in analysis. It provides merely the skeleton of what would constitute a thorough political economic analysis. It leaves both unasked and unanswered many questions which flow from the logic of the analysis that follows.

The premise of this paper is that de-

velopments in the medical care system are but reflections of developments in the larger society, no matter how much seemingly exogenous expertise is imposed upon it. To be more precise, the analysis will attempt to: 1) illustrate how the dynamics of the larger economic system are mirrored in the medical care system; 2) raise the general issue of whether innovations in the medical care system that violate the premises of the larger system can ever be politically viable (can a society which provides little economic security to the average citizen operationalize health care as a "right"?) ; and 3) forecast the likely outcome of the current structural deliberations on the medical care system (national health insurance and health maintenance organizations) in terms of current developments in the banking and financial sector of the American economy.

The Approach

The analytical mode used here will be dialectical.[4] That is, the history of class societies has been a history of evolving social institutions each propelled by its own contradictions, where "the term 'contradiction' [is used] to describe a social process which has been directly generated by a (logically) prior social process and which tends to negate that prior process."[5] The chronological record of these contradictions is what we (ought to) call history; and this approach to the study of history is dialectical. Hence, it is important to recognize and identify the unfolding of the dialectical process and its associated series of contradictions.

Sander Kelman, Ph.D. is Assistant Professor of Medical Economics, Sloan Institute of Hospital Administration, Graduate School of Business and Public Administration, Cornell University.

Some Historical Parallels

This section will discuss, with the use of two historical examples, the dialectical relationship between technology, market structure and social structure. In the following section, this relationship will be applied to the development of the American medical care system in the 20th century.

A capitalist form of economic organization has, essentially, two semi-stable forms of market structure: competition and monopoly.[6] The former is relatively stable where the level of technology is both low and static; and the latter, where technology is ever-rising, irrespective of changes in productivity. Consider what has occurred in recent American agriculture: with the rapid introduction of technological advance and, in this case, substantial increases in productivity have come tremendous declines in farm prices of both dairy products and crops. This has necessitated ever larger scales of agricultural plant both to finance and operate the advancing technology necessary to maintain constant farm incomes in the face of declining prices resulting from the increased productivity of a newer technology. The final consequence, of course, has been an enormous decrease in the number of farm(er)s, as many small operators have been driven off the land by the price squeeze.

A better illustration in terms applicable to the American medical care system is the development of industrial capitalism in cottage-industry-based Elizabethan England. Toward the end of the English feudal period, village life was characterized by small and large landowners and agricultural laborers, common lands for grazing and growing, and yeoman artisans organized into cottage industries. As such, village life was largely self-sufficient and static.

However, with the advent of a rising technology and the development of Empire abroad came the Enclosure Movements, which culminated in the 18th Century. Common lands were first enclosed to en-able the large landowners (the only group with any representation in Parliament at the time) to expand their lands under cultivation and to shift to more efficient modes of production. At the same time, factories were beginning to develop in the cities. The first effect of the enclosures was to drive many small growers and cattle grazers off the land and into the cities to become, at best, wage earners. The effect of the simultaneous development of the factory system was to eventually penetrate the countryside and destroy the yeoman-based agriculture and cottage industry in much the same way that agribusiness is today squeezing out the small American farmers.

Hence, the effect of the emergence of a dynamic technology in the context of rising competitive economic relations was to transform, over a period of several hundred years, a rather stable, self-sufficient yeoman-based village life into an unstable industrial-based system; and turn yeoman farmers and artisans into the precursor of the modern working class, wholly dependent upon large landowners, their tenants, and millowners.[7]

Similarly, if we consider the emergence of a dynamic technology in the competitive American context, we can discover and predict in the same dialectical fashion the history and future of the medical care system.

The Dialectics of American Medicine

From Cottage Industry to
Industrial Capitalism

Before 1910 medical care in the United States was organized in a manner best described as cottage industry. Doctors practiced individually on a rather informal fee-for-service basis—third parties were unheard of, billing was not a highly-developed art, and payment was often in kind. Virtually all of the existing medical technology was contained in the little black bag; and medical education closely approximated the apprenticeship model with training taking as little as one year.

At that time, also, the American Medical Association was an elitist group of doctors interested primarily in medical science. It in no way represented the economic interests of the unorganized, largely competitive practicing physicians. The Flexner Committee, operating through the A.M.A.'s Council on Medical Education and the Carnegie Foundation, investigated medical education and, in 1910, reported that the conditions in medical schools were deplorable, and knowledge of medical science among medical school graduates was very poor. Between 1904 and 1920 the number of medical schools, students and graduates was cut by half; and the scientific content of medical education was greatly increased in the remaining schools.[8]

This emphasis on science is the primary contradiction in the development of the medical care system up to the present day. That is, it is the emphasis on science and the consequent introduction of a dynamic medical technology (this time with no apparent increase in the level of productivity, or even, for that matter, a definition of what medical productivity might mean) that led directly to the disputes and interest group struggles of the past 50 years, that will culminate in the next decade in a system of medical monopoly capital.[9]

Medical science and its consequent technology is characterized as a contradiction in the dialectical sense because it is simply incompatible with the private practice and control of medicine — in just the same manner in which the introduction of technology in late feudal England was incompatible with a yeoman-based, cottage-industry village life. There are two reasons for the contradiction. First, the introduction of science and technology led inevitably to the requirements of an industrial base: in this case the increasing use of hospitals to deliver the latest forms of medical care.[10] The problem is that hospitals as organizations external to the solo fee-for-service practice of medicine become institutions at once increasingly important to the practice of medicine and increasingly difficult to control in the interest of that fee-for-service practice.

Second, the introduction of science and technology also generated the requirement of a substantial financial base for the delivery of medical care. Prior to the era of scientific medicine, medical care was rather inexpensive both in terms of investment by the practitioner and cost to the patient. With the introduction of "industrial" medicine, however, the financial strain on both became quite severe. Once again, this threatens the autonomy of the private practitioner.

To return to the narrative of the early post-Flexner period, the American Association for Labor Legislation in 1915 produced a "Standard Bill" to be enacted by states enabling a compulsory health insurance scheme.[11] The A.M.A.—which was still a group of elitist scientists, not representing private practitioners—appointed a committee of its own to study the desirability of a compulsory health insurance proposal. In 1916 and 1917 the committee issued reports very sympathetic to the principles of social insurance. During World War I, however, all social legislative activities ceased. When, in 1918, the A.M.A. again pressed for medical support of the "Bill," the private practitioners began surfacing. By April, 1920, they had assumed control of the A.M.A.[12] The Association's position was quickly reversed and the issue of compulsory health insurance killed.

The historical importance of these events for the dynamics of the medical profession, then, is that a clear split developed between the practitioners and scientists, with the practitioners assuming control of the A.M.A. for the purpose of protecting their economic interests. The scientists, in turn, moved out of the organization and into the medical schools, research laboratories, and teaching hospitals.[13]

The organization of private practitioners into a strong political and economic group, the defeat of compulsory health insurance, and the subsequent development of a series of licensing arrangements and a host of barriers to entry to the medical profession enabled the A.M.A. to maintain control not only over the profession but also over the administration of hospitals and other medical institutions. It is important to recognize, however, that in an historical sense these developments could only serve to postpone the day when historical forces would eliminate private power over the practice of medicine. These forces could not be reversed without reversing the medical science and technology which generated them.

Interestingly, in the 1930s when both hospitals and physicians felt financially threatened (because patients could not pay their bills), they each set up their own reimbursement (insurance) mechanisms—Blue Cross and Blue Shield—entirely controlled by their own local or state hospital associations and medical societies, with the corresponding national associations being controlled by the American Hospital Association and American Medical Association, respectively.[14]

However, even these insurance systems did not come to terms with the historical forces described above since they not only were controlled by the providers (which satisfied their need for financial support), but also they provided no long run financial security for consumers of medical care. This follows rather directly from the nature of provider-contrived and -controlled insurance. Blue Cross was and is a cost-plus reimbursement mechanism which, in the 1950s—in a period when "charitable" contributions toward hospital expansion were beginning to dry up relative to financial "need"—served as the financial vehicle for hospital expansion, the bill eventually being picked up by Blue Cross premium payers, who are rapidly becoming priced out of the "voluntary" insurance market.

To conclude this sketch of the development of medical industrial capitalism, it is important to follow the "deposed" members of the medical profession into the medical schools, research institutes and teaching hospitals—the nonprofit sector of the medical care system. Like all social and institutional relations in capitalist societies, these institutions, too, operate in a competitive atmosphere, and compete, in part, (like universities) for prestigious faculty and medical staffs. The norms, again like the universities in general, are quality and quantity of research output, where the standards are determined by the profession itself. And furthermore, these academic standards increasingly defined the objectives and development patterns of the large urban-based medical centers (empires[15]). Consequently, in order to attract the prestigious medical staff, the prestige-oriented hospitals were obliged to accumulate the types of research facilities and fancy service units necessary to engage in the current research in vogue. And the cost-plus form of hospitalization insurance made it all possible at the expense of the unwitting consumer and premium payer.

The medical scientists, then, who were "defeated" in the struggle for control of the A.M.A. in 1920, were the ones to prosper from the contradictions of solo fee-for-service in the context of a rising medical technology (which they actually directed). This occurred because of the central role which medical scientists were to play in the industrial base of the medical care system—toward which the system had to gravitate, given the implementation of the Flexner Committee report. Thus, we can read the recent introduction of the "family medicine" specialty as little more than a placebo administered by the scientists to the practitioners.[16]

From Industrial Capitalism to Finance Capitalism

The rise of an industrialized, science-oriented delivery system, *in the context of competitive institutional relations,*[17] led in turn to its own contradictions—and these involved the consumer of medical care. As medical care tended more and more toward the dictates of research-oriented providers, the allocation of medical resources became less and less relevant to consumer needs. Hence, the rise of rather strident demands for consumer control of hospitals and hospital systems among catchment area populations, who viewed the choice of another open-heart-surgery unit over the expansion of needed ambulatory facilities as something of an obscenity. In this case the placebo consisted of specialties in community medicine.

The second contradiction is in the financing system. The dynamics described above, quite apart from any discussion of community versus experience rating, are simply pricing the middle-income consumer out of the market. Blue Cross and private carrier premiums roughly reflect hospital per diem charges, which in turn reflect the rising (research-oriented) overhead expenditures (including not only the capital costs of equipment, facilities, etc., but also the new manpower requirements to operate them). Consequently, there is no way strictly within the private sector for third parties to roll back these costs, since they reflect the prevailing professional dynamics of the delivery system.

And the history of all individuals, corporations, and industries with sufficient political power, who find themselves up against a dialectical wall, is that they seek restitution from the state,[18, 19] or, as it is known in academic circles, the public sector. Thus, we hear said today of national health insurance that "its time has come." For medical care liberals this is a time of rejoicing and the answering of prayers. It should not be, since an understanding of the conditions leading up to "its time has come" should lend some insight into the nature of the outcome.

In his presidential address to the American Public Health Association,[20] Dr. Paul Cornely argued that "[o]urs is not a democracy but rather an economic oligarchy in which powerful economic blocs provide the funds directly or indirectly for the election of our representatives and they in turn pass laws and regulations which benefit these interests."[21] Recently, James Ridgeway has pointed out the comfortable relationship between President Nixon and some leading figures in the insurance industry. His details include not only the quality of personal relationships but also the quantity of campaign contributions in the 1968 presidential election (and a hoped-for repetition in 1972).[22]

At present one of the leading contenders for a national health insurance program is that prepared by the Aetna Life and Casualty Company. Aetna's program would give primary underwriting and administrative responsibilities to the private insurance carriers, who would then come to dominate the financing[23] and delivery of medical care (the latter through the proposal for franchising HMO's, which the carriers would underwrite and set up in competition with each other). The resulting system of national health insurance would become little more than the writing of blank checks by the Social Security Administration to the private carriers, at a rate reflecting the dynamics of the resulting financing and delivery system[24] which the insurance companies would increasingly come to dominate.

Although the impact of such a development on the delivery of medical care can be studied by looking at the internal dynamics of the medical care system, its likelihood cannot be. Instead it is necessary to look at recent developments in the larger financial sector of the American economy. Building upon findings made available by the publication of the House Subcommittee on Banking and Currency *Report on Commercial Banks and Their Trust Activities* (The Patman Report), Robert Fitch and Mary Oppenheimer, in a series of three articles (of which, at this writing, only two are available) document and analyze the increasing control of nonfinancial corporations (even the largest) by commercial banks and insurance companies. Furthermore, they note an extremely rapid concentration within the banking sector itself; the very largest banks appear to be rapidly buying ownership in each other (with obvious anticompetitive implications).[25]

For our purposes the most important finding to come out of the Fitch and Oppenheimer study (via the Patman Report), is a series of proposed mergers to unilaterally link four of the five largest commerical banks (all in New York City and heavily interlocked) with two of the eight largest life insurance companies and the first and third largest casualty companies. "Altogether the four mergers would result in an agglomeration holding over 13 percent of all financial assets in the United States."[26] Moreover, Aetna, the sixth largest life insurance company is slated to merge with Morgan Guarantee Trust, the fifth largest bank in terms of financial assets and the largest in terms of trust assets (through which external control of non-financial corporations is exerted).

What is emerging is a tremendous amount of political and economic power in a very narrow segment of the financial sector of the American economy. This bodes very "well" for a political victory by the insurance companies in their struggle for control of national health insurance.

The current medical care deliberations are even more ironic. Not only has the time for national health insurance come, but so has the time for prepaid group practice in the form of health maintenance organizations. More rejoicing, more answered prayers, more illusions. If the insurance companies succeed in wresting control of the financing mechanisms, they will also succeed in controlling the as yet unclearly defined HMO's through control of their management and information systems.

What is likely, then—in the absence of a major political uprising on the part of the American people—is a medical care delivery system financed through Federal tax revenues, dominated by private insurance companies operating through HMO's and reducing the medical profession to a group of hired professional engineers. Within 10 years we shall be marketing medical care the same way we now market automobiles—and with similar hazards.

Restatement, Exercise, and Further Implications

To summarize, then, the purpose of the above analysis has been to make the case for the use of a distinctly dialectical methodology in the study of the medical care system. "[T]he main structural features of what society can be like in the next generation are already given by trends at work now."[27] Failure to recognize these trends leads easily to the implementation of programs, optimal, perhaps, under a certain, but unstated, set of circumstances; far from optimal under the existing, but unexamined set of circumstances.

An exercise may help to highlight the analysis. It has been argued here that the fundamental contradiction to the solo fee-for-service practice of medicine was the introduction of a dynamic science and technology to the delivery of care in the context of competitive economic relations. The reason, briefly, was that such a change provided the historical necessity of a large financial and industrial base to the delivery of medical care; a base so large, moreover, that private practitioners operating on a fee-for-service basis could not forever provide and control it. In spite of the A.M.A.'s efforts to forestall the eventual decline in its power over the practice of medicine, it has been argued and illustrated that the contradiction was sufficiently strong and that A.M.A. policies constituted no more than holding operations in the face of historical necessity.

Consider, then, what the A.M.A. policies might have been, had they had in their employ a dialectician whose task it was to design a strategy for organized medicine by which it would be possible for M.D.'s to control all aspects of the provision of care, in the context of an increasingly scientific practice of medicine. The strategy, ironically, seems to be prepaid group practice. That is, had the medical profession in 1920 abandoned solo fee-for-service practice and started forming prepaid groups, it would have been able to control not only the actual delivery of care, but also the underwriting of that care and of the institutions in which that care was delivered. Furthermore, its industrial and financial base would have been able to expand at a rate consistent with the increase in medical technology. This, no doubt, would have ushered in an era of increasing corporate concentration in medicine, both horizontally (larger and fewer hospitals) and vertically (sequential stages of production in single corporations: such groups might have encompassed not only hospitals but also hospital supply firms, medical schools, etc.). As a measure of the historical validity of this prognosis, one need only look at the successful economic institutions of today and see that they all embody these same characteristics (save the underwriting, a peculiar necessity of medical care): the auto, steel, aluminum and oil industries. All of these latter are heavily concentrated, both horizontally and vertically. Quite obviously, however, it is too late today for organized medicine to embark upon such a strategy, since 1) it does not have the financial resources to take over the medical care system today, and 2) even if it did, it would not be able to budge newer interests (A.H.A., medical centers, private carriers) which, since the 1920s have become politically entrenched.

The sense in which this strategy is a "solution" needs to be qualified. First, it deals only with the contradictions central to the medical care delivery system. It does not deal with contradictions in the larger system, nor with conflicts which may arise between the delivery system and the larger society. More specifically, it is a strategy for organized medicine *vis à vis* other components in the medical care system. It does not deal with potential conflicts between, say, providers and consumers of care—today a major issue in a much more fragmented system. However, to the extent that the auto industry has been much more successful in parrying assaults from consumer interests, it would appear that the "solution" would lead to somewhat more "desirable" results than those which the hospitals have recently experienced.

Yet this may only be true in the intermediate run, for this brings us to the fundamental contradiction of all capitalist so-

cieties: that they have no control over the allocation of their resources; that, rather, the resources are allocated according to private rationality in the absence of all but trivial necessary conditions for the assumption of Adam Smith's "invisible hand of competition" to be valid.[28] Hence, the "solution" is a solution short of a major confrontation over the social-control-of-resources issue, an issue clearly extending beyond the medical care delivery system.

The second qualification, of course, is that the above analysis is not intended as advocacy of organized medicine's domination over the medical care system. It is simply an exercise in dialectical analysis. Neither is this intended as advocacy of private prepaid group practice. The analysis has shown how the model of prepaid group practice can develop institutionally into an industrial monolith similar to other industries which today are characterized as oligopolistic. Moreover, even though, as was shown, it is now impossible for organized medicine to capture the entire delivery system through the group practice (or HMO) model, it appears, in the context of current deliberations over the health delivery system, that the large private insurance companies together with their large city bank associates are in a particularly advantageous position, both financially and politically, to do so.

This is not a time for rejoicing. Yet, to say so is not to say that national health insurance and HMO's will not provide some modest improvements over the present situation, whatever the nature of their actual implementation. To think, however, that they will eliminate the two-class system of medical care in a society whose very engine is insecurity,[29] is rather naive. To think, moreover, that they will substantially resolve the structural problems in the delivery system is likewise the product of an analytic methodology intent more on technique than on content.

Broadening the Analysis

All exploratory analyses end with some statement to the effect that "more research is indicated," and this is no exception. This paper has concentrated, and only superficially, on the specifics of the delivery system and the interaction of its components. Much more needs to be done in filling out the dialectical analysis of medical care institutions.

More importantly, however, in terms of making explicit the links between the medical care system and the larger system, we must construct a new study of epidemiology. We must begin to develop a meaningful social definition of "health." We must also investigate the ways in which and the extent to which our own social system generates bad health.[30] To the extent that the generation of social classes is inherent in any capitalist society, its implications for health and medical care

are immense.[31] With the incidence of schizophrenia more and more apparent among all social classes, alienation is once again becoming an important term in contemporary social analysis. And with it come substantial implications for mental health care. Which way shall we go? Toward social control consistent with the etiology of schizophrenia,[32] or toward social liberation consistent with the fulfillment of human potential?[33]

These issues lead us, finally, to the ultimate questions that medical care social scientists can address: What are the social, economic, and political conditions necessary for good health and medical care? To what extent does the achievement of the objectives of medical care *liberals* require a transformation of the social order?

References and Notes

1 By "medical care system" is meant nothing more than a collection of institutions and manpower categories to some degree interacting with each other and each somehow related to the delivery of medical care. It should not be inferred that the use of the word "system" throughout the text is intended to confer a notion of a series of rational, functional, organizational relationships. Nor does it, in the context of the current mainstream critique of the medical care "system," assume the absence of them.

2 For an intensive but uncritical discussion of functionalism, see: Martindale, Don. (ed.) *Functionalism in the Social Sciences: The Strength and Limits of Functionalism in Anthropology, Economics, Political Science, and Sociology*, Monograph 5 (Philadelphia: The American Academy of Political and Social Science, February 1965).

3 For a good contemporary critique of Western social science, see: Moore, Barrington, Jr. *Political Power and Social Theory* (Cambridge: Harvard University Press, 1958) chapters 3 and 4. See, also: Chomsky, Noam. "Objectivity and Liberal Scholarship," *American Power and the New Mandarins* (New York: Vintage, 1969). For critiques of contemporary economics, see: Sweezy, Paul. "Toward a Critique of Economics," *Monthly Review*, Vol. 21, No. 8 (January 1970); and Zweig, Michael. "Bourgeois and Radical Paradigms in Economics," Working paper no. 11, Stonybrook, June 1970. For critiques of political science, see: Green, Phillip and Levinson, Sanfor. (eds.) *Power and Community: Dissenting Essays in Political Science* (New York: Pantheon, 1970).

4 However, the case for the application of dialectical analysis in principle will not be given here.

Instead, see: Moore, *Political Power*, chapter 4; Marcuse, Herbert. *Reason and Revolution: Hegel and the Rise of Social Theory* (Boston: Beacon Press, 1960), especially pp. 312-322; Marx, Karl and Engels, Friedrich. *The German Ideology* (New York: International Publishers, 1947); and Mao Tse-tung. *Four Essays on Philosophy* (Peking: Foreign Languages Press, 1968) chapter 2, "On Contradiction."

5 MacEwan, Arthur. "Contradictions in Capitalist Development: The Case of Pakistan," *The Review of Radical Political Economics* Vol. 3, No. 4 (Spring 1971) p. 51, footnote 4.

6 Most economists will argue that there is a third category, namely, oligopoly. However, since most oligopolists recognize the inherent instability of price competition and agree not to compete on the basis of price, yet collaborate closely in political lobbying, it seems more appropriate to consider oligopolists as collective monopolists rather than as a separate market structure category.

7 Trevelyan, George M. *History of England*, Vol. III (Garden City, N. J.: Doubleday, 1953) pp. 141-146.

8 Rayack, Elton. *Professional Power and American Medicine: The Economics of the American Medical Association* (Cleveland: World Publishing, 1967) pp. 66-72.

9 The phrase is borrowed from and intended in the same sense as: Baran, Paul and Sweezy, Paul. *Monopoly Capital* (New York: Monthly Review Press, 1966).

10 Although the introduction of technology was necessary for the shift to hospital-based care, it was not sufficient. Another important characteristic of the first two decades of the 20th century was

an emerging belief in and embellishment of the powers of mass production applied not only in industrial firms, but also in social institutions such as schools and later hospitals (which had previously been used solely for the incarceration of the poor and insane). Clearly this changing attitude was also necessary for hospitals to become the staging area of scientific medicine.

11 Rayack, *Professional Power*, pp. 136-137.

12 *Ibid.*, p. 145.

13 See: Burlage, Robb. *New York City's Municipal Hospitals: A Policy Review* (Washington, D. C.: Institute for Policy Studies, 1967) ; and Burlage, Robb. "The Municipal Hospital Affiliation Plan in New York City: A Case Study and Critique," *Milbank Memorial Fund Quarterly* Vol. 46, No. 1, Part 2 (January 1968). Burlage clearly recognized these two groups of doctors (patricians and practitioners) and their conflicts with each other in the affiliation plan for the municipal hospitals of New York City.

14 Somers, Herman and Somers, Anne. *Doctors, Patients, and Health Insurance* (Washington, D. C.: Brookings Institution, 1962), chapters 15 and 16. Also see: Massachusetts Blue Cross. "Blue Cross Reimbursement Information," February, 1969, p. 6.

15 For a much more detailed discussion of the development of urban medical empires, see: Health Policy Advisory Center. *The American Health Empire: Power, Profits, and Politics* (New York: Random House, 1970) chapters 3-6.

16 The author thanks James Smith of Cornell University for pointing this out.

17 The reason for the qualification is that there appears to be evidence that, in the absence of competitive relations, many of the contradictions which we experience do not occur. See, especially: Horn, Joshua. *Away with All Pests: An English Surgeon in People's China, 1954-1969* (New York: Monthly Review Press, 1971).

18 It is important here to distinguish between the "state" and the "government." The state is the collective use of force and/or coercion to maintain the social order in the interests of the dominant coalition of power in the society. The "government" is the set of particular individuals and institutions who administer the state. Hence, the government may change without changing the basis of state power. See: Miliband, Ralph. *The State in Capitalist Society* (New York: Basic Books, 1969).

19 For an intensive historical analysis of how the Progressive Era of American politics (1890-1910) constituted the conscious use of state power to resolve contradictions in the industries subsequently to be "regulated," see: Kolko, Gabriel.

The Triumph of Conservatism (New York: Free Press of Glencoe, 1963).

20 Cornely, Paul. "The Hidden Enemies of Health and the APHA," *American Journal of Public Health* Vol. 61, No. 1 (January 1971).

21 Cornely, Paul. "What Besides Big is the Medical Care Section?", *Medical Care* 9:105 (March-April 1971).

22 Ridgeway, James. "Hard Times," *Ramparts* (May 1971) p. 4.

23 This is perfectly analogous to the politics of the Overseas Private Investment Corporation (OPIC), a quasi-public corporation created by the 1970 Foreign Aid bill as an investment guarantee program to large American foreign investors against financial losses due to devaluation, changes in taxation, nationalization and other political reversals. OPIC was initially funded with 7.5-billion American taxpayer dollars and is directed largely by the major American foreign investors. The conflict of interest here is rather clear.

24 In a manner precisely identical to the current administration of Medicare.

25 Fitch, Robert and Oppenheimer, Mary. "Who Rules the Corporations? Part I," *Socialist Revolution* 1:98 (July-August 1970).

26 *Ibid.*, p. 104.

27 Moore, *Political Power*, p. 159.

28 From economic theory the necessary conditions for optimal resource allocation under conditions of competition are: 1) universal pure competition (many buyers, many sellers, perfect information, and no barriers to entry) ; 2) rising marginal cost curves; 3) diminishing marginal consumer rates of substitution; 4) no externalities; and 5) social acceptance of the income distribution which results from the competitive process. (1) and (4) and, probably (5) do not hold.

29 Fromm, Erich. *The Sane Society* (New York: Holt, Rinehart and Winston, 1955) chapter 5, "Man in Capitalist Society"; Henry, Jules. *Culture Against Man* (New York: Random House, 1963) ; and Laing, Ronald. *The Politics of Experience* (New York: Pantheon, 1967).

30 Rossdale, Martin. "Health in a Sick Society," *New Left Review* (November-December 1965).

31 University of Michigan, School of Public Health. *Medical Care Chart Book* (1968) pp. 10-23; and U.S. Department of Health, Education and Welfare. *Delivery of Health Services for the Poor* (Washington, D. C.: GPO, 1967) pp. 3-35.

32 Laing, *The Politics of Experience;* and Health Policy Advisory Center. *Health PAC Bulletin*, New York, May 1970.

33 Marcuse, Herbert. *An Essay on Liberation* (Boston: Beacon Press, 1969).

Philip Jacobs

Reprinted with permission of the Blue Cross Association, from *Inquiry:* Vol.XI, No.2, pp.83-97. Copyright © 1974 by the Blue Cross Association.

A Survey of Economic Models of Hospitals

Originally Published in June 1974

The economic models that have been constructed for hospitals can be placed into two categories. The first are those that treat the hospital as an "organism" or entity with its own goals which are usually stated in terms of some aspect(s) of performance, such as quantity and/or quality of output, profits, and so on. Of course, there is frequently a rationale stated, explaining why a particular argument was chosen for the hospital's choice function. But the explicitly formulated model is one in which the hospital's performance is its objective, and so it is "the hospital" which is in effect being identified as the entity with the choice set. Such models will be referred to as "organism" models,[1] since they treat the hospital as a separate organism.

The second type of model identifies those individuals who use the hospital as an organization that functions to enable them to further their own ends. Thus, trustees may wish to provide the needy with medical care, and they will do so through the hospital; or doctors will use the hospital as a place to treat their patients, thus gaining income from their use of it. Whatever the aims of these groups, the hospital serves as an institution that facilitates exchange and/or enables the individuals involved to at-

tain their own goals. This sort of model will be referred to as an "exchange" model. In these models the performance of the firm is a means to an end—the ends of the individuals who use it to achieve their (explicitly stated) goals. The formal model focuses on their behavior.

Nonprofit hospitals are different from most other organizations in that there are "two lines of authority"—medical and managerial. The nonprofit hospital has emerged as an institution where doctors and "management" both are in a position to formulate hospital policies. These two sets of policies need not coincide. The presence of such a schism in the decision-making process (physician and administrator and trustee) is bound to have some effect on hospital resource allocation, and a model of a hospital must come to terms with this fact in one way or another. There are two related points on this issue. First, the models may differ in scope. Doctors have attained a very autonomous position in their role of providing medical services in a nonprofit institution. One can use this autonomous position as a reason, as some analysts have done, for excluding doctors' services entirely from the analysis; one can treat doctors in a peripheral sort of way; or one can attempt to incorporate them into the analysis. Connected with this point is the treatment of doctors' services in hospital cost analyses; some investigators ignore doctors' costs and only a few include them.

Second, there is the question of the hypothesized organizational structure—who makes the decisions? That is, whose utility is to be maximized in the analysis? While this point may sound trivial, it is not trivial even in a profit-making enterprise where there are both a mana-

Philip Jacobs, D. Phil. is a Sessional Lecturer, Department of Economics, Sir George Williams University, Montreal (Quebec, Canada). This paper is based on a chapter of the author's unpublished D. Phil. thesis submitted to the University of York, England, in 1973. The author would like to thank his thesis supervisor, Mr. A. J. Culyer, as well as Professors A. T. Peacock and J. Wiseman, and Mr. M. Cooper, Mr. Panos Filaktos, and Mr. Antonio Zabalza for their help and suggestions. Full responsibility for all errors remains with the author. Financial assistance was provided by the Canada Council.

ger and owners who are not managers.[2] In this case the managers have the opportunity to benefit from on-the-job sources of utility which detract from the owners' profits. In such a case certain policies may be explained better by examining the (utility maximizing) behavior of a salaried manager than by hypothesizing a profit-maximizing "firm"; the point being that even in such a "clear cut" case the theoretical structure of the organization to be used is discretionary. In the case of hospitals, with unpaid trustees, their salaried administrators and doctors, the organizational pattern is much more unclear.

Another point concerns the quality of services. Quality of services is an aspect of medical goods production that has often been stressed in the health care literature.[3] Some hospital models have put their emphasis on quality, ignoring all else. The existence of seldom used open heart surgery machines has captured the fancy of hospital economic model builders everywhere and, so it seems, no model can be without reference to one. Nevertheless, though quality is an elusive trait, it is a peculiarity that must be dealt with in health service analysis.

Finally, the elements of monopoly and competition—the forms of medical market structures—differ from model to model. All this is an unsettled question in the literature and we would expect diversified views. In fact, there has not been widespread attention paid to exchange and market structure facets of the models. What little discussion there has been will be noted.

These are a few points that will appear repeatedly in this survey. They indicate inadequate attention on the part of economists to institutional details that render it difficult to fit a model of the hospital into the usual mold of the theory of the firm. The survey is divided into two parts: organism models and exchange models. The former contain quality and quantity and profit-maximizing models. The latter contain more basic "utility" maximizing models.

Organism Models

Quantity Maximizing Models

The maximization of quantity has been the most frequently suggested objective for a model of a nonprofit hospital.[4] However, formal models are hard to come by in this category. Nevertheless, it is possible to put together a sketch of a model as suggested in the works of P. Feldstein and M. Brown, which is generally along the lines of the usual quantity maximizing model of the firm. Such a model provides a useful starting point because it enables us to highlight certain problems which later models try to meet; such a model, in other words, is useful as a standard by which other models can be compared.

In the views of P. Feldstein and M. Brown, the hospital is much like a firm in any other industry, run by a single administrator. P. Feldstein hints that "this administrator" or "decision-maker" is the actual administrator of a hospital as seen in real life,[5] and not a fictional, composite character made up of trustees, doctors, and administrators. This administrator's job is to "shift around" resources to positions where they are best suited. But medical care also requires doctors who treat the patient and administer or direct the care. Brown[6] attempts to fit the doctor into the hospital organization by giving him the role of "an agent advising a patient." The physician's services to the patient are distinct from those services of the hospital to the patient. In spite of this, however, it is recognized that the physician may exert some influence on hospital policies.[7]

It is the administrator's job to maximize the quantity of output of the hospital.[8] In the hospital industry there is the problem of determining quality, however—a problem of considerable magnitude. Thus, P. Feldstein's assertion that a hospital must "provide a given amount of patient care at minimum cost"[9] is qualified by the statement that "quality is given."[10] Long makes quality a constraint—the care provided must be the "best possible with available equipment and personnel."[11]

Thus, we have a view of a hospital administrator utilizing hospital resources in such a way that quantity of output is maximized (given quality), with the doctor an independent agent of the patient. There is little else of interest to us in these papers except, perhaps, P. Feldstein's assertion[12] that because of restrictions on entry and lack of information the markets facing the consumer are monopolistic.

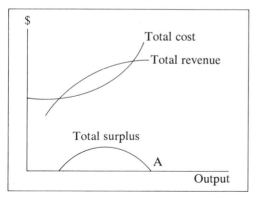

Figure I. Output maximizing firm with no subsidy

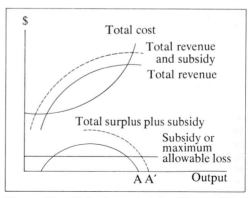

Figure II. Output maximizing firm with a subsidy or permitted loss

Rice[13] provides a complete model of an output maximizing hospital with some modifications to take into account peculiarities in the market for medical services. The model contains an output maximand. Revenues are received from patient care; and assuming that expansion is to be financed out of the surplus of revenues over expenditures, then a minimum surplus is a constraint. In Figure I, Rice's diagrammatic treatment of the theory of the hospital is presented; output will be increased up to the point where the minimum allowable surplus is reached. If no surplus is required for expansion purposes, this will be at point A. One implication of the model is that, if a subsidy or a maximum loss constraint is added, then output can be increased up to the point where the new constraint is reached (OA′ in Figure II). Another implication is that the drive to maximize output leads to minimum costs.

The "standard" uncomplicated model of P. Feldstein and Brown would not depart from these results. Rice does modify his model, however, in an attempt to incorporate institutional characteristics. The final product, health care, is divided into two categories: necessities and supplementary products. Supplementary products are amenities, not strictly necessary for health care. The hospitals maximize profits on these products and apply these profits to the maximization of output on necessary medical services.

It is the physician who coordinates the various inputs (e.g., necessary services, physician services). Physicians, according to Rice, are the true customers of hospital services. Patients should pay physicians and the physicians should pay the hospital; but because of financing problems, the patient pays the hospital directly. It is the physician who is the main producer of medical care, in or out of the hospital.

Rice's emphasis on the physicians' role in the hospital shows a realization of the crucial role of the doctor and represents an attempt to grapple with the issue of the two-headed organization head on—an issue frequently ignored by analysts.[14]

It might be pointed out that this is but one way to treat the problem of the physician-hospital relationship. There are many other possibilities that can be imagined, but the important thing to notice is that Rice does attempt to deal with the issue explicitly, rather than as a feature that need not be considered.

Finally, as to the range of Rice's model, while it contains all of the predictions of any quantity maximizing model, it has little to say about a very important aspect of health care —quality. Also, it infers cost minimization. For the moment, these points will only be noted. As other theories are examined, the position of this theory will become clearer.

Quality Maximizing Models

The next model to be considered, that of M. L. Lee, places heavy emphasis on the quality of care produced.[15] Ostensibly, Lee's is a "manager's" utility maximizing model,[16] the utility function containing, among other elements, "salary, prestige, security, power and professional satisfaction. . . ."[17] The reasons for its being placed in the "organism" category will soon become clear, however.

It is, in Lee's view, the hospital administrator whose utility is being maximized. Doctors are regarded as inputs into the administrators' processes to achieve status. As Lee says:[18]

> . . . the status of the hospital is assumed to vary with the range of services available and the extent to which expensive and highly specialized equipment and personnel (*including M.D.'s*) are available. (emphasis added)

This explanation by-passes many problems and even Lee is not convinced about its completeness, for when he comes to discuss how change is brought about in a hospital, it is not the hospital administrator who is the prime mover within the organization:[19]

> A given hospital may adopt the patterns of inputs utilized by hospitals in higher status groups under a number of circumstances. First, the action may be initiated *by members of the community* (in which the hospital serves) who visualize the desirability of a particular new pattern of inputs and therefore initiate and facilitate the acquisition of such inputs. Second, the action to adopt new inputs may be initiated by the hospital administrator. (emphasis added)

These "members of the community" referred to could be boards of trustees, ignored entirely in Lee's explanation. Yet, if a group other than the administrator leads the hospital, surely it must count in the analysis. Thus, the model suffers from a lack of completeness—events crucial to the model are omitted from it.

Concerning the formalization of the model, Lee in fact turns it into an "organism" model that focuses on an aspect of the hospital's performance—the quality of inputs. Lee says that:[20]

> In addition . . . the salary, prestige, security, power and professional satisfaction of decision makers are dependent on the prestige and status of the organizations with which the decision makers are associated. This implies that the utility of the hospital administrators is a function of the status of the hos-

pitals in which they serve. Thus, it is assumed that the drive for status has become a socially recognized goal among hospital administrators and that this drive plays a *dominant* role as hospital administrators strive to maximize utility. (emphasis added)

Although the model's underlying insight is that administrators seek prestige and that they do this by transforming "their" organization into a prestigious one, the actual model itself is one in which a particular indicator of the hospital's performance is maximized—"prestige"; Lee ties this magnitude to *inputs*.[21] A hospital's status, he contends, is formed by the position, relative to other hospitals, of such characteristics as the range of services available and the more expensive and highly specialized equipment and personnel in the hospital's service. The administrator will seek to maximize an index of inputs that yield prestige, subject to an income constraint.

It is here that the competition element comes in. Prestige is relative. The administrator's perception of his prestige is a function of the prestige (prestigious inputs) of other hospitals. If one hospital moves ahead by acquiring new machinery, presumably others feel they have fallen behind. A new environment is created, and in this new environment their prestige is no longer at a maximum point. New inputs can be acquired which will help to attain this point. Innovation by hospital "A" creates a gap for competitor, hospital "B," between desired and actual prestige.

It might be useful to stress that it is "quality" of inputs that Lee is placing in the hospital's objective function. In a model to be considered presently, "quality" refers to *both* outputs and inputs. While there is no agreement (or even discussion) of this in the hospital economics literature, "quality" of inputs and outputs are quite different concepts.

Continuing with Lee's model, the possibility for a hospital to raise its status comes from increased revenue. Revenue can come from priced services and insurance schemes. Lee's discussion of pricing policies illuminates his model better, however, so they shall be mentioned. Given output, a rise for desired status on the part of the hospital leads to its raising the price for extra revenue.[22] The price elasticity being near zero, this will raise revenue and output will remain about the same. Two problems with this formulation are the inability of the model to say anything at all about output and the lack of specification of a price ceiling. With regard to the first problem, this seems to be a by-product of the hospital's managers' pursuit of prestige:[23]

> Hospitals acquire inputs without adequate regard for the output of services that can be produced with such inputs.

Output, it seems, just happens somehow. With regard to the second problem, prices are determined by "what the traffic will bear."[24] This principle does not work with the perfectly inelastic curve envisaged by Lee, as such a curve would provide a pricing principle only if an upper limit to prices were specified, and no such limit is specified by Lee. In the case where the individual's demand curve has some elasticity, a certain quantity of output for each patient would need to be specified to determine price. The hospital would choose that amount for each patient, and those numbers of patients, which would yield them a revenue point where prestige can be maximized. Put in this way, such a model seems rather cumbersome, and certainly it has not been worked out fully yet.

As with all models, what one gets out depends on what one puts into it. The assumptions of this model are completely quality loaded and, hence, one would expect the implications to have a similar bias. One is not taken by surprise, then, when one learns that some of the major implications include: the inputs used are more than sufficient for those required for the tasks and there will be idle capacity. These imply high costs per unit of output.[25] As well, factor use will be sensitive to factor price. It is accepted that these are characteristics of the hospital scene, but Lee's model explains little else.

The model does not stand up well on exogenous changes. It does not state clearly the sources of change. As well, the principle to determine price and output is incomplete. Finally, there is more to hospital activities than prestige and concomitant price increases. Decision-makers, whoever they are, also make decisions about output—admissions (queues are

a fact of hospital life) and length of stay. There is nothing in Lee's model that would suggest this. It explains a few well-known facts, but in the process omits a lot of others.

Quality and Quantity Maximizing Models

Two models will be examined in this part—those of M. Feldstein and J. Newhouse. Both incorporate maximand elements of both of the previous types examined and, hence, they permit the decision-maker a wider range of choice. The models are quite different owing, perhaps, to the different phenomena that they have been set up to explain. These differences will be briefly pointed out later on, for this comparison will elucidate how the models have been set up to deal with specific phenomena.

In Newhouse's model[26] the "decision-maker" is a monolithic amalgam of trustees, doctors and the hospital administrator which seeks to maximize a weighted function of quality and quantity. All three have stakes in both entities and by some form of bargaining process achieve "some final resolution" among their tastes.[27] The administrator's salary will depend upon the size and prestige of the institution. The trustees' rewards include status, and in this pursuit the institution's prestige plays a key role. The doctors seek to give a high quality of care and professional standing, both of which will be easier obtained in a more prestigious institution. There is a budget constraint limiting the size of the hospital's deficit and, hence, how much of their objectives they can attain.

Newhouse is not clear as to whether it is "quality" of inputs or outputs that is being sought by each group, and, indeed, what this "quality" is. This lack of clarity seems to stem from the absence of a particular reference group that judges quality. "Quality" to doctors and trustees may mean something entirely different, and it is not enough to assume "some final resolution."[28] This issue is crucial at the testing stage. Not having specified what the element "quality" found in the utility function consists of, how can one test for its presence? Such a problem mars much of Newhouse's paper.

Ignoring the possibility of a budget deficit and third-party financing for the moment, the chief budgetary constraint of the hospital de-

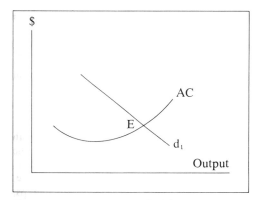

Figure III. Output maximizing firm with fixed quality of product

pends on the ability of the patient to pay the full cost of hospital care. Thus, the hospital's revenue will be calculated according to the individual's demand curves, which shift with quality. The consumer's demand curve is defined as follows:[29]

> Suppose quality is given, say, at the minimum permissible level for accreditation. This determines an average cost curve—call it ACo. At this quality, income and all other relevant variables except price held constant, there is a certain demand at each price which determines a demand curve, call it Do.

Further,[30] when quality is allowed to change, "a higher quality product raises the demand curve." Thus, the general result of a shift in quality is an upward shift in demand.

Given quality, equilibrium is attained where average revenue equals average cost ($AR = AC$). In Figure III such a position is shown at E. The highest quantity that the administrator can produce and sell will be the equilibrium point, for a given quality.

Newhouse assumes the average cost curve to be U-shaped. He further assumes it to shift upwards with an increase in quality. There is, then, at least one equilibrium for every quality: at least one point where $AR = AC$. There may be more. In this event the administrator will choose the combination with the largest quantity each quality has associated with it, an equilibrium point, such as E in Figure III. A trade-off curve is derived, tracing out the maximum equilibrium quantity associated with each quality. The shape of this curve, of course, depends

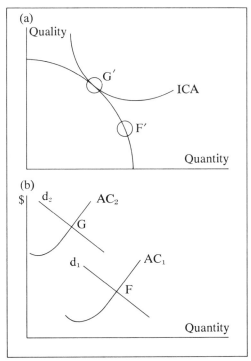

Figure IV. Equilibrium in Newhouse's quantity-quality maximizing model

upon the shifts of the demand and cost curves. The trade-off curve may be upward sloping over some ranges, but eventually will slope downwards as in Figure IV.[31]

The "administrator" is faced with a choice of positions, along the trade-off curve. According to Newhouse:[32]

> The decision-maker will choose the point on this trade-off curve which yields *him* the highest utility. That will be where the curve is tangent to the highest obtainable indifference curve.

The patient, it appears, is one who passively accepts the "decision-maker's" decision.

The decision-maker is a monopolist. "He" appears to have gained his monopoly position because of lack of potential entrants and he is able to keep it because of certain operating advantages the nonprofit firm has over the profit-making firm. Potential entrants are few as entry relies on those with a charitable bent—not profit seekers—to make sufficient outlays. And an increase in demand does not create any incentive comparable with profits to induce entry.[33] This protected status enables less efficient producers to survive.[34] Legal barriers and financial incentives (e.g., philanthropy and favorable tax status) hinder profit-seeking entrants.[35]

If current charges do not cover expenditures —that is, if a deficit is permitted—then the possibilities curve is shifted out and a higher indifference curve can be reached. Little is said about the fund-raising process required to cover the deficit except that:[36]

> The fund-raising drive will be carried on until the marginal benefit to the decision-maker of shifting the trade-off curve out by the amount the marginal dollar would do so equals the marginal cost of raising that dollar.

Little can be inferred from a general statement that any activity is carried on until the marginal cost equals marginal benefits unless one specifies what these costs and benefits are, as well as whose they are. Thus, the revenue side of the picture remains somewhat empty because the "costs" and "benefits" from raising revenue are not specified.

This lack of specification, it is submitted, comes from lumping the various "decision-making" groups into a heterogeneous whole, creating a fictional entity which (who?) is in no way intuitively connected with reality and, hence, whose presence does not readily suggest a more operative specification of these costs and benefits.

Concerning alternative payments methods, "the effect of changing the basis of payment may be merely to alter the location and shape of the trade-off curve and doing that alters none of the conclusions. . . ."[37] Cost or charge reimbursement does pose a problem as logically the possibilities curve can be shifted out without limit unless there is something there to stop it.

A combination of finance and competition assumptions is required for the analysis of cost or charge reimbursement.[38] This sort of reimbursement will lead to a potentially limitless trade-off curve unless some factor is present to limit expansion. One such factor is the influence of the hospital's expenditures on insurance rates.[39] If the hospital's expenditures are an insignificant portion of the fund's total payments to all hospitals (the large-group case),

then the possibilities curve can be shifted out at will. An increase in expenditures will not raise the price of insurance and, hence, will not reduce demand. In the small-group case, the price of insurance is raised and the hospitals will pay more attention to the effects of their increases in expenditures on quality.

One of the implications of Newhouse's model is least-cost production. If a given output could be produced at a lower unit cost, the decision-maker would do so as it would further his aims.

When we drop the assumption that a single quality is produced and permit many different qualities—each with demand and cost curves independent of other qualities[40]—then there is the implication of a bias in favor of higher quality products. If a nonprofit firm can increase quality (given quantity) and cover the cost of it, it will do so regardless of the profit situation. This preference for quality that is built into the utility function ensures this result.[41] In testing his model, Newhouse relies on the usual indications of "quality" in U.S. nonprofit hospitals. However, because of the problem of specification previously noted, what his empirical "tests" actually say is not clear.

Perhaps the major problem with Newhouse's model is its weakness on the "institutional" side. The hospital is placed in a theoretical straightjacket—that of a "firm" with a single head ("the administrator"), with a single utility function. While it is theoretically appealing, such a treatment leaves many problems of application to the real world untouched.

On its predictions, several conclusions are questionable: for example, the explanation of least-cost production[42] and average cost pricing.[43] Thus, one might conclude that, at least in its present form, Newhouse's model is of limited usefulness.

M. Feldstein has produced several models. This survey will only cover a recent one.[44] This model seeks to explain hospital cost inflation. In the explanation, Feldstein relies heavily on the market mechanism—demand and supply are equilibrated by price. Through this mechanism, rising prices are explained.

Hospital utilization is divided into admissions (*ADM*) and average duration of stay (*MS*). Total demand bed days (*BDD*) is equal to the product of the two. For the moment, bed sup-

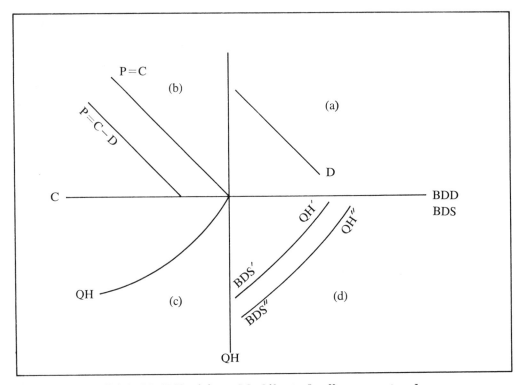

Figure VI.   A deficit in M. Feldstein's model shifts trade-off curve outwards

will assume that $D = O$, so that $P = C$; i.e., there is no philanthropy. Unit cost, C, is equal to $wN + rJ$, where J and N are materials and supplies and labor services per unit of output. With quality (QH) constant, returns to scale will be constant;[46] w and r are the (constant) factor prices.

Maximizing $QH = QH(N,J)$ implies choosing N and J such that C is on the budget frontier. This means that the higher P, the higher C (and hence QH) possible. Thus P will be on the demand curve D at the fixed output; it is the highest price attainable at that output. The market, this implies, is cleared by the price. In Figure V, quadrants a, b and c, we illustrate this short-run equilibrium for two bed supplies, A and B. Given D, the cost-price relationship and the production curve for QH, a quality-quantity trade-off curve can be derived (Figure V, quadrant d). If the quantity of beds is allowed to alter, the investment process becomes one of choosing the optimum bed size and is obtained by maximizing the preference function $U(BDS, QH)$.

This is the skeleton of the model. It is important to note that Feldstein's "utility maximizer" is not clearly identified. The decision-making body appears to be the hospital management. But the "hospital's administration" is reduced to pleasing other groups (medical staff, patients, "other groups"), with its aims unspecified.[47] Such a rationalization, while perhaps yielding an explanation for rising prices, is not suggestive of further hypotheses, not being intuitively connected with the "real world."

Turning to the model's predictions, it has already been seen that a market clearing price is predicted. The model has been set up to explain inflation and does so. An outward shift in the demand function permits a higher price and higher cost of care of a higher quality. A deficit has the same effect—shifting out the trade-off curve (in Figure VI) from $BDS'QH'$ to $BDS''QH''$. A rise in input prices shifts the QH-BDS frontier inwards: the effect on price will depend on the slope of the indifference curves.[48]

As Davis says, it could be doctors or the administrators (take your pick). Pauly and Redisch, on the other hand, are more in line with institutional realities.

According to Pauly and Redisch, the "nonprofit" institution is started by two groups—doctors and equity holders (trustees). In this form of institution there are residual profits, but they go to doctors, not to equity holders.

This, of course, suggests the question of why trustees operate these hospitals and incur these costs, in the first place. As Pauly and Redisch point out, those who provide equity capital for a nonprofit hospital must "be motivated by a desire on the part of contributors to make output available to themselves or those whom they would like to see consume it."[54] Pauly and Redisch do not pursue this line of thinking, however, concentrating almost exclusively on physicians' behavior. Such an analysis, omitting consideration of an important segment of the hospital (trustees), omits treatment of an important source of finance—trustee-raised revenue—and thus omits some important constraints. According to Pauly and Redisch, trustees merely "legitimize the hospital to the local community."[55] The doctors take charge of the process of producing health care.[56]

In assuming this, Pauly and Redisch are explicitly making the complete medical process the product. Whereas the "organism" models considered in the first part of this paper were unclear as to the place (role) of the physician in the hospital and, hence, the scope of the product (i.e., to include or exclude physician services), Pauly and Redisch are explicit about the role of the doctor; and once his role is clarified, so is the scope of the product.

In the formal model, output (Q) is produced by doctors (M), physical capital (K) and other labor (L), and is sold as a unit, to patients, for a price (P_t). Thus P_tQ is gross revenue. This revenue goes to pay non-doctor input expenses, $wL + cK$, which are priced (at P_h) so as to cover costs; i.e.,

$$P_hQ = wL + cK.$$

The residual, $P_tQ - P_hQ = P_tQ - wL - cK$, goes to physicians. Assuming that staff doctors cooperate fully to share profits in some manner,[57] then, given the number of physicians, their

"problem" is to maximize the residual, total profits, subject to production function and demand function constraints. The "solution," in the short run (with M given), is to hire units of L and K until their wages equal their marginal contribution to the value of output. The solution does not discuss how physicians share profits, but the long-run discussion mentions this.

The long-run problem is to determine how many doctors should be admitted to the staff. The solution depends on the assumption made concerning the gains of the marginal physician joining the staff—the lower the payments to them, the fewer the new doctors who will be willing to join the staff. For an individual hospital, long-run physician income is determined by the revenue obtainable by all hospital physicians for their services (their "revenue product"), by the manner in which this revenue is shared, and by their supply schedules. Adding physicians to the staff produces first a rising average revenue product because of scale economies and elastic demand, and later a falling *ARP* curve because of decreasing returns and hence a diminishing *MRP*. Given these conditions, the optimum quantity of doctors (M) at which physician profits are maximized depends on the method of distributing income. In the case of a closed staff, equal income sharing policy, the optimum point will be where the *ARP* is at a maximum—it is the point (C in Figure VII) where average income shared is at a maximum. In the case of discriminatory sharing, on the other hand, physicians will be added

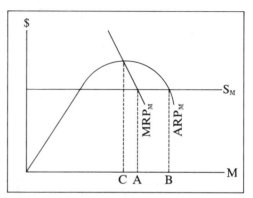

Figure VII. Physician equilibrium in the Pauly-Redisch model

as long as their marginal value exceeds their supply price; each is paid his *MRP*—this is Point A in Figure VII. Finally, in the case of equal sharing with open hiring policies, physicians are hired up to the point where *ARP* equals their supply price (point B); this will be lower than when there is a closed staff policy.

If there are excluded physicians, it may pay them to start a new hospital. In this case, new hospitals will be started "as long as higher incomes can be earned" by doctors who could benefit from a hospital post in a new hospital. There is an entry mechanism; that is, entry is based on doctors' potential profits acting as incentives.[58] This mechanism puts the model in that category of a smoothly-running competitive model, with actors reacting to financial incentives. It ignores barriers to entry, an important consideration in this industry. In fact, in making their model achieve such a smoothly-running state, Pauly and Redisch exorcise all those elements from their model where behavior (e.g., entry) does not respond to financial incentives,[59] and where monopoly hinders adjustment[60]—aspects which are of great importance in understanding how the nonprofit hospital works.

With regard to hospital pricing, Pauly and Redisch claim that average cost pricing, the average price being the lowest price (P_h) consistent with no deficit, will be the price policy followed because any higher price, while raising hospital profits, lowers the doctors' share (residual profits). That is, given P_t, a higher P_h means a lower $P_t - P_h$.

Thus, the pricing policy consistent with maximum physician income is average cost pricing. This notion of prices for hospital services being reduced to a minimum is not consistent with limited evidence from several studies, which show that, although doctors try to reduce hospital "profits," they are only partially successful.[61]

One of the major virtues of the Pauly-Redisch model is its attempt at consistency with institutional factors and its consequent ability to generate explanations in important areas (e.g., staff size). But by concentrating solely on doctors' behavior, some aspects of the hospital's activities (especially those concerning trustee behavior) have been omitted, with the possible result of a reduction in the range of events explainable by the theory, including those in the area of financing.

A General Exchange Model

A more complete framework has been presented by Buchanan and Lindsay.[62] In fact, Buchanan and Lindsay only present a suggestion for a model, but they are more explicit about institutional considerations that affect hospital resource allocation. What Buchanan and Lindsay make explicit are the two lines of authority.

It is inevitable with two lines of authority that conflict must arise between medical and administrative decisions. The outcome of the conflict provides evidence corroborating Pauly and Redisch's construct: "the medical staff usually holds all the aces."[63] The dispute is between hospital administrators and physicians. The trustees "typically exercise only negligible directions of hospital operations." The administrators, who are in charge of the management side, have little stake in opposing doctors. The administrator's "own job security depends far more than on any other factor on his ability to keep the medical staff of his hospital satisfied."[64] The assumption of medical staff domination leads to the conclusion that the hospitals will be run in the doctors' favor. Because doctors have no incentive to keep hospital costs down (indeed, they want high cost equipment and staff slack so that they can economize on their own time), hospital costs will rise quickly. Thus, in the hospital itself there will be some slack and inefficiency.

Buchanan and Lindsay do not develop their model any further, but their placing the hospital in an exchange framework is an advance. Their view of the dominance of the physician and the disinterest of the trustees is challengeable, however. The trustees' interests need not be financial to be strong. They have possible interests in prestige, and there are, as well, externalities of consumption of health care—when the trustees are there to satisfy their demand for others' medical care.[65] In doing so, their interests may be very strong, indeed.

In this sort of exchange model, however, there exists the possibility of deriving testable propositions in the form of the outcomes of various possible sorts of exchange relationships among the different groups. These relationships are not suppressed or presumed, as in the case of "organism" models.

A Trustee-Manager Exchange Model

Another exchange model, from a somewhat different angle, is that of Clarkson,[66] which focuses on differences in behavior between profit maximizing and nonprofit hospitals. These differences are due to property rights differences, with their effects on the relative costs of elements in the managers' utility functions.

Clarkson focuses on trustees (owners) and administrators. The trustees or owners of a profit-making firm have profits as their measure of a manager's success. In a nonprofit firm, additions to wealth are not sought by owners, and hence policies which deviate from the present value (profit-maximizing) rule can be pursued by the managers with a smaller consequent loss, in terms of wealth, to the trustees.[67]

Based on such comparisons, various implications are drawn. It might be pertinent to point out that the assumption that trustees lose less wealth in a nonprofit environment does not mean they lose less in terms of some other sort of benefit by failing to scrutinize the managers. In fact, Clarkson has not identified the sources of gains of trustees, an omission which makes it difficult both to predict policies and to make any statement at all on potential losses by trustees due to a lack of scrutiny.

Clarkson's analysis is based on the fact that the nonprofit environment gives the administrator greater scope to deviate from the present value rule of wealth maximization than does the profit-making environment. One way of deviating is to acquire greater current (nonpecuniary) benefits for himself (the administrator) and the employees of the nonprofit firm (nonproprietary enterprise).

Now trustees will be aware of such potential abuses. They will try to prevent them in several ways. First, they "may appoint authorities [monitors]. . .to prevent them."[68] As well, they will develop a set of rules that will tend to be "different and more explicit"[69] than those found in a profit-making (proprietary) firm. Furthermore, Clarkson concludes both that the prac-

tices of these appointed monitors and the external rules developed by the trustees will tend to be more "heterogeneous" in nonproprietary than in proprietary firms (i.e., they will be less uniform between nonproprietary firms). This will be so partly because the goals of the higher authorities in nonprofit firms will be more diversified (than just "profits" or "wealth") and perhaps less clearly identifiable—hence, more difficult to implement.

It might be interesting to dwell briefly on the subject of the goals or objectives of the trustee of the nonprofit (nonproprietary) firm. According to Clarkson, these goals of the higher authorities are unspecified and perhaps "heterogeneous" (i.e., differing among trustees or firms): "the reasons for becoming non-proprietary non-profit seeking are varied. . . ."[70] This assumption amounts to the absence of a clearly defined trustee objective. It is our contention that attempts to clearly define objectives of trustees of nonproprietary firms, while certainly not an easy task, might also lead to valuable hypotheses. Especially in the hospital context, the clearer identification of trustee goals (as well as constraints, of course), when incorporated in a formal model, will surely shed a good deal of light on the alleged obeisance of the trustees in their relations with doctors (as well as other groups).

Returning to Clarkson's model, some light can be shed on the choices made by managers or administrators, including their choice of inputs. Assuming that police costs (costs to trustees of enforcing policies or policing managers' behavior) prohibit or reduce the effectiveness of the regulating activities of trustees in certain areas; and assuming the reduced loss to owners of nonproprietary firms due to the absence of a residual wealth claim,[71] Clarkson derives implications concerning managerial choice.[72] These include managers choosing (from among the total available choice of activities) those activities that are more pleasant to them (although these activities may be less likely to achieve the trustees' objectives); and managers acquiring information that is less costly (to the manager) to obtain (although it may also be less useful).[73]

In testing his theory, Clarkson rightly stresses the difficulties in obtaining pertinent information. However, despite these problems, he has provided a very useful empirical section on differences in behavior in proprietary and nonproprietary hospitals, which certainly attest to the relevance of his approach.

In conclusion, there seem to be differences in behavior between profit-making and nonprofit hospitals that are caused by property rights attenuation, and the analysis of these differences promises to yield important gains. However, the analysis could be extended by considering alternative possible trustee goals. The analysis would then be made more complete, and could also be used to explain the *existence* of nonprofit firms. Second, doctors do not enter into Clarkson's analysis. While the focus on trustee-administrator exchange certainly is a valuable one, the influence of doctors in the hospital setting is too pervasive to ignore—even in such a "partial" analysis as Clarkson's.

Conclusion

We have, in this paper, surveyed the economic models of hospitals. These models fall into two groups. The first, which treats the hospital as an organism by itself, we have called "organism" models; they focus their attention on some aspect of the performance of the hospital. The second group, more institutional in nature, regards the hospital as an institution designed to serve the interests of the parties connected with it, and hence concentrates on the behavior of these individuals or groups.

In the first group, the emphasis on a "mechanical" choice model which fits the institution has not been successful, probably because the analysts have not been clear about the nature of the institutions they have been writing about. Since the second group of models are more institutionally oriented, they perhaps yield greater gains at a time when institutional understanding is not great. While no analyst has yet come up with a "complete" picture here—one that includes trustees, doctors, administrators and patients—indeed, a model incorporating all of these "trading bodies" simultaneously might prove unwieldly—parts of the picture have been studied with greater consistency and deeper insight with these models. Clarity in institutional matters will have to precede the development of more "mechanical" models of the hospitals.

References and Notes

1 This term comes from A. Downs (*An Economic Theory of Democracy*, New York: Harper, 1957, page 15) who, following James M. Buchanan, classifies models of state decision-making in this way. The terms have been retained to avoid an excessive creation of terms.

2 See: Tullock, Gordon. "The New Theory of Corporations." In: Streissler, Erich. (ed.) *Roads to Freedom* (London: Routledge and Kegan Paul, 1969).

3 Reder, Melvin. "Some Problems in the Economics of Hospitals," *American Economic Review* 56:472–480 (May 1965).

4 See: Long, Millard F. "Efficient Use of Hospitals." In: Mushkin, Selma J. (ed.) *The Economics of Health and Medical Care* (Ann Arbor: University of Michigan Press, 1964); Feldstein, Paul J. "Applying Economic Concepts to Hospital Care," *Hospital Administration* 13:68–89 (Winter 1968); and Brown, Max, Jr. "An Economic Analysis of Hospital Operations," *Hospital Administration* 15:60–74 (Spring 1970).

5 Feldstein, P., *op. cit.*, pp. 71–73.

6 Brown, *op. cit.*, pp. 65–66.

7 *Ibid.*, p. 66.

8 Feldstein, P., *op. cit.*, pp. 75–76.

9 *Ibid.*, p. 74.

10 *Ibid.*, p. 75.

11 Long, *op. cit.*, p. 212.

12 Feldstein, P., *op. cit.*, p. 87.

13 Rice, Robert G. "Analysis of the Hospital as an Economic Organism," *The Modern Hospital* 106:87–91 (April 1966).

14 For exceptions to this (an earlier writer who did stress the importance of physicians), see: Klarman, Herbert. "The Economics of Hospital Service," *Harvard Business Review* 29:71–89 (September 1951); and *Hospital Care in New York City* (New York: Columbia University Press, 1963). See also the section of this paper on "Exchange Models."

15 Lee, Maw Lin. "A Conspicuous Production Theory of Hospital Behavior," *Southern Economic Journal* 38:48–58 (July 1971).

16 *Ibid.*, p. 48.

17 *Ibid.*, p. 49.

18 *Ibid.*, p. 49.

19 *Ibid.*, p. 54.

20 *Ibid.*, p. 49.

21 *Ibid.*, p. 49.

22 *Ibid.*, p. 54.

23 *Ibid.*, p. 52.

24 *Ibid.*, p. 54.

25 *Ibid.*, pp. 54–56.
26 Newhouse, Joseph P. "Toward a Theory of Non-profit Institutions: An Economic Model of a Hospital," *American Economic Review* 60:64–74 (March 1970).
27 *Ibid.*, p. 65.
28 Smith, David B. "The Measurement of Health Care Quality," *Social Science and Medicine* 6:145–155 (February 1972).
29 Newhouse, *op. cit.*, p. 67.
30 *Ibid.*, p. 68.
31 *Ibid.*, p. 68.
32 *Ibid.*, p. 68.
33 *Ibid.*, p. 71.
34 *Ibid.*, p. 71.
35 *Ibid.*, p. 72.
36 *Ibid.*, p. 68.
37 *Ibid.*, p. 73.
38 *Ibid.*, p. 73.
39 *Ibid.*, p. 73.
40 *Ibid.*, p. 69.
41 *Ibid.*, p. 70.
42 See: e.g., Cooper, M. H. and Culyer, A. J. (eds.) *Health Economics* (London: Penguin, 1973) p. 241.
43 See: Davis, Karen. "Relationships of Hospital Prices to Costs," *Applied Economics* 4:115–125 (June 1971); and Kaitz, E. M. *Pricing Policy and Cost Behavior in the Hospital Industry* (New York: Praeger, 1968). Neither study on hospital pricing confirms that price equals average cost.
44 Feldstein, Martin S. "Hospital Cost Inflation: A Study of Nonprofit Price Dynamics," *American Economic Review* 51:853–872 (December 1971). An earlier model, not discussed in our paper, can be found in Feldstein's classic work, *Economic Analysis for Health Service Efficiency* (Amsterdam: North Holland Publishing Company, 1967).
45 Feldstein, M., "Hospital Cost Inflation," p. 855.
46 *Ibid.*, p. 856, note 13.
47 *Ibid.*, p. 855.
48 *Ibid.*, p. 858.
49 See: Cooper, M. H. and Culyer, A. J. *The Price of Blood* (London: Institute of Economic Affairs, 1968).
50 Davis, *op. cit.*
51 *Ibid.*, p. 115.
52 Pauly, M. V. "Notes on a New Model of Nonprofit Hospital Behavior and Investment," July 1969 (processed).
53 Pauly, M. V. and Redisch, M. "The Not-for-Profit Hospital as a Physicians' Cooperative," *American Economic Review* 63:87–100 (March 1973).
54 *Ibid.*, p. 98.
55 See the slightly different version of this paper: Pauly, M. and Redisch, M. "The Not-for-Profit Hospital as a Physicians' Cooperative," unpublished paper de-livered to the Health Economics Section of the Allied Social Sciences meetings, December 1969.
56 Pauly and Redisch, "The Not-for-Profit Hospital," *American Economic Review op. cit.*, pp. 88–89.
57 In a recent paper, George Drakos has questioned the form of cooperative hypothesized by Pauly and Redisch, suggesting that, instead, the hospital should be viewed as a cooperative whose member doctors would be regarded as independent revenue collecting firms which use the hospital as the source of supply of a certain input. See: Drakos, G. "The Not-for-Profit Hospital as a Physicians' Cooperative: A Comment," unpublished paper, Université de Sherbrooke, Sherbrooke (Quebec, 1973). The possibility of experimenting with various forms of cooperatives to explain how physicians organize themselves to deal with hospital trustees, etc., seems to hold some promise.
58 Pauly and Redisch (*A.E.R.*), *op. cit.*, p. 94.
59 See: Culyer, A. J. "The Nature of the Commodity Health Care and Its Efficient Allocation," *Oxford Economic Papers* 23:189–210 (July 1971), esp. pp. 199–207.
60 For some insights on how monopoly elements play a large role in doctors' exchanges with both trustees and patients, see: Kessell, Ruben. "Price Discrimination in Medicine," *Journal of Law and Economics* 1:1–19 (October 1958).
61 Kaitz, *op. cit.*, and Davis, *op. cit.*
62 Buchanan, James M. and Lindsay, C. M. "Financing of Medical Care in the United States." In: British Medical Association. *Health Services Financing* (London: B.M.A., 1970).
63 *Ibid.*, p. 549.
64 *Ibid.*, p. 549.
65 Lindsay, C. M. "Medical Care and the Economics of Sharing," *Economica* 36:351–362 (November 1969); Culyer, A. J. "Medical Care and the Economics of Giving," *Economica* 38:295–304 (August 1971); and Jacobs, P. *A Utility Maximizing Approach to the Analysis of Non-Profit Hospital Behaviour*, unpublished doctoral thesis, University of York, 1973.
66 Clarkson, Kenneth. "Some Implications of Property Rights in Hospital Management," *Journal of Law and Economics* 15:363–376 (October 1972).
67 *Ibid.*, p. 365.
68 *Ibid.*, p. 365.
69 *Ibid.*, p. 365.
70 *Ibid.*, p. 366.
71 *Ibid.*, p. 368.
72 It should be stressed that the absence of a wealth claim is not indicative of a lack of incentive or a reduced incentive to achieve one's goal *unless* wealth is the only goal of the individual.
73 Clarkson, *op. cit.*, p. 369.

Part III

Demand and Supply Analysis

The papers contained in Part II presented the economic and sociopolitical problems of health care, together with a foretaste of the economists' approach to it. Here, in Part III, the emphasis is on empirical economic analyses.

Without question, the most useful way to study the economic problems of health care is to examine them through analyses of demand and supply. Hyman Joseph presents a survey of demand studies of health care conducted in the Sixties. Judith Lave, et al. offer a systematic review of the models used to analyze, as well as to study the results of, the demand for and supply of health manpower and medical care.

The basic economic variable in any demand study is the price and income elasticity of demand. Williams, Ferber and Kovner present direct or indirect estimates of price and income elasticities of demand for hospital and medical care. Wilson and Begun furnish data on the volume (demand) of physicians' services between 1959 and 1974. It is interesting to note that their data definitely support the physician-induced demand hypothesis. From 1969 to 1973, the number of patient contacts per physician actually had increased without interruption as physician supply per population increased.

Analyses of the supply of health care are underrepresented in this collection. Carr and Feldstein estimate that hospitals have a U-shaped (on log paper, on the x-axis) average cost curve, reaching the minimum point at the 200 daily patient census. Whether economies of scale exist in hospitals and other health care and, if so, what its implications are for efficiency, still remain unsettled issues. Since the policy implication of economies of scale is important for health planning, more studies, subsequent to Carr and Feldstein's, clearly are needed.

The major obstacle for research in health economics is lack of a consistent measure of output in the health care industry. Thompson et al. and Berry offer two different bases for measuring hospital output. If output of hospitals is to be measured by the number of cases treated, then weighted by diagnosis-mix, Thompson, Fetter and Mross's study will provide a useful guide. Moreover, Berry's research will be helpful if hospital output is to be measured by the number and type of services provided. Both studies supply a basis for a better gauge of hospital output than the usual measure of patient days or admissions.

Hyman Joseph

Reprinted with permission of the Blue Cross Association, from *Inquiry:* Vol.VIII, No.1, pp.61-71. Copyright © 1971 by the Blue Cross Association.

Empirical Research on the Demand for Health Care

Originally Published in March 1971

The resolution of many of the important problems in the health care industry depends on a knowledge of the demand for health care. The authors of the empirical research studies on the demand for health care that are reviewed in this paper were looking for answers to the following kinds of problems: How much will the demand for health care rise as consumer incomes rise? How do consumers react to reductions in price due to third-party payments? How effective are coinsurance clauses? To what extent do patients shift from uncovered to covered services? The answers to these questions depend on the effect of prices and income on the quantity of health care demanded; and, accordingly, the authors focus their studies on prices and income. This paper examines the answers that the empirical demand studies have provided and suggests what future work needs to be done.

The first section analyzes the important determinants of the demand for health care: own price, prices of substitutes or complements, income, and tastes. The measures of these determinants that are important to economists for policy purposes are described, and potential measurement difficulties are discussed.

Section two critically reviews nine empirical studies of the demand for health

Hyman Joseph, Ph.D. is Assistant Professor, Department of Economics, University of Iowa.
Financial support for this study was provided by Grant # HSM 110-70-17 from the National Center for Health Services Research and Development to the Health Economics Research Center of the University of Iowa. The views expressed in this paper are solely the responsibility of the author.

care. These studies include a variety of data sources from different geographic areas, periods of time, and levels of aggregation.

The third section summarizes the important results of the empirical studies and offers suggestions for future research.

Determinants of Demand for Health Care

Economists usually describe the demand for a good or service as being determined by its own price, the prices of other goods and services, consumer income, and consumer tastes. The emphasis is on economic variables such as prices or income, while all other variables are lumped together under the heading "tastes." The economist attempts to evaluate the impact of the economic variables, while he holds the noneconomic variables constant (perhaps through multiple regression analysis). In contrast, a medical researcher might be primarily concerned with one of the taste parameters (such as the individual's daily cigarette consumption) and he therefore would hold the economic variables and the other noneconomic variables constant.

The demand for a good or service is usually expressed as a quantity per unit of time. Sometimes demand is expressed as expenditures per unit of time. The use of expenditures as the dependent variable has drawbacks that are attributable to the structure of the health care industry. Individuals are sometimes charged different prices for the same product or service.[1] Therefore, variations in expenditures may be due to variations in prices charged as well as to variations in quantities demanded.

The heterogeneity of health services that may be included in an expenditures variable precludes the evaluation of the influence of medical factors on patterns of consumption. And medical factors are probably the most important reasons for health care expenditures.

Own Price

The price of a good or service and the quantity of it demanded will be inversely related if real income is held constant. The responsiveness of changes in quantity to changes in price, as measured by the price elasticity of demand, will help predict the quantitative effect of policies that change the prices of goods or services.

Most sellers of health care are price-setters rather than price-takers. Therefore, prices may remain constant for long periods of time while changes in demand result in changes in rates of utilization rather than in changes in price. This type of seller behavior greatly increases the difficulty of estimating price elasticities of demand. Conceptually, in order to estimate demand curves for a representative individual, we would require a set of data in which roughly similar individuals were charged different prices. The existence of third-party payments for some, but not all, individuals or the existence of different proportions of third-party payments among individuals can help to generate such data.

Survey data of consumer expenditures cannot be expected to be of any help in estimating price elasticities of demand since price information would not be included in such data. In contrast, patient discharge data that contained information regarding different proportions of third-party payments among patients might be useful for estimating price elasticities of demand.

Prices of Substitutes or Complements

The problems that occur in the estimation of own price elasticities of demand also occur in the estimation of cross elasticities of demand. In addition, data that contained own prices (such as patient discharge data) would not contain prices of substitute goods or services that were *not* consumed. Thus we would not expect to find prices of substitutes in empirical estimates of the demand for health care.

Income

The effect of income on the demand for health care can not be predicted with certainty *a priori*. An estimated income elasticity of expenditures greater than unity might imply that the proportion of income spent for health care would rise as income rises, while such an elasticity of less than unity might imply a declining proportion of income would be spent for health care as income rises. However, the effect of medical research (which may discover new diseases), new surgical procedures, and new drugs may be to provide new goods and services for the consumer, thereby increasing health care expenditures over what would be predicted by the estimated income elasticities of expenditures.

The demand for health care may depend on expected future income as well as on current income. Therefore, an estimate of the average of current and future incomes, which is called "permanent income," is sometimes used instead of current income. If only current income is used as a regressor and future incomes are omitted, then the estimated income elasticity of expenditures will usually be biased downwards.

The averaging procedure that is used to obtain an estimate of permanent income may eliminate other important information. If data are averaged for several individuals, then important information about the prices paid by each individual and about the medical condition of each individual would be eliminated. The researcher must make a subjective decision as to whether the loss in information due to averaging is offset by the potential gain in the accuracy of the estimated coefficient of the income variable.

Consumption patterns of individuals may affect their general health and thereby their demand for health care. Individuals with higher incomes may have had better nutrition and better health care in the past, and these factors may lower their current demand for health care. Of course, this would be offset by their ability to buy more health care because of their higher incomes. If individuals with higher incomes are in better health, then this would tend to lower the estimated income elasticities of expenditures.

Tastes

The primary determinant of an individual's demand for health care is the status of his health. For example, an individual's myopia may generate a demand for eyeglasses. His income and the prices of eyeglasses and contact lenses would then affect the amount that he would spend on eyeglasses. But a person with normal vision would not purchase corrective eyeglasses no matter what the price of eyeglasses or his income might be.

Some of the determinants of an individual's physical condition are his health habits (such as cigarette smoking), heredity, age, and urban or rural residence. Residence in an urban or rural place may also affect the available supply of health care facilities.

Other determinants of an individual's tastes may include his educational level (if he is an adult) ; family size (if the household is the unit under consideration) ; and marital status. Finally, the tastes of others, such as his doctor or the hospital administrator, may affect his demand for health care.

Empirical Research

The empirical studies that are critically reviewed in this section were selected to provide results from a variety of data sources that include different geographic areas and various levels of aggregation. Most of the studies utilize multiple regres-

sion analysis to estimate parameters and test hypotheses. None of the included studies involves only data summarization.

M. S. Feldstein Study

M. S. Feldstein[2] analyzed the determinants of hospital admission and length of stay for maternity care cases occurring in 1962 in an area surrounding the city of Oxford, England. He utilized multiple regression analysis on a set of dummy variable regressors. A dummy variable was also utilized .as the dependent variable in the hospital admissions regressions.

The following classes of regressors were included in one or more of the regressions : age, parity (number of previous children), past obstetric history, social class, marital status, hospital proximity, urban-rural, and specialization of attending physician.

Feldstein reported the percentage deviation in mean stay or the percentage deviation in admission probability for each regressor instead of reporting the regression coefficients. The estimate of the standard deviations of the percentage deviations are reported so that the reliability of the estimates can be judged. However, Feldstein correctly noted that the estimates of the standard deviations are biased for the regressions in which the dependent variable was a dummy variable (the admissions regressions).

The regressions indicated that a woman had a higher probability of being admitted to a hospital if she were relatively young or relatively old, if she had no previous children, if she had complications during previous pregnancies (except single miscarriages), if she were in a higher social class, if she were single, if she lived near a hospital, or if she lived in a rural area. These were the important factors that tended to influence the joint doctor-patient decision as to whether the woman should be hospitalized. Economic variables were not included in the analysis because the entire population was covered by the National Health Service.

The regressions indicated that a woman tended to have a longer duration of stay in the hospital if she were in a higher social class, if she were age 40 or older, if she had no previous children, if she had complications during previous pregnancies, if she were single, or if she lived near a hospital. Thus, the decision regarding duration of stay in the hospital appeared to be influenced mostly by medical factors such as age, parity, and previous complications, although social factors, such as social class and marital status, and geographic factors also had some effect. Again, economic variables were not included in the regressions because all of the women were covered by the National Health Service.

P. J. Feldstein Study

P. J. Feldstein[3] utilized 1958 survey data for families in the United States to estimate a series of Engel curves and demand curves. The individual family data were aggregated on a "primary sampling unit basis," which is not defined in the text.

The dependent variables in the multiple regression analysis were alternately: gross medical care expenditures, hospital expenditures, dental expenditures, drug expenditures, gross insurance expenditures, physician visits (total), physician visits (home, office), hospital admissions, hospital patient days, and the percent of families with some insurance. The regressors were: mean family income, age of family head, percent of families with one or more members 65 or over, percent of families with one or more members under five years of age, percent urban, percent of families receiving free or reduced care, percent of family heads with 12 or more years of education, mean family size, percent of single-person families, proportion of bill covered by insurance, and a price variable (to be explained subsequently). Both arithmetic and logarithmic regression results were reported.

The mean-family-income variable had the hypothesized positive coefficient in almost all of the regressions (except where hospital admissions was the dependent variable). The coefficients of the mean-family-income variable were often statistically significant at the 5 percent level. The estimated income elasticities of the dependent variables in the constant-elasticity formulations (the logarithmic regressions) ranged from $-.76$ for the hospital admissions dependent variable to 1.17 for the dental expenditures dependent variable. Most of the estimated elasticities were between .44 and .73. Feldstein thought that these estimates were too low because he believed that some transitory components remained in the income variable even after he averaged it over the families in the "primary sampling units." Therefore, for each regression he switched the dependent variable and the income variable and re-ran the regressions, thereby obtaining another set of income elasticities. The new elasticities ranged from -12.7 to 34.5, but most of them were between 1.32 and 3.96.

Errors in variables cause biased estimates of parameters only when the errors are in the measurement of the independent variable. Therefore, Feldstein's procedure of switching the dependent variable and the income variable is a reasonable one (consistent, but not unbiased estimators are obtained) only if there are errors of measurement in the income variable but not in the dependent variable. However, there are likely to be errors in the expenditures variables because individuals with higher incomes may be charged higher prices (so that the expenditures variable may not measure consumer preferences accurately). It is the opinion of this reviewer that the errors in the measurement of family incomes are more likely to average to zero when the data are averaged on a "primary sampling basis" than are the errors in the measurement of the expenditures variables. Therefore the original, lower, income elasticities will be accepted as being more accurate.

Feldstein developed two price variables. The physician price variable was obtained by dividing net expenditures on physicians by physician visits. The hospital care price variable was obtained by dividing net expenditures on hospital care by the quantity of hospital care. The reasons for the price differences among the 66 "primary sampling units" are not stated in the text. They could be due to differences in supply conditions, for example, in which case the estimates would be subject to simultaneous equation bias. The coefficients of the price variables had the correct signs with low standard errors only when physician visits was the dependent variable. When the dependent variable was one of the expenditure variables, the coefficient of the price variable would be positive with a low standard error. Since expenditures consist of prices times quantities, prices and expenditures would tend to be positively correlated.

The coefficient of the insurance variable had a positive sign except when physician visits was the dependent variable. The proportion of the bill covered by insurance was a statistically significant factor (at the 5 percent level) in the determination of hospital admissions, hospital patient days, and hospital expenditures.

The coefficients of the demographic variables showed no consistent patterns. This may have been due in part to the averaging process by which the family data were aggregated.

Feldstein and Carr Study

P. J. Feldstein and W. J. Carr[4] examined the effect of income on medical care spending for 10 sets of cross-section data. The data were for the years 1960-1961, 1950 (two sets of data), 1944, 1941 (two sets of data), 1935-1936 (two sets of data), 1934-1936, and 1917-1919.

Simple (two variable) regressions of medical care expenditures on family income were run for all 10 sets of data. However, for each set of data, the observations were grouped by income class, and only the class means were utilized in the regressions. Therefore, the number of effective observations was as few as five and only 10 at the maximum.

The income elasticities of expenditures that were computed from the double loga-

rithmic regressions ranged from .496 to .957, with the more recent data yielding elasticities of .683 (1960) ; .706 (1950) ; and .735 (1950).

The authors noted two major problems with the above results. First, measured income was utilized as the regressor instead of permanent income. *Ceteris paribus*, the estimate of the permanent income elasticity of expenditure was biased downward. Second, additional regressors that might explain part of the variation in medical expenditures were omitted. *Ceteris paribus*, the effect of omitting variables that are positively correlated with the included regressor is to bias upward the estimated coefficient of the regressor. The net effect of the two major problems on the estimated income elasticities of expenditure is indeterminate *a priori*.

The authors ran additional regressions with the 1960 data and one of the sets of data from 1950. The data for each set were grouped by city so that the transitory components might tend to average out to zero for each city. Thus the income variable might then be a better approximation to permanent income. Additional regressors were included to take account of factors other than income that might affect medical care expenditures. These additional regressors were: family size, age of head of family, education of head of family, number of family members who were gainfully employed, insurance expenditures, and percent of families insured. The estimated income elasticities of expenditure were .433 for 1960 and 1.065 for 1950.

The authors were unwilling to accept the implication of a low elasticity of expenditures: that medical care expenditures rise less than proportionally to income. Accordingly, the authors accepted the estimate for 1950, but ran additional regressions with the 1960 data. But no matter how they regrouped the 1960 data or omitted variables, they were unable to push the estimated elasticity to unity.

Regressions with health insurance expenditures as the dependent variable were also included in the paper. No variable had an estimated coefficient that was statistically significant at the 5 percent level for both the 1950 and the 1960 regressions.

Joseph Study

In 1970, the author of this review utilized cross-section data by patient from 27 Iowa hospitals to determine the effect of third-party payments on the length of stay in a hospital.[5] The 22 illnesses and conditions that occurred most frequently in the data (excluding the very general categories) were selected for the empirical tests.

Length of stay was the dependent variable in the multiple regression analysis and all of the regressors were dummy variables. The regressors were based on the following characteristics of a patient: whether he received third-party payments, type of accommodation, sex, whether he had complications, his age class, and whether he died. A separate regression was run for each of 22 illnesses or conditions.

The estimates of the coefficient of the third-party payments variable were statistically significant at the 5 percent probability level in seven out of the 22 categories. Third-party payments appeared to have little effect on length of stay for illnesses or conditions that require extensive care or are psychologically unpleasant. However, third-party payments did appear to affect length of stay for the less-serious illnesses or conditions.

The price elasticities of demand that were computed for a representative patient in each of the 22 categories were generally low. Elastic demands were computed only for two categories in which outpatient care might be a reasonable substitute for an extra day in the hospital.

Since patients' incomes were not available in the data, type of accommodation was included as a proxy for income. The regression results showed that patients with higher-priced accommodations tended to

have longer stays. These results are consistent with a positive income effect. The sex of the patient was not a statistically significant determinant of length of stay at the 5 percent probability level in any of the illness categories.

Long Study

S. G. Long[6] estimated several Engel curves based on two sets of household survey data. Both sets of data were obtained from households in the state of Iowa—one set for 1960 and the other for 1966.

Long utilized both total medical expenses paid by households in a year *excluding* insurance costs, and total medical expenses paid by households in a year *including* insurance costs as the dependent variables. The independent variables were: number of children, number of adults, two age class dummy variables, two education dummy variables, a farm dummy variable, a city over 10,000 population dummy variable, third-party payments, an insurance dummy variable, a disadvantaged family dummy variable, and an income variable (either money income or a proxy variable for permanent income, i.e., total household consumption expenditure). Several forms of the regression equation were tested including linear, log-log, semi-log, and per capita regressions. Long chose to report the results from the linear regressions in the main text and the other results in the appendices.

Long discovered statistically significant coefficients (at the 13.36 percent level) for number of adults in household, third-party payments received, the insurance dummy, and income. The number of adults in the household may be considered as a proxy for maternity expenditures and also as a proxy for older relatives living in the household. Maternity expenditures are more likely to occur when a husband and wife live in the same household. Older relatives would tend to require larger medical expenditures than the head of the household. The age class variables that Long used are only for the head of the household, and therefore they do not account for older relatives living in the household.

Third-party payments received is partly a proxy for severity of illnesses and partly a proxy for preferences for risk aversion. A severe illness tends to consume a household's income and assets and makes it more likely to be eligible for welfare or other third-party payments. Households that purchase insurance to avoid risk are more likely to receive third party payments from the insurance carriers than households that do not seek to avoid such risk. Third-party payments is one of the components of the dependent variable and therefore is likely to be correlated with the dependent variable.

Households that had health insurance were found to have significantly higher medical expenditures *including insurance costs* than households that had none. However, when the dependent variable was defined to exclude insurance costs, households that had health insurance were found to have significantly *lower* medical expenditures for one set of data and higher expenditures that were not significant at the 10 percent level for the other set of data. These results neither confirm nor reject the hypothesis that households with health insurance consume more medical goods and services. Instead, the results are a function of how the dependent variable is defined. The income elasticities of demand were positive and less than unity. They ranged from 0.122 to 0.619.

Rosenthal Aggregate Study

G. D. Rosenthal[7] utilized data by state for both the years 1950 and 1960 to estimate the determinants of three hospital variables. The dependent variables were patient days per 1000 population, admissions per 1000 population, and average length of stay. The regressors were charges for a two-bed room, two income class variables, percent hospital coverage, two age class variables, percent of females married, percent male, percent in urban areas, percent over 12 years education,

percent nonwhite, and population per dwelling unit. A linear relationship was assumed for the results that are reported in the main text.

Rosenthal's study does not take into account the fact that the supply of hospital services varies among the states. Therefore, his empirical relationships may be hybrid demand-supply curves and his estimated coefficients for the "demand" relationships may contain simultaneous equation bias.

The coefficients of the two income class variables had the correct signs (assuming that hospital services are a superior good) in 11 out of 12 opportunities. However, only three out of the 11 were statistically significant at the 5 percent level.

The price variables fared better in the 1960 regressions than they did in the 1950 regressions. The coefficients of the variable "charges for two-bed room" had negative signs and were statistically significant at the 5 percent level in all of the 1960 regressions. However, the coefficients of this variable had negative signs in only two of the three 1950 regressions, and neither of the two was statistically significant at the 5 percent level.

"Percent hospital coverage" is also a price variable because insurance coverage lowers the effective price to the consumer. The coefficients of this variable had the hypothesized positive signs in all of the three 1960 regressions, and two of the three were statistically significant at the 5 percent level. However, two of the three coefficients of this variable had the wrong (negative) signs in the 1950 regressions, and the one with the correct sign was not statistically significant at the 5 percent level. Since two price variables were included in the regressions, it is not possible for us to compute the price elasticity of demand for each regression.

The age class variables showed no discernible pattern. States that had higher percentages of people over age 64 did not have significantly higher demand for hospital services.

Both "percent of females married" and

"population per dwelling unit" had negative coefficients in all of the regressions. This suggests that family responsibilities at home and possibly someone at home to care for the sick person may reduce the demand for hospital services.

Rosenthal New England Study

G. D. Rosenthal[8] examined the effect of two alternative price variables on the length of stay of hospital patients. The data consisted of a sample of medical records and financial information from the year 1962 for patients who were in one of 68 New England hospitals.

Rosenthal divided the data into 28 groups, which were each homogeneous with respect to medical or surgical diagnosis, age, and sex. For each of the 28 groups, he regressed length of stay on each of two regressors: cash outlay as a percentage of the total bill, or the average daily room charge.

Since Rosenthal utilized double-log regressions, the estimated coefficient of the independent variable is an estimate of the elasticity of the dependent variable with respect to the independent variable. However, neither of the two independent variables that he alternatively uses is own price. Therefore, the estimated elasticities that are reported in the paper are not price elasticities of demand.

The relative cash variable had a negative-signed coefficient that was significant at the 5 percent probability level in only three of the 28 groups. Average room charge fared better because it had the hypothesized negative-signed coefficient that was significant at the 5 percent probability level in 11 of the 28 groups. Average room charge generally explained more of the variation in length of stay than did relative cash.

Rosenthal found a negative association between length of stay and average room charge. This is consistent with this author's own study, in which third-party payments affected length of stay more for the less-serious illnesses or conditions. In both studies, the patients with more serious conditions were found to be less sensitive to price variables.

Weisbrod and Fiesler Study

B. A. Weisbrod and R. J. Fiesler[9] compared the hospitalization experience of two groups of between 700 and 900 Blue Cross subscribers (plus their dependents) before and after the extension of additional service to one of the groups. The groups consisted of employees of firms in the same industry and both were located in the St. Louis area. Both groups had the "standard" Blue Cross coverage in 1957. One group adopted the more comprehensive Preferred Blue Cross coverage in 1958. The differences between the standard and preferred coverages pertained to ancillary services and private room accommodations.

Weisbrod and Fiesler compared the utilization rates (the number of admissions per 1000 subscribers) and the usage of certain ancillary services and private rooms by the two groups. They found that the utilization rates for both declined for 1958 compared to 1957 and that the decline for the "preferred" group (13.8 percent) was significantly less at the 5 percent probability level than the decline for the "standard" group (20.2 percent). Tabulations of percentage changes in utilization rates by age and by sex indicated that the relatively greater utilization by the "preferred" group occurred among females and among those over 55 years of age.

Under the preferred coverage, ancillary service benefits were greatly expanded, but only on an inpatient basis. Part of the relatively greater usage by the "preferred" group might be attributable to persons who entered the hospital to avail themselves of the free (to them) ancillary services.

The increase in total ancillary service costs per admission for the "standard" group was not statistically significant at the 5 percent probability level, but the increase for the "preferred" group was significant at that level. The extra $2 that was allowed the "preferred" group members did not significantly influence their private room use.

The results of the Weisbrod-Fiesler study are consistent with several hypotheses. First, doctors may have prescribed more ancillary services for patients whose expenses would be paid by Blue Cross. Second, doctors may have hospitalized patients who required extensive ancillary services so that the cost of these services would be paid by Blue Cross.

Wirick and Barlow Study

G. Wirick and R. Barlow[10] examined the determinants of the medical expenditures of a sample of Michigan families during 1957-1958. The statistical technique that was utilized was analysis of variance, which is equivalent to multiple regression when all of the regressors are dummy variables.

The dependent variable was the sum of individual expenditures for medical care (including amounts contributed by sources outside the family and excluding health insurance premiums). The regressors were dummy variables that fell into one of the following seven categories: 1) age of individual; 2) insurance coverage; 3) family income; 4) number of equivalent adults; 5) responses to minor symptoms; 6) education of family head; and 7) where family head grew up. The data were divided into two parts based on the sex of the individual.

For both males and females, all of the regressors together explained only about 8 percent of the variation in each group. The age class variables accounted for about one-half of the explained variation for males and about three-quarters of the explained variation for females. Medical expenditures was thus shown to be positively related to the age of the individual.

Unfortunately, no measures of reliability, such as standard errors, t-values, or F-values, were given in the study. It is therefore difficult to assess the importance of each of the regressors.

Summary of Results and Suggestions for Future Research

Own Price

Price appears to explain a relatively small amount of the variation in the demand for health care. The Rosenthal New England study found statistically significant coefficients for price variables in only a minority of the groups analyzed. The author's own study, which utilized Iowa data, found generally low price elasticities of demand except for two illness categories in which outpatient care might be a reasonable substitute for an extra day in the hospital. Both of these studies found that patients with more serious conditions were less sensitive to price variables.

Neither the P. J. Feldstein study nor the Rosenthal aggregate study contradicts the above results. However, these two aggregate studies are difficult to assess as to the effect of price on quantity demanded. Both contain two or more price variables in each regression equation so that it is difficult to interpret the coefficients of these variables. Both neglect the role of supply among the regions under study and, therefore, may have estimated a mixed supply-demand curve instead of a demand curve.

The Weisbrod and Fiesler study indicated that "free" ancillary hospital services increased their usage and possibly increased the admissions rate so that the patients could avail themselves of these "free" services.

Income

The studies show that health care expenditures increase as consumer income increases. The income elasticity of expenditures was usually estimated to be less than unity. A notable exception was the income elasticity of dental expenditures in the P. J. Feldstein study. People may consider many dental expenditures, such as for orthodontia, as elective rather than crucial and may not make these expenditures unless their income is sufficiently high.

Tastes

Several noneconomic variables were included in the various studies. The age of the individual was shown to be an important determinant of the demand for health care in those disaggregated studies (M. S. Feldstein, Joseph, Wirick and Barlow) in which it was included. The studies that utilized the age of the head of the household and/or aggregated the data usually did not show age to be a statistically significant variable. However, it is the age of the *patient* that is relevant, not the age of the head of the household or some average age. Therefore we should assign much more importance to the evidence of the disaggregated studies.

The author's own study indicated that the sex of the patient was not a statistically significant determinant of the demand for hospital care for those conditions that were common to both sexes. The other studies did not test for differences in demand that were based on the sex of the individual.

The studies did not generate much evidence regarding the roles of other taste variables, such as urban-rural residence, marital status, or education level of adults.

Suggestions for Future Research

Prices and incomes are the important economic variables that are affected by changes in public policies or institutional structures. The responsiveness of the demand for health care to changes in prices or incomes (as measured by elasticities) may be used to predict the impact of alternative public policies or institutional structures.

Estimated price elasticities of demand are needed for states in addition to Iowa and for categories of health care in addition to hospital services. Data by individual, as opposed to aggregated data, would appear to be potentially more fruitful for obtaining estimates of price elasticities. It would be desirable if estimates of income elasticities of demand could be made from the same sets of data. Individual or family income for several past years would be required in the data in order to generate a permanent income series. Such a series would allow estimation of permanent income elasticities of demand without averaging the data in such a way as to make it impossible to obtain estimates of price elasticities of demand in the same regression equations.

Future demand studies should utilize only one own price variable per regression. Otherwise it becomes impossible to estimate price elasticities of demand. The empirical studies have verified an inverse relationship between price variables and quantity demanded. Now efforts should be directed toward estimating the quantitative relationship between own price and quantity demanded.

Estimates of demand by category of illness could be a useful input into new price indices of medical care in which treatments rather than individual items form the base. It can be argued that the costs of treatments for illnesses in contrast to the cost of individual items of medical care are the relevant costs that should be included in a price index of medical care. Demand studies by category of illness could provide information regarding the quantities of items that should be in the different treatments that are included in a new price index of medical care.

Estimates of cross-elasticities of demand are needed to show preferences among different types of facilities, such as between hospitals and nursing homes. These estimates could be useful for policy decisions regarding the items that should be covered in insurance contracts.

Future demand studies might give more consideration to supply conditions. This is especially important in cross-section studies that include diverse geographic areas. Perhaps demand and supply curves might be estimated jointly.

References and Notes

1 Kessel attributes this price discrimination to profit maximization, while Ruffin and Leigh attribute it to utility maximization and charity. See Kessel, R. A. "Price Discrimination in Medicare." *Journal of Law and Economics* pp. 20-53. (October 1958); and Ruffin, R. J. and Leigh, D. E. "Charity, Competition, and Pricing of Doctor's Services." Unpublished paper, Iowa City, Iowa, 1969.

2 Feldstein, M. S. *Economic Analysis for Health Service Efficiency.* (Amsterdam: North Holland Publishing Co., 1967) Chpt. 8.

3 Feldstein, P. J. "The Demand for Medical Care." In: The Commission on the Cost of Medical Care. *General Report, Vol. I.* (Chicago: American Medical Association, 1964)

4 Feldstein, P. J. and Carr, J. W. "The Effect of Income on Medical Care Spending." *American Statistical Association: Proceedings of the Social Sciences Section.* (1964)

5 Joseph, H. "Hospital Insurance and Moral Hazard." *Journal of Human Resources.* Forthcoming.

6 Long, S. G. "Demand for Medical Care." Ph.D. dissertation, University of Iowa, 1969.

7 Rosenthal, G. D. *The Demand for General Hospital Facilities.* (Chicago: American Hospital Association, 1964)

8 Rosenthal, G. D. "Price Elasticity of Demand for Short-Term General Hospital Services." In: Klarman, H. E. (ed.). *Empirical Studies in Health Economics.* (Baltimore: Johns Hopkins University Press, 1970)

9 Weisbrod, B. A., and Fiesler, R. J. "Hospital Insurance and Hospital Utilization." *American Economic Review* 51:126-132. (March 1961)

10 Wirick, G. and Barlow, R. "The Economic and Social Determinants of the Demand for Health Services." In: Mushkin, Selma J. (ed.). *The Economics of Health and Medical Care.* (Ann Arbor: Bureau of Public Health Economics, University of Michigan, 1964)

Judith R. Lave
Lester B. Lave
Samuel Leinhardt

Medical Manpower Models: Need, Demand and Supply

Reprinted with permission of the Blue Cross Association, from *Inquiry:* Vol.XII, No.2, pp.97-125. Copyright © 1975 by the Blue Cross Association.

Originally Published in June 1975

As planning has moved into center stage in health care delivery, Comprehensive Health Planning and other agencies have sought advice in estimating the extent of manpower shortages and in finding policies to remedy existing ones. We propose a framework for examining these questions and summarize the literature that bears on them.

We begin by looking at expectations of the medical care delivery system and at what it can provide. We then discuss a range of models used to forecast physician requirements, demand for physicians, and the distribution of physicians, and examine their implications for the formulation of public policy. Given the nature of the topic, more questions are raised than answers provided.

Some Issues in Health Care Delivery

The goal of a medical care system is to improve the health status of the population served. One of the first questions that results from this assumption is: What is the effect on the health of the population of having more physicians? In other words, what is the health effect of an increase in the physician/population ratio?

Judith R. Lave, Ph.D. is Associate Professor of Economics and Urban Affairs, School of Urban and Public Affairs; **Lester B. Lave, Ph.D.** is Professor and Head, Department of Economics, Graduate School of Industrial Administration; and **Samuel Leinhardt, Ph.D.** is Associate Professor of Sociology, School of Urban and Public Affairs, Carnegie-Mellon University (Pittsburgh, PA 15213). Their names appear in alphabetical order.

Financial support for this study was provided by the Department of Health, State of California, through a contract with the Rand Corporation, and by grant #1 R01 HS01529-01 from the National Center for Health Services Research, DHEW.

But this question contains a question: How should health be measured?[1] Health status encompasses mortality, morbidity, disability, restricted activity, bed-days, hospital days, patient anxiety, and the level of satisfaction with the medical care delivery system. There are conceptual difficulties in formulating what is to be measured; and there are methodological difficulties in measuring and combining each of the components so that an acceptable, reliable health status index results. Yet, as we argue in more detail later, there is no reasonable alternative to using a quantitative output measure of the medical care delivery system. The major policy issues require such measures as inputs in the search for a solution.

Suppose there were a health index, the next question that arises is: What is the most effective way of improving the health status of a population? Is it through personal health services, through public health services, through educational programs aimed at altering personal habits with respect to diet, exercise, and smoking? A fundamental paradox in the development of public medical care policy is that medical care obviously does save specific lives, it does lessen disease, and it does prevent or repair disability; yet, it appears that increases in medical care expenditures have little effect on overall mortality rates[2]—the whole is less than the sum of the parts due to competing risks or simply aging. Indeed, more of a good thing can be harmful if iatrogenic disease—that due to drug reactions, mistaken therapies and unnecessary surgery—is considered. It is difficult to get the right mix and amount of medical care to all groups, especially those most in "need" of care—the poor and other disadvantaged groups. Although additional personal health services do not seem to improve health, save for those most in need of care, additional expenditures on public health and improved personal habits do improve health.

If we knew which health services were efficacious, we would have to raise another question: What is the most effective way of producing them? Traditionally, a physician visit has required a physician, a secretary, and possibly an office nurse. A richer set of resources can be used. For example, paraprofessionals working under a physician's direction can handle a great part of the traditional patient visit. In particular, patients with chronic diseases can be monitored without routine involvement of the physician.[3]

Assuming we knew the "right" way to produce physician services, we would then want to know how physicians should be distributed geographically. Equally distributed, physicians in urban areas would probably be much busier than those in rural areas, both because urban residents would find it easier to get to physicians and because they have different perceptions about when care is needed. Those physicians in areas with a heavy concentration of older residents would be busier because the aged seek more care than the young.

Do remote areas, those with low population density, have unique problems? An area with a population density of less than one person per square mile, located far from a metropolitan area, is extremely difficult and costly to serve. Non-acute care can be provided by transporting the patient to the physician or vice versa, but providing emergency care is difficult. Given threshold requirements for practices, can one expect a "sufficient" number and diversity of physicians to choose to locate in these areas? The problem of serving remote and highly dispersed populations is probably the most difficult one in health care delivery, and is not likely to be handled by policies that provide financial incentives for relocation.

Such questions are usually raised individually and, in effect, we examine demand and supply independently; but we must also look at their interaction. To what extent is the demand for medical care amenable to manipulation by physicians; that is, to what extent can physicians increase or decrease the demand for their services?

One of the most important public policy trends has been to lessen or remove price as a mechanism for rationing the allocation of care. This trend has made the monetary cost of care zero or very small for a significant proportion of the population (because of government programs or insurance). As a result, access costs (travel time, waiting time, transportation cost, etc.) have become one of the most important means of rationing care. We can expect this trend to continue since an increased proportion of the population will soon be facing a negligible price for medical services. Thus, in the future, access costs will increase in importance.

We raise these general issues to provide a framework within which to consider demand and supply models. If the reader has a feeling of unease or dissatisfaction, we have no immediate antidote to offer. Later in this paper we will provide a more structured framework for handling these issues and then examine policy issues.

Models Used to Forecast Physician Requirements

What will be the *demand* for, the *need* for, and the *supply* of physicians at a given time and place? What is the gap (if any) between estimated requirements and estimated supplies? What actions, if any, does a gap suggest? The concepts of need and demand are quite different and are often confused. Since they play an important role in motivating the development of forecasts, we discuss them briefly before considering various approaches.

A population's *need for medical services* has been defined by Jeffers, *et al.*, as "that quantity of medical services which expert medical opinion believes ought to be consumed over a relevant time period in order for its members to remain or become as 'healthy' as is permitted by existing medical knowledge."[4] Need is thus a "normative" concept and is identified with the amount of preventive care medical professionals believe the population should have, as well as the amount of care they believe will bring the best medical knowledge to bear on the population's illness problems. These standards are flexible, and as Hiestand has pointed out: "Such standards will always advance in front of what can exist in fact. In a progressive, increasingly affluent society this is perfectly reasonable."[5]

A related concept is "wants." According to Jeffers, *et al.*, a population's *wants for medical services* may be defined as "that quantity of medical services which its members feel they ought to consume (at zero price, zero lost wages, zero waiting time, zero access constraints, etc.) over a relevant time period based on their own psychic perceptions of their health needs." Thus, wants are quite distinct from needs and vary among different groups. Some care that may be deemed "needed" by professionals may not be "wanted" by the population; preventive medical care and, especially, preventive dental care are examples. Other care, such as visits for the common cold, may be "wanted" by the lay population, but not deemed "needed" by physicians.

Demand is yet another related concept. Jeffers defines *the demand for medical services* as the "multivariate functional relationship between the quantities of medical services that its members desire to consume over a relevant time period at given levels of prices of goods and services, financial resources, size and psychological wants of the population as reflected by consumer tastes and preferences for (all) goods and services." Thus, the demand for medical care will depend on the underlying health status, perceptions of the efficacy of medical care, and the cost of medical care. "Demand" will be less than "need" because seeking care involves out-of-pocket costs, travel and waiting time, lost wages, discomfort, and emotional or psychic costs.

There are, therefore, important differences between need and demand: A person may not demand needed medical care because it is not perceived to be effective (not wanted or demanded at a zero price) or because, relative to the desirability of other goods and services (which compete for the individual's scarce money, income and time), it is not valued highly. In addition, price, waiting time, travel cost, or psychic costs may be so high that the

individual demands no care, even though physicians believe it is needed and the individual wants it.

We consider next some of the approaches developed for forecasting manpower requirements and indicate the strengths and weaknesses of each approach. It should be clear that this analysis is closely related to the analysis of the concept of "physician shortage," which will be discussed in a later section. Note that here we are considering how to forecast future physician requirements; we are not concerned with the precision of the forecasts, an issue that will also be discussed later.

Approaches Based on Professionally Defined Standards

The classic approach to developing manpower estimates based on professional standards or estimates of a population's medical *needs* was developed by Lee and Jones in 1933.[6] The approach consists of four steps: 1) determining the frequency of occurrence of illness by type in a population; 2) polling experts to determine the amount of services required to diagnose and treat each illness type; 3) estimating the average number of services rendered per hour by a provider; and 4) securing professional opinion on the average number of hours that a provider spends per year in caring for patients. Applying their method, Lee and Jones estimated that the need for individual preventive services and the need for the diagnosis and treatment of diseases and defects— i.e., all medical services—required 135 physicians per 100,000 population instead of the 126 per 100,000 existing when the study was performed.[7]

The Lee and Jones study was not replicated until the study by Schonfeld, *et al.* in 1972.[8] They interviewed practicing internists and pediatricians and determined what these professionals thought constituted good primary care. They then collected morbidity data from the National Health Survey, and, assuming that pediatricians worked 2,227 hours and internists 2,198 hours per year, they estimated that 133 physicians per 100,000 population were required to give good *primary* care (not including dental, mental health and obstetric care, nor routine physical examinations for adults). This estimate implies that a substantially greater gap between need and supply exists in the 1970s than Lee and Jones estimated existed in 1933, since it reflects only a portion of primary care, whereas the Lee and Jones estimate was for total medical care.

Even if we accept the concept of need as the relevant criterion, these estimates suffer from many drawbacks. We detail some of these here:

1 The standards used represent only averages. Neither Lee and Jones nor Schonfeld, et al., indicated the range of appropriate treatment patterns identified by physicians. If there is little agreement among professionals, so that the variation in individual estimates is large, then the need concept is not very meaningful for policy purposes.

Another difficulty derives from the fact that the approach does not take account of substitution for physician services in the delivery of primary care. Although independent "practice" for paramedics and nurse practitioners is still being debated, few would argue that they cannot perform, under supervision, many of the services currently performed by physicians.[9] It would thus appear, as Huebscher notes, that the number of physicians required to render primary medical care is "fluid."[10]

2 This approach does not include an evaluation of the health outcomes implied by the standards. How do morbidity and mortality rates compare between groups receiving care at the professional standards level and groups receiving much less care? Is there a noticeable difference, and can it be attributed to the level of care? Evidence indicates that the relationship is far from straightforward. For example, the Kaiser Health Plan (which is often cited as an ideal health plan where high quality medical care is believed to be provided) has less than half the number of "needed" primary care physicians (34 internists, 10 generalists and 16 pediatricians) available per 100,000 subscribers.[11] These questions must be considered if the standards approach is to be taken seriously.

3 The approach is excessively narrow because it regards "need" strictly from a professional viewpoint. Do people demand this much medical care? It is not altogether clear that, under the best circumstances, patients behave as physicians would have them. For example, Jacobs,[12] in criticizing the Schonfeld, et al., study, noted that in his community of 200,000 there were 122 primary care physicians (less than half the standard). He pointed out that although these doctors provided more inclusive care (e.g., routine medical examinations) and the community was very wealthy, the physicians were underemployed. Should the patients be "educated" to demand more care? Surely that depends on the answer given to the question of the preceding paragraph.

4 The approach fails to consider alternatives. It emphasizes physician-based personal medical services, but what priority should the government place on the provision of personal medical services? If resources were available to provide medical care meeting professional standards, then surely the share of national income going to personal medical services would increase enormously. Should such an allocation of national income be preferred to one of more recreation, books, housing, and the like? If the goal of public policy is to improve health, we must determine—or at least consider—whether that goal will be better met by providing enough personal medical services to meet professionally determined standards or by the provision of other services such as nutritional programs or education?[13]

These criticisms are quite general and apply equally well to other studies where the estimates of need are based on professional standards. Professional standards and, indeed, all normative approaches should be used for manpower planning purposes only after careful evaluation of alternative approaches.

Approaches Based on Evidence in Comprehensive Prepaid Group Practice

A number of observers have argued that the observed demand for manpower in specific

Table 1. Average number of physicians per 100,000 population served in six medical groups providing prepaid medical services, by specialty

Specialty	Average number of physicians	
	Mean	Median
Internal medicine	45.2	44.9
Allergy	1.6	1.4
Dermatology	2.8	2.5
Pediatrics	18.0	15.8
Obstetrics	9.1	8.0
Orthopedics	3.2	3.0
Ophthalmology	3.7	3.3
Otolaryngology	4.6	3.5
Surgery	6.5	6.7
Urology	1.9	1.5
Radiology	4.4	4.0
Physical medicine*	1.3	1.0
Anesthesiology*	1.5	1.5
Pathology*	1.8	1.6
Neurology*	1.0	1.0
Psychiatry	2.8	1.5
Total**	109.4	----

* Physical medicine based on three groups; anesthesiology based on two groups; pathology and neurology based on four groups. These services are provided in the remaining groups in other ways.
** Exclusive of interns and residents in hospitals.
Source: *Health Manpower Perspective*, 1967. U.S. Public Health Service, Bureau of Health Manpower, Washington, D.C., 1967, Appendix Table 6, p. 75.

prepaid group practice plans is the best guide for general manpower planning. They have argued that this mode of practice is ideal (supporters of prepaid medical practice often ignore the effect of access costs). It is presumed that the plan provides members with all needed medical care and that this care is of high quality. Whatever one's beliefs about prepaid group practice, we doubt that the staffing ratios observed in these groups could serve to forecast the need for specialist or primary care manpower.

In Table 1 we show the distribution of physicians by specialty averaged across six prepaid group practices. In interpreting the data presented in the table, one should note that the numerator includes only active physicians engaged primarily in clinical care and that the average masks a considerable amount of variation.

The Kaiser System, for example, is com-

posed of numerous different local plans. The number of physicians per 100,000 members varies across the different plans. There were 96.6 physicians per 100,000 Kaiser member in 1970. This ranged from 76 in the Colorado plan to 105 in the Northern California plan. In plans with over 100,000 members, the range was from 82 to 105.[14] Before one uses estimates derived from such prepaid group practice programs, several questions must be answered. For example: What factors generated the between-plan manpower ratio differences? Are the populations served different? Is more use made of outside physicians in some plans? Are there more paramedical personnel in some plans? Are the health levels of the groups different? These questions have not been answered, but the variability across plans is striking. This variability is strong evidence that fixed manpower ratios make little sense.

Even if these questions are answered, it is still not clear whether these prepaid comprehensive group ratios should be used in determining manpower requirements for the nation. The data are of doubtful relevance and are likely to underestimate the physicians needed for the following reasons:

1 The plans in the Kaiser System are tightly administered. The total number of physicians is administratively determined and does not necessarily represent a physician/population ratio that would be observed in fee-for-service practice. The number of patients to be seen per hour and the length of the work week are defined; physicians are closely monitored for such aspects of care as ordering lab tests and hospitalization of patients; patients must often wait substantial periods to have a scheduled visit with their physician.

2 The distribution of physicians by specialty type is determined administratively. Supposedly, intensive peer review is practiced, and referral and hospitalization rates are closely monitored, resulting in lower rates than in fee-for-service practice. Without the organization of the prepaid comprehensive plan, it is hard to see why their utilization patterns would generalize. Note also that this kind of medical system represents a

Table 2.   Non-federal physicians by census region and activity, December 31, 1970

Census region	Total physicians*		Patient care	
	Number	Percent	Number	Percent
Total non-federal	281,344	100.0	255,027	100.0
Northeast	87,641	31.2	77,928	30.6
New England	20,391	7.2	17,802	7.0
Middle Atlantic	67,250	23.9	60,126	23.6
North Central	66,993	23.8	61,451	24.1
East North Central	48,162	17.1	44,281	17.4
West North Central	18,831	6.7	17,170	6.7
South	70,178	24.9	64,031	25.1
South Atlantic	37,560	13.4	33,871	13.3
East South Central	12,155	4.3	11,200	4.4
West South Central	20,463	7.3	18,960	7.4
West	54,043	19.2	49,368	19.4
Mountain	10,368	3.7	9,500	3.7
Pacific	43,675	15.5	39,868	15.6
Possessions	2,489	0.9	2,249	0.9

* Excludes 19,621 inactive physicians and 358 not classified.
Note: Percentages may not add due to rounding.
Source: Haug, J. N.; Roback, G. A.; and Martin, B. C. "Distribution of Physicians in the United States, 1970," (Chicago, American Medical Association, 1971).

type of practice that currently serves only 5 percent of the population. The members themselves selected this type of system (all had a fee-for-service alternative) and are not a representative subsample of the national population. They tend to be actively employed, middle-class individuals whose level of income and knowledge leads to better health, less need for prolonged hospitalization, and fewer complicated illnesses. In 1970, for example, about 4.5 percent of the members of the Kaiser plans were over 65 and 1.5 percent were on Medicaid. To put these figures in perspective, in 1970, 9.8 percent of the United States population was over 65 and about 10 percent had incomes below the poverty level.

3 At least in the past, Kaiser patients had incentives quite different from those of other patients; monetary costs were low and access costs could be substantial. Indeed, many patients sought care outside the system at a substantial monetary cost rather than accept the nonmonetary costs within the system. Subtle rationing is associated with the centralized clinic ambulatory practice which leads to greater travel time and cost. A final factor is the emphasis placed on educating subscribers to recognize disease that

is not helped by medical care and to improve personal habits, such as not smoking, getting exercise, and avoiding obesity.

Although the data from the Kaiser System do provide a minimum reference point, they are unlikely to be of direct relevance for planning in the absence of significant structural change in the nation's medical care delivery system.

Manpower Planning Using the Ratio Approach

There is considerable variation in the ratio of physicians to population among various geographic regions. In Table 2, the 1970 distribution of M.D.s by region is presented. The Northeast and West have proportionately more physicians per capita than the South and North Central regions; the variation among states is much greater than that among regions. For example, in 1970 for the country as a whole, there were 171 physicians per 100,000 population, with a range of 83 per 100,000 in Mississippi to 238 per 100,000 in New York. The District of Columbia had 385 physicians per 100,000. There is some indication that these regional differences are becoming larger. In 1950, Mississippi had 66 physicians per 100,000 and New York had 201; thus, between 1950 and 1970, the gap between the state with the highest and lowest number of physicians per 100,000 population rose from 135 to 155. There is also some evidence that these trends favor the coastal states at the expense of those that are more inland.

Within states there are great differences between rural and urban physician/population ratios. In 1970, there were 173 physicians per 100,000 population in the urban areas, but only 80 physicians per 100,000 in rural areas. Within the state of California, physician/population ratios across the planning areas ranged from 220 per 100,000 in the San Francisco Bay area to 99 per 100,000 in Superior, California. Even within urban areas, the variability in the local supply of physicians is great. Physicians are usually concentrated in only a few census tracts, while most census tracts have none.

We explore spatial distribution of physician manpower more extensively in the next section. Here, we consider an approach to planning for medical manpower that makes use of physician/population ratios. In it, some present physician/population ratio is considered a minimum requirement for the future. This approach has a number of variations involving the selection of the ratios:

☐ The minimum required physician/population ratio at some future time is taken as the average ratio existing now in the United States.

☐ The minimum required physician/population ratio at some future time is taken as that now existing in the states with the highest physician/population ratios (the criterion ratio).

☐ The minimum required physician/population ratio is calculated for each demographic group in a place where the population is deemed to be "adequately" served. To determine the number of physicians required, it is then necessary to forecast the expected population growth and the future demographic characteristics of the population. For example, if the aged need more physicians and if the mean age in the population is rising, then to ensure continued access to physicians similar to that of today, the overall physician/population ratio will have to rise.

Ignoring for the moment the problems that can arise in forecasting, we address the strengths and weaknesses of forecasting requirements on the basis of existing physician/population ratios.

1 Of these planning techniques, the first ratio approach seems to require the least information. Projections that incorporate expected changes in the demographic composition of the population (the third method) will provide more reliable insight than projections based simply on total population.

2 There is an implicit, but untested, assumption that the base ratio is adequate and needed; that is, a reduction in the ratio would be adverse. It is often assumed that the more physicians, the better. However, there is evidence that adding physicians to an area may simply lead to unnecessary medical care or to underemployment of physicians. Thus, the criterion ratio approach (second method) is likely to set future requirements too high.

3 In the absence of structural changes in the delivery system, the ratio approach will provide reasonable forecasts of *demand* over the short term. Changes in organization, medical technology, immunology, treatment, financing and payment mechanisms, or mode of practice, for example, are likely to invalidate manpower projections based on current utilization patterns.

4 Using national ratios hides a great deal, e.g., variability in physician distribution by state, county, and type of practice. The wide variation in local physician/population ratios is shown in Table 2. Suppose, for example, that enough physicians are trained to raise the United States physician/population ratio to the level of the highest 10 states (as of 1975). There is little reason to believe that these newly produced physicians will choose to concentrate in states with relatively fewer physicians, or in areas within states that have the lowest ratios. Indeed, we would predict that the difference between areas would increase as a result of training these additional physicians, as it did between 1950 and 1970. However, all states had more physicians per capita in 1970 than in 1950; thus, the

poorer states were better off in absolute terms, even though they were worse off in relative terms.

5 If the numerator is to indicate the availability of physician services, it should be derived with respect to full-time-equivalent active physicians engaged in providing clinical services as opposed to teaching, research, public health, and other activities, and it should take account of physicians who work part time.

6 The ratio approach ignores all changes in physician productivity and assumes that physicians are used in fixed proportions in delivering medical services. Existing data indicate that the way in which physicians allocate their services to patients is predictable; for example, more tasks are delegated to allied health personnel when the physician/population ratio is low.[15] The volume of services provided by physicians is not fixed and physician productivity has been increasing over time. Klarman[16] presents a number of estimates of increases in physician productivity; the mean estimated increase is about 3 percent per year. The ratio approach also takes no account of changes in medical technology and public health practice or the introduction of new health manpower.

In all fairness, it should be pointed out that these criticisms are acknowledged by researchers who have used this approach. It should also be pointed out that without a good deal of clairvoyance it is impossible to forecast some of these trends. However, these arguments suggest that the system is more fluid than the ratio approach implies and that policies should encourage flexibility, not fixed ratios.

Economic Models

In developing an economic model of demand, the question is: What will utilization (use of physicians' services or other aspects of medical care) be at some future time? This question is approached by estimating a demand function, a relationship between the amount of care sought and its cost, access constraints, and other factors. To predict the future level of services that will be sought, the future value of each factor in the demand function is estimated and the estimated parameters are used to predict future utilization.

Economists have tended to neglect access costs, which are becoming more important than direct payment to the provider. Acton and Richardson[17] have investigated some of the effects of access costs. Costs due to scarcities in rural areas were investigated by Marshall, et al.[18] Their finding—that dissatisfaction over travel time to get to a physician in rural Kansas was great and was likely to have adverse effects on patient behavior—is corroborated in a study by Weiss and Greenlick,[19] who analyzed the behavior of urban and suburban patients in the Kaiser program. However, Weiss and Greenlick noticed that distance did not have a constant effect on all types of patients. Instead, they detected an interaction effect, which led them to conclude that patients in upper socioeconomic status (SES) groups were little affected by distance, while lower SES groups were led either to delay seeking care until symptoms became quite severe or to substitute emergency room encounters for routine appointments with medical staff. Such findings have been reported elsewhere[20] and have been incorporated into most current theories of patient illness behavior.[21]

The demand for medical care (and physician services) is derived from the demand for health.[22] Medical care is a service than can be bought to improve or maintain health "stock." The demand for medical care is thus dependent upon an individual's underlying health status, perception of the efficacy of medical care, and cost of getting medical care, where cost is a vector consisting of time costs, money costs, and psychological costs. To determine the demand relationship, this theoretical formulation must be made specific and then estimated with empirical data.

Investigators may use age as a surrogate for underlying health status, education as a measure of awareness, reported money income as a measure of both earned and unearned income, sex as another indication of the underlying health status, distance to facilities as a measure of time cost, and insurance and Medicaid coverage as a measure of the difference between the "market" price and actual price to the individual. Demand functions have been estimated using individuals, groups of individuals, and states as the basic unit of observation.[23] Single equation demand models have been estimated as have general systems (with demand as one part).

Economists have focused their attention on determining the income and price elasticities of the demand for medical care and physician services. Income elasticity is defined as the percentage change in quantity bought due to a 1 percent change in income, and price elasticity is defined as the percentage change in quantity bought due to a 1 percent change in price. The former is a measure of the responsiveness of demand to a change in income, and the latter is a measure of responsiveness of demand to a change in price.

In estimating income elasticities, economists distinguish between earnings and wealth. Separating earned income from unearned income is particularly important where the time price is high, such as in medical care. As earnings rise, other things equal, the value of time rises, and it is assumed that people are willing to substitute money for time. This may explain why employed men and women are more alike in their demands for care than employed women and homemakers, income level held constant.[24]

The empirical estimates of income elasticity have been varied. The range of these estimates is presented in Table 3. The Fein estimate indicates that a 1 percent increase in income will generate at .21 percent increase in physician visits.

The price elasticity of the demand for physician care has also been estimated. The estimates range from −.1 to −.36.[25] Some recent attention has been directed to estimating nonprice costs and their effect on services demanded. Both waiting time and travel time are shown to have high elasticities.[26]

These results indicate that as the monetary price (to consumers) of medical care falls and as income rises, the quantity of medical services demanded will also increase. As access costs to medical care drop, demand will also rise.

Table 3. Several measures of income elasticity of demand for physician expenditures or services*

Source	Income elasticity
Fein[1] (visits)	.21
Feldstein, P.[2]	
visits	.62
expenditures	.56
Gorham[3] (expenditures)	.33
Andersen and Benham[4]	
visits (observed income)	n.v.
visits (permanent income)	.01
expenditures (observed income)	.41
expenditures (permanent income)	.63
Fuchs and Kramer[5] (visits)	.04–.57

* This table is adapted from Klarman, H. E. "Economic Aspects of Projecting Requirements for Health Manpower," *The Journal of Human Resources* 4:360–376 (1969).

[1] Fein, R. *The Doctor Shortage* (Washington, D.C.: The Brookings Institution, 1967).
[2] Feldstein, P. J. "The Demand for Medical Care," in: Commission on the Cost of Medical Care. *General Report*, Vol. I (Chicago: American Medical Association, 1964).
[3] Gorham, W. "A Report to the President on Medical Care Prices," (Washington, D.C.: U.S Department of Health, Education and Welfare, 1967).
[4] Andersen, R. and Benham, L. "Factors Affecting the Relationship between Family Income and Medical Care Consumption," in: Klarman, H. E. (ed.) *Empirical Studies in Health Economics* (Baltimore: The Johns Hopkins Press, 1970).
[5] Fuchs, V. R. and Kramer, M. J. *Determinants of Expenditures for Physicians' Services in the United States 1948–1968*, DHEW Publication No. (HSM) 73-3013 (Washington, D.C.: DHEW, HSMHA, December 1972).

However, if the time costs of medical care rise, the number of services demanded will fall, particularly for those with a high opportunity cost for time.

Some investigators have argued that the demand curve may be affected by the supply of physicians.[27] In this conceptualization, the physicians themselves are thought to influence the number of visits people make by suggesting patterns of care (which include revisits) through follow-up recommendations, and by lobbying for the construction of medical institutions. The crux of the physician-induced demand argument is that the pattern of recommended care may vary with the physician load. That is, in areas with many physicians, physicians can maintain their income by recommending more visits—visits that may be of marginal medical efficacy.

Some major work on the demand for and supply of physicians has been done by Fuchs and Kramer.[28] They estimated a five equation model using state data that contained a demand function (number of visits per capita), a supply function (number of doctors per 100,000 population), an output per physician function (number of visits per thousand), an insurance benefits function, and two identities—the quantity demanded of physician services equals the quantity supplied, and one defining net price. Since it is a simultaneous system, two stage least squares was used to estimate the parameters.

Fuchs and Kramer hypothesized that one of the factors affecting the number of visits demanded per capita was the number of M.D.s per capita. This variable was included because it was argued that physicians were able to generate a demand for their services without lowering price. Fuchs and Kramer suggest that when physicians are abundant, they may order care that is not medically indicated (unnecessary surgery), or of marginal importance (numerous post-operative visits, follow-up visits, or overzealous well-baby care); when physicians are scarce, patients may lower their expectations and handle minor complaints themselves. They also suggested that when physicians are plentiful, the nonmonetary costs of care (waiting time, time to get an appointment, and travel costs) are likely to be lower. In the statistical results, the M.D. variable (physicians per capita) was the one with the highest elasticity and with the highest level of significance, presumably indicating that the supply of physicians had the most influence on the demand for care.

Although the number of M.D.s per capita may be a surrogate for nonmonetary costs, Fuchs and Kramer believe that the importance of the variable stems from physicians' ability to control demand. They quote Ginzberg:[29]

The supply of medical resources has thus far effectively generated its own demand. Much unnecessary surgery continues to be performed. . . . There is substantial over-doctoring for a host of diseases, including, in particular, infections of the upper respiratory tract. . . . [Physicians] usually have wide margins of discretion about whether to recommend that a patient return to the office for one or more follow-up visits.

It could be argued that Fuchs and Kramer have uncovered a simultaneous equation problem rather than physician-induced demand. If physicians moved their practice to areas where the most care was needed, the data would show a close association between supply and demand. Although many of the characteristics expected to lead to increased need are included in the analysis, the possibility remains that the result reflects the altruistic nature of physicians rather than their artificially induced demand. Results similar to those obtained by Fuchs and Kramer were found in a study in Canada. Examining physicians in British Columbia, Evans[30] argued that a strong case could be made for supplier-induced demand. These results are open to question (and have been questioned). Nonetheless, they do have very important implications for manpower planning.

Systems Models of Health Care

A number of theoretical systems models of health care delivery have been proposed, but only two have been fully specified and estimated. The first is actually a series of models developed by Martin Feldstein.[31] These are econometric models with about half a dozen equations (and endogenous variables). For example, in his analysis of the effects of Medicare, the endogenous variables are the proportion of enrollees with supplementary insurance, the hospital admissions rate, the rate of extended care admissions per hospital admission, and the hospital insurance benefits per hospital episode. These variables are modeled as being determined by demographic variables, such as the proportions of white enrollees, male enrollees, those living in large cities, the ratio of enrollees over 75 to total enrollees, and per capita income. Other variables include the proportion of the population under 65 with health insurance, the proportion of enrollees for which the state government declines to pay premiums (and who are indigent), short-term beds per capita, private physicians per capita, per capita state expenditure for the aged on health, the number of months the state had participated in Medicaid, extended care beds per capita, and hospital cost per patient day. The equations were estimated by an instrumental variables technique (similar to two stage least squares) on observations for each state. Since the model was designed to explain the variation among states in the dependent variables, it has little to do with the sort of behavior one would expect to observe in individual patients, physicians, and hospitals. In this sense, it is a "macro" model and ignores the details of an individual's behavior, assuming it to be unaffected by the policy variables except as summarized in the macro variables. The other conceptual difficulty is the lack of an output measure, but we return to this difficulty after discussing the second model.

Yett, *et al.*,[32] have developed an elaborate model of the medical care sector that uses more than 100 equations (and endogenous variables) to characterize almost every aspect of the system. There are a number of sub-models, concerned with manpower, hospitals, and so on, that are joined by some interaction equations. The rationale given for each of the behavioral equations is that of the decisions to be made by an individual and the factors affecting them. Thus, the Yett, *et al.*, model is different in orientation, as well as in complexity, from the Feldstein models, but data are not available to estimate the relations. The best that Yett, *et al.*, can do is to use state observations to get most of the variables. Even so, it is impossible to obtain the relevant measures of insurance coverage and other factors. Given the size of the model and the quality of the data, the authors choose to estimate the equations individually, using ordinary least squares. This means that the parameter estimates are inconsistent compared with estimates generated by, for example, two stage least squares, although, given the quality of the data, their choice of an estimating technique is appropriate. Unfortunately, the good intentions of constructing a model to reflect individual behavior are not realized because of the lack of data for estimating the model.

Yett, *et al.*, have attempted to spell out the implications of their model using simulation techniques. Using the parameter estimates gained from ordinary least squares regression on state data, the authors vary one or another parameter and use simulation to explore the resulting change in the equilibrium of the model. For a model of this size, there is no alternative way of investigating the system influences of a change in a set of parameter values. For example, their manpower planning subsystem uses the forecast demand for services, the production relations for these services and the equations determining the supply of manpower. The output is then a forecast of the number of physicians that would be required to meet the demand, as well as an estimate of the number of hours per week they would work and their income.

The Feldstein and Yett, *et al.*, models share the problem of not having a measure of the output of the medical care sector. They determine the conventional measures of utilization, available manpower, and cost, but have no explicit measure of output. One might continue to use utilization and input measures (number of patient visits, inpatient days, etc.) as surrogates for output, but the implications in a model of this sort would be that more and more resources should be put into medical care delivery. Although these models can be helpful in exploring the structure of the medical care system, they are inherently limited by their lack of an output measure. Policy implications must be drawn cautiously from a model when it cannot be known whether increasing the number of patient visits will have a positive or negative effect on health (much less on social welfare). The models do tell us the implications of parameter changes, such as those that might result from a particular type of national health insurance. If one knew whether an increase in one aspect of utilization was good or bad, such models might be used to determine what parameters ought to be altered to achieve a desirable result.

We have constructed a model with these properties[33] and are currently attempting to estimate its parameters. Summary inputs and outcomes in the model consist of physician hours, hospital days, physician visits, total cost, and several health status measures. The underlying health status of the population and an individual's health status at any point is the primary factor determining whether care will be sought or prescribed treatment compliance will occur. Since health status is treated explicitly in the model, there is no alternative to specifying spontaneous rates of improvement or deterioration in health, and the efficacy of some contact with the health care system in improving health status. We regard the model as giving many insights, but we must stress the obvious difficulties in getting health status measures and in estimating how these change spontaneously or with medical care.

Summary and Critique of the Models

The ratio model has the advantage of being simple and will predict utilization accurately insofar as the underlying conditions determining demand and supply do not change (no major changes in medical knowledge, organization, or financing of medical care). However, since the ratios reflect the current system, their use presupposes a future system where utilization is similar to the current one. In contrast, the Lee and Jones[34] approach is more of an attempt to get at ideal requirements. Its principal problem is that the actual level of medical care demanded is far less than that predicted by the model (since not everyone who needs care seeks it, nor do people adhere to their prescribed regimen). Thus, manpower policies based on the ratio approach will tend to preserve the current system, while policies based on the Lee and Jones approach would lead to an oversupply of physicians. Both approaches ignore the substitution possibilities in producing care and increasing productivity.

The simple economic models go far in allowing one to gain insight into the factors that affect physician utilization. They allow one to predict what effect changing socioeconomic or demographic characteristics of the population will have on the demand for medical care and what the effects will be of increasing population or the amount of insurance. However, many of the crucial variables, such as travel time and waiting time, are necessarily the result of interactions between supply and demand. Since these models look only at the demand side of the picture, they cannot determine the level of these access variables and so are conceptually incomplete (although one might guess at future values of these parameters).

Two models of medical care delivery that look at the simultaneous interaction of supply and demand have been described briefly. However, they are unsatisfactory in two important ways. First, they were estimated using aggregate (state level) observations. Second, they had no output measures associated with them. Thus, one knows only that by manipulating the system one can change the number of patient visits or hospital visits, but one cannot know whether these changes increase or decrease the public welfare.

To construct a model capable of predicting demand after a structural change (such as that represented by national health insurance or reorganization into health maintenance organizations), to take account of the simultaneity of supply and demand, and to estimate the social welfare implications of changes, one must have a model of the health care system like the two presented, but having the additional property that output is included directly. This is the crucial issue; however, in addition, the system must be estimated using disaggregated data so that it reflects individual consumer and physician preferences while acknowledging that there are other ways of providing care.

Models of the Supply of Physician Services

Physician services might be measured by the number of hours of service by physician specialty and location. Thus, one must know the current stock of physicians; changes in the stock due to deaths, retirements, and new graduates; factors affecting choice of specialty; factors affecting the number of hours a physician devotes to medical care; and factors affecting geographical location (by region, by rural versus urban area, and by location within an urban area). While there have been insightful discussion of these issues,[35] there has been little formal modeling and empirical investigation.

In this section we examine research findings

that bear on physician supply. These studies have focused predominantly on the maldistribution of physician services. Determining maldistributions, measuring their extent, and studying the factors associated with them are central policy issues since many government agencies have reacted to perceived local scarcities by elaborate, and often expensive, intervention into the local delivery system. Unfortunately, this research area is filled with contradictory results; thus, one must look carefully at the underlying data base and analytical methods to resolve the contradictions.

Approaches to Studying Physician Supply

Three techniques have been most commonly used to study maldistribution and the factors causing it. By far the most common involves a simple tabular comparison of physician/population ratios. Variability across the units of analysis is often presumed to be sufficient evidence of a maldistribution of physicians. The extent of this maldistribution is identified with the range of the ratios. Thus, DeVise[36] argues that coastal regions have a comparative advantage over inland regions; and Fahs, *et al.*,[37] argue that the central states lose medical graduates to the western states. Comparisons of this sort inevitably show that the more heavily urbanized states have more physicians than the rural states, and, within the states, urban counties have more physicians than rural counties. However, these findings while suggestive are not definitive. The studies suffer from an absence of control for other factors known to be important determinants of physician location. For example, the coastal states with the greatest number of physicians are also highly urbanized states; is the coastal location or the urbanization the true cause of the movement? What aspects of urban or coastal environments attract physicians? What qualities of rural communities repel them? For purposes of policy formulation, such simple comparisons represent only first steps.

The second most common approach employs multivariate statistical analysis and represents an improvement over tabular comparisons. Studies using these methods attempt (at levels of aggregation such as regional, state, county,

or census tract) to relate the physician population of a locality to qualities of the locality that are presumed to act as positive or negative inducements to physicians. These studies are often predicated on a well-formulated model of physician spatial behavior. Typically some form of regression is used to estimate the relation. In their classic study, Rimlinger and Steele[38] used least squares techniques to estimate a linear model relating physician/population ratios for 200 county groups that constituted the United States to characteristics of these areas in 1959. Their findings indicated that income, leisure, and mobility were significant explanatory variables; and they argued that such factors are positively associated with urbanization. The power of the multivariate approach is that it has the potential of allowing the investigator to examine the influence of a host of variables simultaneously and to estimate the individual effect of each. Since some of these variables are amenable to policy manipulation, the technique can provide a basis for choosing among alternative policies.

Although this approach is superior to cross tabulations, it has many pitfalls. Ordinary least squares (OLS) has predominated in these analyses, but it may not be an appropriate estimation technique because of multicollinearity or simultaneous influences among the variables. This is often the case when ratios are used as dependent variables.[39] Often the relevant variables are so closely associated in the observed data that it is impossible to distinguish among them.[40] Other problems in the applicability of OLS lie in the assumptions that must be made concerning independence and normality in the distribution of errors and linearity of the equation. Thus, estimation techniques such as two stage least squares, ridge, Tobit, and Poisson regression may be required to give accurate estimates of relationships.

The third approach, and one that is becoming more common, involves surveying physician opinion. Here, researchers attempt to ascertain from physicians themselves the factors regarded as most important in the choice of a practice location. This approach has the potential of uncovering factors that may be neglected by analysts who have little personal experience with the practice location decision. Clearly, the outcome of such studies may be input to more elaborate econometric analyses of aggregate data. For example, Cooper, *et al.*,[41] report the results of a survey conducted by the American Medical Association in an attempt to ascertain the conditions under which particular physicians decide to locate in rural or urban areas. Attitudinal surveys focus on preferential differences among physicians, whereas spatial models focus on extant differences among localities. Both are useful for policy formulation. On the one hand, surveys help determine which background qualities of physicians make them better long-term choices for rural locations. On the other hand, spatial models may reveal whether professional amenities lead more physicians on average to choose a particular type of locale.

These three approaches are not exhaustive of those used to investigate physician distribution but they do typify the bulk of the reported research. In general, the questions that have been phrased are these: Where are the physicians? What are the characteristics of the areas they favor and of those they shun? What are the characteristics of physicians in areas where there are scarcities? The underlying assumption of the research is that by understanding the attractive factors or the personal predispositions of physicians, policies can be instituted to modify or equalize the availability of medical care. We proceed to review this literature first in terms of the choice between urban and rural settings and then between sites within cities; we consider the role of the foreign medical graduate; and last, we examine what has been learned regarding the initial location decisions of recent medical graduates.

In Table 4 we have categorized factors that have been the subject of research and indicated the direction of their apparent influence on physicians. Some effects, such as that of loan forgiveness programs, are debatable. But in the absence of further research the displayed effects seem reasonable. The results emphasize the attractive nature of urban areas and the physician's personal acquaintance with a particular area or type of area. Although the table summarizes the most relevant research,

we shall briefly consider some of the studies from which it was constructed.

The Rural-Urban Choice

The discussion of rural-urban differences in physician manpower is commonplace in state medical journals.[42] Generally, the opinion surveys indicate that those physicians who chose to locate in small communities did so simply because they or their spouses like these locales. Yett and Sloan[43] report that physicians tend to set up practice in areas near their place of rearing or medical training. These findings and the associated finding that most small town practitioners were reared in small towns suggest that, of those physicians practicing in small towns, personal life-style preferences rather than professional issues predominate.[44] Physicians who report that professional considerations predominate find urban locations most attractive. These physicians give a high priority to proximity to colleagues and supporting medical facilities, the ability to have a varied practice, and the possibility of joining a group practice—qualities associated with urban locations. Non-urban physicians report heavy workloads, while higher pay scales and more readily scheduled activities are reported by urban physicians. The surveys also indicate that young physicians are more anxious than older physicians to join group practices and that they are tending more often to choose financially secure and readily scheduled positions on academic or medical staffs and in other institutional settings. These findings imply that extant urban-rural differences are likely to increase as older physicians are replaced.

The regression studies have addressed the issue of life-style variables and urban versus rural location at many levels of data aggregation. In their analysis of state level data, Fuchs and Kramer[45] used two stage least squares techniques to estimate a model of physician distribution for 33 states in 1966. The most important variables they identified were per capita income, the presence of medical schools, the price of care, and the number of hospital beds. However, the relevant variables were so closely associated that they could not separate the various hypotheses. They concluded by

Table 4. Factors affecting physician location*

Dependent variable	Relationship	Independent variable
Number of physicians	+	Per capita income in state
	+	State educational expenditures
	+	Per capita income in county
	+	Construction of hospital in community
	+	Median income in community
	+	Population of area
	+	Physicians' price practices, based on per capita income of area
	+	Failure rate of licensing examination
	+	Physician income in state
	−	Lack of recreational facilities
	−	Contruction of hospital in rural county
	−	Cyclic variations in income levels in area
	+	Presence of commercial activity
Practice in urban areas	+	Graduation from certain medical schools
	+	Graduation from urban medical school
Practice in rural areas	+	Rural background
	+	Participation in loan forgiveness program
Practice in same state	+	Internship and residency training in state
Ability to attract physicians	+	Mobility of community residents
	+	Educational level of population
	−	Percent population in agriculture
Number of primary care physicians	+	Percent population white
	+	Percent population 0–5 years old and 65+ years old
	−	Inadequate cultural and recreational resources in community
Number of specialists	+	Educational level of population
	+	Number of supportive institutions
	+	Number of general hospital beds per 1000 population
	+	Medical school in community
	+	Presence of high concentrations of commercial activity
	+	Presence of university medical facility
Presence of physician	+	Economic growth rate of town

* This table is adapted from Cooper, J. K.; Heald, K,; and Samuels, M. "The Decision for Rural Practice," *Journal of Medical Education* 47:939–944 (December 1972).

suggesting that, in general, professional convenience and urban "life-style" factors were attractive to most physicians. Lave and Lave[46] performed a similar analysis on 1950 and 1970 state data in which they included variables meant to characterize urban qualities more precisely. The urbanization effect was strong in both 1950 and 1970. In a follow-up study to their 1963 report, Steele and Rimlinger[47] reported the results of county level analyses for 1949 and 1959. Although some specific results seemed at odds with their earlier findings, the general results from both studies were similar. Family income was less important as an explanatory variable in 1959 than in 1949, while the amenities that the authors associated with an "urban environment" became more important over time.

Marden's[48] study of physician location in 369 metropolitan counties was particularly important because he grouped physicians as either specialists or general practitioners. The following characteristics of the metropolitan areas were included: educational attainment, age composition, racial composition, and number of hospital beds in the counties. Race and age composition were found to be the most important explanatory variables, with hospital beds important only for the smallest cities. However, Marden's analysis was replicated by Joroff and Navarro[49] with contradictory results. Examining 299 cities and using 10 independent variables, they did not find race to be important once the presence of a medical school and the population's educational attainment were taken into account. Additional important factors were hospital beds and the population's age distribution. Lankford's[50] analysis supported the predominance of population as a determinant of physician location.

Further support for the role played by medical facilities or professional amenities is provided in two Ph.D. dissertations using state level data. Weiss[51] reported that physicians were attracted to states in proportion to the number of medical centers they contained; and Sloan[52] reported that high physician/population ratios were associated with high income, low cyclical economic variability, high capital stock, and high numbers of medical students (a likely surrogate for the medical center effect detected by Weiss). Finally, Benham, et al.,[53] performed analyses on 1930, 1940, 1950, and 1960 levels of physicians and dentists in the states and found that, over time, increasing importance was being placed on high per capita income, population, and medical training facilities.

These results for the effects of population and medical facilities on physician distribution have received widespread support. Income seems no longer to be the most important factor.[54] Instead, it would appear that physician salaries are currently so high that the lure of still higher income influences few. Physicians seem now to be more concerned with cultural, environmental and professional amenities. These include leisure time (attained by a not overly-demanding practice and the effectiveness of non-price rationing procedures[55]), medical resources, interesting case variety, income security, colleagues, and other qualities associated with large populations or dense urban areas. In this vein, Parker, et al.,[56] found that most physicians who chose to practice in small towns could be readily distinguished from other physicians in that they did not share the views about urban and professional qualities. Instead, they were often originally from small towns, had a preference for this life-style, and claimed to be unconcerned about urban-rural physician income differentials.[57] These findings indicate that as the bulk of physicians come from urban backgrounds and as they pass through the medical education system, they acquire a set of values that reinforces their predisposition to choose an urban location for their practice. Thus, urbanization, medical specialization (leading to greater dependence among physicians on cooperative activities), dependence on hospital-based technological care, and the rise of staff positions in institutional medicine seem to be the primary processes influencing the contemporary national spatial distribution of physicians.

Intra-Urban Location Decisions

The state, metropolitan, and county level studies provide some information on the factors affecting the spatial distribution of physicians in the United States. They also suggest variables that may be relevant to intra-urban spatial research. The research we have reviewed indicates that physicians tend to gravitate toward areas that satisfy their own personal objectives in terms of life-style and professional behavior, and that factors such as the racial composition of the population do not appear to be very important.

The processes affecting regional distribution seem readily understood, although precision and knowledge of interactions need to be improved. On the local level, however, the situation is not as clear-cut. Because of the affected urban population groups—the poor, the aged, and the nonwhite—local maldistributions may be as significant as regional maldistribution. Adverse conditions are likely to lead here to patterns of behavior accentuating the severity of an illness episode and frustrating the efficient delivery of therapeutic medical services.[58]

There is a copious literature bearing on local distribution. Chicago, New York, and Boston have been the sites of extensive investigations. Some other cities have been studied.[59] We concentrate on recent studies of the three major sites, detailing others only when relevant.

Lepper, *et al.*,[60] performed a study of physician/population ratios in Chicago's OEO-defined poverty areas. Their conclusion that physicians were fairly scarce in these locales was also reached by Rees, by DeVise and Dewey, and by Dewey.[61] In his two studies, Rees examined the exodus of physicians from Chicago to the surrounding suburbs. He chose an extremely gross unit of analysis (three concentric zones or a few neighborhoods) and, consequently, only vague conclusions could be drawn. Thus, he could only determine that the numbers of physicians setting up practice in the Chicago suburbs appeared to outpace those starting up in the city. DeVise and Dewey summarize the Dewey study. Decennial data on physician/population ratios for 1950, 1960, and 1970 were contrasted with data on race, population, retail buying power, and hospitals. Again, physicians were found to be fleeing the inner city for the more affluent white suburbs; physicians were seen to seek office locations near expensive residential tracts so as to minimize their own travel time to the office; socioeconomic levels were the most influential qualities of a locale; suburban shopping centers and office buildings were observed to have high attractive potential for physicians. Unfortunately, these conclusions must be viewed cautiously because the coarse nature of the zone boundaries used in the analysis confuses the influence of many variables, some of which may be important and unrelated to locale, affluence, or racial characteristics.

Elesh and Schollaert[62] used data describing conditions in Chicago census tracts in 1960. In this study, general categories of physicians were regressed on population, commercial activity, hospitals, age distribution, education, and racial composition. The results indicated that physicians avoid black areas, are attracted to populated areas, commercial activity, hospitals, the central business district (CBD), older populations, educated populations, and high income areas. However, the explanatory power of the models was low (R^2 never exceeded .4), indicating that important variables influencing physician distribution had not been included in the models. Furthermore, several variables were entered in the analysis (such as hospitals) in a questionable fashion.

In a similar though less ambitious study, May[63] analyzed the distribution of physicians in Brooklyn, New York, in 1960. In contrast with Elesh and Schollaert, May did not find that race was important. Using both ratios and counts of physicians in tracts, he found median years of education to be the only important socioeconomic variable, while population size and hospitals were other crucial variables. May's findings also contradict the observation of Piore and Sokal[64] that New York City physicians avoid low income areas because of their obvious poverty-stricken character. Roemer[65] also drew this conclusion in his description of conditions in Los Angeles—and, regardless of the publication of seemingly contradictory evidence, it is the viewpoint most often represented when local "doctor shortages" or "physician maldistributions" are discussed.[66]

The true complexity of the situation, though, is best illustrated by the work reported by Dorsey and by Robertson on conditions in Boston, and by Hambleton's analysis of 15 SMSAs.[67] Dorsey examined data for census tracts in Boston and Brookline between 1940–1961. He observed the growth of an increasingly specialized population of physicians. Using income, occupation, and education in a composite indicator of socioeconomic status (SES), he determined that the changing physician mix over time had left low SES tracts with few primary care physicians. However, Robertson drew quite different conclusions in a study of Boston census tracts covering the same period, 1940–1960. He observed that because of a tendency for physicians to cluster together, simple longitudinal analyses are likely to be erroneous. This would be due to any lagged effect introduced by clusters of physicians attracting physicians. To avoid this problem he used a differential equation model of change originally described by Coleman.[68] Socioeconomic status was found not to be important for the location of general practitioners, but it was related to the distribution of internists and pediatricians. All three types of physicians tended to concentrate in areas characteristically high in a factor identified with low owner-occupied housing and low median income. Robertson concluded that in Boston between 1940 and 1960, medical practice had become more specialized and physicians had clustered into a few locales that were characterized by office buildings and proximity to hospitals. This clustering had proceeded with little regard to changes in other local conditions. The result was that although some few areas were well served by locally available primary physicians, this was generally accidental. Because of clustering, physicians were located near only a small portion of the population.

Hambleton's study[69] is in accord with these conclusions. Studying local distribution in 15 SMSAs in 1960, he found that clusters of physicians in the central business districts and in other inner city areas left predominantly poor or nonwhite groups with locational advantages over other areas. This was especially true for specialists, who, he argued, tend to cluster in the central business district more than do general practitioners because they have a city-wide market orientation. Poor and black residents near business districts were close to medical offices, which, it appeared, had been located without regard to neighborhood, race or income characteristics. However, Hambleton raised the cautionary note that proximity did not guarantee accessibility. Hambleton's conclusions were similar to those drawn by Kaplan and Leinhardt[70] in a multivariate study of physician location in Pittsburgh. Census tract data on commercial activity, hospital beds, and socioeconomic and demographic composition were used; and physicians were found to be attracted to professional facilities, giving little regard to local socioeconomic or racial conditions.

The importance of professional factors seems well documented. Physicians are not uniformly distributed within cities but instead are concentrated in areas that can provide professional amenities. Although this provides no overt advantage to the middle class, there are subtle advantages. The middle class can more easily travel the distances and deal with the centralized medical system than can the poor.

The Role of the Foreign Medical Graduate

A large portion of the current physician supply in the United States and the one most amenable to short-term policy-induced variation is the group that has received training outside of the United States. Some of these foreign medical graduates (FMGs) are U.S. citizens who sought training in foreign countries. Most, however, are foreign citizens who have come to the United States for a period of years to improve their training or to immigrate. These FMGs represented approximately 20 percent of the active physicians and about 33 percent of the hospital interns and residents in 1970[71]. Between 1960 and 1970 the influx of FMGs increased at a faster rate than the domestic production of new physicians. In 1968–1970, FMGs made up 29 percent of newly-licensed physicians. Of all physicians admitted as immigrants in 1970, 70 percent (approximately 6,300 physicians) came from Central and South America, Asia, and Africa. Between 1962 and 1971, nearly 29,000 FMGs immigrated to the United States. During the same period, 46,812 FMGs came to the United States under the two-year exchange visitor physician program, and most of these have stayed.

This flow of skilled manpower from underdeveloped areas to the United States poses important questions for international relations and represents a form of reverse foreign aid that may be quite detrimental to the source countries.[72] However, United States policymakers view FMGs as a significant aid in alleviating the presumed physician shortage. Indeed, such thoughts led, in 1970, to legislation making it fairly simple for an FMG to convert a visitor visa to permanent-resident status. But the growing dependence of the United States on a manpower source over which U.S. policymakers have little control should not be accepted without question. Although, by evidence of their increasing numbers of applications, there is currently a large and anxious stock of FMGs seeking entrance to the United States, there is no way of assuring continuity in this supply. The health needs of other nations are certainly as great as those of the United States, and it is unclear how long these nations will permit skilled manpower to be drained off by the incentives of the U.S. market for physicians.

Another issue concerns the effect of this increasing supply of FMGs on the general distribution and availability of physicians within the United States. If one assumes that a nonuniform distribution of physicians is detrimental, then, clearly, the initial locational choice decisions of FMGs and their migratory propensities within the United States can work either to alleviate or to aggravate this maldistribution. Although important research on this topic is limited, Marguiles and Bloch[73] indicate that, at the state level, FMGs tend to concentrate in urbanized areas. An extensive investigation of FMGs has been performed by Butter and Schaffner.[74] Addressing spatial distributional effects, they used 1968 data from the AMA giving physician/population ratios for states and counties. They compared deviations from a uniform distribution of physicians first excluding FMGs and then including FMGs. They argued that state and urban-rural differences in physician/population ratios were exacerbated by the addition of FMGs.

FMGs appear to distribute themselves selectively, and although they add to the aggregate physician supply, they probably increase the disparity between states and between urban and rural areas. Several factors may explain this finding. FMGs may be dependent on institutional support, probably desire cosmopolitan environments, are likely to have urban backgrounds, and may desire to serve urbanized ethnic groups. Unless urban FMGs are viewed as replacements for U.S. trained physicians who are thus freed to serve rural communities (an unlikely assumption), they should not be considered as a force with which to arrest the growing rural-urban disparity in physicians.

In a second study, Schaffner and Butter[75] examined the interstate geographic mobility of FMGs. They questioned whether the regional mobility of FMGs would act to equalize the selectivity of their initial locational decisions. Using data from the AMA's 1966 and 1968 physician census, they computed FMG in- and out-migration rates for 36 states (95.4 percent of all FMGs). As surrogate measures for determining the relative physician shortage in a given state, they used the physician/population ratio, the five-year rate of change of physician income, and the state level of physician income (this assumes that physician income is responsive to demand and that relative increases in income indicate increases in demand without concomitant increases in supply, i.e., shortage). Only 8 percent of all FMGs moved between states during the period and the mobile FMGs tended to move to only those states that ranked low in terms of their measures of medical manpower shortage. Thus, the mobility of FMGs appeared to add to the disparity between the states. However, these conclusions must be viewed with caution. Only 36 states were included in the study, a period of only two years was analyzed, and the AMA records on FGMs are likely to be incomplete. An adequate study of initial locational propensities of FMGs, their migratory patterns, and the factors influencing their local spatial distribution would require a longer time span, a lower level of aggregation, controls for factors likely to attract or repel FMGs, and data detailing residency location, specialty, and subjective characteristics. Nonetheless, informed planning must take into consideration the large and increasing FMG physician population.

New Physicians

Understanding the locational decisions of physicians can be decomposed into two related issues: 1) the decision to locate and initiate a practice, and 2) the decision to move a practice. Presumably, different factors influence these decisions. Physicians making their initial locational decisions will be younger and less experienced, and their families will be at a different stage of development than physicians considering a move from one locale to another. This latter decision is often tied to the issue of changes in type of practice or specialty type.[76] Although an important distinction, few analyses of physician location or migration have attempted to distinguish between physicians who have relocated and those who are locating practices for the first time.[77] Clearly, just as with FMGs, if different concerns motivate these two groups of physicians, specific policies to take advantage of them might be formulated. The works that have made this distinction have focused on the behavior of new physicians. These studies detail the effectiveness of programs that have been instituted during residency to alter the specialty and geographic distribution of physicians.

Sloan and Yett have performed several studies investigating the behavior of recent medical school graduates. Sloan has examined choice of specialty and practice mode, and Yett and Sloan have modeled spatial distribution.[78] Their findings suggest that earnings differentials do not account for the strong trends away from general practice in favor of careers in specialty medicine. Elasticities based on lifetime earnings coefficients for most specialties were near zero and, although there was a significant positive effect in some regression results, the effect of the income variable was always small. The number of FMGs in a specialty was significant in several estimates, but it always had a negative coefficient. In other words, medical students are attracted to those specialties that have higher relative lifetime incomes and fewer FMGs, but neither effect is very great. Indeed, the negative FMG coefficient may indicate that FMGs are allocated into residual categories, i.e., they fill up positions domestic medical graduates shun.

On choice of practice, Sloan's report[79] is descriptive, presenting the results of a survey of residents carried out by the *Hospital Physician*. Partnerships and groups were clearly preferred and even academic medicine was preferred to solo practice. Although practice mode decisions are made fairly late in the medical education process, the decision to engage in academic medicine seems to be made while the physician is still a medical student.

In an extensive investigation of a 1966 survey carried out by Medical Economics, Inc., Yett and Sloan[80] studied the effect of several variables on the spatial distribution of new physicians across states. Variables describing the following general factors were included: previous attachment to the state, income, population growth, barriers to entry (using licensure failure rate as a proxy), opportunities for professional development, general environmental conditions, and level of effort required to establish a satisfactory practice. Previous attachment to a state (through birth or attendance at a medical school, internship, or residency program) was found to be an attractive factor. Income levels and environmental conditions were significant, too. But the only action a state could take to increase its physician supply (besides attachment) that is predicted to have a strong effect is to lower the failure rate on licensure examinations.

Summary of the Planning Implications of Current Supply

The supply of physician manpower seems best explained by behavioral theories that emphasize decision-making by individual physicians in which the role of pecuniary incentives has diminished over time. Although fee-setting by physicians may involve profit-maximizing behavior, locational and specialty choices do not. Instead, professional and personal amenities and conveniences seem most important, with income security rather than income maximization gaining in importance. These findings suggest that physicians will be more, rather than less, ready to accept staff positions in institutional facilities and they will become more, rather than less, ready to accept paraprofessional substitution. Increasing concentration in group practice also indicates that there is an increasing readiness for the individual physician to relinquish some control over decision-making.

Policies that aim at reducing distributional inequities must build on these results if they are to succeed. Other policy effects that can be manipulated are the propensity of physicians to delay decisions until the time of residency and to emphasize life-style qualities in the locale they choose. Possible alternatives include programs to reduce the difficulty of entering practice in locales that are attempting to gain physicians, to reduce the differentials in insurance programs that pay "prevailing rates," to promote the social and organizational integration of FMGs, to attempt to motivate residents to choose certain areas, and to entice students from areas with few physicians to choose medicine as a career and to take training in their own state.

Concept of a Physician Shortage

In preceding sections we examined models of the demand for physicians and looked at physician supply. Here, we consider the following questions: Under what conditions does the interaction of supply and demand factors lead to a condition requiring government intervention? How is a physician shortage to be detected? Answering these questions will require a recapitulation of some of our earlier arguments. The six most important criteria for a physician shortage are as follows:

1 Professional standards: A shortage is said to exist if the number of physicians available at a given place and at a given time is inadequate to meet some professionally defined standard of medical care. We noted a number of methods that had been used to develop professional standards and argued that such measures were unlikely to help policymakers determine whether action should be initiated to change a situation. We also noted that in almost all areas, the amount of manpower available will be much less than that necessary to meet professionally defined standards, and that, by these definitions, shortages are perpetual.
2 Comparative ratios: A shortage is said to exist in all those states (or counties) with a physician/population ratio lower than the mean ratio across states (or counties), or with a physician/population ratio lower than that of the "best" areas—defined, for example, by the areas with the highest ratios. Since it is extremely unlikely that physicians will be uniformly distributed across regions, such a definition will always imply a shortage in some areas. As noted earlier, these ratios make no sense unless the numerator is full-time-equivalent physicians providing patient care, and the denominator is adjusted

for age, sex, and race. Consider, for example, a situation in which one county has a physician/population ratio of 75/100,000 and another has a physician/population ratio of 150/100,000. Assume that half the physicians in the latter county spend their time in teaching, research, and administration, and in staffing a hospital that provides specialty care to citizens of the entire state, while some of the remaining physicians are retired or treat patients living in other counties. If, in the former county, all physicians are engaged in full-time patient care, strict manpower ratios would grossly overestimate the differential availability of physician services.

These ratios suffer the same problems as the professional standards approach. There is little reason to believe that additional physician services would be used, no assurance that additional physician services would improve the health of the populace, and no reason to believe that additional physicians would choose to settle in "underserved" areas.

3 Demand/supply differential: A shortage is said to exist if, at current prices, the demand for medical care exceeds the supply of medical care. This is a strict economic definition of a shortage. Consider, for example, the market for rental apartments. An economist would argue that a well-functioning market would equate the quantity supplied to the quantity demanded (and determine an equilibrium price). If the demand for apartments suddenly expanded or some event curtailed the supply, the rental price might rise a great deal, but this would not be considered a shortage. According to this interpretation, a shortage is possible only if the market is not functioning. For instance, in the apartment rental example, if an apartment owner cannot or will not raise prices but customers want more apartments than the owner can supply, an economic shortage would be said to exist. However, from an economic viewpoint, this shortage is artificial and created by the constraint on price. As with rent control in New York City, the pernicious effects of keeping the market

from clearing include curtailing future supply, increased litigation, and immobility. When such constraints occur in the market for medical care, they give rise to economically defined shortages. In such situations, the rationing role played by price is replaced by nonmonetary rationing devices.

Constraints on the supply of physicians lead, in a well-functioning market for medical care, to a high price per patient visit and high incomes for physicians. If physicians cannot or will not raise prices then the market would tend to equilibrate (i.e., ration services among those demanding them) through the use of nonmarket rationing. In the delivery of physician services the most common rationing devices are: 1) service unavailability (physicians refuse to see a new patient); 2) long waits for service (a delay of several weeks for an appointment); 3) deterioration in the product or service itself (a long wait to see the physician once one arrives, a small amount of time with the physician, a less than thorough examination, and perhaps little effort by the physician to be reassuring and friendly); and 4) other increased difficulties in gaining access (such as a greater distance to travel, less convenient office hours, and a general way of putting more burden on the patient and having the service take more of the patient's time and effort).

Much current evidence indicates that such shortages for some kinds of physicians exist. The market for medical care is not well functioning, since numerous factors prevent price from playing a rationing role. Some institutions commit themselves to deliver care at zero price to the patient, but they do not hire the manpower necessary to deliver that care. Physicians traditionally take an oath not to deny care to those who cannot pay for it; Blue Shield and other review mechanisms often set an effective upper bound on the price that physicians can charge (to specified groups); the welfare associated with medical care tends to induce strong expectations in the physician and patient that the price of care be related to the ability of each individual patient to af-

ford it. Thus, high prices are not considered a socially acceptable way of rationing medical care. Nonetheless, price may have an important role to play as an incentive.

4 Rate of return: A related way of detecting a physician shortage is to determine whether there is a high rate of return to physicians at a given time or place. A high rate of return across regions could indicate that physicians were able to create an artificially high demand for their services or that supply constraints existed. The latter is a market signal to attract more people into medical professions. Thus one could determine the rate of return to physician education at different locations (or equivalently, look at physician incomes and education costs at different places). This technique is likely to yield evidence that is contrary to the assumption of a general shortage. In addition, urban areas, which have the highest physician/population ratios and, therefore, should have relatively low prices and low physician incomes, have the highest prices and highest (hourly) incomes.

5 Health levels: A more difficult (but more objective) way of determining the existence of a shortage involves surveying the health of a population. Correcting for age, race, sex, and income, such a survey would determine the rates of mortality, acute disease, chronic disease, disability, and bed days. If one assumes that medical care is a principal factor influencing health, this approach could be used to identify the need for more physicians.

An alternative to a health survey is based on the assumption that a shortage of physicians leads individuals to seek care only when they are very ill. If so, looking at the mortality rate and at the severity of patient presentations to physicians in an area would provide an estimate of the population's health status.

6 Community satisfaction: A final measure of shortage involves surveying a population to determine whether there is general satisfaction with local medical services. The level of satisfaction need have little correspondence to the physician/population ratio. If

the health status indices indicate a shortage of physicians, but people are satisfied with the level of service and there is no indication of nonmarket rationing, it would make little sense to provide additional service since it would go unused. Alternative policies are required in this instance to motivate the use of extant supply. Note that if nonmarket rationing is important, the provision of extra services would be reasonable and the services would probably be used (since non-market rationing is an indication that current demand exceeds current supply at current price).

Discussion

We have described six methods of determining whether a physician shortage exists. Professional standards and ratios have little to recommend them other than their simplicity; there is no guarantee that additional services would be used or, if they were, that they would be efficacious. Examining the existence of non-market rationing of physician services is relevant because of the many constraints that prevent price from equilibrating supply and demand. This approach has the virtue of indicating that at current prices people desire more medical services than are being supplied. A similar approach, although a more costly one, is to survey the population regarding the satisfaction with the medical care system. Clearly, the best approach is to survey the health status of a population and determine whether additional physicians would be efficacious. This approach, together with one indicating unsatisfied demand, would indicate not only that additional physicians would be used, but that the additional services would be efficacious.

Accuracy of Forecasts

The demand and supply models described earlier imply that there is a physician shortage. Even more important, they indicate that this shortage is likely to become worse over time. Analysts have forecast population, number of physicians, and the requirement for physicians. On the basis of forecasts that we are in the midst of a worsening shortage, it has been argued that government policies influencing the supply of physician services must be rethought and that new policies, such as expanding the number and size of medical schools, must be established. However, as indicated in the earlier sections, we do not accept the conclusions that derive from the models that have been used to estimate physician requirements or supply. In this section we detail why we lack confidence in these estimates. Table 5 presents selected forecasts that have been made in the past for population, physician supply, and physician requirements. The notes to the table spell out the assumptions underlying each forecast. The table shows the shortages that were expected and the actual population and physician levels.

In general, these results indicate that: 1) the population estimates covered a wide range, and the smallest estimate exceeded the actual population of the United States (and its outlying territories) in 1970; and 2) the estimates of physician supply covered a wide range with the highest estimate lower than the actual number of physicians existing in 1970. Clearly, forecasting is not a science and is subject to considerable error. The table indicates that forecasters should make their assumptions clear, and instead of generating a single estimate they should present a range of possibilities.

In Table 6, we present some estimates that have been made for 1975 (in the notes to the table, the assumptions underlying the projections are given). The projections, made in 1966, indicate that, once again, a large doctor shortage is expected.

The forecasts of both physician supplies and population are poor. By 1970, we had more physicians than were predicted by the Bane Committee Report for 1975. By 1971 (according to the AMA), there were 344,823 physicians. Little has changed in forecasting techniques and it is very likely that again all forecasts of physician supplies will be under-estimates.

It should also be noted that these forecasts do not take increases in productivity into account. If one assumed that physician productivity were to increase at 4 percent per year, the available "effective" supply in 1975 would be

Table 5. Projections from various sources of physician supplies and requirements for 1970*

Sources	Date of projection	Population (in thousands)	M.D.s and osteopaths (active and inactive)	M.D.s only	M.D.s and osteopaths	Difference
			Supply		**Requirement**	
A	1958	209,380		273,474	276,458 (b) (c)	2,984
				274,469 (b)	286,938 (d)	12,469
B	1959	213,810	294,900 (a)		299,000 (e)	4,100
			296,500 (f)			2,500
C	1959					
		213,810		279,000 (g)	283,000 (h)	
D	1960					
E	1964	214,570	327,900 (j)			
			324,900 (k)			
			319,900 (m)			
F	1966	212,683	335,000 (n)			
			340,000 (p)			
G	1966		306,954 (q)			
			326,915 (r)			
H	1966	208,576	332,700			
Actual	1970	207,976	348,300			

* This table is adapted from Butter, I. "Health Manpower Research: A Survey," *Inquiry* 4:5–41 (December 1967).
(a) Present production rate. (b) Increase graduates of U.S. schools. (c) Maintaining 1955 physician/population ratio. (d) Increase graduates sufficiently to maintain 1955 ratio of graduates to population. (e) To maintain 1959 ratio. (f) Recent growth rate. (g) Graduates at levels currently predicted. (h) Increase graduates to maintain 1957 ratio. (j) At current planned growth, increase graduates (1,600 foreign graduates licensed annually). (k) 1,000 foreign graduates annually. (m) No foreign graduates licensed after 1965. (n) Low estimates of U.S. graduates and new foreign unlicensed, stable new foreign licenciates. (p) High estimates of graduates and foreign unlicensed, stable new foreign licenciates. (q) Based on HMP growth in 1950–60, 4½ percent per year. (r) HMP growth rate, 5½ percent per year.
Sources:
A Perrott, G. S. and Pennell, M. Y. "Physicians in the United States: Projections 1955–1975," *Journal of Medical Education* 33:638–644 (September 1958).
B U.S. Surgeon General's Consultant Group on Medical Education. "Physicians for a Growing America," USPHS Publication 709, Washington, D.C., 1959.
C *Health Manpower Source Book*, Section 9, "Physicians, Dentists, Nurses," (Washington, D.C.: DHEW, Manpower Analysis Branch, 1959).
D Stewart, W. H. and Pennell, M. Y. "Health Manpower, 1930–75," *Public Health Reports* 75:274–280 (March 1960).
E *Health Manpower Source Book*, Section 18, "Manpower in the 1960's," (Washington, D.C.: DHEW, Manpower Analysis Branch, 1964).
F Ruhe, C. H. W. "Present Projections of Physician Production," *Journal of the American Medical Association* 198:168–174 (December 1966).
G Weiss, J. H. "The Changing Job Structure of Health Manpower," Ph.D. dissertation, Harvard University, Cambridge, July 1966.
H Fein, R. *The Doctor Shortage* (Washington, D.C.: The Brookings Institution, 1967).

about 390,000, and the projected deficit would disappear.

Concluding Comments

Government agencies have taken on the role of planning the delivery of health care and consequently find themselves confronted with defining "need." How many physicians, hospital beds, ancillary health personnel and other health facilities are needed in an area? What policies will serve to increase the supply of these health resources when they are needed? An earlier paper[81] examines this set of questions for hospitals, focusing on the financing of new facilities. This study attempted to answer these questions for physicians.

Based on the criteria in the literature discussed, there is contradictory evidence on the overall shortage of physicians. There are significant problems with maldistribution of phy-

Table 6.   Summary of physician projections for 1975*

Projection study	Requirements (I)	Supplies (II)	(−) Deficit (+) Surplus (III)
Bane Committee Report[1]	30,000 (minimum)	(i) 312,800	−17,200
		(ii) 318,400	−11,600
Fein[2]	(i) 340,000 to 350,000	361,700	+21,700 to +11,700
	(ii) 372,000 to 385,000		−10,300 to −23,300
U.S. National Advisory Commission on Health Manpower[3]	(i) 346,000 (minimum)	360,000	+14,000
U.S. Bureau of Labor Statistics[4]	390,000	360,000	−30,000
U.S. Public Health Service[5]	(i) 400,000	360,000	−40,000
	(ii) 425,000		−65,000

* This table is taken from Hansen, W. L. "An Appraisal of Physician Manpower Projections," *Inquiry* 7: 102–113 (March 1970).

Notes: Physicians include both M.D.s and D.O.s, except for Line 2, which excludes D.O.s. Column III equals column II minus Column I.

Sources:

[1] U.S. Surgeon General's Consultant Group on Medical Education. "Physicians for a Growing America," USPHS Publication 709, Washington, D. C., 1959.
Column (I) Table 2, p. 3.
Column (II) Table 2, p. 3.
Column (III) Calculated.
Requirements based on assumption that 1959 represents minimum rates to maintain health of population. Supply: Continuation of physician growth rate.

[2] Fein, R. *The Doctor Shortage* (Washington, D.C.: The Brookings Institution, 1967).
Column (I) (i) Based on 12–15 percent increase due to population growth above.
(ii) Based on 22–26 percent increase due to all factors. See pp. 134–135.
Column (II) Table III-9, p. 87.
Column (III) Calculated.
Requirements based on the demand for physician services at 1965 prices given anticipated changes in population composition expected by 1975. (i) shows estimated effect only accounting for population change; (ii) shows the effect of a whole range of factors.
Supply takes into account expected increase in medical school graduates as well as the immigration of foreign trained physicians.

[3] U.S. National Advisory Commission on Health Manpower. *Report*, Vol. 1 (Washington, D.C.: GPO, 1967).
Column (I) (i) Based on 13.5 percent increase in total visits by 1975. See p. 243.
Column (II) Table 4, p. 235.
Column (III) Calculated.
Methodology for determining requirements and supply similar to Fein.

[4] U.S. Bureau of Labor Statistics. *Health Manpower 1966–1975, A Study of Requirements and Supply* (Washington, D.C.: GPO, 1967).
Column (I) Page 18.
Column (II) No figure is given. We assume National Advisory Commission on Health Manpower Supply figure of 360,000 is appropriate to use.
Column (III) Calculated.
Requirements taken into consideration: population changes, increased demand for services across all age groups and need for an expansion of physicians engaged in research.

[5] U.S. Public Health Service, "Health Manpower Perspective: 1967," USPHS Publication 1667, Washington, D.C., 1967.
Column (I) (i) and (ii), Table 8, p. 15, and accompanying text.
Column (II) Same as Column II, line 4.
Column (III) Calculated.
Requirements: (i) is based on the application of "professional standards"; namely, the utilization rate for members of prepayment group practice plans to the entire 1975 population; and estimate (ii) applies the highest physician utilization rate among the four major regions of the United States to the entire 1975 population.

sicians, both by geographic area and by specialty. No simple policies to equalize the distribution of physicians are likely to be successful. However, it is not reasonable to assume that an area has a physician shortage just because some other area has a higher physician/population ratio. Instead, one must gather evidence of non-price rationing or of unsatisfactory health indices (mortality ratio, morbidity ratio, or disability days).

Although the overall number of physicians does not seem to warrant changes in govern-ment policy, locational problems are important. The research has implications for determining whether an area is underserved and what might be done to increase the supply of physicians. A major unsolved problem is the provision of services to rural areas distant from major cities.

In view of past attempts to solve medical care delivery problems by intervention, we would caution that good intentions are not enough. If funds are not to be wasted or to have a pernicious effect, careful data collection and analysis are necessary.

References and Notes

1 Berg, R. L. *Health Status Indexes* (Chicago: Hospital Research and Educational Trust, 1973).

2 See: Auster, R.; Leveson, I.; and Sarachek, D. "The Production of Health: An Exploratory Study," *The Journal of Human Resources* 4:411–436 (Fall 1969); and Stewart, C. T. Jr. "Allocation of Resources to Health," *The Journal of Human Resources* 6:101–122 (Winter 1971).

3 See: Lave, J. R.; Lave, L. B.; and Morton, T. E. "Paramedics: A Survey of the Issues," in: Stein, B. and Miller, S. M. (eds.) *Incentives and Planning in Social Policy* (Chicago: Aldine Publishing Co., 1973) and "The Physician's Assistant—Exploration of the Concept," *Hospitals* 45:42–51 (June 1, 1971). Also see: Sadler, A. M.; Sadler, B. L.; and Bliss, A. A. *The Physician's Assistant Today and Tomorrow* (New Haven: Yale University Press, 1972).

4 Jeffers, J. R.; Bognanno, M. F.; and Bartlett, J. C. "On the Demand versus Need for Medical Services and the Concept of 'Shortage'," *American Journal of Public Health* 61:46–63, Part 1 (January 1971).

5 Hiestand, D. L. "Research Into Manpower for Health Service," *Milbank Memorial Fund Quarterly* 44:146–179, Part 2 (October 1966).

6 Lee, R. I. and Jones, L. W. *The Fundamentals of Good Medical Care* (Chicago: University of Chicago Press, 1933).

7 Lee and Jones were aware of the difference between need and demand. They noted that people were not aware of the need for preventive care. In addition, they pointed to the fact that there was a wide distribution in the physician/population ratios across the states and emphasized that if the supply of physicians were increased the new doctors would probably locate in doctor "surplus" areas. They stressed the need for education and for changes in in the way medical care was financed and organized.

8 Schonfeld, H.; Heston, J.; and Falk, I. "Numbers of Physicians Required for Primary Medical Care," *The New England Journal of Medicine* 286:571–576 (March 16, 1972).

9 See: Lave, Lave, and Morton, "Paramedics," *op. cit.*, and "The Physician's Assistant," *op. cit.*

10 Huebscher, J. "Letter to the Editor," *The New England Journal of Medicine* 286:1164 (May 25, 1972).

11 Somers, A. R. *The Kaiser-Permanente Medical Care Program* (New York, The Commonwealth Fund, 1971).

12 Jacobs, G. "Letter to the Editor," *The New England Journal of Medicine* 286:1164 (May 25, 1972).

13 Other studies following the Lee and Jones method have been reported. Daitz [Daitz, B. D. "The Challenge of Disability," *American Journal of Public Health* 55:528–534 (April 1964)] proceeds by estimating that 74 million people had a chronic condition in 1960; of those, 10 million people had an incipient or manifest functional impairment associated with chronic disease, injury or congenital defects that require medical care to prevent further deterioration of functional capacity or to restore functional capacity. He then assumes that each of these 10 million people requires a minimum of 40 hours of professional care services per year, of which five should be physician time. This leads to an estimated need of 25,000 physicians to care for chronically ill patients. Knowles [Knowles, J. H. "The Quantity and Quality of Medical Manpower: A Review of Medicine's Current Efforts," *Journal of Medical Education* 44:81–118 (February 1969)] reports on responses he received from letters sent to the executive secretaries of the various specialty boards to determine what they thought the manpower needs were in their respective specialty. One executive secretary assumed that there would be one operation per 13 people per year and that the annual caseload of an anesthesiologist could be 800; he estimated that 37,000 anesthesiologists were needed. There are only 7,011 in practice. The estimate of needed anesthesiologists is based on what seems to be a small caseload (about four operations per day for a 200 day work year), and it neglects the fact that many anesthetics are given by nurse anesthetists. In addition, since Americans have many more operations (per person per year) than Western Europeans (or even Americans enrolled in prepaid group practices),

one may also want to question the assumed rate of surgical procedures.

14 Williams, G. *Kaiser-Permanente Health Plan—Why it Works* (Oakland, California: Henry J. Kaiser Foundation, 1971).

15 Riddick, F. A.; Bryan, J. B.; Gershenson, M. I.; and Costello, A. C. "Use of Allied Health Professionals in Internists' Offices," *Archives of Internal Medicine* 127:924–931 (May 1971).

16 Klarman, H. E. "Economic Aspects of Projecting Requirements for Health Manpower," *The Journal of Human Resources* 4:360–376 (1969).

17 See: Acton, J. P. "Demand for Health Care Among the Urban Poor with Special Emphasis on the Role of Time," (New York: The Rand Corporation, April 1973); and Richardson, W. C. "Ambulatory Use of Physicians' Services in Response to Illness Episodes in a Low Income Neighborhood," Center for Health Administration Studies Research Series 29 (Chicago: University of Chicago Press, 1971).

18 Marshall, C. L.; Hassanein, K. M.; Hassanein, R. S.; and Paul, C. L. "Time and Distance—Rural Practice: Dissatisfaction with Travel Distance to the Physician in a Rural Area," *Journal of the Kansas Medical Society* 70:93–96 (March 1969).

19 Weiss, J. E. and Greenlick, M. R. "Determinants of Medical Care Utilization: The Effect of Social Class and Distance on Contacts with the Medical Care System," *Medical Care* 8:456–462 (November–December 1970).

20 Lave, J. R. and Leinhardt, S. "The Delivery of Ambulatory Care to the Poor: A Literature Review," *Management Science* 19:78–99, Part 2 (December 1972).

21 Shannon, G. W.; Bashshur, R. L.; and Metzner, C. A. "The Concept of Distance as a Factor in Accessibility and Utilization of Health Care," *Medical Care Review* 26:143–161 (1969).

22 See: Grossman, M. "The Demand for Health: A Theoretical and Empirical Investigation," Occasional Paper 119 (New York: National Bureau of Economic Research, 1972) and "On the Concept of Health Capital and the Demand for Health," *Journal of Political Economy* 80:223–255 (March–April 1972).

23 The ratio model that projects current utilization ratios into the future, keeping them constant for each socioeconomic demographic group [an approach explored by: Fein, R. *The Doctor Shortage.* (Washington, D.C.: The Brookings Institution, 1967)] is a variant of this approach.

24 Newhouse, J. P. and Phelps, C. E. "Price and Income Elasticities for Medical Care Services," (Santa Monica: The Rand Corporation, R-1197-NC, 1972).

25 Fuchs, V. R. and Kramer, M. J. *Determinants of Expenditures for Physicians' Services in the United States 1948–1968*, DHEW Publication No. (HSM) 73-3013 (DHEW, HSMHA, December 1972).

26 See: Acton, J. P. "Demand for Health Care When Time Prices Vary More than Money Prices," (New York: The Rand Corporation, May 1973) and "Demand for Health Care Among the Urban Poor," *op. cit.* Also see: Weiss, J. E.; Greenlick, M. R.; and Jones, J. F. "Determinants of Medical Care Utilization: The Impact of Spatial Factors," *Inquiry*

8:50–57 (December 1971); and Richardson, "Ambulatory Use of Physicians' Services," *op. cit.*

27 See: Ginzberg, E. *Urban Health Services* (New York: Columbia University Press, 1971); Fuchs and Kramer, *Determinants of Expenditures for Physicians' Services, op. cit.*; Evans, R. G. "Supplier Induced Demand: Some Empirical Evidence and Implications," paper prepared for the International Economic Association Tokyo Conference on Economics of Health and Medical Care, April 1973; and Stevens, C. M. and Brown, G. D. "Market Structure Approach to Health-Manpower 'Planning'," *American Journal of Public Health* 61:1988–1995 (October 1971).

28 Fuchs and Kramer, *op. cit.*

29 Ginzberg, E. *Men, Money and Medicine* (New York: Columbia University Press, 1969).

30 Evans, R. G. "Supplier Induced Demand," *op. cit.*

31 See the following works of Feldstein, M. S. "An Aggregate Planning Model of the Health Care Sector," in: Paelink, J. (ed.) *Programming for Europe's Collective Needs* (Amsterdam: North Holland Publishing Co., 1970); "An Econometric Model of the Medicare System," *The Quarterly Journal of Economics* 85:1–20 (February 1971) and "Hospital Cost Inflation: A Study of Nonprofit Price Dynamics," *American Economic Review* 61:853–872 (December 1971).

32 See the following works of: Yett, D. E.; Drabek, L.; Kimbell, L.; and Intriligator, M. "The Development of a Micro-Simulation Model of Health Manpower Supply and Demand," in: *Proceedings and Report of Conference on a Health Manpower Simulation Model* (Washington, D.C.: U.S. Public Health Service, Bureau of Health Manpower Education, December 1970); "A Macroeconometric Model for Regional Health Planning," *Economic and Business Bulletin* 24: 1–21 (Fall 1971) and "Health Manpower Planning: An Econometric Approach," *Health Services Research* 7:134–147 (Summer 1972).

33 Lave, J. R.; Lave, L. B.; and Leinhardt, S. "A Model of Medical Care Delivery," in: Perlman, M. (ed.) *The Economics of Health and Medical Care* (London: The Macmillan Co., 1974).

34 Lee and Jones, *The Fundamentals of Good Medical Care, op. cit.*

35 Fein, *The Doctor Shortage, op. cit.*

36 DeVise, P. "Physician Migration from Inland to Coastal States: Antipodal Examples of Illinois and California," *Journal of Medical Education* 48:141–151 (February 1973).

37 Fahs, I. J.; Ingalls, K.; and Miller, W. R. "Physician Migration: A Problem in the Upper Midwest," *Journal of Medical Education* 43:735–740 (1968).

38 Rimlinger, G. V. and Steele, H. B. "An Economic Interpretation of the Spatial Distribution of Physicians in the U.S.," *The Southern Economic Journal* 30:1–12 (July 1963).

39 Lankford, P. M. "Physician Location Factors and Public Policy," *Economic Geography* 244–255 (July 1974).

40 Fuchs and Kramer, *Determinants of Expenditures for Physicians' Services, op. cit.*

41 See: Cooper, J. K.; Heald, K.; and Samuels, M. "The Decision for Rural Practice," *Journal of Medical Education* 47:939–944 (December 1972). A

more recent analysis is found in: Cooper, J. K.; Heald, K.; Samuels, M.; and Coleman, S. "Rural or Urban Practice: Factors Influencing the Location Decision of Primary Care Physicians," *Inquiry* 12: 18–25 (March 1975).

42 See: Stine, O. C. "Changes in the Supply of Physicians Giving Office Medical Care to Children," *Maryland State Medical Journal* 17:66–69 (January 1968) and "The Number of Children and the Supply of Physicians in Maryland Since 1940," *Maryland State Medical Journal* 19:51–55 (June 1970); Reas, H. W. "The Distribution of Physicians in Northwestern Ohio: 30 Years' Trends," *The Ohio State Medical Journal* 68:524–527 (June 1972); MacQueen, J. C. "A Study of Iowa Medical Physicians," *Journal of the Iowa Medical Society* 58:1129–1135 (November 1968); Baker, A. S.; Bishop, F. M.; Hassinger, E. W.; and Hobbs, D. J. "Distribution of Health Services in Missouri," *Missouri Medicine* 64: 925–926, 929 (November 1967); Martin, E. D.; Moffat, R. E.; Falter, R. T.; and Walker, J. D. "Where Graduates Go," *The Journal of the Kansas Medical Society* 69:84–89 (March 1968); Royce, P. C. "Can Rural Health Education Centers Influence Physician Distribution?" *Journal of the American Medical Association* 220:847–849 (May 1972); and Matthews, H. A. "The State of Franklin: A Physician Opinion Survey," *North Carolina Medical Journal* 32:242–246 (June 1971).

43 Yett, D. E. and Sloan, F. A. "Migration Patterns of Recent Medical School Graduates," *Inquiry* 11: 125–142 (June 1974).

44 Parker, R. C.; Rix, R. A.; and Tuxill, T. G. "Social, Economic and Demographic Factors Affecting Physician Population in Upstate New York," *New York State Journal of Medicine* 69:706–712 (March 1969).

45 Fuchs and Kramer, *Determinants of Expenditures for Physicians' Services, op. cit.*

46 Lave, J. R. and Lave, L. B. "The Hospital Construction Act: An Evaluation of the Hill-Burton Program, 1948–1973," (Washington, D.C.: American Enterprise Institute for Public Policy Research, 1974).

47 Steele, H. B. and Rimlinger, G. V. "Income Opportunities and Physician Location Trends in the United States," *Western Economic Journal* 3:182–194 (Spring 1965).

48 Marden, P. G. "A Demographic and Ecological Analysis of the Distribution of Physicians in Metropolitan America, 1960," *American Journal of Sociology* 72:290–300 (1966).

49 Joroff, S. and Navarro, V. "Medical Manpower: A Multivariate Analysis of the Distribution of Physicians in Urban United States," *Medical Care* 9:428–438 (September–October 1971).

50 Lankford, "Physician Location Factors," *op. cit.*

51 Weiss, J. E. "The Effect of Medical Centers on the Distribution of Physicians in the U.S.," Ph.D. dissertation, University of Michigan, Ann Arbor, 1968.

52 Sloan, F. "Economic Models of Physician Supply," Ph.D. dissertation, Harvard University, Cambridge, 1968.

53 Benham, L.; Maurizi, A.; and Reder, M. W. "Migration, Location, and Remuneration of Medical Personnel: Physicians and Dentists," *Review of Economics and Statistics* 50:332–341 (August 1968).

54 See: Marshall, C. L.; Hassanein, K. M.; Hassanein, R. S.; and Marshall, C. L. "Principal Components Analysis of the Distribution of Physicians, Dentists and Osteopaths in a Midwestern State," *American Journal of Public Health* 61:1556–1564 (August 1971); and Terris, M. and Monk, M. A. "Recent Trends in the Distribution of Physicians in Upstate New York," *American Journal of Public Health* 46: 585–591 (May 1956).

55 Sloan, F. A.; Cleckner, J. E.; and Wayne, J. B. "Non-Price Rationing of Physicians' Services," University of Florida, Gainesville, September 1973.

56 Parker, R. C., *et al.*, "Social, Economic and Demographic Factors," *op. cit.*

57 Nonetheless, Steinwald and Sloan (Steinwald, B. and Sloan, F. A. "Determinants of Physicians' Fees," American Medical Association, Chicago, and University of Florida, Gainesville, July 1973) argue that income is still important since a profit-maximizing model of physician fee-setting dominates alternative models. But this conclusion does not conflict with individual location choice based on non-income considerations.

58 Shannon, G. W., *et al.*, "The Concept of Distance," *op. cit.*

59 See the following: Kaplan, R. S. and Leinhardt, S. "Determinants of Physician Office Location," *Medical Care* 11:406–415 (September–October 1973); McMillan, A. W.; Gornick, M. E.; Rogers, R. R.; and Gorten, M. K. "Assessing the Balance of Physician Manpower in a Metropolitan Area," *Public Health Reports* 85:1001–1011 (November 1970); Fine, E. M. "Urban Health Challenge: Survey of Physician Manpower in Metropolitan Baltimore," *Maryland State Medical Journal* 20:67–71 (October 1971); and Terris and Monk, "Recent Trends in the Distribution of Physicians," *op. cit.*

60 Lepper, M. H.; Lashof, J. C.; Lerner, M.; German, J.; and Andelman, S. L. "Approaches to Meeting Health Needs of Large Poverty Populations," *American Journal of Public Health* 57:1153–1157, Part 2 (July 1967).

61 See: Rees, P. H. "Movement and Distribution of Physicians in Metropolitan Chicago," Chicago Regional Hospital Study, Working Paper I.12, June 1967, and "Numbers and Movement of Physicians in Southeast Chicago: 1953–1965," Chicago Regional Hospital Study, Working Paper I.13, July 1967; De Vise, P. and Dewey, D. "More Money, More Doctors, Less Care," Chicago Regional Hospital Study, Working Paper I.19, March 1972; and Dewey, D. "Where the Doctors Have Gone," Illinois Regional Medical Program, Chicago Regional Hospital Study, Research Paper, 1973.

62 Elesh, D. and Schollaert, P. T. "Race and Urban Medicine: Factors Affecting the Distribution of Physicians in Chicago," *Journal of Health and Social Behavior* 13:236–250 (September 1972).

63 May, L. A. "The Spatial Distribution of Physicians —The Special Case of the City," B.A. Honors Thesis, Harvard University, Cambridge, March 1970.

64 Piore, N. and Sokal, S. "A Profile of Physicians in the City of New York Before Medicare and Medicaid," (New York: Urban Research Center, 1968).

65 Roemer, M. I. "Health Resources and Services in

the Watts Area of Los Angeles," *California's Health* 23:123–143 (February–March 1966).

66 Lave, J. R. and Leinhardt, "The Delivery of Ambulatory Care to the Poor," *op. cit.*

67 See the following: Dorsey, J. L. "Physician Distribution in Boston and Brookline, 1940 and 1961," *Medical Care* 7:429–440 (November–December 1969); Robertson, L. S. "On the Intraurban Ecology of Primary Care Physicians," *Social Science and Medicine* 4:227–238 (1970); and Hambleton, J. W. "Determinants of Geographical Differences in the Supply of Physician Services," Ph.D. dissertation, University of Wisconsin, Madison, 1971.

68 Coleman, J. E. "The Mathematical Study of Change," in: Blalock, H. M. Jr. and Blalock, A. B. (eds.) *Methodology in Social Research* (New York: McGraw-Hill, 1968) pp. 428–478.

69 Hambleton, J. W. "Determinants of Geographical Differences in the Supply of Physician Services," *op. cit.*

70 Kaplan and Leinhardt, "Determinants of Physician Office Location," *op. cit.*

71 Dublin, T. D. "The Migration of Physicians to the United States," *The New England Journal of Medicine* 286:870–877 (April 1972).

72 Bowers, J. Z. and Rosenheim, L. "Migration of Medical Manpower," *Journal of the American Medical Association* 214:2039 (December 1970).

73 Marguiles, H. and Bloch, L. S. *Foreign Medical Graduates in the United States* (Cambridge: Harvard University Press, 1969).

74 Butter, I. and Schaffner, R. "Foreign Medical Graduates and Equal Access to Medical Care," *Medical Care* 9:136–141 (March–April 1971).

75 Schaffner, R. and Butter, I. "Geographic Mobility of Foreign Medical Graduates and the Doctor Shortage: A Longitudinal Analysis," *Inquiry* 9:24–32 (March 1972).

76 Crawford, R. L. and McCormack, R. C. "Reasons Physicians Leave Primary Practice," *Journal of Medical Education* 46:263–268 (April 1971).

77 Although there are several surveys of medical school graduates [Martin, *et al.*, "Where Graduates Go," *op. cit.*, and Weiskotten, H. G.; Wiggins, W. S.; Altenderfer, M. E.; Gooch, M.; and Tipner, A. "Trends in Medical Practice. An Analysis of the Distribution and Characteristics of Medical College Graduates, 1915–1950," *The Journal of Medical Education* 35:1071–1121 (December 1960)], these are usually descriptive studies of the current character of various past graduating classes. They typically fail to distinguish initial from subsequent decisions or to look closely at the behavior of recent graduates.

78 See: Sloan, F. A. "Lifetime Earnings and Physicians' Choice of Specialty," *Industrial and Labor Relations Review* 24:47–56 (1970) and "Supply Responses of Young Physicians: An Analysis of Physicians in Residency Programs," (Santa Monica: The Rand Corporation, R-1131-OEO, March 1973); and Yett and Sloan, "Migration Patterns," *op. cit.*

79 Sloan, "Supply Responses of Young Physicians," *op. cit.*

80 Yett and Sloan, "Migration Patterns," *op. cit.*

81 Lave and Lave, *The Hospital Construction Act, op. cit.*

Robert Williams

Reprinted with permission of the Blue Cross Association, from *Inquiry*, Vol.III, No.3, pp.28-42. Copyright © 1966 by the Blue Cross Association.

A Comparison of Hospital Utilization and Costs by Types of Coverage

Originally Published in September 1966

The following study examines the relationship of full pay, deductible, and co-pay coverage to utilization and costs in five Blue Cross plans. In each of these Plans full pay plus one of the other forms of coverage were offered so it was possible to compare hospital usage and costs between members under different coverages within a single, homogeneous Plan. The findings indicate that coverage alone is not solely responsible for the observed differences and the omission of one-day cases might have a strong effect on admission rates and average lengths of stay. The summary makes recommendations for the design of further studies in this area.

A widely held practice among prepayment agencies is to offer hospital cost coverage under a variety of payment schedules. The most common forms of these schedules are full payment, deductible, coinsurance, co-payment, and indemnity. One assumption behind these various types of schedules is that different forms of coverage payment, like different degrees of coverage, yield specific patterns of hospital utilization and costs. Another aim of various payment schedules is to keep the monthly scope of covered services within a specific dollar range. The purpose of this study was to analyze and interpret findings on hospital utilization and benefits paid in several Blue Cross Plans as

Robert Williams is Research Assistant, Division of Research and Planning, Blue Cross Association.

they related to various payment schedules.

Before reviewing the research already accomplished in this area it seems relevant to describe the schedules under consideration as they are applied to Blue Cross. Full payment, possibly the most common form of hospital prepayment coverage, provides full payment for all services and/or care received by the subscriber (and his dependents) which are covered under his contract with Blue Cross. This means that benefits specified in the contract (or not specifically excluded) are paid for by the covering Plan.

Deductible payments are specific dollar amounts payable by the subscriber (or dependent) upon each hospital admission or on a yearly basis for all admissions. Blue Cross is responsible only for expenses in excess of the deductible amount paid by the subscriber and which are covered by his contract. If, for example, the deductible payment was $25 per admission the Plan would pay only for those covered benefits costing more than the first $25.

Under coinsurance payment the Plan pays a specific percentage of the total hospital bill covered by the contract while the subscriber pays the rest. Unlike deductible coverage, coinsurance is not a fixed amount but varies with the size of the total covered bill.

Co-payment requires the subscriber to pay a fixed dollar amount per day of hospital stay. Just as the amount paid by the coinsured subscriber varies with the size of his hospital bill, so the amount paid by those with co-pay coverage varies with the length of hospital stay.

Indemnity payment coverage fixes the maximum amount of the covered bill that a Plan must pay. The rest is paid by the subscriber. The maximum paid by the Plan is not a percentage of the covered bill but a specific dollar allowance. None of the Plans used in this study had a complete indemnity contract, but several applied indemnities to specific items such as X-rays and room allowances.

PREVIOUS STUDIES

Of the payment schedules described here, all but full pay coverage involve some amount of personal expense to the subscriber in addition to his regular monthly (or quarterly) coverage costs each time he goes to the hospital. It is such personal expenses that are assumed to exercise some control over hospital utilization and Plan costs for coverage of such use. Many believe that if an individual has to pay more than a token amount for each hospital admission or day of stay he will be less likely to use his hospital coverage unnecessarily. This restrained usage should produce lower utilization by the subscriber and lower coverage cost for the Plan. Although this is an apparently popular belief, few studies have appeared in the literature on it, and what has appeared has frequently been contradictory and inconclusive. Statements supporting deductible forms of hospital coverage focus their assumed controlling effects on admission rates:

> "We have found when local operating personnel realize the first dollar of a loss is not going to be paid by the insurance company but by them, they increase their efforts to avoid losses."[1]

[1] *The National Underwriter*, No. 28 (July 12, 1963), p. 2.

Diokno,[2] in surveying 65 insurance companies found only six which definitely felt that neither deductibles nor coinsurance were effective utilization controls. Over half the opinions favored one or the other form of personal expenses as a control on hospital use and costs. As Diokno pointed out:

> ". . . the deductible clause was designed for a two-fold purpose: 1. To eliminate small claims which the insured can meet from his regular income without undue hardship [since] the handling of such small claims results in disproportionately high costs which made the insurance expensive and inefficient. 2. To curb abuse and make the insured more prevention conscious."[3]

Diokno was cautious about his recommendations on the use of deductibles and coinsurance. He felt that their value had been shown in limiting utilization but feared their indiscriminate application might affect " . . . needed utilization. as well as that which represents inappropriate use of services and facilities."[4]

This last point raises an important question about the effect of deductibles and coinsurance on *needed* care. While it may be a correct assumption that these types of clauses eliminate utilization abuses, they may also inhibit individuals from seeking needed care. *The Report of the State of Maryland Commission to Study Hospital Cost* made the following point:

> "Those who argue against it believe that the 'deductible' merely shifts the cost of illness out of the insurance premium paid by the policyholder in the form of payment at time of sickness; hence, while it

[2] A. W. Diokno, "Studies on Prepayment and Insurance" in Walter J. McNerney *et al.*, *Hospital and Medical Economics* (Chicago: Hospital Research and Educational Trust, 1962).
[3] *Ibid.*, p. 1093.
[4] *Ibid.*, p. 1112.

offers an illusory lower premium rate it does not lower cost to him of the care needed. To the claim that less medical care is demanded, they reply that denial of needed care is not a satisfactory answer."[5]

The report stated also that deductible clauses would have little effect on inpatient utilization charges since only a very small proportion of these charges were under even $50 (a moderately high deductible charge).

Reginald Dabney of the Maryland Hospital Service (Blue Cross) contributed to the report by pointing out that deductible coverage is usually held by younger, "good risk" people while full pay coverage is taken by older, "poor risk" individuals. He also felt that even a deductible of $75 would not have any appreciable effect on hospital admission rates and total utilization.[6]

Dabney's conclusions were supported by the findings of a study conducted by the Columbia University School of Public Health and Administrative Medicine.[7] These investigators found that there were essentially no major differences between three representative types of health coverage. Admission rates, patient-days, and average length of stay—three of the most common measures of hospital utilization—were found to be about the same for deductible, full pay, and group practice coverage, indicating that the type of coverage had little bearing on hospital utilization.

While the Columbia study found no major differences between types of hospital coverage offered by three *different*

programs, Ackart did discover at least one difference within a *single* Blue Cross Plan offering both deductible and full payment coverage to a homogeneous population.[8] His major finding was in the area of admission rates where he showed that individuals who paid $50 for each hospital admission had a rate 6.7 percent *lower* than that of those who had full pay coverage. Of course part of this difference might have been due to the fact that admissions with deductible coverage whose hospital charges were $50 or under (one-day stays) were, from the point of view of the Plan data, never recorded as being admitted to the hospital at all. No bill would have been sent to the Plan. This fact should be kept in mind when examining data on deductible covered people as reported by Blue Cross Plans—lower admission rates for this group in part reflect the absence of one-day stays as well as a lower rate of entering the hospital. This is especially true where the deductible is large ($50 or more). Co-insurance and co-payment coverage admission rates are not affected by such selective recording.

The absence of some one-day stays for deductible covered cases in the Ackart data possibly accounts for the difference between the lengths of stay for deductible and full pay members. The average length of stay for the deductible covered cases was 0.07 of a day longer than that for full pays. If, in fact, some one-day stays were not counted in the deductible population and were counted in the full pay, this might account for the difference, rather than because deductible cases really stayed longer than full pay cases.

CHARACTERISTICS AND SCOPE OF THIS STUDY

From the foregoing it is apparent that the research literature is rather

---

[5] *Report of the State of Maryland Commission to Study Hospital Costs* (Baltimore, 1964), p. 92.

[6] *Ibid.*, pp. 93-4.

[7] Josephine J. Williams *et al.*, "Family Medical Care under Three Types of Health Insurance" (New York: The Foundation, 1962). This is a report on a survey conducted for The Foundation on Employee Health, Medical Care, and Welfare, Inc. by the School of Public Health and Administrative Medicine, Columbia University, with the cooperation of the National Opinion Research Center of the University of Chicago.

[8] R. J. Ackart, "Deductibles and Co-insurance," *Virginia Medical Monthly*, Vol. 88 (July, 1961), pp. 276-277.

sparse and often not comparable in its data on utilization and costs of hospital care by type of payment coverage. While the present study is by no means conclusive, it is felt that the data presented here will contribute to the increasing knowledge of hospital coverage payment in at least two respects: this study used a large population, and it compared several types of payment coverage within geographically homogeneous Blue Cross Plans.

Analyses were made in terms of payment coverage and the age and sex of the utilizing members. Information about diagnoses, socio-economic levels of the membership, and other demographic characteristics were not included in the original data and therefore could not be included in the analysis. Intra-Plan data were assumed to be at least geographically homogeneous but no division between urban and rural membership could be made. Payment coverage was matched as far as possible by the number of days of coverage per admission and the benefits available.

Description of the Sample and Procedures Used

The data used in this study were taken from a survey of Blue Cross Plans made in 1964. This survey included information on Plan enrollment and utilization by age and sex of the membership. The current study is one of several planned involving these data.

Five Blue Cross Plans distributed across the United States which submitted data complete with appropriate age-and sex breaks for their membership, as well as comparable information on enrollment and utilization, were selected for the present study. Some Plans with less than complete data in some areas were used because they offered particular kinds of coverage, such as co-payment, which were rarely found on major certificates. Only data from the first most widely held and most comprehensive certificates were used, as they generally included two distinct forms of coverage and/or encompassed the majority of the Plan membership. (In some Plans the second most widely held certificate was frequently the Plan's most comprehensive certificate and vice versa.)

The Plans studied gave from 30 to 150 days of coverage per admission. Deductible charges, when present, ranged from $20 to $25 per hospital admission. Plans offering co-payment coverage paid all of the daily covered bill in excess of $4.

Data were obtained for group enrollment and inpatient utilization only. The measures of utilization were admissions per 1,000 members, average length of stay, patient-days per 1,000 members, benefits per day, and benefits per admission. The term "benefits" refers to the amount of money paid by a Plan on the covered portion of the total hospital bill. Only paid claims data for such care were reported by the Plans, thus only their portion of the actual hospital bill was known. Benefits per day and per admission should not, therefore, be construed as representing an actual total average cost for care but only the expenses borne by the Plans.

Whenever possible, utilization data were adjusted for differences in the age and sex composition of the membership between Plans and different coverage classes. This was done by redistributing Plan enrollment according to the age and sex distribution of the total United States population as of July, 1964. When utilization figures were recomputed according to this age-sex adjustment, they were referred to as "adjusted" utilization. Raw utilization figures were called "unadjusted." The advantage of using age-sex adjusted utilization figures was to equalize the age and sex distributions between Plans and categories. Once this was done, observed differences were not merely reflective of utilization trends correlated with peculiar age and sex distributions.

FINDINGS

The findings of the present study are presented according to the various measures of utilization and by coverage classification. Since most of the data were adjusted for age and sex distributions, little attention was given to detailing age and sex trends in utilization. In general, these trends followed typical utilization patterns.

Admissions per 1,000 Members

Data were obtained from three Plans that offered both full pay and deductible inpatient group coverage. The adjusted average admission rates for both full pay and deductible covered members are shown in Table 1.

TABLE 1

Admission Rates per 1,000 Members in Plans Offering Both Full Pay and Deductible Coverage for Inpatient Group Services

	Adjusted		
Plan	Full	Ded.	Percent Difference
A	195	171	−12.3
B	184	169	− 8.2
C	116	137	18.1

The most noteworthy characteristic about Table 1 is that all members with deductible coverage had *lower* admission rates than members in the same Plan with full pay coverage, except for Plan C. In Plan C the opposite relation between full pay and deductible admission was observed. This apparent contradiction to both hypotheses and observations of similar Plans resulted from the fact that Plan C, unlike the other Plans offering both full pay and deductible coverage, did *not* offer the same benefits on both certificates. The deductible certificate gave more generous room allowances as well as additional services not available under full pay coverage. The additional benefits seemed to outweigh the necessary deductible cost for each admission.

Of the two Plans, D and E, offering both co-pay and full payment hospital coverage, Plan D provided very complete data. Plan E provided analysis of membership by sex but not by age. Plan D had an adjusted average co-pay admission rate of 136 per 1,000 members while the adjusted rate for full pay covered members was 156 admissions per 1,000. As in Plans offering deductible and full pay coverage, this Plan showed a higher rate of admissions by members with full pay coverage than it did for those with co-pay coverage.

While Plan E did not provide nearly as much detailed information, the unadjusted average admission rates for all ages indicated that women under both types of coverage in this Plan had higher average admission rates than did men, and the unadjusted average rate for co-pay covered members was lower (135 admissions per 1,000) than that for members with full pay coverage (144 admissons per 1,000) at all ages and for both sexes.

Comparison of co-pay and full pay covered admissions in these two Plans showed that, in general, co-pay admission rates were lower than those for members with full pay coverage. From a purely intra-Plan point of view it can be said that co-pay admissions appeared to be lower than full pay admissions, both on an adjusted and unadjusted basis, indicating that type of coverage did have some effect on admission rates.

Average Length of Stay

When the distribution of the average lengths of stay by age and sex for the three Plans was examined for both full pay and deductible coverage, it was found that length of stay tended to increase linearly with age for both male and female cases. Under both kinds of coverage, however, women after the age of 55 appeared to have a longer length of stay than men of the same age.

Table 2 gives the distribution of average adjusted lengths of stay in Plans offering both full pay and deductible hospital coverage.

TABLE 2

Distribution of Length of Stay for Group, Inpatient Cases for Plans Offering Full Pay and Deductible Coverage

Plan	Adjusted		
	Full	Ded.	Percent Difference
A	6.2	6.6	6.4
B	6.9	7.6	11.3
C	7.4	7.3	− 1.4

The above table shows that, generally, admissions with deductible coverage had a slightly longer average length of stay than did those with full pay coverage. As already mentioned in the introduction, it was quite possible that some one-day stays reported for full pay covered cases were not reported for deductible ones because their covered costs did not exceed the maximum deductible amount. If this was so, the net effect would be a lower admission rate and a higher average length of stay. The reversal of this trend found in Plan C was probably due to the more liberal benefits offered by it under its deductible certificate. The more services covered, the greater the likelihood that one-day deductible cases would be covered and therefore reported.

Assuming the differences in lengths of stay between full pay and deductible covered cases were the result of the omission of some uncovered one-day stays among the deductibles and that each of these one-day stays represented one admission per 1,000 members, the effect of such omissions on the admission rate can be computed using the following equation:

$$(adm/m - odc)(los) = pd/m - odc$$

where adm/m = admissions per 1,000 full pay members

odc = one-day cases not covered by deductible amount per 1,000 full pay members

los = length of stay for deductible covered members

pd/m = patient-days per 1,000 full pay members

Using this equation it was found that the expected admission rate for Plan A deductible covered members was 185.3 per 1,000 if only uncovered one-day cases were responsible for the difference in admission rates. The actual rate of 171 indicated that uncovered one-day cases possibly accounted for slightly more than 40 percent of the observed difference.

In Plan B it was found that applying this equation to the adjusted data, 100 percent of the difference between full pay and deductible admission rates could be explained by the omission of one-day cases.

Since the admission rate for deductibles exceeded that of full pays in Plan C, this equation, of course, was meaningless to apply.

Plans D and E, which offered full and co-pay coverage, showed the same kind of distribution of length of stay by age and sex as did the Plans offering full pay and deductible coverage. Only Plan D had enough data to permit age-sex adjustments, however. It was found that the adjusted average lengths of stay for this Plan for the two types of coverage differed by only 0.1 of a day, with cases under full pay coverage having an average stay of 8.4 days and cases with co-pay coverage staying 8.3 days. The unadjusted figures for Plan E were also similar—6.3 days for full pay cases and 6.5 days for co-pays.

It is interesting to note that these Plans offering both co-pay and full pay hospital coverage showed only small differences between the lengths of stay of cases under the two types of coverage, unlike those cases in Plans that offered deductible and full pay coverage. It has been remarked before, however, that it was possible that some deductible cases with only one day of stay were not reported because their cost did not exceed the basic deductible amount. In cases with co-payment, one-day stays would, of course, be counted. The findings on length of stay for co-pay versus full pay lent support to the belief that the difference in stay between deductible and full pay cases resulted, in part, from the omission of some one-day stays in the former coverage class.

Average Benefits per Day

The three Plans offering full pay and deductible coverage for group, inpatient hospital care all showed a higher daily cost for deductible covered cases than for those with full pay coverage, as can be seen from the adjusted figures in Table 3.

As with average length of stay, average benefits per day excluded certain cases not under deductible coverage but which were included under full pay coverage, namely, cases in which the total covered hospital charges were under $20 or $25. Judging by the average daily benefits for full pay covered cases, all three Plans did have such average charges below $20 or $25 for a typical one-day stay. With the exclusion of all cases costing $20 or $25 or less (usually, one-day stays), it is not surprising to find average benefits per day higher for deductibles than for full pay covered cases, just as it was not surprising to find longer lengths of stay for this coverage class. It was not possible to calculate how much of the difference was due to omission of some one-day cases since the amount of benefits per case-day could not be determined. This could, in theory, have ranged from under $1.00 to $20.99 or $24.99.

The distribution of benefits per day by age and sex did not display any regular trends under either type of coverage. In some Plans the maximum average daily benefit was achieved at the 19 to 34 age level while in others the peak cost was reached at later ages, including 65 and over. In all three

TABLE 3

Average Benefits per Day for Four Plans Offering Full Pay and Deductible Coverage

Plan	Adjusted	
	Full	Ded.
A	$23.06	$26.91
B	20.73	24.35
C	19.02	27.63

Plans the average daily benefit was higher for male cases than for females under both forms of coverage. The lack of any definite kind of distribution of benefit per day by age category may have reflected the variability of diagnoses among different age groups and the consequent differences in the cost of treatment and care. While it is safe to assume that as one becomes older more time is required to recover from sickness or injury, it cannot be assumed that the cost of such recovery is a direct function of time only.

In the two Plans offering both full and co-pay coverage it was found that the daily average benefit was higher for full pay cases than for co-pay covered ones. In Plan D the adjusted benefits were $31.11 for full pays and $29.44 for co-pays. In Plan E the unadjusted figures were $23.24 and $20.06 for full and co-pay cases respectively. These findings were the reverse of what was seen among Plans offering deductible and full pay coverage. They possibly resulted from the inclusion of cost for one-day stays among the co-pays as opposed to the omission of such stays for deductibles. The difference in benefits per day between full and co-pay cases in both Plans, in fact, was almost $4, the amount of the daily co-payment.

Age and sex trends of daily benefits were a bit more regular between and within the two types of coverage. The overall tendency showed an increasing cost with age up to 44 or 54 years, then a slight reduction by ages 65 and over. Both men and women displayed this pattern under full and co-payment coverage, although female cases tended to reach their maximum daily benefits at younger ages (19 to 34) than did male cases (45 to 54). Men under co-pay coverage did not appear to have as sharp a decrease in daily benefits as women under the same type of coverage at the ages of 65 and over.

Average Paid Benefits per Admission

So far, the utilization measures reported here have not been *directly* related to each other (although certain indirect relationships will be discussed later). Average paid benefits per admission, however, is the product of two distinct utilization measures — length of stay and paid benefits per day. Benefits per admission differs from these two measures in that it helps to bring into focus the total covered charges for each admission. Paid benefits per day may be misleading as an index of total hospital charges paid if length of stay is very long. By combining these two factors it is possible to estimate the average effect of the type of coverage on the total covered charges for each case. Table 4 shows the adjusted average paid benefits per case for the Plans that offered both full pay and deductible coverage.

TABLE 4

Average Paid Benefits per Admission for Plans Offering Both Full Payment and Deductible Coverage

Plan	Adjusted	
	Full	Ded.
A	$143.56	$178.06
B	145.03	186.39
C	140.46	200.52

Table 4 reflects both the higher daily benefits and longer lengths of stay for deductible covered admissions whose benefits per admission were higher than those for the full pay covered cases in all the Plans. The observed differences in benefits under the two forms of coverage must, in part, be ascribed to the omission of some one-day stays under deductible coverage while such short stays and their cost were included under full pay coverage.

The distribution of benefits per case by age showed a positive linear relationship within the three Plans and under both types of coverage. As the admitting age increased so did the benefits per case.

In two of the Plans (A and C) the average benefits per case were higher for men than for women under the same kind of coverage, both for deductible and full pay. Also, in these Plans the benefits paid per female admission 65 and older tended to be greater than the paid benefits for male admissions in the same age group. In Plan B the benefits paid per case for women were higher under both kinds of coverage and there, too, female cases over the age of 34 tended to cost more than male cases in the same age categories.

The average paid benefits per admission for the two Plans providing data on both full and co-pay coverage utilization showed that each average full pay case cost the Plans more than did the average co-pay case. The adjusted paid benefits per case for Plan D were $261 per full pay case and $245.80 per co-pay case. The unadjusted cost for Plan E was $169.02 per full pay covered case and $139.23 per co-pay case. These findings reflect earlier ones regarding the lower average daily paid benefits for co-pays in these two Plans, as well as the similarity of their lengths of stay with those covered by full pay certificates.

Both types of coverage showed age and benefits per admission to be positively related with a slight tendency of benefits to level off at 65 and older. Benefits paid for male admissions were greater than those for women under full pay in both Plans and under co-pay in Plan D. In Plan E, however, the average benefit for female admissions under co-payment coverage was higher than for men under the same coverage.

Patient-Days per 1,000 Members

Patient-days per 1,000 members, like benefits per admission, is the product of two independent utilization measures—admissions per 1,000 members and average length of stay. This rate provides an average of the total number of hospital days used per 1,000 members, which the separate measures of admissions and average lengths of stay do not give. Thus, if a group had high admissions and short stays or low admissions and long stays, they would have a lower patient-day rate than a group with both high admissions and long stays. Table 5 shows the distribution of patient-days for the Plans offering both full pay and deductible coverage.

TABLE 5

Patient-Days per 1,000 Members for Plans Offering Full Pay and Deductible Coverage

Plan	Unadjusted		Adjusted		Percent Change
	Full	Ded.	Full	Ded.	
A	1,049	951	1,213	1,133	−6.6
B	1,202	1,236	1,269	1,289	1.6
C	799	1,001	858	993	13.6

It can be seen from Table 5 that the adjusted patient-day rates were lower for deductible covered members in one of the three Plans, about equal in one Plan, and somewhat higher in the third Plan. The third Plan (C) is, of course, the one that provided more comprehensive care under deductible coverage than it did under full pay. The differences among the other Plans can generally be ascribed to their lower admission rates, since neither form of coverage showed any sizeable differences in average lengths of stay (see Table 2). In fact, the lengths of stay for deductible covered cases were generally longer than those for full pays, probably because of the omission of uncovered one-day cases among the deductibles.

Looking at the distribution of patient-day rates by age and sex it was observed

that this was similar to the pattern of average length of stay for most Plans, except that it rose more steeply for older members (55 and over) than did the average length of stay for members these ages. In all Plans the rates for patient-days tended to be, on the whole, higher for females than for men, except in the youngest age group (under 19).

The patient-day rate for the two Plans offering co-pay and full pay coverage was higher for full pays both for Plan D with the adjusted rates of 1,310 for full pay and 1,129 for co-pay, and Plan E whose unadjusted rates were 915 and 875 patient-days per 1,000 full pay and co-pay members, respectively. The lower patient-day rates for co-pay covered members reflected their relatively lower admission rates rather than any appreciably shorter lengths of stay.

Plan D provided information on patient-day rates by age and sex claimants. Generally, this rate showed a gradual increase with age until the ages of 65 and over when it took a steep rise for both sexes. The pattern of patient-days for males and females examined separately revealed itself to be similar to that for admission rates—there was a sharp increase in the rate at ages 19 to 34 which gradually tapered off until a second, higher increase occurred at age 65 and over. Female claimants had a higher patient-day rate than did males at ages 19 to 54 while males had a higher rate for the youngest and oldest age categories. The age-sex pattern was obtained for both full pay and co-pay claimants and differed only in magnitude between them.

Benefits per 1,000 Members

This measure is also a composite of two distinct utilization measures—admissions per 1,000 and benefits per admission. Like other composites, benefits per 1,000 members reveals more than its components. While admissions may be high, the total average benefits paid

TABLE 6

Benefits per 1,000 Members for Plans Offering Both Full and Deductible Coverage

Plan	Unadjusted		Adjusted	
	Full	Ded.	Full	Ded.
A	$24,035	$25,181	$27,948	$30,467
B	32,311	30,462	26,679	31,615
C	16,307	27,434	15,230	27,832

under one form of coverage may be less than those of another form, depending on the total enrollment, number of admissions, and benefits per admission. Table 6 gives the rate of benefits per 1,000 paid by Plans offering full and deductible coverage.

In no Plan was the adjusted benefit rate lower for deductible covered members than for others. This rate for deductible covered members was from 8 percent to 45 percent higher than the full pay rate. With the exception of Plan C, the Plans all had a lower admission rate for deductible covered members than they did for full pays (see Table 1). The average benefits per admission (Table 4) were all higher for deductibles than they were for full pays. As previously mentioned, costs for deductibles tended to be higher probably because of the omission of some one-day cases. This finding about benefits paid per 1,000 members indicates that although deductibles had fewer admissions, the expense of these admissions was not solely due to the absence of one-day stays. It would appear that deductible admissions, in general, were more expensive than full pay admissions. While there were no data to confirm it, the average amount of benefits paid for the two kinds of coverage indicates that deductible admissions were more seriously ill and/or had illnesses of a different nature than did full pay admissions. In support of these hypotheses are the distributions by age of enrollment, cases, days, and paid benefits for the Plans. Table 7 shows the percentage distribution of these Plans

for ages under 65 (generally inexpensive hospital admissions) and 65 and over (generally expensive hospital admissions).

In Plan B the 65 and over group constituted a larger portion of cases and used a greater percentage of days and benefits among the deductibles than they did among the full pay members. The distribution for these variables was about equal by age for both forms of coverage in Plan A; in Plan C the reverse was obtained. It would seem therefore, that the proportion of 65 and over claimants with deductible coverage in these Plans was not especially responsible for some of the higher benefit costs found under this type of coverage.

In the two Plans offering both full and co-pay coverage the benefits paid per 1,000 members were less for co-pay covered members than for full pays. In Plan D the adjusted benefit rates were $40,667 for full pays and $33,383 for co-pays. The unadjusted rates for Plan E were $24,375 and $18,833 for full and co-pay members, respectively. This was consistent with the previous findings of lower admission rates, benefits per day, and benefits per admission found for co-pay covered members.

Surprisingly, the percentage distribution of members by ages under 65 and 65 and over in these Plans was similar to that found for Plans with full and deductible coverage. The 65 and over age co-pay group had a higher percentage of enrollment and admissions and utilized more days and benefits than did the full pay members in the same age category. It would appear that payment of a fixed dollar amount per day of stay was effective in keeping down total average cost for these Plans.

SUMMARY

The Relation of Deductible and Full Pay Coverage to Utilization

The admission rates for members with deductible coverage were lower

TABLE 7

Percentage Distribution by Age of Enrollment, Cases, Days, and Paid Benefits for Plans Offering Both Full Pay and Deductible Coverage

		Unadjusted							
		Enrollment		Cases		Days		Benefits	
Plan	Age Group	Full	Ded.	Full	Ded.	Full	Ded.	Full	Ded.
A	Under 65	95.5	96.4	90.3	91.8	84.2	86.6	86.2	87.5
	65 & over	4.5	3.6	9.7	8.2	15.8	13.4	13.8	12.5
B	Under 65	NA*	NA*	92.4	90.4	86.8	81.2	87.4	82.5
	65 & over	NA*	NA*	7.6	9.6	13.2	18.8	12.6	17.5
C	Under 65	94.4	93.9	86.5	89.9	78.8	83.8	79.8	84.0
	65 & over	5.6	6.1	13.5	10.1	21.2	16.2	20.2	16.0

* Not available.

than those for members with full pay coverage when the degree of coverage was the same. In one Plan where deductible coverage was superior to that of full pay, admissions were higher for deductible covered members. This finding indicates that the effect of a deductible upon admission rates is tempered by the benefits available under such coverage.

Length of stay for members with deductible coverage was somewhat longer in the two Plans that offered the same benefits under both forms of coverage. It was a fraction longer for deductible covered members in the Plan that provided more benefits under that form of coverage. The slightly longer length of stay in the former two Plans suggests that this was due to the absence of one-day cases/stays whose service costs did not exceed the maximum deductible. By assuming that the differences in admission rates and lengths of stay between deductibles and full pays were due to the omission of some one-day cases the expected admission rates for the two kinds of coverage were calculated. It was found that the omission of one-day cases accounted for 40 percent of the observed difference in admission rates in one Plan and 100 percent of these differences in another.

While it might be argued that the cost of a one-day stay in most hospitals is typically higher than most deductible costs, it should be remembered that the costs referred to here are *covered* costs and not total average hospital charges. As was shown earlier (Table 3), the average daily covered costs paid by these Plans for full pays was *not* larger than their deductible amount.

The patient-day rate for two of the three Plans was slightly higher for deductible covered members. In one Plan, which had the lowest percentage difference between deductible and full pay admission rates, the patient-day rate was lower. Since the patient-day rate is a composite measure of utilization, this finding reflects a low admission rate combined with a longer length of stay for one Plan with a rate higher for deductibles than for full pays, and a high admission rate combined with a minutely shorter length of stay for deductible covered members in the other Plan. Again, an important factor to remember here is the absence of some one-day stays.

The Relation of Deductible and Full Pay Coverage to Paid Benefits

Benefits per day were higher for deductible covered members in all three Plans providing full pay and deductible coverage. The exclusion of the first $20 or $25 of hospital costs probably produced this difference, in spite of the somewhat longer lengths of stay usually associated with lower daily costs.

Benefits paid per admission were also higher for deductible covered members. The higher daily benefits paid offset the lower admission rates in two of the Plans, and in the third both a higher admission rate and a higher daily benefit rate produced a large difference in benefits per admission between deductible and full pay covered members.

Finally, benefits per 1,000 members were higher for deductible covered members in all three Plans offering the two types of coverage. This measure, a product of admissions per 1,000 members and average benefits per admission, showed (in two Plans with lower deductible admission rates) the degree to which higher benefits per admission can offset low admission rates.

Age did not seem to be an important factor in utilization or benefits paid under either form of coverage, at least in terms of ages 65 and over and under 65. Only one Plan had more deductible covered admissions 65 and over who used more days and dollars than did full pay covered members. "Poor risks" seem to have been fairly distributed between the two types of coverage, at least in terms of age.

The Relation of Co-pay and Full Pay Coverage to Utilization

Admission rates for the two Plans offering both co-pay and full pay coverage were lower for the co-pay members. The benefits provided under both types of coverage and in both Plans were the same and so it was not possible to determine what effect improved benefits for co-pay coverage might have on admission rates.

The average length of stay for the two forms of coverage was not consistent between the two Plans. In one, co-pay stay was shorter while in the other it was longer. Considering the small amount of the difference without knowledge of the distribution of lengths of stay for the admissions, it was not possible to say whether or not these variations were statistically random or if they represented meaningful differences.

Patient-days per 1,000 members were lower for co-pay covered admissions in both Plans. The slightly longer length of stay in one Plan was not sufficiently large to offset the low admission rate.

The Relation of Co-pay and Full Pay Coverage to Benefits Paid

The most striking observation about the difference in benefits paid per day of stay was that the cost of the co-pays was almost $4 less than that of the full pay— the amount of the co-payment. Considering the similarity in lengths of stay, that figure may have reflected the actual co-payment cost paid by the hospitalized members.

Benefits paid per admission were likewise lower for co-pay covered admissions than for full pays in both Plans. This figure represented both the lower admission rate of this group and the lower daily benefits paid for their care.

The benefits paid per 1,000 members were also lower for members with co-pay coverage than for those with full pay. This followed from the lower benefits per admission and lower admission rate. Interestingly, the distribution of members, admissions, days, and dollars by the ages 65 and over and under 65 showed the co-pays to have a higher proportion than did the full pays of members 65 and over in all of these categories. It would seem that risk, as reflected by the proportion of 65 and over members, did not play an important role in either utilization or benefits paid in these two Plans.

CONCLUSIONS

From the foregoing data it would seem that deductibles had a minimal effect in reducing utilization, and practically no effect in reducing the amount of benefits paid by the Plans involved. Their chief effect seemed to be in reducing the admission rate, but this may have been partially accomplished by the elimination of uncovered one-day stays. The absence of some one-day stays also contributed to the somewhat longer lengths of stay for deductible covered admissions. A longer length of stay for deductibles appeared to be more responsible than admission rates for higher patient-days and paid benefits in one Plan offering both deductible and full pay coverage.

The distribution of members and admissions age 65 and over did not seem to have a noticeable effect on either utilization or benefits.

One important difference noted in a Plan offering both full and deductible coverage was the effect the degree of coverage had on utilization and benefits. In one Plan deductible coverage provided more services than did full pay coverage and it was found that utilization and benefits for deductibles consistently exceeded those for members with full pay coverage. Because more services were covered by the deductible certificate in this Plan it seems that fewer uncovered one-day cases were omitted, the one-day cases that probably contributed to the lower admission rates found for deductibles in the other Plans.

The data on co-pay coverage in two Plans was far more consistent. Both utilization and benefits were lower for those with co-pay coverage. Not only did co-payment seem to reduce the amount of benefits paid by these Plans, it also showed some effect in keeping down admission and patient-day rates. The effect of co-payment on length of stay was negligible. The most surprising fact about the co-pays was that they contained a higher proportion of people 65 and over than did the full pays.

Among deductible covered people, the assumed absence of uncovered short-term or one-day cases would seem to explain both their low admission rates and longer lengths of stay when compared with members under full pay coverage receiving the same benefits. It would be valuable to quantify this variable in more exact terms. A distribution of hospital admissions by the number of days in the hospital would show what percentage of full pays have covered short stays and what percentage of deductible covered admissions have similarly short stays.

Another important variable that impinges on utilization and costs is diagnosis. Certain diagnoses require longer and/or more expensive care than others. How admissions for members under different coverages are distributed by diagnoses would be useful information, as would knowledge of the distribution of costs for each admission.

Perhaps the best approach to the study of the relationship of different types of coverage to hospital use and Plan costs would be to examine the utilization and benefits of a population that has been covered under two forms of coverage during a given period of time; for example, a Plan membership that has gone from full pay coverage one year, to deductible coverage the next, or vice versa. Of course, such a change should not have been the result of a change in utilization or Plan cost nor should there have been any marked changes in the size or characteristics of the membership. Under such circumstances greater experimental control would be present. Instead of having two distinct populations under two forms of coverage, one would have one population going from one form of coverage to another.

While the current study has not produced final answers to the problem of the relationship of type of coverage to hospital utilization and Plan costs, it has suggested several lines of important research in these areas.

Bernard Ferber

The Relationship of Multiple Health Insurance Coverage and Hospital Utilization

Originally Published in December 1966

The hospital utilization experience of 1,025 Pittsburgh patients discharged from a large general hospital in 1963 was studied to determine the possible relationship of the type and extent of hospital use to insurance coverage. The primary concern was to ascertain if there were differences in the number of previous hospital admissions, type of hospital accommodation, average length of stay, and the number of services received by individuals with one hospitalization insurance and those with multiple insurance coverage. Except for a higher percentage of those with more than one insurance coverage receiving private accommodations, there were generally no significant differences evident for the two groups of insured concerning the factors under study. It was also noted that for approximately 30 percent of the individuals with single hospitalization coverages, full payment of the hospital charges was not made by the insuring agencies.

Concomitant with and possibly as a result of the rapid and dynamic growth of voluntary health insurance and the broadening of benefits has been the increase in the number of insured individuals with multiple insurance contracts. In 1963, approximately 78 percent of the civilian population of the United States or nearly 147.2 million had some form of health insurance coverage. This number of insured people represented an increase of about 92 percent over 1950. During the same time period, the number of individuals with multiple health insurance contracts rose from 5.4 million to nearly 22.6 million; a 318 percent increase.[1] From data compiled by the Health Insurance Institute, it is estimated that approximately 15 percent of the individuals insured for health protection have more than one contract.[2] The present study was undertaken to ascertain the possible effect of this increase in multiple insurance on the use of the hospital.

Multiple insurance is defined here to include coverage for similar or different benefits by more than one insurance contract or agreement which are generally intended to supplement one another in terms of services or benefits. Multiple insurance may result in duplicate or excess coverage when essentially the same benefits are available.

The possession of more than one health insurance policy is a result of an individual's right to choose both the extent to which he will protect himself against the cost of medical care and the method of achieving his objective. In exercising this prerogative, multiple insurance is usually obtained from more than one source. In many instances it takes the form of two family contracts

Bernard Ferber was formerly Manager, Research Department, Blue Cross of Western Pennsylvania (Pittsburgh). Currently Director of Continuing Studies Program, Division of Research and Planning, Blue Cross Association.

---

[1] Adapted from *Source Book of Health Insurance Data, 1964* (New York: Health Insurance Institute), p. 12; *Ibid.*, 1965, p. 12.
[2] *Ibid.*

when working wives are covered both through their places of employment and their husbands' places of employment. In other cases, the husband is protected by his employer and secures added family protection on an individual or nongroup basis. In addition, multiple coverage can result if the husband has two jobs.

To the extent that multiple insurance covers a different type or class of medical care expense it is highly desirable. It is similarly desirable if such insurance, although essentially covering the same benefits, results in more completely meeting the medical and nonmedical costs of health care. In these instances, it seems logical to assume that there will be little or no financial deterrent to obtaining comprehensive medical care at the earliest possible time. However, when protection against a given expense is obtained from two or more sources and the benefits payable exceed the amount of the health and health related expenses, it can be considered overinsurance and it is wasteful. Accordingly, multiple coverage may not be in the best interest of the individual, the providers of medical care, and prepayment organizations.

A small sample study conducted by the Health Insurance Council and covering the period 1956-58 reported that for individuals with multiple hospital expense coverage, aggregate benefits of $1.41 were paid for every $1.00 of hospital expense incurred.[3] As the proportion of individuals with health insurance protection increases and benefits are broadened and extended, it can be expected that the percentage of individuals with multiple coverage and the amount of possibly excess payments will increase substantially.

In a report to the National Association of Insurance Commissioners jointly prepared in 1960 by the Blue Cross, Blue Shield, and the Health Insurance Association of America, some of the ways in which multiple insurance and more specifically overinsurance is believed to be contrary to the public interest were listed.[4]

1. "Unnecessarily increasing premiums due to its effect on claim frequency and costs.

2. "Encouraging the insured patient to demand unnecessary or luxury services and care.

3. "Encouraging patient demands on the practicing physician for unnecessary hospital confinements and unjustified prolonged hospital stays.

4. "Destroying the individual's incentive to return to work, thereby adversely affecting the constructive influence of rehabilitation services and ultimately impairing the individual's productivity.

5. "Complicating the hospital credit and collection practices in insured confinements in those instances where multiple coverage results in the submission of multiple claim forms and overpayment of the hospital bill through the use of assignments.

6. "Frequently providing greater benefits for procedures than are customarily charged by the physician or surgeon.

7. "Diverting premium resources to purchase excess coverage when such resources might be used more effectively and economically to fill other needs in the insured's overall insurance program or other necessary living expenses."

As Luck[5] notes, "some of the above points represent assumptions or hypotheses rather than tested conclusions."

---

[3] Health Insurance Council, "A Survey of Multiple Hospitalization Coverage," September, 1959 (Processed), cited by Elizabeth Luck, "The Problem of Duplicate Coverage and Overinsurance," Inquiry, Vol. 1, No. 1 (August, 1963), p. 28.

[4] John P. Hanna and Artemas C. Leslie, "Status Report on Overinsurance for the Non-Profit Hospital and Medical Service Association Committee of the National Association of Insurance Commissioners," May, 1960 (Processed), cited by Luck, Ibid., pp. 22-23.

[5] Luck, Ibid., p. 22.

Accordingly, the primary purpose of this paper is to investigate those items relevant to the admission patterns, length of stay, and the number of services received by individuals with multiple hospital insurance coverage compared to individuals with no insurance and individuals with single contracts. In the following analysis, observed differences among the three groups were considered statistically significant only if the results met the criterion of the .01 level.

METHODOLOGY

This study to determine possible differences in hospital utilization by various insurance classifications is part of an intensive investigation to study the effect of socioeconomic status and hospital insurance on the use of the hospital for Pittsburgh, Pennsylvania residents during 1963. Of the 23 hospitals included in the undertaking, one hospital recorded and verified all insurance coverages for their patients. This hospital listed for each admission, the name of the insurer, type of coverage, and a summary of the major benefits available (including exclusions). Accordingly, it was feasible to compare the hospital experience of individuals with no insurance, those with one hospital insurance contract, and those with more than one contract.

This hospital is a large voluntary nonprofit general hospital with psychiatric care facilities. It is a fully accredited institution having available nearly all the services and facilities listed in the 1964. Guide Issue (Part Two) of *Hospitals.*

Initially, lists were prepared containing the names and addresses of each patient (excluding newborns) who was discharged during 1963, from hospital admission books for 1962 and 1963. From this, a sample of one out of every eight patients was selected. Since the study related to Pittsburgh residents, patients with out-of-city addresses were deleted. All addresses were checked against the *Census Tract Index to Pittsburgh Streets and House Numbers* compiled by the Department of Public Safety in Pittsburgh. A total of 1,056 individuals were chosen.

For each study participant, the medical and business office records were pulled. From the medical records, the following data were abstracted: accommodation at time of discharge, birth date, age at time of admission, hospital coverage, marital status, employment status, length of stay, living arrangements, prior hospitalization in the same hospital within one year of the current admission, discharge status, all diagnoses, the presence of complications, all operative procedures, and the number and type of diagnostic and therapeutic services received, exclusive of drugs. From the business office ledger cards, the number of hospital contracts in force, the total hospital bill, and the sources and amounts of payments were recorded. In addition, the hospital accommodation and certain services which were abstracted from the medical record were checked against the ledger card.

DATA LIMITATIONS

Although the business office staff conscientiously verified each insurance source at admission, or shortly after, there was limited verification if an individual stated he had no insurance protection. Therefore, it is possible that some individuals classified as having no insurance actually had some coverage. In discussions with the assistant comptroller, it was his feeling that the number of such individuals would be very small, since in most instances the business office, knowing the name of the employer, would also know (by experi-

TABLE 1

Number of Patients by Hospital Insurance Category and Major Source of Payment

Insurance Category— Major Payment Source	No.	Percent
Total*	1,025	100.0
No Insurance	353	34.4
Patient (self-pay)	78	7.6
Workmen's Compensation	13	1.3
Government	57	5.6
Service	141	13.8
Other†	64	6.2
One Insurance‡	555	54.1
Patient	29	2.8
Blue Cross	417	40.7
Commercial	88	8.6
Union	9	0.9
Government	2	0.2
Service	2	0.2
Other	8	0.8
Two or More Insurances§	117	11.4
Patient	1	0.1
Blue Cross	105	10.2
Commercial	10	1.0
Union	1	0.1

* Excludes 31 individuals for whom insurance status could not be ascertained.
† Includes write-offs, and open balances (unpaid) where these constitute major portions of the total hospital charges.
‡ There were 10 individuals with Blue Cross for whom this coverage was not the major source of payment. In addition, there were 31 individuals with commercial insurance for whom such coverage did not constitute the major source of payment.
§ There were three individuals with Blue Cross for whom this coverage was not the major payment source.

ence) if insurance protection was generally available at that company. If insurance coverage was available and the patient reported no coverage, this would be checked further.

Similar checks were instituted for individuals claiming one insurance but who might have additional coverages. In addition, all patients and/or family members were informed that divulging all insurance sources would facilitate the processing of duplicate copies of the hospital bill and any correspondence with the insuring agency.

An individual was classified as having single or multiple insurance only if the name of the insuring organization and

most of the major benefits available were listed on the ledger card and/or some payment was received from a prepayment organization. It was felt that only with these procedures could a high degree of classification accuracy be achieved. Nevertheless, there were eight individuals who met the verification criteria, but for whom assignment forms were not honored. Presumably this was so because the insurance coverage was not currently in force. There were an additional 21 individuals who had insurance but from whom notice was received from the insuring agency that such coverage was not available for the current admission due to certain diagnostic exclusions, waiting periods, or exhaustion of benefit days. These 29 individuals comprised about 2.7 percent of the total study group and were classified as having no insurance.

In no instance did the business office ledger card list two Blue Cross coverages. An investigation of this fact revealed that in the few cases where two Blue Cross agreement numbers were furnished by the patient, only one number was recorded.

FINDINGS

Insurance Coverage and Major Source of Payment

Of the 1,056 individuals in the study, insurance status could not be determined for 31 patients since business office ledger cards were not available for them (Table 1). Of the 1,025 individuals for whom the necessary information was obtained, 353 or 34.4 percent had no insurance coverage, 555 or 54.1 percent had one hospital insurance contract, and 117 or 11.4 percent had two or more hospitalization contracts.

The fact that 353 or about 34 percent of the patients did not have any insurance coverage is of interest. Somewhat more than half of these individuals (198) were primarily service (free) or government cases. In addition, nearly all of the 64 individuals with major (primary) sources of payment[6] other than those listed in the table were classified by the hospital social service department as medically indigent. For these cases a major portion of the hospital bill was written off or remained open with little expectation of payment. A further check of the 78 self-pay patients did not reveal any additional information concerning insurance coverage. It is possible that some of these individuals did have insurance coverages, although there were no requests for copies of the hospital bill (for insurance purposes). However, the original bill possibly could have been submitted by the patient for reimbursement.

Approximately 65 percent, or 672 patients, had some insurance coverage. This percentage cannot be directly compared with the percentage of individuals having hospital insurance protection in the general population. This is primarily so because of possible differential hospital utilization for those with and those without hospital insurance, differences in the characteristics of the population and area served, and the type of administrative policies and procedures followed by the hospital. Of the 30 individuals with insurance protection and who made major payments concerning their hospital charges, 19 had some additional payments made to the hospital by Blue Cross or commercial insurance companies, while the remaining 11 individuals elected to pay their own bills and have detailed copies of such statements submitted to their insurance companies.

Type of Insurance Coverage

Table 2 shows the number of individuals with insurance coverage. Thus, of

[6] Major payment source is defined as the individual, organization, or agency paying the largest amount of the hospital bill.

TABLE 2

Number of Patients by Hospital Insurance Category and Extent of Insurance Payment

Insurance Category— Extent of Insurance Payment	No.	Percent
No. of Individuals with Insurance	672	100.0
One Insurance	555	82.6
Blue Cross— full payment*	340	50.6
Blue Cross— part payment	87	12.9
Commercial†— full payment	40	6.0
Commercial†— part payment	77	11.5
Commercial—unknown	11	1.6
Two or More Insurances‡	117	17.4
Blue Cross and Commercial	108	16.1
Commercial§ only	9	1.3

* Full payment includes complete payment of the total hospital bill and those instances where $15 or less was not paid by the insuring agency. Part payment includes those cases where more than $15 was not paid by the insuring organization.

† Includes a few individuals insured through their union.

‡ Extent of payment, in most instances, could not be determined.

§ Includes individuals with two or more commercial insurances only and those individuals insured through their union and also having additional commercial coverage.

the 672 patients with insurance, 427 had Blue Cross only, 137 had commercial only (one or more than one contract) and 108 had Blue Cross and commercial coverages. For those with one insurance having Blue Cross, their coverage resulted in full payment for 340 or nearly 80 percent of the individuals. Full payment was defined to include complete payment of the total bill and those instances where $15 or less of the bill was not paid by the prepayment organization. The $15 amount was chosen because in most instances this figure represented telephone and/or rental of television charges. Accordingly, for 20 percent of the Blue Cross patients, amounts in excess of $15 were not paid by their coverage. Of the 128 individuals with one commercial contract a similar comparison could be made for 117 individuals. Based on this number, full payment as defined above was made for 40 or about 34 percent of the individuals, and 66 percent (77 persons) had only partial payments. A comparable analysis could not be made for individuals with more than one hospital insurance.

Overall, of the 544 individuals with one insurance and for whom extent of insurance payment could be determined, full payments were *not* made for 164 or approximately 30 percent of the patients. It would seem that for those individuals there were deficiencies in coverage resulting in failure to meet current hospitalization needs.

Age and Sex

The average age of the uninsured males was approximately 44.3 years. For those with single insurance policies and those with multiple contracts, the comparable averages were 41.0 years and 44.5 years, respectively. These age differences were not statistically significant.

For females, no significant difference in average age was noted for those with single insurance (41.8 years) as compared to those with multiple insurance (42.5 years). However, the average age of the uninsured females (49.4 years) was significantly higher than that for the insured groups.

Diagnosis

Depending on the primary diagnostic reason for hospital admission (final diagnosis), the patients included in the study were categorized as to type of illness; acute, chronic, and mental. These diagnostic groups were based on a similar classification used by Ciocco and his associates in a study of illness and the receipt of medical services.[7]

[7] A. Ciocco, S. Graham, and D. J. Thompson, "Illness and Receipt of Medical Services in Pittsburgh (Arsenal), and Butler County," *Pennsylvania Health*, Vol. 17, No. 8 (October-December, 1956), pp. 8, 13.

For males with one insurance and those with multiple coverages, no significant differences in diagnoses were noted. However, the diagnostic composition of the uninsured males differed significantly from those with insurance. Part of this difference was attributed to the higher percent of uninsured with mental illnesses. Similar results were noted for the females.

Socioeconomic Status

As part of the larger investigation involving 23 voluntary hospitals in the Pittsburgh area, census tracts for the city of Pittsburgh were classified into four socioeconomic categories: high, median high, median low, low. These designations were based on education, occupation, and income data available from the 1960 census. Before final adoption of the classification, it was tested and found adequate using study data for six hospitals. A patient was assigned a socioeconomic classification depending upon the census tract of his residence.

For the present study, the four socioeconomic classifications were collapsed into two—high and low (Table 3). Socioeconomic status was reviewed in order to explain, at least partially, differences in admission patterns, length of stay, and the number of services among the three groups of individuals. Approximately 56 percent of those with multiple insurance were classified as having high socioeconomic status. The comparable figures for those with one insurance and those with none were about 51 percent and 31 percent, respectively. No statistically significant difference in socioeconomic status was noted for individuals with one or more than one insurance contract. However, a statistically significant higher percent of those insured individuals (single or multiple contracts) were of high socioeconomic status as compared to those with no insurance. This latter finding

TABLE 3

Number of Patients by Hospital Insurance Category and Socioeconomic Status

Insurance Category	Socioeconomic Status					
	Total		High		Low	
	No.	Percent	No.	Percent	No.	Percent
Total*	1,025	100.0	457	44.6	568	55.4
No Insurance	353	100.0	108	30.6	245	69.4
One Insurance	555	100.0	284	51.2	271	48.8
Two or More Insurances	117	100.0	65	55.6	52	44.4

* Excludes 31 individuals for whom insurance status could not be ascertained.

was to be expected because, as previously noted, there were a large number of service, government, and medically indigent individuals among those with no insurance.

Admission Patterns

As listed in Table 2, 117 or 17.4 percent of the 672 admissions with hospital insurance had multiple coverage. This is higher than the 15 percent estimated from the Health Insurance Institute data.[8] It is difficult to determine statistically whether or not the difference between the 17.4 percent observed and the 15 percent estimated represents excessive hospital admissions, since there is no reliable information available regarding the expected number of hospital admissions for individuals with multiple coverage. It cannot be assumed that since 15 percent of the individuals with insurance have multiple coverage the same percent of insured admissions should have multiple insurances. It is highly likely that individuals securing multiple insurance contracts expect to use the hospital more frequently than other groups. On the other hand, it can also be argued that people who secure multiple coverage may be more concerned about their health. Accordingly, they will seek needed medical attention at the earliest possible time; possibly obviating the need for inpatient care.

[8] *Op. cit.*

It was possible, however, to compare the number of previous hospital admissions within a one-year period to the same hospital for individuals with no insurance coverage, individuals with one contract, and those with two or more policies (Table 4). Approximately 18.8 percent of those with multiple coverage had prior hospital admissions. For individuals with no insurance, the percentage was 19.6; while that for individuals with one contract was 15.5. These differences were not statistically significant. In addition, the three groups were essentially similar in regard to the average number of previous admissions. As a result there was no evidence that those with more than one hospitalization agreement had a possible "excess" number of prior hospitalizations in the same hospital within a one-year period of the current admission.

Hospital Accommodation

In Table 5 the individuals in each of the three categories are classified according to accommodation at time of discharge. As might be expected, most of the individuals (82 percent) without hospital insurance had ward accommodations. For those with one insurance, approximately 7 percent had private, 63 percent had semiprivate, and 30 percent had ward facilities. About 17 percent of the individuals with two or more insurances had private, 62 percent had semiprivate, and 21 percent

TABLE 4

Number of Patients by Hospital Insurance Category and Prior Hospital Admission*

| Insurance Category | Total | | Prior Hospital Admission | | | | | |
| | | | None | | One or More | | Unknown | |
	No.	Percent†	No.	Percent	No.	Percent	No.	Percent
Total‡	1,025	100.0	843	82.7	176	17.3	6	—
No Insurance	353	100.0	283	80.4	69	19.6	1	—
One Insurance	555	100.0	465	84.5	85	15.5	5	—
Two or More Insurances	117	100.0	95	81.2	22	18.8	—	—

* Prior admission to the study hospital within one year of current admission.
† Percentages are based on the number of cases for whom previous hospital admission could be determined.
‡ Excludes 31 individuals for whom insurance status could not be ascertained.

had ward accommodations. It is of interest to note that the percent of individuals using semiprivate facilities was approximately the same for the two groups of individuals having hospitalization contracts. Therefore, the differences noted for these individuals related to private and ward accommodations.

When the two groups having insurance were compared, the differences in accommodations were statistically significant. Thus, there was evidence that individuals with multiple insurance coverages requested and received private accommodations more frequently than those with single insurance coverage. Although individuals with multiple coverage more frequently occupied private rooms, the fact that only 17 percent obtained such accommodations, while 83 percent did not, is of interest.

Possibly patient preferences, the number of private rooms available, and hospital policy account for this finding.

Average Length of Hospital Stay

The average length of stay by sex is shown in Table 6. For males with no insurance coverage, the average length of stay was 15.2 days. The comparable average for those with one insurance was 11.7 days, 1.1 days longer than the length of stay for those with multiple coverages (10.6 days). The differences noted for those with insurance coverages were not significant; however, the average length of stay for patients with no insurance coverage was significantly higher than that for all individuals with insurance.

For females, the average length of

TABLE 5

Number of Patients by Hospital Insurance Category and Hospital Accommodation*

| Insurance Category | Total | | Hospital Accommodation | | | | | |
| | | | Private | | Semiprivate | | Ward | |
	No.	Percent	No.	Percent	No.	Percent	No.	Percent
Total†	1,025	100.0	72	7.0	470	45.9	483	47.1
No Insurance	353	100.0	15	4.2	48	13.6	290	82.2
One Insurance	555	100.0	37	6.7	350	63.1	168	30.3
Two or More Insurances	117	100.0	20	17.1	72	61.5	25	21.4

* At time of hospital discharge.
† Excludes 31 individuals for whom insurance status could not be ascertained.

TABLE 6

Number of Patients by Hospital Insurance Category, Average Length of Stay (Days), and Sex

Insurance Category	No.		Average Length of Stay
	Patients	Patient-days	
Male			
Total*	436	5,568	12.8
No Insurance	153	2,323	15.2
One Insurance	232	2,706	11.7
Two or More Insurances	51	539	10.6
Female			
Total†	589	6,383	10.8
No Insurance	200	2,237	11.2
One Insurance	323	3,445	10.7
Two or More Insurances	66	701	10.6

* Excludes 13 individuals for whom insurance status could not be ascertained.
† Excludes 18 individuals for whom insurance status could not be ascertained.

stay for those with one insurance (10.7 days) was about the same as that for individuals with multiple coverage (10.6 days). These averages were only slightly lower than those with no insurance (11.2 days). These differences were not statistically significant. When obstetrical admissions were omitted, little difference was noted in the average length of stay for the two insurance groups. However, the noninsured females had a significantly longer average length of stay than their insured counterparts.

Overall, the average length of stay for those included in the study was 11.7 days, somewhat higher than that of the average length of stay for all general hospitals in the city of Pittsburgh in 1963 (10.1 days). In all probability, this difference is mainly due to the type of sample taken (i.e., only Pittsburgh residents) and to the administrative policies and practices of the study hospital.

Services

Table 7 indicates the total number of services excluding administration of drugs, such as laboratory tests, X-rays,

EKG's, received by each sex. For males with one insurance, the number of services per case was 16.9 while that for multiply insured individuals was 17.9, a difference which was not statistically significant. However, the 20.3 services per uninsured individual was significantly higher than the comparable average number of services for both types of insured individuals. In all probability, this is due, in large part, to the longer average length of stay of uninsured individuals.

Because of the wide variation in the number of services received by patients with mental illnesses, comparisons of the average number of services per patient were made excluding this diagnostic entity. The resulting findings, however, were similar to those noted above.

When length of stay was taken into consideration in the analysis, the number of services (per day) for uninsured males (1.3) was about the same as that for males with one insurance (1.4). However, those with multiple coverage had 1.7 services per day, significantly higher than that for the other two groups. When mental illness admissions

TABLE 7

Number of Patients by Hospital Insurance Category, Number of Services, and Sex

	No.			Average No. of Services	
Insurance Category	Patients	Patient-days	Services	Per Patient	Per Patient-day
Male					
Total*	436	5,568	7,932	18.2	1.42
No Insurance	153	2,323	3,101	20.3	1.33
One Insurance	232	2,706	3,919	16.9	1.45
Two or More Insurances	51	539	912	17.9	1.69
Female					
Total†	589	6,383	9,366	15.9	1.47
No Insurance	200	2,237	3,131	15.7	1.40
One Insurance	323	3,445	5,240	16.2	1.52
Two or More Insurances	66	701	995	15.1	1.42

* Excludes 13 individuals for whom insurance status could not be ascertained.
† Excludes 18 individuals for whom insurance status could not be ascertained.

were excluded, no significant difference in the number of services per day was noted for each of the three groups. The same finding was evident when separate analyses were made for males with acute and those with chronic diseases.

For females, the findings regarding the number of services received were somewhat different from those observed for the males. Thus, the number of services per case was lowest for those with multiple coverage (15.1), and highest for those with single insurance policies (16.2). For the uninsured females, the average number of services per case was 15.7. Again, these differences were not statistically significant. When females with mental diagnoses were excluded, no significant difference in the number of services was observed for the two insurance categories. However, as was also noted for the males, the number of services received for the noninsured was significantly higher than that received by the insured.

When length of stay was incorporated into the analysis, there was no significant difference in services received (per day) for females with one insurance (1.52), and those with multiple insurance coverages (1.42). However,

both insurance groups combined received a significantly higher average number of services than those with no insurance (1.40). When mental illness was excluded, females with single coverage had a significantly higher average number of services per day than each of the other two groups. It is of additional interest to note that after excluding mental illnesses, those with no insurance had a significantly higher number of services per day than those with multiple coverages. Females with multiple insurance coverage had significantly lower average numbers of services than did the females with one insurance contract when acute and chronic diseases were considered separately.

Maternity (Delivery) Admissions

The total number of cases available for study was too small to do an analysis by specific detailed diagnosis. Nevertheless, maternity admissions without complications, believed to be sensitive to possible over hospital utilization related to multiple insurance coverage were studied. No significant difference in accommodations was noted between the two insurance groups. However, as expected from previous findings, there was a significant difference in accommodations between the uninsured and the two groups of insured individuals. This was due to the higher percentage of the former group being assigned ward facilities.

Although maternity admissions with multiple insurance coverages had a slightly longer average length of stay (5.8 days), compared to those with one insurance (5.6 days) and those with no insurance (5.5 days) these results were not significant and could have been due to random fluctuations. Similarly, there was little if any difference in the average number of services per patient or per day received by individuals with insurance coverage. On the other hand, the uninsured maternity admissions with a somewhat shorter average length of stay received a significantly higher average number of services. This was due to hospital policy, which dictated certain diagnostic tests be administered more frequently to service and medically indigent maternity patients; major components of the uninsured group.

SUMMARY AND CONCLUSIONS

The present investigation of the hospital utilization experience of 1,025 Pittsburgh patients discharged from a large, general hospital in 1963 was undertaken to determine the possible relationship of the type and extent of hospital use and insurance coverage. The number of previous hospital admissions, the type of hospital accommodations, the average length of stay, and the average number of services received were analyzed for patients with no insurance, those with single hospitalization insurance, and those with multiple hospitalization contracts.

At the inception of the study, it was recognized that the number of individuals in each classification is generally determined by existing admission policies and practices and would vary widely by hospital. This could affect the percentage of admissions with insurance coverage and the percent of insured admissions with multiple coverages. Nevertheless, it was felt that the type and extent of hospital utilization of the two groups of insured individuals, once admission was accomplished, would not be altered significantly by admission and possibly other practices. Accordingly, after appropriate analysis any differences noted in the variables under study for the insured groups could be attributed, in large part, to the number of insurance coverages.

Approximately one-third or 353 of the hospital admissions did not have any hospitalization coverage, while the remaining 672 had one or more contracts currently in force. This high percentage of noninsured, mostly service, government, and medically indigent cases, is a reflection of the characteristics of the population and area served and the expressed aims and purposes of the hospital included in the study. About 17.4 percent of the insured patients had more than one hospital expense policy. As noted above, this percentage of multiply insured individuals can be expected to fluctuate among hospitals.

The basic patient characteristics of those without insurance, related to hospital use, was expected to be significantly different from the other groups of patients. Nevertheless, the noninsured were included in all analyses undertaken, although major emphasis was restricted to comparisons between the two insured groups.

The two groups of individuals with insurance coverage were essentially similar in regard to age, diagnosis, and socioeconomic status. On the other hand, significant differences in these variables were noted for the noninsured as compared to the insured.

For the three groups of patients, there were no significant differences in the percent of individuals having prior admissions to the study hospital within a one-year period. Similarly, there were no significant differences noted in the average number of prior admissions.

Individuals with multiple insurance received private rooms significantly more frequently than those with single insurance coverage. However, it was not possible to determine if such assignments were medically indicated and thus in the best interest of the patients. On the positive side, the more frequent use of private facilities may result in the alleviation of possibly crowded semiprivate and ward accommodations.

With one exception, the average length of stay and the number of services received for both groups of insured individuals were essentially similar. The exception was that the average number of services per day for females with single insurance exceeded the comparable average for those with more than one insurance. In most instances, the average length of stay and the average number of services for the uninsured were significantly higher than the comparable averages for the insured.

In summary, except for the differences noted in hospital accommodations, there was no statistical evidence that those with multiple insurance used the hospital more extensively than those with one insurance. However, the comparisons listed below between individuals with multiple insurance coverages and those with single insurance, although not statistically significant, must be kept in mind. If the relationships observed persist with a larger number of study cases, significant findings would be obtained:

1. A higher percent of individuals with multiple insurance coverage had prior hospital admissions within a one-year period to the study hospital.
2. The average number of previous hospital admissions was higher for the multiply insured.
3. The average number of services per case for multiply insured males was higher.
4. Maternity admissions with multiple insurance had a longer length of hospital stay.

On the other hand, the case for multiple or supplementary insurance coverage is strengthened when it is realized that for about 30 percent of those with single health insurance policies there were gaps in coverage resulting in failure to meet most of the total hospital charges. If hospital costs continue to rise and prepayment organizations do not initiate indicated changes in benefit structure, the percent of individuals with coverage deficiencies can be expected to increase.

Further studies involving more patients and permitting comparisons of differential admission rates are needed. With an expanded number of cases, various subgroups of the noninsured such as self-pays, can be analyzed in detail. In addition, for a thorough evaluation of the effect of multiple coverage on hospital use, the complete medical and medically related costs resulting from hospital confinement must be ascertained.

Joel W. Kovner
L. Brian Browne
Arnold I. Kisch, M.D.

Income and the Use of Outpatient Medical Care by the Insured

Reprinted with permission of the Blue Cross Association, from *Inquiry:* Vol.VI, No.2, pp.27-34. Copyright © 1969 by the Blue Cross Association.

Originally Published in June 1969

For present and future health planning, both governmental and voluntary, the determination of whether a relationship exists between income and the use of outpatient medical services for the insured is most important. If use is related to income, the organization and administration of delivery systems for outpatient care should reflect awareness of such a fact. Many studies have thoroughly examined the relationship between income and the use of ambulatory care for populations consisting of both insured and uninsured persons. None, however, has precisely or extensively investigated the relationship between income and use for insured populations only; it is the purpose of this paper to present such an analysis.

Previous Studies

The studies that have analyzed the relationship between income and the use of outpatient medical services for populations consisting of both the insured and uninsured have reached essentially similar conclusions. On a nationwide basis, the National Health Survey[1] indicates a positive relationship between income and use. For the state of Michigan, McNerney, et al.,[2] present similar findings. In a more precise manner, Stigler[3] has pointed out that the income elasticity of demand (the percentage change in the quantity of medical services taken by buyers associated with a 1 percent change in income) is less than one for physician services, but nevertheless positively dependent. He further concludes that the income elasticity appears to increase as income levels increase. Paradiso[4] presents essentially similar results, but implies that the elasticity is greater than one. Paul Feldstein[5] also opts for positive dependence but sets the elasticity at 0.6. For insured populations only, there are several studies[6, 7] that have considered the relationships between use and various demographic parameters; however the relationship between use and incomes has, with one exception, not been investigated. The empirical study by Darsky, et al.,[8] on Windsor Health Services does present data on income versus per capita use for the insured only. However, income is not considered in its most sensitive form, per capita income; and use is in terms of the number of physician office and home visits, an aggregation that could hide many substantial relationships (e.g., the use of preventive services versus income). Additionally, and unfortunately, although the Darsky data would allow one to conclude that there seems to be a trend between increasing income and decreasing per capita use of physician home and office visits, the relationship is neither extensively considered nor quantified.

Joel W. Kovner, Dr. P.H. is Health Plan Economist, Kaiser Foundation Health Plan, Southern California Region, and Lecturer, School of Public Health, University of California at Los Angeles. **L. Brian Browne, M.A.** is Public Administrative Analyst, School of Public Health, and **Arnold I. Kisch, M.D.** is Assistant Professor of Preventive Medicine, School of Medicine, UCLA.

This research was supported by a grant from the Ford Foundation. Co-principal investigators under the grant are Milton I. Roemer, M.D. and Arnold I. Kisch, M.D.

Methodology of the Present Study

The Study Populations

Two populations served as the data bases for this study: 1) longshoremen and their dependents in Stockton, California, and 2) employees of the Los Angeles Department of Water and Power and their dependents. Within these populations, the segments selected for study were the longshoremen covered under the health plan offered by the San Joaquin Foundation for Medical Care, and the employees of the Department of Water and Power enrolled with the Ross-Loos Medical Group. Among the longshoremen in Stockton there were approximately 500 subscribers to the health plan. All of these, together with insured dependents, were included in the study. In Los Angeles, a study group was selected by random sampling within a much larger population.

The two health insurance plans represented in this study, the Ross-Loos Medical Group and the San Joaquin Foundation for Medical Care, have both been extensively described in the literature.[9, 10] Both offer comprehensive coverage with the quality of insured care monitored through a continuing audit program. Ross-Loos provides services through a multispecialty group practice of physicians located in a large home office and in 13 branch offices throughout the Los Angeles area. The plan serves a population of about 140,000 subscribers and dependents.

The San Joaquin Foundation, sponsored by the San Joaquin County Medical Society, provides services through physicians primarily in a solo or single specialty practice setting. There are approximately 300 affiliated physicians (representing over 95 percent of the members of the County Medical Society). A population of approximately 100,000 persons, covered by a variety of health insurance contracts, receives care through the Foundation.

An attempt was made to interview each health plan subscriber in the study populations: 426 interviews were completed in

Los Angeles; 282 in Stockton. For the 395 subscribers in Los Angeles and the 264 subscribers in Stockton who gave permission, both their own and their dependents' medical records at the respective health plan were reviewed to ascertain the total quantity of insured services received by each individual in the period July 1, 1966 to June 30, 1967. In all, 1,025 records were examined in Los Angeles; 858 in Stockton.

In interviewing the subscribers, questions relating to the total dollar expenditures for insured services were asked, as well as questions on family size and income.

Because of the wide differences in the demographic characteristics of the two populations and in the respective medical care delivery systems, the Ross-Loos and Stockton populations will be considered separately.

Quantification of the Variables

Although many previous studies have considered income in terms of family income, the most sensitive measure of disposable income streams is per capita income; hence, income will be in terms of per capita income. For the San Joaquin population, per capita income ranged from $0 to $17,000; for the Ross-Loos group, the range was $72 to $45,000.

Where the data permitted, outpatient medical care was measured by a system developed by one of the authors (JWK).[11] It was felt that such an analysis was preferable to other indices presently applied because of its specificity.

Kovner disaggregates ambulatory health services into five broad subsets: 1) office visit services, 2) laboratory services, 3) minor surgical services, 4) radiological services, and 5) all other services. The first three subsets are further divided into distinctive elements. For office visit services these elements are: a) initial office visit for acute or chronic illness, b) follow-up office visit for acute or chronic illness, c) office visit for severe accidental injury, d) initial office visit for mild accidental injury, e) follow-up office visit for mild accidental injury, f) physical examination, child (age less than 12) with no presenting illness, g) physical examination, child (age less than 12) *with* presenting illness, h) physical examination, adult (age more than 12) with no presenting illness, i) physical examination, adult *with* presenting illness, j) telephone consultation, k) visit with only nurse seen, and l) visit for injection or immunization. For laboratory services, the elements are: a) routine blood count, b) blood chemistry, c) serology, d) other blood examinations, and e) urinalysis. For minor surgical services the elements are: a) initial visit for minor surgery, and b) follow-up visit for minor surgery. All of these subsets and elements are easily identifiable and therefore quantifiable. Further, they represent distinct types of patient services.

For purposes of this paper, utilization was measured by cumulating incidence in each of the above categories of ambulatory services. Volume indices (e.g., dollar value per category of services delivered) would of course have been a more accurate measure of utilization. However, incidence does reveal trends in utilization and constraints on time and data collection further recommend it in this case. Categories with fewer than 10 incidences of use were not included in the analysis. Thus the "blood serology" and "all other service" categories were eliminated, leaving 19 categories. The disaggregation outlined above could only be applied to insured services in the present study. Only for such services could data be retrieved from patient medical records.

For uninsured outpatient services (those services which the plans did not cover or for which they did not reimburse any dollar amounts to the individual) utilization was considered in terms of dollars spent, and data were obtained from subscriber recall. Such care was disaggregated into four categories of dollar expenditures: 1) all laboratory, X-ray, and diagnostic

services, 2) physician visits, 3) ancillary care (nurses, chiropractors, etc.), and 4) appliances, glasses and artificial limbs.

Essentially the same type of outpatient services are insured under both plans. One important exception is initial office visits for dependents, which are covered by Ross-Loos, but not by the San Joaquin Foundation. Relative to Ross-Loos, this constraint results in some shifting of utilization by dependents in the San Joaquin plan toward follow-up office visits (which are insured). Nonetheless, the percentage of uninsured services received per person (the dollar value of uninsured services/the estimated dollar value for all outpatient services) is similar for both plans.

Statistical Analysis

Two methods of analysis were utilized. First, the correlation coefficient, r, between per capita income and the utilization of each of the 23 categories of outpatient services (19 insured and 4 uninsured) was computed. The correlation coefficient indicates the standardized relationship between the covariance of the two variables being considered. Values for r lie between and include -1 and $+1$, with $+1$ indicating perfect dependence (or correlation), -1 perfect negative dependence, and 0 independence.

Unfortunately, r does not allow for the detailed analysis which the income elasticity of demand provides. Hence, using least squares estimation, utilization of each of the categories of services was regressed against per capita income. From the $b_{y_i x_i}$ (where y equals the category of service and x per capita income), income elasticities of demand are usually computed as the product of $b_{y_i x}(\overline{x}/\overline{y}_i)$.

A slight methodological problem is presented in testing for the significance of $r_{y_i x}$ and $b_{y_i x}$. Twenty-three variables or categories are being tested and the level of significance should take this into consideration. This problem is obviated by use of the multiple contrast method in

Table 1. Correlation coefficients between the use of outpatient medical services and income

Insured services

Category	San Joaquin Foundation	Ross-Loos
Initial office visit for acute or chronic illness	+ .051	+ .013
Follow-up office visit for acute or chronic illness	+ .071	+ .040
Office visit for severe accidental injury	− .009	− .037
Initial office visit for mild accidental injury	− .042	− .028
Follow-up office visit for mild accidental injury	− .009	− .028
Physical examination, child (age less than 12) with no presenting illness	− .008	− .026
Physical examination, child (age less than 12) *with* presenting illness	− .013	− .024
Physical examination, adult (age more than 12) with no presenting illness	− .010	+ .056
Physical examination, adult (age more than 12) *with* presenting illness	+ .111	− .003
Initial visit for minor surgery	+ .012	+ .038
Follow-up visit for minor surgery	− .006	− .006
Telephone consultation	− .013	− .020
Visit with only nurse seen	+ .005	− .015
Visit for injection or immunization	+ .015	− .004
Routine blood count	+ .003	+ .014
Blood chemistry	+ .076	+ .032
Other blood examinations	+ .020	+ .025
Urinalysis	+ .046	+ .031
X-ray	− .001	+ .045

Uninsured services

Category	San Joaquin Foundation	Ross-Loos
All laboratory, X-ray, and diagnostic services	+ .048	− .002
Physician visits	+ .001	+ .094
Ancillary care (nurses, chiropractors, etc.)	− .003	+ .072
Appliances, glasses and artificial limbs	− .039	+ .109

Table 2. Income elasticities for outpatient medical services

Insured services

San Joaquin Foundation	Ross-Loos
All categories approach zero except physical examination, adult *with* presenting illness = .816	All categories approach zero

Uninsured services

Category	San Joaquin Foundation	Ross-Loos
All laboratory, X-ray, and diagnostic services	Approaches zero	Approaches zero
Physician visits	Approaches zero	.7401
Ancillary care (nurses, chiropractors, etc.)	Approaches zero	1.2336
Appliances, glasses, and artificial limbs	Approaches zero	1.7590

which the $\alpha = .1 - \alpha_1$, where $\alpha =$ the level $\overline{2m}$ of significance used, $\alpha_1 =$ the predetermined level of significance, and $m =$ the number of categories tested.

Results

The correlation coefficients r_{y_1x} between the use of each of the 23 categories of outpatient services and per capita income are found in Table 1; the income elasticities in Table 2.

Considering insured services first, the r_{y_1x} for all outpatient services provided to members at the Ross-Loos plan appear independent of income (tabled $r_{.05,1025} = .104$). For members of the San Joaquin Medical Foundation Plan, all services appear independent (tabled $r_{.05,858} = .123$), with the exception of physical examination for adult with presenting illness which (r = .111) approaches dependence.

Similarly, the income elasticities will approach zero (as r approaches zero, b approaches zero; hence, the income elasticity approaches zero) for all insured services in the Ross-Loos population. In the San Joaquin Foundation population, the income elasticities all approach zero, with the exception of physical examination, adult *with* presenting illness, which at .816 approaches significance $(b_{y_ix} / (b_{y_ix})$ = 3.29; tabled t $_{05,858}$ = 3.291).

When uninsured services are examined, the r_{y_ix} for three of the categories of service appear dependent or approach dependence in the Ross-Loos population: physician visits (r = .094) and ancillary care (r = .072) approach significance, while appliances (r = .109) is significant. For the San Joaquin Foundation population, the r_{y_ix} for all uninsured services appear independent.

Similarly, the income elasticities for the three above-mentioned services in the Ross-Loos population do not approach zero: for physician visits, the income elasticity is equal to .7401 and approaches significance $(b_{y_ix}/(b_{y_ix})$ = 3.02); for ancillary care, the income elasticity is 1.234 and also approaches significance $(b_{y_ix}/(b_{y_ix})$ = 2.35). For appliances, the income elasticity is 1.759 and is significant $(b_{y_ix}/(b_{y_ix})$ = 3.56).

In the San Joaquin Foundation population the income elasticities for all uninsured services approach zero.

Discussion

When insured populations utilize insured outpatient services (regardless of the comprehensiveness of coverage), it appears that: 1) an independent relationship exists between use and income, and 2) the income elasticities for outpatient health services approach zero (i.e., changes in income have no effect on consumption). This finding applies equally in two different health insurance plans.

For uninsured outpatient services, the results of the two sample populations are dissimilar. The population at the San Joaquin Foundation exhibits an independent relationship between use and income, with income elasticities approaching zero. The Ross-Loos population results, by contrast, suggest that for three out of the four categories of uninsured services, income and use are dependent, with income elasticities of over .7 for each.

Insured Services

The income elasticities approach zero and income and use are independent, with one exception, for all insured services. The one exception, physical examination for an adult *with* a presenting illness, would seem to be atypical in the light of results on all other insured care. The finding is explicable perhaps by the fact that only 44 such services occurred for the full year's period. More importantly, when correlation coefficients and income elasticities are computed for only those individuals that used insured services, physical examination, adult *with* presenting illness, becomes independent of income, and the income elasticities approach zero.

The possible reasons for the above findings are numerous. The most plausible, however, is that since the apparent market price of an outpatient service approaches zero when that service is insured, price no longer acts as a rationing device and income will not, of itself, have any effect on the demand for medical services. Although it can be correctly argued that coverage for the insured service is not complete and that considerable opportunity costs are involved in obtaining the care, it is clear from a reading of the insurance contracts for both plans that the price of the insured service is being reduced to a considerable extent.

Another possible explanation might be that involvement in a prepaid plan convinces many individuals that they are "losing money" if they do not use the services for which they have paid. Since the insurance premium does not discriminate against income groups, this would also result in independence between income and use.

The similarity of results for insured services in the two plans is especially noteworthy because the two medical care delivery systems involved are fundamentally different. One might suspect that the above conclusions can be generalized to still other populations covered by health insurance.

Uninsured Services

Unlike insured services, the relationship between use and income are different for the San Joaquin Foundation and Ross-Loos populations.

Considering the Ross-Loos population first, use and income were dependent for physician visits, ancillary care, and appliances; with income elasticities of .74, 1.23, and 1.76, respectively. The income elasticities for the three services demonstrate that changes in income do affect changes in demand for these uninsured services. For appliances, the consumer will increase his demand at a greater percentage rate than his increase in income; for ancillary care, at a percentage only slightly higher than the increase in income; for physician visits, at a percentage somewhat less than the increase in income.

The reasons for the differing levels of these income elasticities are the same reasons applicable to any study of this measure: the different prices of the three services, the price of competing goods, and personal preference patterns.

The Ross-Loos results are especially relevant and intuitively appealing because they approximate what other investigators, such as Paradiso and P. Feldstein have found to be the relationships between income and use for the general population (where the majority of outpatient care is uninsured). Most noteworthy, perhaps, is the finding that the income elasticity for physician visits is .74, which is close to the income elasticity computed by Feld-

stein (.6) from 1958 household interview data.

Parenthetically, a regression of each of the three services against per capita income in its linear and squared form suggests that the income elasticity for each of the services starts at high levels and declines as income increases. This is in contradiction to Stigler's work, and suggests that further study of income elasticities for medical care products in the national marketplace is called for.

Considering the San Joaquin Foundation population, it would be consistent to assume that data for uninsured services would be similar to both the Ross-Loos results on uninsured services and estimates provided for the general population. However, as can be seen, such is not the case. As with insured services, income and use are independent and the income elasticities approach zero in this population.

The primary reason for this finding are the financial constraints applicable to obtaining insured services in Stockton and the already demonstrated independent relationship between use and income for insured services. The most important of the financial constraints involves a dependent's coverage for physician office visits. From an analysis of the San Joaquin Foundation insurance contract for the study population, it appears that in order for a dependent to be covered for physician office visits (excluding visits resulting from accidental injury) an initial visit must first be fully paid for by the patient. As a result the Foundation provides, under insurance, a heavy preponderance of follow-up office visits. Approximately 52 percent of the total output provided per person in the San Joaquin plan is composed of follow-up visits as opposed to 16 percent of the output per person at Ross-Loos.

Given then an independent relationship between income and use for insured services and also given the fact that in many cases uninsured services are utilized to obtain eligibility for insured care, it seems logical that in Stockton the pattern of utilization for uninsured services should closely mirror that for insured care. If, on the other hand, the use of uninsured services had no effect on the ability to receive insured care, such a relationship would not be expected.

An example of the latter situation is found at Ross-Loos. Here, in our sample population, the consumption of uninsured services has no bearing on an individual's ability to obtain insured care. Hence it is reasonable to expect that income elasticities for uninsured services will approach national levels—and such is indeed the case.

Speculations from Results

The results of this study suggest the following generalizations. First, income elasticities of demand for outpatient uninsured care will approach zero in any insurance scheme in which the use of uninsured care is undertaken to enable the individual to obtain insured care. Such behavior by the patient (or system) implies, however, that the dollar imputed benefits received from the insured care considerably offset the cost of the uninsured services necessary to qualify for insured care. In the San Joaquin Foundation population such apparently is the case. Under other insurance plans this might not necessarily follow, however.

Second, and conversely, where use of uninsured services bears no relationship to insured services, it is reasonable to expect that the income elasticities for outpatient uninsured service will approach the general market conditions (where presently the majority of outpatient care is not compensated for by health insurance).

Summary

The relationship between income and the use of outpatient medical care services in two insured populations has been analyzed. Income is considered in terms of per capita income, services in terms of 23 discrete categories of outpatient care. Using correlation coefficients and income elasticities, it has been found that for insured services, there is an independent relationship between income and use. Given the large differences in the delivery systems of the two insurance plans under study, it has been hypothesized that such a relationship could extend to all insured populations.

For uninsured services, it has been found that a dependent relationship exists between income and use in one plan, but not another. In the plan where the dependent relationship exists, the income elasticities approach levels found for the general population. In the plan where an independent relationship exists between income and use of uninsured services, it has been suggested that this is because the use of such services is necessary in order to obtain valuable insured services and because the income elasticities of insured services approach zero.

References

1 U.S. National Center for Health Statistics. Vital and Health Statistics, Series 10, No. 18, June, 1965, "Volume of Physician Visits, United States, July 1963-June 1964" (Washington, D.C.: U.S. Public Health Service, 1965).

2 McNerney, Walter J., *et al. Hospital and Medical Economics*, 2 Vols. (Chicago: Hospital Research and Educational Trust, 1962).

3 Stigler, George J. *The Theory of Price* (New York: Macmillan, 1952).

4 Dewhurst, Frederic J., *et al. America's Needs and Resources* (New York: The Twentieth Century Fund, 1947).

5 Feldstein, Paul I., and Severson, Ruth M. "The Demand for Medical Care," in *Report of the Commission on the Cost of Medical Care*, Vol. 1 (Chicago: American Medical Association, 1964).

6 Columbia University School of Public Health and Administrative Medicine. *Family Medical Care*

Under Three Types of Health Insurance (New York: 1962).

7 Anderson, Odin W., and Sheatsley, Paul B. *Comprehensive Medical Insurance—A Study of Costs, Use, and Attitudes Under Two Plans.* Research Series 9 (New York: Health Insurance Foundation, 1959).

8 Darsky, Benjamin J., *et al. Comprehensive Medical Services Under Voluntary Health Insurance. A Study of Windsor Medical Services* (Cambridge, Massachusetts: Howard University Press, 1958).

9 Sasuly, Richard, and Hopkins, Carl E. "A Medi-

cal Society-Sponsored Comprehensive Medical Care Plan. The Foundation for Medical Care of San Joaquin County, California," *Medical Care*, Vol. 5, No. 4 (July-August, 1967).

10 Kisch, Arnold I., and Viseltear, Arthur J. *The Ross-Loos Medical Group*, Medical Care Administration—Case Study No. 3 (Washington, D.C.: U.S. Public Health Service, 1967).

11 Kovner, Joel W. *A Production Function for Outpatient Medical Facilities* (unpublished Ph.D. dissertation, University of Michigan, 1968, available University Microfilms).

Glenn Wilson
James W. Begun

Trends in Physicians' Patient Volume

Reprinted with permission of the Blue Cross Association, from *Inquiry:* Vol.XIV, No.2, pp.171-175. Copyright © 1977 by the Blue Cross Association.

Observers of the national health care delivery system have long held the hope that improvements in physician productivity will alleviate pressures for increasing the supply of physicians. The federal government has argued that since "we shall never have all the physician manpower we need," improvements in physician productivity are essential.[1,2,3] Several studies review and evaluate various methods of increasing physician productivity.[4,5,6,7] Fein has argued that "Improvement in America's consumption of health services requires increases in productivity."[8] By "increases in productivity," the federal government and researchers usually refer to increases in the quantity of patients seen by physicians in a given amount of time. Observers generally assert that in recent decades physician productivity, as measured by numbers of patient visits, has increased.[9,10,11]

This paper will present data on patient visits from 1959 to 1974 which question the assertion that physicians' patient volume has increased in the long run. The data then will be examined in the context of the macro-level model shown in Figure I. The variables in Figure I, shown as causes of physicians' patient volume, technology and support workers per physician, derive from economic theory of manpower productivity. The variable "physician income" is, of course, only one outcome of physicians' patient volume. It is a particularly relevant one in economic terms, because physicians' earnings have been increasing at a fast pace.

Glenn Wilson, M.A. is Professor of Medical Economics and Associate Dean of the School of Medicine, and **James W. Begun** is a doctoral student at the University of North Carolina (Chapel Hill, NC 27514).

The variable of main concern here is "physicians' patient volume." Data measuring this variable are presented in the next section.

Trends in Patient Volume

Estimates of total visits to physicians in the United States are prepared annually based on household interview data from the National Health Survey; these data are commonly used to examine trends in physician visits per person. The data, however, also are valuable as a longitudinal indicator of the quantity of outpatient contacts by physicians, since data on patient visits from the National Health Survey are available, for selected years, from 1959 to the present. The data are collected from a representative sample of the civilian, non-institutionalized population. A physician visit is defined as a consultation in person or by telephone with a physician for examination, diagnosis, treatment, or advice. The service can be provided either by the physician himself or by a nurse or another person acting under the physician's supervision.

Problems of reliability and comparability of the data over time are discussed in several National Health Survey publications.[12] Sampling errors for the data used here are very small because of the large size of the estimates. Respondent error in reporting physician visits does exist, but ". . . reporting of physician visits is subject to substantial underreporting as well as overreporting, which, to an undetermined extent, tend to compensate for each other."[13]

Changes have been made over time in data collection methods which make the physician visit data not perfectly comparable. In 1964, a few more "recall" questions were employed than in 1959, which probably increased the

Table 1.   Estimated patient contacts of non-federal patient care physicians, selected years 1959–1974

(1) Year	(2) National Health Survey Visits	(3) Inpatient Days	(2) + (3) = (4) Total Patient Contacts	(5) Total Non-federal Patient Care Physicians	(4) ÷ (5) = (6) Total Patient Contacts per Physician
1959	813,412,000	168,526,800	981,938,800	198,489	4,947
1964	844,347,000	200,099,900	1,044,446,900	216,473	4,825
1967	829,622,000	224,000,400	1,053,622,400	230,827	4,565
1968	815,324,000	229,118,400	1,044,442,400	238,481	4,380
1969	839,605,000	234,508,200	1,074,113,200	247,508	4,340
1970	926,926,000	239,866,400	1,166,792,400	255,027	4,575
1971	999,289,000	241,136,000	1,240,425,000	263,730	4,703
1972	1,016,548,000	243,138,300	1,259,686,300	269,095	4,681
1973	1,031,010,000	247,735,800	1,278,745,800	272,850	4,687
1974	1,025,340,000	256,955,400	1,282,295,400	278,517	4,604

Sources: Column 2 data are from: United States National Center for Health Statistics. "Current Estimates from the National Health Survey," *Vital and Health Statistics* Series 10, No. 52 (p. 24), No. 60 (p. 22), No. 63 (p. 23), No. 72 (p. 25), No. 79 (p. 26), No. 85 (p. 26), No. 95 (p. 26), No. 100 (p. 25); and "Physician Visits," *Vital and Health Statistics* Series 10, No. 18, p. 13. Column 3 data are from: American Hospital Association. *JAHA Guide Issue*, 1975 edition, p. 18, and 1960 edition, p. 365. "Inpatient days" is number of admissions multiplied by average length of stay for non-federal, short-term general and other special hospitals. Column 5 data are from: American Medical Association. *Distribution of Physicians in the U.S.* (Chicago), 1964–1974 editions. Physician totals are dated 12/31. 1964 and 1967 totals are decreased 7.4% from published figures due to 1968 classification change in non-federal patient care physicians in the U.S., from 257,674 to 238,481. See Theodore, C. N., Haug J. N., Balfe B. E., et al. *Reclassification of Physicians, 1968* (Chicago: American Medical Associaton, 1971), pp. 158–177. 1959 figure estimated at 76.2% of 6/30/60 total physicians (260,484) from 1973 edition of *Distribution of Physicians in the U.S.*, p. 37. 76.2% is percentage of total physicians in 1964 counted here as non-federal patient care. Actual 12/31/59 total of non-federal patient care physicians is probably somewhat lower, and thus "total patient contacts per physician" somewhat higher. Patient care physician totals for 1970–1974 are underestimates—see footnote 16.

reported numbers of physician visits.[14] After 1964 more specific questions were asked regarding the date of the physician visit, eliminating some reported visits.[15] The differences are not great enough, however, to affect the trend in patient contacts discussed here.

Table 1 shows that the volume of patient visits has increased about 26% between 1959 and 1974, while at the same time the number of patient care physicians has expanded some 40%.[16] But before concluding that the quantity of patient contacts per physician has declined, the National Health Survey data should be supplemented, because the National Health Survey definition of "patient visit" excludes inpatient hospital contacts with physicians. Inpatient hospital contacts by physicians can be estimated by assuming one physician visit for every inpatient hospital day in short-term hospitals in the United States. Table 1 provides the resulting estimate of total patient contacts, both in- and outpatient, for years for which data on pa-

tient visits are available from the National Health Survey. The data in Table 1 indicate that since 1959 there definitely has been no trend toward a higher volume of patient contacts per physician. It should be noted that the trend exhibited in Table 1 would not be upward even if the assumption of one-half, or two, or three physician visits per inpatient day had been made.

The Department of Health, Education and Welfare recently has taken note of the decline in N.H.S.-reported visits per physician for the years 1971 to 1974. HEW refers to this as a decline in "primary care" by the average physician and speculates that it could be due to an "increase in the average time duration of physician contacts, or to a shortening by physicians of the average number of hours devoted to ambulatory patient contacts."[17] The 1959–1974 data in Table 1 indicate that the absence of an increase in patient contacts per physician is a longer range trend.

What the Findings Indicate

Three factors would lead us to anticipate that patient contacts per physician would have increased, rather than decreased, over the past several years. First, allied medical personnel per 100,000 population increased from 92 to 261 between 1950 and 1970, much faster than physicians per 100,000 population. The number of allied medical personnel per physician has grown substantially, from 0.64 to 1.65, over the same time period. Nursing personnel per 100,000 population also have shown increases much larger than that of physicians per 100,000 population. Thus, the number of registered nurses per physician rose from 1.71 to 2.16 between 1950 and 1970.[18]

Second, medical technology has grown significantly in recent years. New drugs, modes of therapy, chemical tests, machines, and procedures have been developed in the past 20 years. Traditional economic theory argues, and it has historically been the case, that new technologies commonly result in time-saving or labor-saving changes in production.

The third reason which might suggest that patient contacts per physician should be increasing is that physician earnings have risen faster than the cost of living. This third factor we would expect to be a result, not a cause, of increased patient contacts per physician. Between 1960 and 1970 the Consumer Price Index averaged a 2.7% annual increase, compared to 5.2% for self-employed physicians' earnings.[19] Between 1950 and March, 1974, the Consumer Price Index rose by 98%, compared to 170% for its medical care component and 168% for the physicians' fees part of the medical component.[20] Again, traditional economic theory would argue that increased compensation is often a result of increased service.

As Table 1 indicates, however, the number of patient contacts by the average physician has not shown an increase. This trend, along with the trends in physician earnings and allied health manpower, can all be explained by the argument that the technological sophistication and specialization of care has more than offset any improvements in physicians' patient volume.

First let us examine the case of increased earnings of physicians. Because medicine has a recognized status in America as an independent profession, internal professional controls are expected to determine prices, in response to supply and demand. The demand for medical care has hardly been saturated thus far, though, so physicians are able to increase fees with little danger of reducing demand. Thus, physicians who feel that the quality of their services is improved by more specialized knowledge and technology can be expected to have no hesitancy about raising fees.

Why have not increased numbers of allied medical personnel per physician increased the patient volume of the average physician? First, it is significant that the vast majority of the occupations classified as "allied medical" are located primarily in hospitals, such as dieticians, physical therapists, and radiologic technicians. A large percentage of the nursing personnel, of course, also is concentrated in the institutional sector. In 1930, less than one-third of health workers were located in hospitals or other institutions; today nearly two-thirds are.[21] Hospital personnel per 100 census have increased from 178 in 1950 to 326 in 1974.[22] The proliferation of job categories among these workers is even more astounding. More than 600 primary and alternate job titles for health professions are listed in the 1974 edition of *Health Resources Statistics*.[23] The following brief report illustrates the point:

> Greater New York Blue Cross . . . recently sent a form to its member hospitals asking them to enter the number of people in different jobs. The form listed 280 titles, excluding physicians. A typical medium-sized, general-care hospital with 300 beds employs 1,000 people. If the 280 job titles were equally distributed among this workforce, there would be fewer than four people in each category. Even with the technological complexity of modern medicine, one is hard put to imagine 280 different and distinct tasks to be performed. There is necessarily considerable overlap in the work done by different people with different titles, incomes and status.[24]

Due to the institutional concentration and role specialization of allied health workers, the

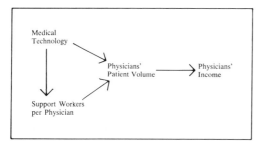

Figure I.   Conceptual model for discussion of patient volume trends

increased ratio of support workers to physicians has not contributed to greater efficiency (time-wise) in the delivery of patient visits. Instead, the personnel are contributing to the delivery of more technical and specialized medical care.

Finally, let us turn to the technological improvements in health care delivery. Again, an emphasis on technical specialization over quantity of services is evident. Facilities and services which were rare or non-existent in 1950, such as the electroencephalograph, renal dialysis and open heart surgery, are now available in large numbers and require substantial additions of manpower. In most industries new technologies often decrease costs and increase the quantity of goods produced, but in the health care sector this does not seem to be the case. Health care does not resemble a "mass production" industry in this respect.

Conclusions

Data on patient contacts per physician from 1959–1974 have been presented. Based on the simplified conceptual model shown in Figure I, we would have expected patient volume to increase. Contrary to expectations, patient volume has not increased. Our discussion suggests that any increases in patient volume have been more than offset by increases in the specialization of care.

It is difficult to draw implications from changes in the macro-level data and from the conceptual discussion presented here. Nevertheless, the data add weight to the contention that Americans have been paying for more specialized care rather than increased availability of basic primary care. The data also suggest that efforts to increase physician "productivity" in terms of the volume of patient visits may be more than offset by advances in technology that increase the specialization of care rendered. The decrease in patient contacts per physician between 1959 and 1974 represents a "loss" of the services of the equivalent of about 21,000 full-time physicians in 1974.

It is very likely that the increased specialization of care has resulted in higher quality service to the consumer of healh services. At some point, however, the trade-off between cost and specialization of care must be addressed. We suggest that this point is not only with us now but has been for some time.

References and Notes

1 Stewart, William H. "Medical Education and the Community," *Medical Annals of the District of Columbia* 35:417 (August 1966).

2 U.S. Department of Labor. *Manpower Report of the President* (Washington: Government Printing Office, March 1972), p. 131.

3 U.S. Department of Health, Education and Welfare. *Toward a Systematic Analysis of Health Care in the United States* (Washington: Government Printing Office, October 1972), pp. 11–14.

4 Hiestand, Dale L. "Research into Manpower for Health Service," in John B. McKinlay, ed., *Economic Aspects of Health Care* (New York: PRODIST, 1973), pp. 223–256.

5 Kehrer, Barbara H. and Zaretsky, Henry W. "Utilization of Allied Health Personnel in Medical Practice,"

in Robert J. Walsh *et al.*, eds., *The Profile of Medical Practice* (Chicago: American Medical Association, 1972), pp. 127–133.

6 Reinhardt, Uwe E. "Manpower Substitution and Productivity in Medical Practice: Review of Research," *Health Services Research* 8:200–227 (Fall 1973).

7 Golladay, Frederick L., Miller, Marianne, and Smith, Kenneth R. "Allied Health Manpower Strategies: Estimates of the Potential Gains from Efficient Task Delegation," *Medical Care* 11: 457–469 (November–December, 1973).

8 Fein, Rashi. The Doctor Shortage (Washington: The Brookings Institution, 1967), p. 149.

9 *Ibid.*, p. 92.

10 Klarman, Herbert E. *The Economics of Health* (New York: Columbia University Press, 1965), p. 81.

11 The number of patient visits per physician is not really a measure of physician productivity because it takes into account only one dimension of that multi-dimensional concept. In particular, the quality of the patient visit is completely ignored. Therefore the work "productivity" will not be used in the discussion of patient visits per physician below.

12 U.S. Department of Health, Education and Welfare. "Physician Visits," *Vital and Health Statistics* Series 10, Nos. 18, 75, 97.

13 *Ibid.,* No. 97, p.3.

14 *Ibid.,* No. 18, p.2.

15 *Ibid.,* No. 75, p. 3.

16 1959-1974 growth in patient care physicians is probably underestimated due to 1969—1974 increase in the number of physicians "not classified," from 0 to 20,343. Many of the "not classified" physicians are probably patient care. See American Medical Association, *Distribution of Physicians in the U.S.* (Chicago), 1969—1974 editions.

17 U.S. Department of Health, Education and Welfare. *Forward Plan for Health, FY 1977—81,* DHEW Publication No. (OS) 76-50024 (Washington: Government Printing Office, August 1975), p. 11.

18 Russell, L. B., Bourque B. B., Bourque D. P. and Burke, Carol S. *Federal Health Spending* 1969—1974. (Washington: National Planning Association, 1974) p. 27.

19 U.S. Department of Health, Education and Welfare. *Medical Care Expenditures, Prices, and Costs: Background Book.* DHEW Publication No. (SSA) 74-11909 (Washington: Government Printing Office, 1973), pp. 54—55.

20. U.S. Bureau of the Census. *Statistical Abstract of the U.S.: 1974* (Washington: Government Printing Office, 1974), pp. 68, 411—412.

21 Caress, Barbara. "Health Manpower," *Health/Pac Bulletin* 62:8, (January—February, 1975).

22 American Hospital Association. JAHA *Guide Issue,* 1975 edition (Chicago, 1975), p. 18.

23 U.S. Department of Health, Education and Welfare. *Health Resources Statistics, 1974,* DHEW Publication No. (HRA) 75-1509 (Washington: Government Printing Office, 1974), p. 3.

24 Caress, "Health Manpower," p. 8.

W. John Carr
Paul J. Feldstein

The Relationship of Cost to Hospital Size

Reprinted with permission of the Blue Cross Association, from *Inquiry*: Vol.IV, No.2, pp.45-65. Copyright © 1967 by the Blue Cross Association.

Originally Published in June 1967

The primary purpose of this study is to estimate the net, or independent, effect of hospital size upon the cost of providing care. In the process, estimates of the approximate effects of a number of other factors upon cost are also derived. The results indicate that, other things being held approximately equal, average cost per patient day falls initially as size is increased because of the economies associated with the use of specialized personnel and equipment and then probably rises at very large size levels due to increased managerial problems of communication and control. Apparently, the greater the capability of a hospital to provide a wide range of diversified services, the more rapidly average cost initially falls with increased size.

The study was undertaken by applying multiple regression analysis to data from 3,147 U.S. voluntary short-term general hospitals collected by the American Hospital Association. The variables utilized in the study were: total cost, hospital size, number of services provided, number of outpatient visits, whether or not the hospital had a nursing school, number of

student nurses, number of different types of internship and residency programs, number of interns and residents, whether or not the hospital was affiliated with a medical school, and average wage rate. An initial analysis was undertaken by using data from all of the hospitals in the study. Separate analyses were then conducted for five groups of hospitals in order to determine the effect of differences in the capability of hospitals to provide a wide range of service upon the cost-size relationship.

An enormous amount of work has already been dedicated to the achievement of an efficient distribution of hospital facilities. But this is a task that can never be completed. Shifts in the size and distribution of the population, variations in the prevalence of disease, disability, and pregnancy, and changes in medical technology continuously alter the optimum number, size, and geographic distribution of hospitals.

At first glance, it may appear that each case for areawide planning demands a unique approach since conditions in individual communities, and even in the same community over time, are of such a varied nature. Although it has been recognized that hospital planning is best undertaken on a local level, enough common ground has been found, however, to make the development of general guidelines and principles worthwhile.[1]

W. John Carr is Research Associate, John Fitzgerald Kennedy School of Government, Harvard University, and **Paul J. Feldstein** is Associate Professor, Program in Hospital Administration, the University of Michigan.

The work on which this article is based was performed by the American Hospital Association under a contract with the U.S. Public Health Service, Division of Hospital and Medical Facilities. Funds were also provided by Community Health Project Grant #CH-00236-01. The authors would like to thank Ann Morton for her editorial assistance.

[1] For this reason, the American Hospital Association and the U.S. Public Health Service have issued reports embodying principles ap-

The major purpose of this study is to describe and estimate one of the fundamental relationships which underlies the apparent diversity of individual planning situations—namely, the effect of hospital size upon the cost of providing care. Because our results can be most meaningfully understood and applied within the more comprehensive theoretical structure of areawide planning, we shall devote some attention to determining their position within this broader framework.[2] In this brief discussion, emphasis will be placed upon planning as it relates to the inpatient care functions of hospitals while matters of outpatient care, teaching, and research will be largely ignored.

THE RELATIONSHIP OF HOSPITAL COST TO AREAWIDE PLANNING

When viewed from a comprehensive standpoint, the areawide planning prob-

lem can be divided into two major parts. First, what is the need or demand for hospital services in a given area, and, second, what distribution of facilities and personnel will most efficiently provide the care to be utilized.[3]

It has been increasingly recognized that certain socio-demographic and economic characteristics of the population have an important effect upon both the need and demand for hospital care and ought to be taken into account in planning. Quantitative estimates of the independent effects of these factors may be applied to projected population measures in order to forecast levels of need or demand for an entire planning area.[4]

Given the level of demand or need, one is faced with the problem of determining the optimal distribution of hospital resources. This problem may be divided into three interrelated parts: (1) what is the best distribution of various types of personnel and facilities among hospitals, (2) what are the optimal sizes (and number) of these institutions, and (3) what is the optimal locational pattern for hospitals. Finding the answer to any one of these questions involves the simultaneous determination of the answers to each of the others and, in addition, the simultaneous de-

plicable to the organization and operation of areawide planning agencies. See, particularly, Joint Committee of the American Hospital Association and Public Health Service, *Areawide Planning for Hospitals and Related Health Facilities* (Public Health Service Publication No. 855 [Washington, D.C.: U.S. Government Printing Office, 1961]), and U.S. Public Health Service, *Procedures for Areawide Health Facility Planning, A Guide for Planning Agencies* (Public Health Service Publication No. 930-B-3 [Washington, D.C.: U.S. Government Printing Office, 1963]).

[2] Economic characteristics of the medical care field which suggest the need for planning (or some other form of market intervention), as opposed to substantial reliance upon market mechanisms to allocate resources among hospitals, are pointed out in M. W. Reder, "Some Problems in the Economics of Hospitals," *American Economic Review*, Vol. 55, No. 2 (May, 1965), pp. 472-480, and Burton A. Weisbrod, "Some Problems of Pricing and Resource Allocation in a Nonprofit Industry—The Hospitals," *Journal of Business*, Vol. 38, No. 1 (January, 1965), pp. 18-28.

It should be noted that hospital care is only one of many components, or factors, used in the production of medical care and that to some extent these components are substitutable. This means that hospital planning should not be considered in isolation from the rest of the medical care system. See Paul J. Feldstein, "Research on the Demand for Health Services," *Milbank Memorial Fund Quarterly*, Vol. 44, No. 3, Part 2 [Health Services Research 1] (New York: The Milbank Memorial Fund, July, 1966), pp. 128-165.

[3] By demand, we mean the amount of care for which persons are willing and able to pay. Given the distribution of income, need may be defined as the amount of service (including prepayment or insurance) which fully informed, or knowledgeable, consumers would purchase plus any amount arising from external benefits to other members of society. The use of a need criterion of this sort within the context of hospital planning raises certain practical problems. In particular, although it may be possible to reduce demand which exceeds need by some means, such as the establishment of utilization review committees, building facilities to serve needs which are not reflected in demand may only result in underutilization.

[4] Empirical estimates of the net effects of various socio-demographic and economic characteristics upon hospital utilization may be found in Gerald D. Rosenthal, *The Demand for General Hospital Facilities* (Chicago: American Hospital Association, 1964), and Rosson L. Cardwell, Margaret G. Reid, and Max Shain, *Hospital Utilization in a Major Metropolitan Area* (Chicago: Hospital Planning Council for Metropolitan Chicago, 1964).

termination of the quantity demanded or needed.[5] Since no satisfactory method for the simultaneous solution of this problem is yet available, and because of their limited powers to initiate change, areawide planners have proceeded by seeking the optimal solutions to a series of partial alterations in the systems for which they are responsible. While there is no guarantee that this process will converge upon an optimum distribution of resources for the entire system, some inefficiencies should be avoided.

The Cost-Size Relationship

For the present, we shall ignore these difficulties and concentrate our attention upon the effect of hospital size and other factors on the cost of providing care and, in turn, upon the general relationship of these considerations to the optimal distribution of facilities and personnel among hospitals and the determination of optimal hospital sizes and locations. Let us first consider the independent effect of size upon cost, given the capability of a hospital to produce "products" (diagnoses and treatments) of various sorts and the mix and quality of products actually produced.

Economists have distinguished certain factors which make the production of products and services more economical as the size of an organization is increased and others which cause efficiency to decline with larger size. Two important factors which make large scale production of products and services more economical are the gains obtained from the use of more highly specialized personnel and the economies associated with the more extensive use of large or specialized equipment.[6] Off-

FIGURE I

Cost per Patient Day in Relation to Hospital Size

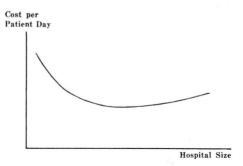

setting these advantages is the greater proportion of time and effort required to coordinate and control work in large organizations.

In general, for sufficiently small outputs, efficiency increases with size because the advantages that accrue from the use of specialized labor and equipment far outweigh the increased cost of management. As size increases, however, the reduction in per-unit cost afforded by greater and greater specialization begins to decline and is eventually outweighed by increased costs of coordination and control.[7] Other things being equal, hospital cost per patient day may thus be expected to decline initially and then rise as size is increased as shown by the U-shaped curve in Figure I.

---

[5] This is the case because, according to the above definitions, the quantity of care demanded or needed is dependent upon economic factors, including price (which, in turn, should reflect cost).

[6] In addition, dealing with large quantities of supplies may result in savings from low record handling costs, quantity discounts, re-

duced per-unit freight costs, and relatively low inventory requirements.

To some extent, small hospitals may circumvent the various diseconomies associated with their size by purchasing auxiliary services from outside firms. For example, 40 percent of voluntary short-term general and other special hospitals with less than 200 beds had their laundry service provided by cooperative ventures and outside firms whereas only 11 percent of similar hospitals with 200 or more beds entered into such arrangements. Source: *Hospitals*, Vol. 38, No. 15, Part 2 (August 1, 1964), p. 516.

[7] For an extensive discussion of factors affecting the cost-size relationship, see E. A. G. Robinson, *The Structure of Competitive Industry* (Chicago: University of Chicago Press, 1958).

FIGURE II

Cost of Basic Care and of a Specialized Service per Patient Day in Relation to Hospital Size

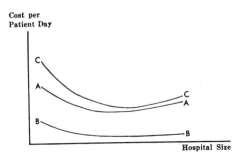

FIGURE III

Hospital and Travel Cost per Patient Day in Relation to Hospital Size

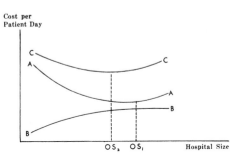

Service Capability and Cost

Let us now turn to the question of the effects of differences in the capability of hospitals to produce different types of care and in the mix of services they actually provide upon cost. For simplicity, we may conceive of a hospital as producing both a component of basic care (room, board, and routine nursing care) and a number of distinct, specialized services. In general, there may be economies associated with the large scale production of each individual service as well as with the provision of basic care. In Figure II, line AA indicates the cost of providing basic care in relation to hospital size and line BB the cost of providing a fixed average number of units of a given specialized service per patient day in relation to size. From line CC, which indicates the sum of these costs, we may infer that, other things being equal, the greater the number of specialized services provided: (1) the higher the level of average cost per patient day at any given size and (2) the more rapidly over-all average cost initially falls with increased size.[8]

A second factor affecting the relationship between the provision of individual

services, average cost, and the degree of economies of scale is the extent to which each service is utilized, on the average, by hospital patients. In general, more extensive utilization of a service per patient day will result in higher average costs at any given size level. However, it is not possible to determine the effect of the degree to which services are utilized upon the rapidity of the fall in average cost as size increases without knowledge of the shapes of the relevant cost curves.

Costs External to the Hospital

Determination of the optimum allocation of hospital resources involves consideration of both the costs incurred by hospitals themselves and the costs associated with hospitalization which are borne by patients, visitors, and the hospital staff. Perhaps the most obvious external cost is travel cost, measured in terms of both dollar outlay and the psychological cost of time consumed.

In any given community, average travel cost per patient day will depend upon a complex array of factors such as the geographic distribution of hospitals of various types, the distribution and characteristics of the population, and the configuration of travel routes. In general, however, it is safe to assume if the sizes of hospitals were increased (with constant utilization rates), their geographic service areas

---

[8] The provision of additional services may also accentuate the rise in average cost due to managerial problems at large size levels because of the greater organizational complexity involved.

would expand and, consequently, average travel cost would rise.[9] In Figure III, line AA represents the relationship of average cost per patient day incurred by the hospital to the size of the institution, line BB represents average travel cost, and line CC indicates their sum. Note that the optimum size of a hospital is reduced (from OS_1 to OS_2) when travel cost is taken into account.

From the foregoing discussion, it is evident that both the scope of services offered and the cost of travel affect the optimum size (and, thus, number and location) of hospitals and ought to be taken into account in planning.[10] In this study, only the costs incurred by hospitals, and reflected in their accounts, will be analyzed.[11] Once the relationship between hospital costs and size is known, however, the effects of other factors can be readily brought into consideration.

[9] In addition to travel cost, account should be taken of possible increases in morbidity and mortality arising directly from the time it takes to get to hospitals.

[10] In addition, the relationship of costs to short-run variations in demand should be considered by those engaged in areawide planning. To some extent, the cost of maintaining "standby" facilities and personnel may be offset by delaying or discouraging admissions, releasing patients sooner than usual, shifting patients or "swing beds" among departments within a hospital, or by centrally allocating patients to hospitals. See Millard F. Long, "Efficient Use of Hospitals" in *The Economics of Health and Medical Care* (Ann Arbor, Mich.: The University of Michigan, 1964), pp. 211-226. Each of these methods will affect the cost-size relationship and thus the optimum hospital size as determined by the above analysis. A study in which consideration was given to the effect of both hospital size and short-run variations in demand on hospital and travel cost (for obstetric care in the Chicago area) may be found in Millard Long and Paul Feldstein, "The Economics of Hospital Systems: Peak Loads and Regional Coordination," *American Economic Review* (May, 1967).

[11] A number of other hospital cost studies, with varying objectives, data, and methodologies, have been conducted in the last few years. See Ralph E. Berry, "Returns to Scale in the Production of Hospital Services," to be published in *Health Services Research;* Harold A. Cohen, "Variations in Cost Among Hospitals of Different Sizes," *Southern Economic Journal*, Vol. 33, No. 3 (January, 1967), pp. 355-366; Robert E. Coughlin, *Hospital Complex Analysis: An Approach to Analysis for Planning a Metropolitan System of Service Facilities* (unpublished Doctoral Dissertation, University of Pennsylvania, 1965); Martin S. Feldstein,

METHODOLOGY

Factors Affecting Hospital Cost

In the previous section, we have outlined the basic theory of the cost-size relationship and have pointed out how variations in service capability affect it. A number of additional determinants of hospital cost must, however, be taken into account if statistical measures of the independent effect of size on cost are to be obtained. For the purposes of this study, we need only consider those factors that have a potentially important nonrandom effect. After selecting and classifying these, we shall be better able to adjust for their influence on hospital cost.

The primary long-run determinants of hospital costs, other than size, can be divided into three major groups:

(1) variation in the capability of a hospital to provide different types of care and in the mix of "products" actually produced;

(2) differences in the prices paid for the factors used in production (except to the extent that such prices are affected by size);

(3) variation in the efficiency with which hospitals operate (except to the extent that efficiency depends upon size).

"Hospital Cost Variation and Case-Mix Differences," *Medical Care*, Vol. 3, No. 2 (April-June, 1965), pp. 95-103; Paul J. Feldstein, *An Empirical Investigation of the Marginal Cost of Hospital Services* (Chicago: Graduate Program in Hospital Administration, University of Chicago, 1961); Thomas Fitzpatrick, Symond Gottlieb, and Grover Wirick, "The Nature of Hospital Costs," (Ann Arbor, Mich.: Bureau of Hospital Administration, The University of Michigan, 1964 [mimeo.]); Mary Lee Ingbar and Lester D. Taylor, *Hospital Costs: A Case Study of Massachusetts* (Cambridge, Mass.: Harvard University Press, 1967); and Kong Kyun Ro, *A Statistical Study of Factors Affecting the Unit Cost of Short-Term Hospital Care* (unpublished Doctoral Dissertation, Yale University, 1966); John F. Deeble, "An Economic Analysis of Hospital Cost," *Medical Care*, Vol. 3, No. 3 (July-Sept., 1965), pp. 138-146.

A critical discussion of most of these and some additional cost studies may be found in Judith R. Lave, "A Review of the Methods Used to Study Hospital Costs," *Inquiry*, Vol. 3, No. 2 (May, 1966), pp. 57-81.

1. Mix of Products—There are considerable differences in the type of patient care which hospitals are capable of producing and in the distribution of types of cases for which they normally provide care. This distribution reflects the aggregate demand for various kinds of care in an area and, more importantly, the way in which this demand is apportioned among different hospitals. Also, there are differences in the quality of care hospitals provide for the same medical conditions, both in terms of medical outcomes and in the degree of amenity provided to patients, and these variations affect the costs incurred.[12]

Hospitals operate a number of patient care programs in addition to inpatient service that may have a significant effect upon cost. The most pervasive of these is general outpatient services, but other programs, such as home care, may be of importance in a few cases. Research and educational activities, such as nursing education and internship and residency programs, may also have a fairly substantial effect upon costs, particularly in large institutions.

2. Prices Paid for Factors Used in Production—The prices paid for the factors of production used in providing hospital services can be divided into two major groups: labor inputs and materi-al inputs. The wages paid to hospital employees vary considerably from one region to another and between urban and rural areas.[13] There would appear to be much less variation in the prices of material inputs, although differences in transportation cost may affect the prices of supplies and equipment.

3. Efficiency—Finally, the factors of production may be combined with varying degrees of efficiency to produce a given mix of products. The efficiency attained will depend, in large part, upon the managerial competence of a hospital's administrative staff, the techniques and methods passed down from previous generations of management, the activities of the medical staff, and the nature of the physical plant. In addition, the level of efficiency attained may be affected by the pattern of incentives associated with the form of organization under which the hospital operates (i.e., proprietary, voluntary, governmental).

These three factors — product mix, factor prices, and efficiency—constitute, together with size, the basic categories of long-run cost determinants. In the following statistical analysis, we have used eight measures of service capability and product mix variation because of their potential importance and because of the number of different types of data available. Because of lack of data, the number of factor-price measures used was limited to one—the average wage rate. In view of the relatively small variation expected in material price, however, a price variable covering these factors probably would not have contributed much to the accuracy of the estimates of the cost-size relationship. We were unable to find adequate measures of efficiency for use in the statistical analysis, but this should not be a serious shortcoming. All of the hospitals included in this study are of a single organization type (voluntary nonprof-

[12] In studies of a number of diagnostic conditions based upon data from England and Wales it was found that case-fatality rates are usually higher in non-teaching hospitals. See J. A. H. Lee, S. L. Morrison, and J. N. Morris, "Fatality from Three Common Surgical Conditions in Teaching and Non-teaching Hospitals," *Lancet*, 2 (London: Proprietors, The Lancet, Ltd., October 19, 1957), pp. 785-790, and J. A. H. Lee, S. L. Morrison, and J. N. Morris, "Case-fatality in Teaching and Non-teaching Hospitals," *Lancet*, 2 (London: Proprietors, The Lancet, Ltd., January 16, 1960), pp. 170-171; and L. Lipworth, J. A. H. Lee, and J. N. Morris, "Case-fatality in Teaching and Non-teaching Hospitals 1956-59," *Medical Care*, Vol. 1, No. 2 (April-June, 1963), pp. 71-76. These differences, no doubt, reflect both the distribution of medical resources among hospitals and advantages that arise directly from the educational process. It appears plausible that hospital size and a number of other factors may also affect the quality of care, but it would be very difficult to put weights (e.g. dollar values) on the resulting quality differences even if they were known.

[13] For empirical evidence on the extent of wage rate differences, see Harold A. Cohen, *op. cit.*

it). Thus, to the extent that variations in efficiency are not dependent upon size, they can be considered as largely random in nature.

The Measure of Size

In a study of this type, the variable used as a measure of size is of critical importance. If hospital sizes are over-stated or understated, incorrect conclusions may be reached about the effect of size on cost.

The most obvious measure of hospital size that comes to mind is bed capacity. However, this is not an adequate standard, if size is defined as the average number of patients for whom care can be provided in an optimal manner. Since hospital admissions (and discharges) are to a large extent randomly distributed in time, a hospital administrator must operate his institution, on the average, at a level of occupancy somewhat lower than maximum capacity in order to provide enough space for unforeseen variations in demand. Because the relative degree of variation in census level is greater for small hospitals than it is for large institutions, small hospitals must operate at lower average occupancy than large hospitals to maintain the same probability of having available beds.[14] Thus, using number of beds to measure hospital size overstates the size of small hospitals.[15]

One solution to this problem is to use an adjusted bed size measure, which may be determined by subtracting the average number of unoccupied beds at each size level from reported bed capacity figures. Another solution is to use average daily census (i.e., actual output) as an estimate of size.

Each of these variables is subject to some degree of error as a measure of the capacity of a hospital to provide care for a given average number of patients in an optimal manner. The use of average daily census as a size measure involves the implicit assumption that all of the factors used in producing care, such as building space, equipment, and personnel, have been adjusted to a level appropriate to each hospital's average output. Since utilization cannot be predicted perfectly and because there is an inevitable time lag between changes in average output and the quantity of productive factors utilized, some hospitals will be operating at average output levels for which they were not designed and incurring costs which differ from long-run optimal values.[16] To this extent, average daily census will provide an imperfect measure of size.

Measures based upon the adjusted values of reported bed capacity are also subject to error, however, because of the well-known variations in the criteria which hospitals use in determining what shall be counted as bed capacity. Since yearly average data will be used in the

---

[14] The optimal average occupancy rate also depends upon other considerations such as the number of patient care units into which a hospital is divided and among which patients are not normally transferred. See Mark S. Blumberg, " 'DPF Concept' Helps Predict Bed Needs," *Modern Hospital*, Vol. 97, No. 6 (December, 1961), pp. 75-81.

[15] The standby cost associated with the relatively high proportion of normally unoccupied beds in small hospitals provides an additional reason to expect the existence of economies of scale.

[16] If an output measure which primarily reflects very short-run changes (such as daily census or average daily census computed on a monthly basis) is used, hospitals operating at abnormally high levels of output will have below normal per-unit costs and *vice versa* because of delays in the adjustment of factor inputs. This phenomenon, which is a variant of the so-called regression fallacy, was pointed out by Milton Friedman in "Discussion" in *Business Concentration and Price Policy* (Princeton, N. J.: Princeton University Press, 1955), pp. 230-238. It is discussed further in J. Johnston, *Statistical Cost Analysis* (New York: McGraw-Hill, 1960), pp. 188-192, and A. A. Walters, "Expectations and the Regression Fallacy in Estimating Cost Functions," *Review of Economics and Statistics*, Vol. 42, No. 2 (May, 1960), pp. 210-216. On the other hand, if an output measure covering a relatively long time period is used, hospitals operating at higher than optimal levels of average output may incur average costs that are either above or below the amounts which obtain at optimal average output levels because in short-run equilibrium the factors of production utilized are combined in nonoptimal proportions.

empirical part of this study and because most hospital costs are incurred for factor inputs, supplies and personnel (rather than capital consumption), which can be adjusted over this time span, it appears that average daily census will provide a reasonably accurate measure of size. This variable will therefore be used in the empirical analysis to follow.[17]

Method of Analysis

We have used the statistical technique of multiple regression analysis to estimate the net, or independent, effect of hospital size upon cost per patient day. Estimates of the net effects on cost of each of the other factors included in the analysis were also obtained from application of the regression technique.[18]

In essence, multiple regression analysis consists of deriving estimates of the coefficients of an equation relating a dependent variable (in our case, total cost) to a number of independent variables (in our case, size and other factors believed to affect cost).[19]

---

[17] The wide range of values of size utilized relative to the expected amount of error in average daily census as a measure of size suggests that any biases in measures of the cost-size relationship arising from this source are likely to be relatively small.

Analyses were conducted using adjusted bed capacity as a measure of size, with a separate measure of output variation, but the results (available from the authors upon request) did not differ materially from those based upon the average daily census measure of size.

[18] An introduction to regression analysis can be found in Mordecai Ezekial and Karl A. Fox, *Methods of Correlation and Regression Analysis: Linear and Curvilinear* (3rd edition; New York: John Wiley & Sons, 1959). A more advanced treatment of regression methods, with particular attention to the problems encountered in applying them to economic data, is contained in J. Johnston, *Econometric Methods* (New York: McGraw-Hill, 1963).

[19] Total, rather than average, cost was used in the regression analyses of this study primarily in order to avoid spurious correlation that may arise when data are ratios. Under certain conditions, however, this may not be a very serious problem in cost studies based upon cross-section data. See John R. Meyer and Edwin Kuh, "Correlation and Regression Estimates when the Data Are Ratios," *Econometrica*, Vol, 23, No. 4 (October, 1955), pp. 400-416.

In the analyses to follow, we will utilize an equation of the form:

$$TC = a + b \ (ADC) + c \ (ADC)^2 + d \ (OPV) + \ldots,$$

where TC = total cost, ADC = average daily census, and OPV = number of outpatient visits. Given values of TC, ADC, OPV, and the other variables included in the equation for each of the hospitals included in the analysis, the regression technique, when properly applied, yields estimates of the coefficients (e.g., a, b, and c) which best represent the average net effects of each of the independent variables upon total cost. For example, if the d coefficient turned out to be $6.50, we could say that, on the average, each additional outpatient visit adds about $6.50 to total cost.

There are a number of considerations which should be kept in mind in order to increase the likelihood that application of the regression technique will provide accurate, unbiased measures of the relationships considered. One of these is that each of the factors having a potentially important effect upon the dependent variable (total cost) be included in an equation which correctly represents the relationships which are hypothesized to exist. For example, in the section on the cost-size relationship, we hypothesized that cost per patient day would initially fall and then rise as hospital size increases. In order to determine whether the above equation is capable of representing a relationship of this type, both sides may be divided by (365 × ADC) in order to convert the dependent variable to total cost per patient day (i.e., average cost):

$$TC/PD = (a/365) \ (ADC)^{-1} + b/365 + (c/365) \ ADC + \ldots.$$

Now, if a, b, and c are each positive, the value of the $(a/365) \ (ADC)^{-1}$ term of the equation will fall at a decreasing rate as ADC increases, the value of the b/365 term will remain constant, and the value of the (c/365) ADC term will

FIGURE IV

Relationship of Total Cost per Patient Day to Hospital Size Described by the Terms of a Hypothetical Regression Equation

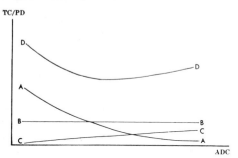

increase at a constant rate, as shown by the lines AA, BB, and CC, respectively, in Figure IV. The sum of the values of these terms of the equation is represented by the U-shaped DD curve in Figure IV, indicating that it is possible for the above total-cost equation to represent the hypothesized relationship between average cost and size.[20] The other variables utilized, and their relationship to total cost will be introduced in the section on empirical analysis.

Another important consideration affecting the accuracy of the regression coefficients is the possibility of errors in the independent variables. This matter has already been discussed with respect to the measure of size, but it should be kept in mind that similar considerations may affect the other variables included in the analysis.

Finally, the regression coefficients derived may differ randomly from their "true" values because they are affected by random errors in the cost data. If all of the important independent variables have been measured with little error and included in a correctly specified mathematical model, however,

meaningful measures of the potential degree of error in the regression coefficients may be calculated. These measures will be introduced in the empirical-analysis section to follow, and conditions which may effect both their accuracy and the efficiency of the regression technique (in terms of minimizing potential random errors in the regression coefficients) will be pointed out.

THE EMPIRICAL RELATIONSHIP OF COST TO HOSPITAL SIZE

Two sets of analyses relating cost to hospital size were conducted. In the first analysis, data from all of the hospitals in the study were used in calculating the coefficients of a regression equation. In the second stage of the study, hospitals with different numbers of facilities, services, and programs were grouped together according to service capability and each group was then analyzed separately in order to detect any substantial differences in the degree of economies of scale. Our expectation was that the greater the capability of a hospital to provide a wide range of diversified services, the more rapidly average cost would initially fall with increased size.

Analysis Based on all Hospitals

The following cost-affecting factors were included in the regression analysis as independent variables.[21]

(1) Hospital size, as measured by average daily census (ADC). In addition, average daily census squared (ADC)[2] was included to

[20] We have implicitly assumed, here, that all of the costs associated with the a term of the total cost equation may be attributed to inpatient care and that none of the other variables included in the equation represent part of the cost-size relationship (i.e., that size is measured exclusively in terms of inpatient care).

[21] Our analyses use 1963 data on 3,147 United States short-term voluntary general hospitals registered by the American Hospital Association and taken from the A.H.A. annual survey of hospitals accepted for registration. Some additional information, relating to internship and residency programs, was derived from the American Medical Association's report on internships and residencies.

allow for the possibility that average cost first falls and then increases with hospital size.

(2) The number of facilities and services available (S).[22] In addition, the number of facilities and services available times average daily census (S × ADC) was included in the regression equation. These measures were intended to reflect a component of long-run cost associated with the provision of specialized services which is relatively constant regardless of size and a component which is relatively constant per patient day, respectively.[23]

(3) The number of outpatient visits (OPV).

Five additional variables were added in order to hold constant the costs associated with operating important research and educational programs:

(4) Existence of a hospital-controlled professional nursing school (NS).

(5) Number of student nurses (N).

(6) Number of types of internship and residency programs offered (IRP).[24]

(7) Number of interns and residents (IR).

(8) Affiliation with a medical school (MS).

In addition to the variables listed above, the level and structure of wage rates may have an important effect upon hospital cost. Because detailed information on geographic differences in the wage rates of hospital employees throughout the United States is not available, it was necessary to use the differences between the average wage rate of the employees of each hospital and the average wage rate of all hospital employees as a basis for adjustment. The adjustment was accomplished by multiplying the number of full-time-equivalent employees in each hospital by the average yearly wage rate paid by all hospitals in order to obtain an adjusted payroll cost figure. This amount was then added to nonpayroll cost to obtain the adjusted total cost (ATC) measure used as a dependent variable in this study.[25]

In addition to taking account of geographic wage-rate differences, this method will effect an adjustment for variations in the average skill level of employees among hospitals. Therefore,

---

[22] This variable consists of a count of the number of facilities and services present in a hospital out of the first 28 listed in *Hospitals*, Vol. 38, No. 15, Part 2 (August 1, 1964), p. 14.

[23] The following qualifications need to be made about variable 2:

(1) Using a count of the number of facilities and services available as a variable involves the assumption that the costs associated with them are approximately equal.

(2) In counting the number of services, we have also made the implicit assumption that the variety of services provided within each service classification and the degree of utilization of each service is constant among hospitals of different sizes. However, it appears plausible that the variety and perhaps the amount of service per patient day rendered within each classification increases with hospital size.

(3) Some of the services listed by the American Hospital Association are not inpatient care units. However, to the extent that their output is correlated with hospital size, the costs incurred in operating them should be adequately held constant by the services variable utilized.

[24] To form this variable, the existence of internship programs, regardless of the number of types, was counted as one and added to a count of the number of different types of residency programs in a hospital out of the 28 listed in *Directory of Approved Internships and Residencies* (Chicago: American Medical Association, 1964), p. 129. In addition, the existence of a cancer program approved by the American College of Surgeons was counted as one and added to the total.

[25] As noted above, we could not make an adjustment for price differences in the other important factors of production (e.g., supplies) because of lack of data. A more refined analysis would also take account of the possibility that differences in the relative prices of the factors of production may cause the proportion in which they are used to vary among hospitals. For an elegant mathematical treatment of this idea, see Marc Nerlove, "Returns to Scale in Electricity Supply," in Carl F. Christ, *et. al., Measurement in Economics* (Stanford, Calif.: Stanford University Press, 1963), pp. 167-198.

there are a few qualifications associated with its use:

(1) The optimal average skill level of employees may be affected to some extent by hospital size. For example, a large hospital may require a greater proportion of supervisory personnel who are paid at above average wage rates. On the other hand, it is also probable that in a large institution there is a greater opportunity to save money by delegating tasks requiring lesser knowledge and skill, thus making more effective use of supervisory and professional manpower. Although these differences are probably small, and will tend to cancel, ideally no adjustment should be made for wage rate differences resulting directly from size.

(2) The optimal average skill level of employees will also be affected by the mix of products produced by a hospital. We would generally want to hold costs associated with variations of this type constant in estimating the cost-size relationship. However, this will result in biases in the coefficients of variables reflecting product-mix variation because, when adjusted, they will indicate only those cost differences resulting from nonpayroll factors and the number of full-time-equivalent personnel utilized.[26]

The results of the regression analysis based upon data from all hospitals are as follows (the size measure has been converted from average daily census to patient days, PD, for ease of comprehension):[27]

$ATC = -\$307,568$

$+ \$0.0000351 \ (PD)^2$
$(\$0.0000029)$
$- \$0.31 \ (S \times PD)$
$(\$0.07)$
$+\$23,188 \ (NS)$
$(\$31,593)$
$+ \$5,034 \ (IR)$
$(\$617)$
$+ \$34.70 \ (PD)$
$(\$1.19)$
$+ \$33,827 \ (S)$
$(\$3,619)$
$+ \$4.81 \ (OPV)$
$(\$0.34)$
$- \$1,805 \ (N)$ $+ \$55,347 \ (IRP)$
$(\$295)$ $(\$5,480)$
$+\$174,796 \ (MS)$
$(\$43,744)$

The following interpretation may be made of the results obtained:

(1) An increase of one patient day raises predicted long-run cost by about $34.70 plus an amount associated with the $(PD)^2$ measure. The coefficient of the $(PD)^2$ measure was statistically significant, suggesting that the relationship between adjusted total cost and size may be curvilinear.

---

[26] In general, we would expect the coefficients of variables representing products which require a high level of skill to be biased downward and *vice versa*. This expectation was borne out in a comparison of regression analyses using total cost and adjusted total cost as dependent variables (available from the authors upon request), but the dependent variable utilized did not substantially affect the estimate of the cost-size relationship.

[27] The regression coefficients shown may differ randomly from their "true" values because of random errors in the cost data. An estimate of the degree of potential error in each regression coefficient arising from this source is indicated by the standard error measure shown in parentheses below it. Subject to the quali-

fications mentioned below, and in the methodology section, we may say, with a 95 percent chance of being correct, that the estimated effect of each variable upon total cost plus or minus about two standard errors describes a range encompassing the true effect.

In general, as hospital size rises, the degree of absolute error in the total cost measure will increase and this condition (a case of heteroscedasticity) will bias the standard errors of the size-related regression coefficients downward. (It will not bias the regression coefficients themselves.) More importantly, heteroscedasticity will result in a loss of efficiency in the estimation of the size-related regression coefficients as compared with estimation based upon average cost data (or, more properly, by means of weighted least squares). For regression analyses covering a rather wide range of sizes, however, the loss of efficiency in terms of the resulting increase in the true standard errors of the regression coefficients will not be inordinately great. See the examples given in J. Johnston, *Econometric Methods* (New York: McGraw-Hill, 1963), pp. 207-211.

The proportion of variation in the dependent variable, adjusted total cost, accounted for by the independent variables is indicated by the coefficient of determination (R^2). For this equation $R^2 = 0.947$.

(2) The average constant component of cost associated with each additional facility or service was estimated at $33,827. However, the coefficient of the (S × PD) measure, which was intended to represent the average increase in cost per patient day per additional service was apparently significantly negative. This unexpected result may have arisen from the high degree of correlation between the (S × PD), PD, and (PD)² measures accompanied by errors in these variables.[28] The average amount of service rendered per patient day no doubt increases with hospital size. Thus, to the extent that errors in the (S × PD) measure may be relatively greater than errors in the PD measure, we would expect the cost of providing a given number of services per patient day to be partly reflected in the coefficients of the PD and (PD)² variables, and, thus, to bias them upward. This phenomenon may also account for the fact that the constant term of this regression equation was, unexpectedly, negative.[29]

(3) On the average, each outpatient visit apparently added about $4.81 to total cost.

[28] The correlation coefficient of (S × PD) and PD was 0.986 and of (S × PD) and (PD)² was 0.898. This condition of high correlation between independent variables (known as multicollinearity) when accompanied by errors in the independent variables, may result in possible errors in the associated regression coefficients that are larger than those indicated by their respective standard errors. See the discussion of case III multicollinearity in J. Johnston, *Econometric Methods* (New York: McGraw-Hill, 1963), pp. 206-207.

[29] Suppose, for example, that three types of hospitals have total cost curves as described by the lines AA', BB', and CC' of Figure V. The height of each curve at any given size level depends upon the service capability and product mix produced by each type of hospital. Assume that hospitals of type CC' tend to be larger than those of type BB', which, in turn are generally larger than those of type AA' (hypothetical observations from each type of hospital are represented by the a's, b's, and c's, in Figure V). A simple regression equation based upon these data (indicated by the line RR') may have a negative constant term (OR) even though the constants of the "true" cost equations (OA, OB and OC) are positive. A similar phenomenon will occur in multiple regression analyses if the adjustment for service capability and product mix is not completely adequate.

Hypothesized Actual and Measured Relationship Between Total Cost and Hospital Size

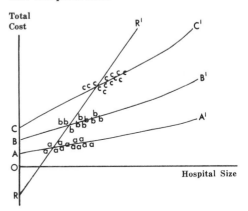

(4) The variable representing the existence of a hospital-controlled professional nursing school (NS) was intended to reflect the constant costs associated with nursing education. The coefficient of this variable turned out to be positive, but it was not statistically significant. The coefficient of the student nurse variable (N) was intended to account for the average incremental cost associated with each additional student-nurse year. This would normally include the cost of training and of food, housing, and other living expenses. These costs would of course, be offset somewhat by the value of the students' clinical experience to the hospital. Unexpectedly, the coefficient of N turned out to be very significantly negative, indicating that total costs were about $1,805 lower per additional student-nurse year. A discussion of the possible reasons for this result is deferred to the summary and conclusions section.

(5) The IRP variable was intended to take account of the educational, research, and increased patient care costs associated with the operation of internship and residency programs. The coefficient of this variable indicated an average increase in cost of about $55,347 per program. The number of interns and

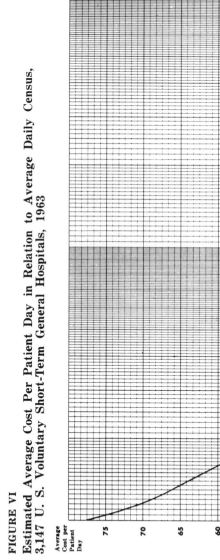

FIGURE VI

Estimated Average Cost Per Patient Day in Relation to Average Daily Census, 3,147 U. S. Voluntary Short-Term General Hospitals, 1963

FIGURE VII
Estimated Average Cost Per Patient Day in Relation to Average Daily Census,
3,147 U. S. Voluntary Short-Term General Hospitals by Service-Capability Group, 1963

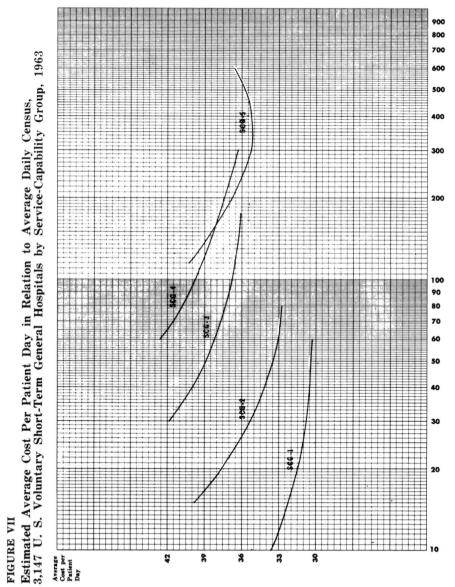

residents was included as a variable (IR) to hold approximately constant the additional cost associated with their presence. This amount turned out to be about $5,034 per person.

(6) An average incremental cost of $174,796 was shown by the coefficient of the variable representing affiliation with a medical school. It should be recognized that this estimate reflects only those cost differences which exist after the costs associated with internship and residency programs and other foregoing factors have been taken into account.

The main findings of the analysis based upon all hospitals were those related to the cost-size relationship itself. The regression results, stated in terms of adjusted total costs, were converted to adjusted average cost (AAC) by assuming the presence of the mean number of services (14.15) and the absence of all the other cost-affecting characteristics (e.g., nursing school, interns and residents). In order to obtain estimates of average cost at various size levels, the relevant terms of the regression equation were divided by patient days, to yield the following equation:

$$\text{AAC} = \$171,085 \ (\text{PD})^{-1} + \$30.31 + \$0.0000351 \ (\text{PD})$$

The relationship between adjusted average cost and size (measured in terms of ADC) described by this equation is portrayed graphically in Figure VI.

The results indicate that as hospital size increases, average cost declines until it reaches a minimum level at about 190 ADC and then begins to rise. However, to the extent that the constant term of the regression equation may be biased downward and the coefficient of the (PD)^2 term biased upward, as noted above, the degree of the initial decline in cost will be underestimated and the amount of the rise in cost at large size levels will be overestimated.[30] There-

fore, we decided to carry out a second series of analyses that would account more satisfactorily for the influence of the number of facilities and services upon the cost-size relationship.

Analyses by Service-Capability Group

For these analyses, the hospitals were divided into five service-capability groups (SCGs) according to the number of facilities, services and programs they provide as shown in Table 1. A separate regression equation was then fitted to the data from hospitals in each group.

As in the case of the all-hospital analysis, we decided to use adjusted rather than reported total cost as the dependent variable in order that geographic wage differences and wage variation associated with product mix could be held approximately constant. Of the independent variables used in the all-hospital analyses, only (S), the number of facilities and services, was not included. The differences in constant cost associated with facilities and services were largely accounted for by the division of the hospitals into service-capability groups. However, an (S × PD) variable was included to reduce the degree of possible bias in the PD and (PD)^2 regression coefficients and, thus, in the constant term.

The results of the regression analyses based upon the five service-capability groups are presented in Table 2. Positive constant terms that become greater as service capability increased were estimated, suggesting that the initial decline in costs is more rapid with greater service capability. The results were

to be attached to them have been presented. Although such measures would be subject to the potential biases noted above, and it is not presently clear as to just what type of measures would be most useful for areawide planning purposes, it should be possible to calculate them from the means and joint confidence regions of the regression estimates. See, for example, H. Gregg Lewis, "On the Distribution of the Partial Elasticity Coefficient," *Journal of the American Statistical Association*, Vol. 36, No. 215 (September, 1941), pp. 413-416.

[30] It should be noted that no measures of the degree of economies of scale or confidence limits

TABLE 1
Hospitals by Service-Capability Group

Service-Capability Group	Number of Facilities, Services and Programs (S)	Number of Hospitals	Mean Average Daily Census (ADC)
SCG 1	0 through 9	680	26
SCG 2	10 through 12	693	46
SCG 3	13 through 16	729	93
SCG 4	17 through 19	490	170
SCG 5	20 through 28	555	294

converted to average cost per patient day by a method similar to the one described in the all-hospital analysis. The estimated relationships between average cost and size, for the range of sizes encompassed by the regression analyses, are shown in Figure VII.

Economies of scale in the provision of care appear to exist over a wide range of sizes in each of the service-capability groups. As the number of services increases, the size level at which a relatively low level of average cost is attained apparently increases. Possible diseconomies of scale were indicated only for hospitals in the upper size range of the highest service capability group.

In the analyses of service-capability groups 1 through 4, the coefficients of the $(S \times PD)$ measure were positive. This suggests that product-mix variation was more adequately taken into account in the analyses by service-capability group than in the all-hospital analysis. The fact that the $(S \times PD)$ coefficient decreases with increased service capability suggests that the less commonly available services cost less per patient day on the average, no doubt because they are utilized less intensively on a patient-day basis.[31]

The following interpretations may be made with respect to the other variables

included in the service-capability-group analyses:

(1) The lower cost per outpatient visit in hospitals in the lower service-capability groups appears to be a result of the type of care typically provided in the outpatient clinics of those hospitals. Such care consists primarily of normal emergency and clinic services of lower cost per visit than the more specialized services available in the referral programs of hospitals in the higher service-capability groups.

(2) The effect of the nursing-school variable on hospital cost was generally insignificant, perhaps because the relatively constant cost of operating a nursing school is likely to be a small percentage of total hospital cost. The presence of student nurses generally appears to have a negative effect on total cost; that is, total cost decreases with increased numbers of student nurses. This result is particularly apparent for hospitals in the highest service-capability group, which are those with the largest number of student nurses.

(3) As expected, total cost increases with the operation of internship and residency programs and the presence of interns and residents. However, the increased cost of having interns and residents is smaller in hospitals of higher service capability. Since the average number of interns and residents in these hospitals is relatively high, a possible explanation for this is that there may

[31] The variation in the coefficients of the PD, $(PD)^2$, and $(S \times PD)$ measures may also be partially explained by the high degree of correlation among these measures.

TABLE 2
Regression Coefficients, Adjusted Total Cost in Relation to Patient Days and Other Characteristics, 3,147 Voluntary Short-Term General Hospitals, by Service-Capability Group, 1963

	Service-capability group				
	SCG 1	SCG 2	SCG 3	SCG 4	SCG 5
Number of hospitals	680	693	729	490	555
R²	0.844	0.861	0.875	0.850	0.896
Constant	13,422	55,003	83,756	134,677	570,398
Variable	Regression coefficients				
PD	21.36	9.58	27.76	36.19	27.25
	(3.06)	(4.50)	(4.49)	(6.85)	(5.25)
$(PD)^2$	−0.0000182	0.0000667	0.0000146	−0.0000149	0.0000370
	(0.0000515)	(0.0000294)	(0.0000165)	(0.0000148)	(0.0000069)
S × PD	1.1151	1.8130	0.4301	0.0270	−0.0479
	(0.3260)	(0.3835)	(0.2849)	(0.3671)	(0.2152)
OPV	1.78	1.29	2.36	1.86	6.20
	(0.47)	(0.69)	(0.83)	(0.69)	(0.85)
NS	239,157	−129,390	−70,969	−83,077	5,404
	(71,728)	(63,977)	(41,698)	(59,329)	(104,622)
N	−1,456	3,260	234	−52	−2,621
	(918)	(891)	(585)	(591)	(760)
IRP	6,075	86,147	8,374	11,085	70,491
	(17,661)	(30,308)	(17,533)	(15,459)	(12,705)
IR	34,767	21,547	18,578	7,928	4,157
	(9,387)	(5,482)	(3,744)	(3,099)	(1,315)
MS	*	✧	−34,707	127,469	171,734
			(96,867)	(86,670)	(107,551)

* None of the hospitals in these groups were affiliated with medical schools.

be economies of scale in the operation of internship and residency programs.

(4) Although the results for costs of affiliation with a medical school are not statistically significant, they indicate that such costs are rather small. This may be because some medical school costs are reflected in the accounts of other organizational entities (e.g., a university), or because they are partly reflected in the internship and residency variable or in other variables.

SUMMARY AND CONCLUSIONS

The main purpose of this study has been to estimate the net relationship between patient-day cost and the size of hospitals. It was hypothesized that, according to economic theory, average cost would initially decline as size is increased—primarily because of the gains resulting from specialization—but that, after some point, average cost would begin to rise because of increased problems of internal control and communications. If the net relationship of cost to size could be determined, hospital construction plans could be appropriately adjusted and great savings could be made.

Two approaches were used to empirically estimate the independent effect of size on cost. In the first analysis, data from 3,147 U. S. voluntary short-term general hospitals were used to relate total hospital cost to hospital size and a number of other variables by means of multiple regression analysis. Although the primary reason for the inclusion of the other variables was to eliminate their effect on hospital cost, estimates of their independent effects on cost were also derived. The additional variables utilized were the number of services in the hospital, the number of outpatient visits, the presence or absence of a nursing school, the number of student nurses, the number and types of internship and residency programs, the number of interns and residents, and affiliation or non-affiliation with a medical school.

The major finding of the first analysis was consistent with our hypotheses. Average cost initially declined with increased hospital size but, after a point, began to increase with size. However, the results of the all-hospital analysis were not considered conclusive because the adjustments for variations in the services provided by hospitals of different sizes were apparently inadequate.

Therefore, in a second series of analyses, the effect of the amount of specialized service provided upon cost was partially held constant by dividing the hospitals into five categories according to the number of facilities and services provided. Regression coefficients were then calculated for each group of hospitals, using essentially the same variables as in the first analysis. The results confirmed the general relationship determined in the previous all-hospital analysis. For hospitals with a given number of services, economies are associated with increased size. As the number of services increases, a relatively low level of average cost is reached in hospitals of successively larger size. Only for the largest hospitals in the highest service-capability group were diseconomies of scale indicated within the size range covered by the regression analysis.

Additional studies of hospital cost

could provide more refined knowledge of the cost-size relationship. For instance, in future studies, the extent of economies of scale could be determined for individual services and facilities; then the interrelationships of different services could be ascertained to determine what facilities and services should be provided together in the same hospital. In addition to making possible a more accurate estimate of the over-all cost-size relationship, such a study would make it possible to determine the number of hospitals that should provide certain facilities and services in any given area.

In any case, our findings on the net relationship of cost to size are useful as they stand. They provide estimates of the independent effect of size upon cost and, more broadly, they indicate the range of practicable hospital sizes.

Our findings suggest that small hospitals with high service capability should not generally be built because they are likely to be of uneconomic size. Large hospitals having low service capability are also likely to be uneconomic, since there are few or no additional economies associated with increased size to offset the greater transportation costs incurred.

The most interesting of our findings relating to variables other than size concerned nursing education. The coefficient of the student-nurse variable (N) was negative in both the analysis based on all hospitals and in the separate analysis of service-capability group 5. In each of these cases, the student-nurse coefficient was statistically significant in the sense that the associated standard error measure was relatively small.

These results are broadly consistent with the relationships found for 1951 and 1952 in the study of the Commission on Financing Hospital Care. At the time of that study, average expense per patient day was found to be 11 percent lower in small hospitals with nursing schools than it was in similar hospitals without such schools.[32]

These findings are surprising in view of the available evidence showing that the cost of maintaining and educating student nurses substantially exceeds the value of the services they provide during their clinical training. In a recent analysis of the costs associated with diploma programs in nursing, it was found that the average gross cost incurred by the parent institution was about $2,400 per student-year. The average value of the students' clinical experience to the parent institution was estimated at $600 per student-year.[33] This leaves an estimated net cost to the hospital of $1,800 per student-year.

One explanation for this apparent contradiction may be that the lower cost per patient day in hospitals with nursing students is a reflection of factors other than the direct value of students to hospitals. For example, the National League for Nursing study suggested that hospitals which operate nursing schools have an advantage in the recruitment of professional nursing personnel.

In conclusion, we should like to make a few comments about factors affecting optimal hospital size that may not be reflected in the results of our statistical analyses.

[32] See John H. Hayes, ed., "Factors Affecting the Costs of Hospital Care," *Financing Hospital Care in the United States*, Vol. 1 (New York: The Blakiston Company, 1954), pp. 119-120.

[33] See National League for Nursing, "Cost of Basic Diploma Programs," *Study on Cost of Nursing Education*. Part I (New York: National League for Nursing, 1964), particularly pp. 68-70.

First, it should be pointed out that hospitals operating above the lowest levels indicated on the least-cost curves are not necessarily inefficient. For example, certain teaching and research programs may require a hospital large enough to furnish a certain number of medically specialized cases, even though this size level would be uneconomic if only the patient care operations of the hospital were considered.

Another factor—mentioned earlier in this paper—that may affect optimal size is travel cost, including both the monetary and non-monetary costs associated with distance. Now that an estimate has been made of the magnitude of internal economies of scale, we are in a better position to determine in later studies the "trade off" between the increased travel costs involved in having fewer, larger hospitals and the loss of economies of scale involved in having more but smaller hospitals closer to prospective patients.

Finally, it should be recognized that our analyses are based upon historical costs as they are reflected in hospital accounting records. The costs relevant for planning purposes, on the other hand, are often those associated with new facilities. And they are always those which will be incurred in future time periods. More generally, all planning activity is directed toward the future, and statistical studies based upon past data (as they must be) have value, in this context, only to the extent that they allow us to draw inferences about expected future relationships.

John D. Thompson
Robert B. Fetter
Charles D. Mross

Case Mix and Resource Use

Originally Published in December 1975

Reprinted with permission of the Blue Cross Association, from *Inquiry:* Vol.XII, No.4, pp.300-312. Copyright © 1975 by the Blue Cross Association.

This study deals with two specific aspects of hospital performance: 1) the effect of an institution's diagnostic mix on its use of resources; and 2) the application of diagnostic-specific case groups as the preferable units of output (products) upon which selected aspects of hospital performance and costs could be analyzed and monitored, and for which the hospital would, in many instances, be reimbursed. This research, then, attempts to extend and refine the Lave and Lave[1] observations that a hospital is a multiple product firm as reflected by its case mix. The planning, quality and control, and administrative implications of case mix and resource use, as well as an extensive bibliography, are explored in another report;[2] this paper focuses on the economic and payment implications of the study.

In the Lave and Lave article cited, three approaches were identified as bases for defining a hospital's case mix: 1) to define groups of patients by the amount and types of resources expended to treat them; 2) to aggregate patients

John D. Thompson is Professor of Public Health and Chief of Health Services Administration, Department of Epidemiology and Public Health, Yale University School of Medicine (60 College Street, New Haven, CT 06510).

Robert B. Fetter, D.B.A. is Professor, School of Organization and Management and the Institution for Social and Policy Studies, Yale University (56 Hillhouse Avenue, New Haven, CT 06520).

Charles D. Mross, M.P.H. is Assistant Director, Ochsner Foundation Hospital (1516 Jefferson Highway, New Orleans, LA 70121).

This work was completed under U.S. Public Health Service Research Grant HS-00163-07, as part of the Health Services Research Program, Institution for Social and Policy Studies, HS-00090-05.

by clinical service (pediatrics, obstetrics, etc.) and define case mix in terms of the proportion of patients in these groups; and 3) to classify patients by various ICDA groupings and define case mix by the percentage of patients within these diagnostic groups. Our paper utilizes the first and third approaches through defining patients by diagnoses-related categories and, further, into isoresource groups.

The first step in such an approach is to define the hospital's output as the total care given to patients within a meaningful and manageable number of diagnostic-specific product groups, based both on the utilization of some definable resource (in this case patient days) and by the kind of medical specialty primarily concerned with their treatment. The study then examines these product groups across 18 hospitals to determine whether a different pattern of these diagnostic-related groups is being treated and, consequently, different outputs being produced among the hospitals.

When the literature is examined for approaches to the next logical step in considering a hospital's diagnostic mix, i.e., the effect of that mix on a hospital's costs or on a proposed prospective reimbursement rate, one encounters only indirect approximations of the influence of the patterns of diagnoses treated.

Two approaches have been utilized in an attempt to measure the effect of mix on costs by factoring various characteristics of the hospital itself,[3-5] rather than the medical characteristics of its patients. Such institutional characteristics as the teaching/non-teaching function, the size, the categorization of its medical staff, or the relative percentage of patients treated in its various clinical services have been utilized as a surrogate for mix. A less common approach has been to cost the treatment of one or two diseases and infer from cross-hospital comparisons of these costs the pattern of costs for the total institution.[6] The real problem is that the failure to merge the individual patient's medical abstract, which provides the diagnostic and salient medical information, with the patient's account, which records the resources consumed in treating that patient, precluded the development of an input-output model for these diagnostic groups.

This study attempts to determine the resources expended by the same diagnoses-related groups used in delineating the hospital's diagnostic mix, to price these resources, and to explore the implications of these different expenditures.

This research will be presented in five steps:

1 Devise diagnostic-related product groups for hospital inpatients on the non-maternity services that account for a high proportion of the caseload of the 18 hospitals in the study;
2 Test the study hospitals for case mix differences in these diagnostic groups;
3 Demonstrate the relationship of these diagnostic groups to overall non-maternity special service costs;
4 Price out the groups using the billed charges from another hospital;
5 Explore the implications of these prices and the patterns of resource use in the 18 hospitals.

The Study Setting

The study was carried out in 18 of the 35 acute general hospitals in Connecticut that were subscribers of the Professional Activities Study (P.A.S.), and in one additional hospital that served as the pilot institution for the development of the Connecticut Utilization and Patient Information System. No claim is made that these hospitals in any way represent the totality of hospitals in Connecticut or in the United States.

The 18 study hospitals, as a subset of the 35 acute general hospitals in Connecticut, are all voluntary hospitals with an average annual capacity of 277 beds for the treatment of non-maternity cases. The largest hospital had a capacity of 561 such beds, while the smallest hospital reported 61 beds assigned to non-maternity cases. Although this latter figure was from the smallest hospital in the state, and in spite of the fact that the two largest institutions (845 and 697 non-maternity beds) were not represented in the study sample, the average size of the study hospitals was slightly larger than the average of all 35 hospitals, which was 260 in 1970. The study beds were experiencing an 86 percent occupancy as compared to the 85 percent occupancy of all hospitals. The length of stay of the 18 hospitals was 8.75 days, while the 35 hospitals' weighted average length of stay for non-maternity patients was 8.73 days in 1970.

None of the study hospitals could be categorized as a major teaching hospital in 1970, although seven of them were in the process of negotiating formal affiliations with medical schools during the study year. Ten of the hospitals were located in multi-hospital towns, while the remaining eight were the only hospital in their community. Although the larger hospitals (those above the median of 247 beds) tended to be in multi-hospital towns, two of the sole hospitals were in the larger size range while three of the smaller hospitals were in multi-hospital settings.

In other words, these 18 hospitals were, in the main, all performing about the same role in their communities within a small, relatively wealthy state with no isolated geographic sections.

One unusual feature of the study hospitals is the Connecticut Hospital Association-centered statewide standard accounting system by which reasonable comparative and consistent costs for each of the hospitals can be derived. The Connecticut Hospital Association has further refined its costing analysis into routine costs (room and board), and special service costs (radiology, laboratory, operating room, special drugs, etc.), again on a per patient day basis. By 1960, these two classifications of costs were further subdivided into three service categories: non-maternity, maternity, and newborn costs.

The costs per non-maternity patient day for the 18 hospitals in 1970 were $84.87, compared with $85.38 for all hospitals in the state;

Table 1.   Classification of 34 diagnostic groups using Connecticut P.A.S. data

Diag-nostic group	Diagnosis
1	Parasitic and other infective diseases
2	Acute myocardial infarction
3	Diseases of gallbladder and biliary ducts
4	Diseases of the male genital organs
5	Functional heart disorder, congestive heart failure and others (age 40–99)
6	Cerebrovascular disease (thrombosis, cerebral embolism and others)
7	Other diseases of circulatory system
8	Diseases of the eye
9	Diseases of liver and pancreas except diabetes mellitus
10	Bronchitis, emphysema and other diseases of the respiratory system
11	Arteriosclerotic heart disease
12	Congenital anomalies
13	Diseases of the urinary system
14	Fractures, dislocations and sprains
15	Acute appendicitis, inguinal and umbilical hernia, femoral hernia (no obstruction)/age 36–66—lipoma, hydrocele, no secondary diagnosis
16	Diseases of breast—partial mastectomy/benign neoplasm of breast or no secondary diagnosis
17	Arthritis and rheumatism
18	Acute appendicitis, inguinal and umbilical hernia, femoral hernia (no obstruction)/age 10–35—no secondary diagnosis
19	Other diseases of intestines and peritoneum
20	Osteomyelitis and other diseases of bone and joint
21	Diseases of upper gastro-intestinal system
22	Diseases of the skin and subcutaneous tissue
23	Other diseases of musculo-skeletal system
24	Diseases of oral cavity, salivary glands and jaws
25	Wounds and burns
26	Injury to internal organs
27	Diabetes mellitus
28	Other cerebrovascular disease
29	Hypertrophy of T&A, tonsillectomy, adenoidectomy or no surgery
30	Disorders of menstruation or benign neoplasm of uterus/D&C or no sugery/infection of cervix or no secondary diagnosis
31	Diseases of the ear
32	Psychotic and psychoneurotic disorders
33	Adverse effects of chemical substances and other trauma
34	Acute respiratory infections

Source: Original P.A.S. data from the Connecticut Hospital Association, 1970.

special service costs were $35.42 per non-maternity day against $35.78 for the state. Within the study hospitals, costs per day for these kinds of care varied from a high of $95.71 to a low of $72.70; special service costs varied from $43.00 down to $28.19 per non-maternity day.

Diagnostic-Related Product Groups

As an aid to insure more meaningful hospitalization utilization review, a patient classification system (AUTOGRP)[7] was developed at Yale University that groups patients into diagnostic categories based on significant differences in the utilization of hospital resources, consider-ing such additional features as age, sex, presence or absence of specified surgery and complications. Although AUTOGRP could classify patients using length of stay and dollar value of grouped or selected special services, or preoperative length of stay as the resource consumption variables, this study used length of stay as the dependent variable for diagnostic groupings when applied to the Professional Activities Study (P.A.S.) data on the 18 hospitals. At the time of this research, the study team of physicians and other personnel had completed the classification of 174 diagnostic groups utilizing the Connecticut P.A.S. data. Thirty-four of these groups were selected for further study on the basis of their substantial contribution to the non-obstetrical workload of each of the 18 hospitals. As previously mentioned, this study is concerned with the non-maternity patients; therefore, all maternity and newborn patients were eliminated from consideration. A list of the 34 diagnostic groups appears in Table 1.

These patient groups comprised 65.3 percent of all non-maternity patients treated in the study hospitals and accounted for 63.5 percent of all patient days in these services. Table 2 displays the average percent of patients treated and patient days for each group for the 18 study hospitals. The differences in the mean percent of patients treated and patient days is, of course, due to the different lengths of stay among the diagnostic groups. Group #2 (acute myocardial infarction), for instance, accounts for an average 1.85 percent of patients treated and 4.11 percent of patient days, while Group #29 (hypertrophy of tonsils and adenoids) makes up 4.78 percent of all patients and only 1.04 percent of patient days. The average length of stay for the 34 groups was slightly lower, 8.53 days, than the length of stay for all non-maternity patients in the study hospitals, which was 8.75 days.

The fairly tight values of the coefficients of variation in the length of stay among the hospitals is not surprising since the groupings were based on length of stay clusters.

Differences in Case Mix

The concept of diagnostic mix has then taken on two definitions: 1) the number of patients treated in certain specific categories; and 2) the number of patient days experienced by the patients in these same categories. In order to explore the patterns of the diagnostic mix in the study hospitals, two matrices were generated, with the diagnostic categories on the vertical axis forming the columns, and the hospitals on the horizontal axis forming the rows. The number of patients treated or hospital days utilized in diagnostic group *i* and in hospital *j* was entered into cell *i,j* of the appropriate matrix. Since this paper is mainly concerned with diagnostic mix among patients treated in different hospitals and not with variations in length of stay, it is the first of these matrices that will be discussed. The length of stay findings will be examined later in this presentation, where its

Table 2. Average percent distribution of patients and patient days in 34 diagnostic groups, average length of stay and coefficient of variation, 18 study hospitals, 1970

Diagnostic group	Mean percent of patients treated	Mean percent of patient days	Average length of stay	Coefficient of variation
1	1.32	0.92	6.27	.2160
2	1.85	4.11	18.94	.1138
3	2.26	3.20	12.18	.0919
4	1.80	1.78	8.69	.2210
5	2.03	2.73	11.91	.1437
6	0.95	2.08	18.87	.1783
7	4.27	5.27	10.96	.1302
8	1.99	1.38	6.16	.1476
9	0.86	1.46	14.74	.1162
10	1.57	2.04	11.63	.1655
11	2.18	3.18	13.17	.1700
12	1.32	1.05	6.96	.2003
13	3.62	2.72	6.56	.2054
14	4.98	7.07	12.58	.1624
15	1.12	0.87	6.63	.1203
16	1.12	0.40	3.04	.1096
17	0.98	1.25	11.60	.2177
18	1.02	0.62	5.16	.1124
19	3.15	2.86	7.98	.1538
20	2.82	3.57	11.11	.1777
21	2.44	2.79	10.30	.1950
22	1.77	1.35	6.46	.2806
23	1.08	0.57	4.66	.2799
24	1.32	0.40	2.37	.4097
25	1.71	1.37	7.31	.2199
26	2.36	1.69	6.32	.2378
27	0.58	0.80	12.11	.1885
28	0.62	0.83	11.73	.1524
29	4.78	1.04	1.78	.2532
30	2.74	0.79	2.31	.2903
31	1.07	0.44	3.52	.3046
32	1.19	1.39	11.61	.3330
33	1.54	1.17	6.62	.1587
34	1.59	1.10	5.82	.1987
Total weighted mean	65.31	63.52		

Average length of stay, all groups: 8.53
Average length of stay, all non-maternity patients: 8.75

Source: Original data from the Connecticut Hospital Association, 1970.

influence on the choice of reimbursement schemes will be discussed.

The patient matrix was submitted to the Friedman test based on ranking the percentage of each diagnosis group's admissions to each hospital. The result revealed that there was no pattern in the rankings across the 18 hospitals. In order to determine in detail this lack of consistency in the relative number of cases across

Table 3. Indicators of patient mix* by diagnostic group for 18 study hospitals (A through R)

Diagnostic group	A	B	C	D	E	F	G	H	I	J	K	L	M	N	O	P	Q	R
1	+1.75				−0.84				−0.99	−0.73		−0.74	−0.64		+2.86	+1.85	+1.60	
2		+2.41			+2.82				−1.00							+2.72	−1.22	
11	+2.69	−1.42	−1.35	−1.36					−1.74	−1.70	−1.41	+3.48			−1.65	−0.75		
5		+2.65				+3.65	+4.11		−1.43		+4.01		−0.58		−1.13	+3.23		
7			+7.54			+2.76	−3.44		−3.67				−3.60		−3.79			−1.08
6								−0.46		−0.62								
28						+3.05						+1.23	−0.51		−0.24		−0.34	
3		+2.65										−0.32	+1.48		−1.91			
9																		
21				+3.16		+3.18			−1.90		+4.01	−1.69						
19		+4.73		+4.77							+4.34						+2.90	
27				+0.93		+0.93		−1.66										+3.80
13	−2.38		−2.81	+4.95			+5.09			−2.37	−2.58	−3.04				+4.35	−2.31	
18							−0.70					+1.50						
15					+1.53	−0.69			−0.83			+1.50						
16		−2.00						+2.13		+1.50		+1.42			+1.71			
17		+1.40						−0.38		+1.72		−0.47	−0.75		+1.91		−1.74	+1.29
20				−1.98			+1.39		+4.31				−0.68		+1.58			
23			−0.98	+3.30			+3.93		−0.87		+2.28	−0.73						+2.05
34			−0.82							−1.02	−0.56				+2.75			+1.87
10															−1.08			+1.94
12	+1.83								+1.77			+2.04						
14	−3.83	−3.44		−3.46				−2.50	−3.26	+7.64	+6.12		+6.25	+8.65				−3.63
33				+1.92						+2.31					−1.00			
25		−0.98	+2.75	−0.69					−1.27			−1.01						
26			+3.41	−1.67				−1.26	−1.64		+3.65	−1.27					+2.43	+3.13
24	−0.79		+2.38		−0.69	−0.76	−0.57		+3.55		−0.93		−0.90			−0.87		
4	−1.23							+3.47										
29	+6.70			−2.15			−2.89	+5.51			−2.84			+2.82				
30		−2.21	−2.71		−1.74	−1.56		+6.95	−3.57	−3.18		−3.87	+9.36	+6.91	+6.77		−1.90	−1.44
31	−0.84	+1.96	−2.20			−0.35			+5.51	−1.96	−0.34	−2.04	−2.23	−1.74	+4.59	−0.71	+1.72	−0.72
32	−0.32	−0.23	−0.76	+2.43	−0.54		+2.92		+2.60	−0.39	−0.41	+1.69	−0.87				+2.04	−0.38
8		−1.21	+3.39								+2.39	+1.70		−0.94	−0.35		+3.10	−1.14
22		+2.16	+2.84	−1.31	−0.54	−1.30			−1.22	+2.36		+2.50	−1.31					
Total signs	10	15	13	14	6	10	9	9	18	13	14	19	13	5	15	7	11	12

* Cells show percent of patients treated in each diagnostic group. A *plus* indicates when more patients than expected were actually treated; a *minus* indicates when fewer patients than expected were actually treated. Chi square < .01.
Source: Original data from the Connecticut Hospital Association, 1970.

hospitals, each cell was examined to determine if the number of patients treated in the cell's hospital was higher or lower than expected when compared with the proportion of patients treated in that category by all the study hospitals. A chi square value of < .01 was used to determine significant differences. The number of these differences in the cells was so high that the presentation of the chi square matrix itself would only be confusing.[8]

A rearranged matrix was prepared for this presentation (Table 3) in which each cell where a significant difference was found is identified with the direction of the difference (a *plus* when more patients than expected were actually treated and a *minus* when fewer patients than expected were treated). In addition, in order to illustrate the magnitude of this variation, the *percent* of patients treated was entered in those cells. The diagnostic groups were then rearranged according to the body system affected and two subclassifications were marked; i.e., those diseases most likely to be the result of trauma, and those diseases considered the province of the less common specialties. For example, patients with acute myocardial infarction (diagnostic group #2) contributed 2.82 percent of the patients treated in Hospital E and only 1.00 percent of patients in Hospital I. The number of patients treated in these hospitals was significantly different than expected—in the first instance, more patients, and in the second, fewer. Two other hospitals (B and P) treated more patients than would be expected with these diseases, and another (Hospital Q) treated fewer such patients than expected. There was only one disease category (diseases of liver and pancreas, excluding diabetes mellitus, #9) in which there were no differences in the relative number of patients treated in all hospitals; while two groups (psychotic and psychoneurotic disorders, #32, and disorders of menstruation, #30) generated significant differences from the grouped experience in 13 out of the 18 hospitals.

It could be maintained that some of these differences are artificial, that some may be due to different styles of using the diagnostic nomenclature between hospitals. Whether a patient has arteriosclerotic heart disease or a functional heart disorder may be a moot point,

depending on the training of the physician. In selected diagnostic groups this indeed may be true. If all the cardiovascular categories (groups 2, 5, 7, and 11) are considered as one group, the relative differences in this overall classification do flatten somewhat. However, around a mean of 10.3 percent, one hospital reported 7.8 percent of its patients in these four categories, and another, 13.1 percent—still a considerable difference. Such an explanation could not account for the substantial differences in inter-hospital patient mix within these diagnostic groups, where such confusion of diagnoses does not make medical sense.

There is one inescapable conclusion from Table 3; there is a substantial difference in the diagnostic mix of patients treated in hospitals that are seemingly delivering the same product and fulfilling the same role in their communities. Additional insight into these findings is gained by the observations that the differences are especially marked in selected areas of medical and surgical subspecialties, and in the relative number of patients treated with those diseases and conditions related to trauma whose usual mode of entry into the hospital is through the emergency room.

A common characteristic of the former type of patient groups is that the majority of these diagnoses fall in the category of "elective" admissions; i.e., that their period of treatment can be scheduled. More efficient use of facilities is possible with such diagnoses than with those diagnoses that tend to come in a non-predictable mode through the emergency room. Such a payoff is probably a marginal consideration. The main rationale is more likely to be an attempt to increase overall occupancy and thereby produce more patient days. Whether or not such a strategy is effective depends on how the costs of these patients compare with those of other options. It is, therefore, necessary to examine the cost implications of the differences in mix of all diagnostic groups.

Relationship between Diagnostic Groups and Special Service Costs

In order to determine whether or not certain diagnoses affect hospital costs, a multiple regression analysis was undertaken using special service costs as the dependent variable and the

Table 4. Summary of multiple regression analysis

Diagnostic group	Diagnosis	Patients treated R^2	Number of patient days	
			Diagnostic group	R^2
17	Arthritis and rheumatism	0.1358	17	0.1197
33	Chemical substances and other trauma	0.8333	33	0.6562
15	Acute appendicitis, etc. (36–55)	0.8653	14	0.7106
14	Fractures, dislocation, sprains	0.8718	15	0.7449

Source: Original data from the Connecticut Hospital Association, 1970.

number of patients treated for selected diagnoses as the independent variable. The same procedure was followed using costs and patient days. The results of these analysis are shown in Table 4.

The results of the multiple regressions were quite dramatic. Approximately 87 percent of the variation in special service costs was explained by the number of patients treated in four diagnostic groups, and 74 percent of this cost variation was explained by the number of patient days the hospital experienced in these same diagnostic categories. The residuals were plotted and the fit was considered satisfactory. The diagnostic groups were selected on the basis of their explanatory contribution to the variation in the cost per patient day, whether by number of patient days or number of patients treated in the diagnostic groups by each hospital. In all cases, the first two groups entered in the step-wise regression program in the same order.

The four diagnoses are interesting: they are fairly common and together they comprised, on the average, 8.6 percent of the patients treated and accounted for 10.4 percent of the patient days in the study hospitals. One was a medical diagnosis, one surgical, and the other two were emergency-room related. All were discrete diagnoses not likely to be classified in other categories.

A word of caution—although the purpose of the exercise was achieved, i.e., a relationship was identified, the limitations of the data prevent too much further elaboration of the findings. The data were for one year's experience only and the number of observations (N = 18) are minimal. It was for this reason that further development of the results in the area of deriving predictive equations, for example, was not attempted. Since this study is primarily concerned with an input-output model and with the resource allocation implications of the diagnostic mix, another approach at exploring the relationships between diagnostic mix and use of specific resources was undertaken.

Pricing the Diagnostic Groups

The Connecticut Utilization and Patient Information System accepted in its information requirements and operating logic the necessity of linking admitting information, the medical abstract, and the hospital bill into a single record covering one period of hospitalization. The developmental work was carried out in a single Connecticut hospital. This hospital's data were not included in the study group, even though the linkage had been accomplished. The pilot hospital had an average capacity of 262 beds, close to the average size of 259 beds for non-maternity services in all 35 hospitals. Its per diem costs were lower than average, $78.21 against a mean of $85.38, which was reflected both in routine costs, $49.24 against an average $49.60, and special service costs of $28.97 compared with an overall mean of $35.78. Its overall ratio of costs to charges was 1 : 1.13 for special services.

In this one hospital, then, the record abstracts were used to classify patients based on length of stay into the diagnostic groups used in the first part of this paper. The dollar value of special service charges was then utilized to "price" each diagnostic group. Some editing of the dollar value distributions was done and an average special service "price per case" was obtained from these distributions of patients' bills. The "price per case" of this one hospital

Table 5. Special service price per case and per patient day, 34 diagnostic groups, pilot hospital, 1970

Diagnostic group	Price per case	Mean length of stay	Price per patient day
1	$592.88	12.75	$ 46.50
2	587.64	21.10	27.85
3	568.70	10.62	53.54
4	506.85	7.89	64.24
5	456.16	11.37	40.12
6	450.35	20.35	22.13
7	432.32	10.63	40.66
8	407.69	6.21	65.65
9	403.31	11.68	34.53
10	390.60	9.76	40.02
11	388.97	12.02	32.36
12	354.80	5.44	65.22
13	349.27	5.94	58.80
14	348.79	9.46	36.87
15	348.45	6.34	54.96
16	344.55	2.66	129.43
17	341.10	8.92	38.24
18	337.56	5.37	62.86
19	327.54	6.69	48.96
20	324.22	8.60	37.70
21	318.41	7.54	42.23
22	299.73	5.21	57.53
23	295.78	3.16	93.60
24	284.45	2.15	132.30
25	281.48	5.41	52.03
26	266.34	4.68	56.91
27	256.39	10.17	25.21
28	250.81	10.82	23.18
29	246.94	2.31	106.90
30	243.71	2.11	115.50
31	235.37	4.58	51.39
32	219.89	7.32	30.04
33	199.89	4.21	47.48
34	119.56	3.78	31.62
Mean	346.49	7.88	54.89
Median	339.33	....	50.18
Standard deviation	107.79	4.48	28.43
Coefficient of variation	.31	....	.52

Source: Original data from the Connecticut Hospital Association, 1970.

was then accepted as a surrogate resource use indicator per case for each of the 34 groups. Surrogate resource use per patient day was then obtained for these same groups by dividing the pilot hospital's diagnostic specific length of stay into the price per case. A list of these prices appears in Table 5.

This table first reveals that when considering "cheap patients" and "expensive patients," one must first define whether these adjectives are modifying case costs or per diem costs; there is very little relationship between the two measures. Two of the least expensive prices on a case basis are for diagnostic groups #29 and 30 (T&A and disorders of menstruation), yet these cases are the fourth and third highest per diem prices. Diagnostic group #2 (acute myocardial infarction) with the second highest case price ranks 31st in the per diem price. The price per day is so dependent on the length of stay ($r = -.672$) that it suppresses strongly the variability in price per case.

The variation in the price per case is relatively less (coefficient of variation $= .31$) than the value of .52 found in the price per day. The average price per case is also heavily influenced by the modal group (diagnostic groups #12 through 20), where there is a spread of but $30.00 over these nine groups that account for 20.1 percent of patients treated and 20.4 percent of the days of care offered in the 18 study hospitals. There is no similar strong indicator of central tendency in the price per day display.

If, indeed, hospitals would attempt to use their patient mix to lower their overall cost per patient day, an effective strategy is obvious from this table. Those diagnostic groups where the largest difference in mix was demonstrated are the very groups that would selectively increase undifferentiated costs per day. Groups #4, 8, 24, 29, 30, and 31 are among the most expensive in terms of per diem prices, ranking 8, 7, 1, 4, 3, and 16 from the highest prices. And these are among the diagnostic groups demonstrating the most marked variation between hospitals. On the other hand, the emergency room diagnostic groups (#13, 25, 26, and 33 rank 25, 15, 12, and 19) place collectively at the median rank of prices per patient day and, therefore, have minimal influence on costs so measured.

Special Service Prices

Since the main thrust of this paper is to relate hospitals' diagnostic mix and their utilization of different kinds of special service resources, special service prices were subdivided into five different categories: laboratory, diagnostic radiology, operating room, pharmacy, and mis-

Table 6. Average price of selected services by diagnostic group per case, pilot hospital, 1970

Diagnostic group	Laboratory	Diagnostic radiology	Operating room	Pharmaceuticals
1	$181.88	$140.25	$113.22	$35.06
2	187.36	75.96	.84	26.29
3	92.71	115.33	135.19	40.46
4	106.75	77.16	152.12	22.33
5	131.55	79.02	5.34	22.05
6	74.04	114.16	.20	20.35
7	97.79	87.70	96.09	27.53
8	51.48	12.54	203.43	24.72
9	152.30	124.85	10.39	34.57
10	85.10	98.96	19.52	17.27
11	111.79	81.62	3.12	16.94
12	53.09	36.34	139.70	11.47
13	82.57	122.84	56.90	12.36
14	56.00	90.53	56.82	13.81
15	45.28	19.65	144.99	23.14
16	97.99	23.86	122.43	8.59
17	75.10	108.65	41.74	11.69
18	48.75	6.28	144.35	28.57
19	66.57	100.22	54.59	20.54
20	59.59	58.82	80.84	8.68
21	80.07	145.67	8.14	12.44
22	64.81	18.86	109.41	23.81
23	55.11	8.56	134.52	6.51
24	48.39	23.30	118.82	12.79
25	49.60	66.33	61.02	17.31
26	46.75	135.43	4.53	13.20
27	109.12	61.52	4.98	13.02
28	65.14	92.94	3.14	8.54
29	40.08	10.27	109.88	9.24
30	49.62	4.45	107.36	2.08
31	45.44	52.72	58.58	14.34
32	64.19	79.05	5.20	8.27
33	59.53	28.03	11.70	17.59
34	38.97	23.05	.60	13.23

Source: Original data from the Connecticut Hospital Association, 1970.

cellaneous prices. All of these are self-explanatory but for the last two. Pharmacy price includes those drugs that are not included in routine prices but are ordered for a specific patient, such as injectables, antibiotics, and expensive oral medications. The miscellaneous price includes special nursing care, such as intensive care and postoperative recovery room, and the less common special services, such as electrocardiography, medical and surgical supplies, etc. This section of the study concentrates primarily on the first four categories since special care units were the province of a previous paper.[9] These first four categories comprised 68.2 percent of the total special service price at the pilot

hospital. The prices of the four subgroups are listed by diagnostic group in Table 6.

What is of interest here is not so much the variation across diagnostic categories of each subset of prices, but the overall pattern of the different kinds of resources that are being utilized for patients within each group. This is particularly true in the first three subsets of prices. There is, for example, a negative correlation ($r = -.516$) between diagnostic radiology and operating room prices over these 34 diagnostic groups, while a less obvious positive correlation ($r = +.487$) exists between radiology and laboratory prices.

The trends must, in the future, be refined by stating these services in more exact terms than prices. It is probable that the pricing policies of the pilot hospital may have influenced the findings of Tables 5 and 6. Even with this imperfect instrument, however, an indication can be gained of the complexity of differing resource consumption by the different products (diagnostic groups) the hospital is producing.

Resource Use of Diagnostic Groups in 18 Hospitals

In order to explore further the effect of diagnostic mix on the use of these resources in the 18 study hospitals, some standard diagnostic-specific surrogate for such use must be generated. Based on one underlying assumption that cannot be proven—that the quality of diagnostic work-up and treatment of patients in the pilot hospital approximated those in the study hospitals—we can accept the operating assumption that the prices generated in each diagnostic group in the pilot hospital should reflect the resource use that would be experienced for these same groups in the other 18 hospitals.

The mechanics of the derivation of surrogate special service use per case for each of the 18 hospitals then becomes relatively simple. A standard (surrogate) diagnostic-specific price is multiplied by the number of patients treated with that diagnosis in each hospital. The product then represents the value of all special services utilized by all the patients within that diagnostic group in each hospital. For example, there were 112 patients treated in Hospital K with the diagnosis of acute myocardial infarction. The surrogate special resource used for this group was priced at $587.64. Hospital K was then assigned the expenditure of $65,815.68 for the cost of special services used in the treatment of these patients, and the relative contribution of each of the subsets of special services to this total was derived. This same procedure was repeated for all 34 diagnostic groups in each of the 18 hospitals. Each hospital's surrogate special service resource use was the total of its 34 diagnostic categories.

This calculation, in essence, standardizes the resource use of each hospital's case mix to that of the pilot hospital. Thus, the variability exhibited is due solely to case mix differences. This further demonstrates the importance of disaggregating case costs to the level of individual resources in order to understand this variability.

The surrogate resource use per stay for three selected services is displayed in Table 7. It can be noted that the variations in hospital averages for these three services follow the pattern these same services demonstrated in the diagnostic-specific prices displayed in Table 6. Operating room and radiology costs vary more than laboratory costs in both instances. A strengthening of the negative correlation between operating room prices and radiology prices results from the application of prices to caseloads. In this context, it can be interpreted that some of these hospitals (Hospital H, for example) are treating more surgical patients among these 34 groups, while others are varying their mix with a higher relative number of medical patients (Hospital F) who require more diagnostic radiology services. Laboratory costs between hospitals show the smallest variation of the three average surrogate costs, just as they demonstrate less price variation among diagnostic groups. The negative coefficient of correlation, −.51 between operating room surrogate costs and radiology in the diagnostic display, is increased to −.92 in the hospital comparison (see Figure I). This difference in resource use is due to the difference in diagnostic mix of the hospitals.

These results support previous empirical observations that there are "medical" hospitals and "surgical" hospitals and further delineates the different kind of resource expenditures implicit in such a categorization. Variations in special service costs by ancillary departments

Table 7. Average surrogate costs per case for selected special services

Hospital	Surrogate operating room costs per case	Surrogate radiology costs per case	Surrogate laboratory costs per case
A	$73.07	$68.36	$75.60
B	71.27	72.15	78.46
C	72.65	72.90	76.22
D	63.26	74.87	77.21
E	69.22	71.40	77.62
F	66.94	75.51	78.25
G	65.02	74.37	77.72
H	83.17	60.34	75.30
I	76.12	65.02	71.80
J	72.12	69.81	74.41
K	65.68	73.59	76.78
L	74.66	68.92	76.58
M	73.02	67.41	70.68
N	67.95	72.88	73.55
O	76.85	68.26	74.74
P	69.12	72.86	79.58
Q	71.88	70.60	74.53
R	69.94	73.17	74.99
Mean	71.22	70.69	75.78
Standard deviation	4.67	3.74	2.25
Coefficient of variation	.07	.05	.03

Source: Original data from the Connecticut Hospital Association, 1970.

are far more sensitive indicators of hospital function and specific resource expenditures than overall charges or even average special service charges.

Discussion

There are three unequivocal findings of the study: 1) the number or percentage of patients treated within four of the 34 diagnostic groups explains a substantial percentage of the variation in actual special service costs experienced by 18 hospitals in Connecticut; 2) there are significant differences in case mix among these same hospitals within all but one of the 34 diagnostic groups; and 3) there are marked differences in the kinds of resources used to treat patients in the 34 diagnostic categories and, by extension, used by the hospitals caring for these patients.

We suggest that diagnostic-specific (product-centered) case costs could be derived based on resource utilization and would be preferable both as a measure of hospital output and as a

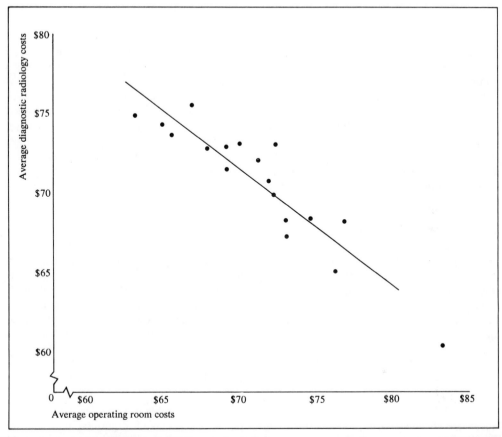

Figure I. Average surrogate costs, diagnostic radiology versus operating room, for 34 diagnostic groups in 18 Connecticut hospitals

basis for reimbursement than the undifferentiated patient day. Patient days, generated in a diagnostic-specific mode must be retained as the basic data for utilization review and can be aggregated in various ways to obtain meaningful occupancy rates.

There are two meaningful issues in this approach to pricing diagnostic groups: the first is the propriety of using charges rather than costs as the basis for the pricing; and the second is the limitation of pricing only special services and not routine services. Research now under way at Yale University is focused on the examination of these two issues.

Hospital charges have always been considered as rather arbitrary expressions of what the hospital administration felt a selected market would bear; and furthermore, they reflected internal "Robin Hood" factors where some special services were priced to make up for losses in routine services or in other special services. Although their importance was thought to be diminishing as more and more third parties sought cost-based reimbursement, such a conceptual frame was probably quite fitting in the past. There are indications at this time, however, that as more attention is paid to uniform costing and revenue systems—mandated under Public Law 93-641—the conversion from charges to costs is indeed attainable.

In Connecticut, at the present time, we are approaching the problem in two ways—the application of departmental ratios of cost to charges (RCC), and the use of standard relative value units across which both costs are allocated and charges based. The American Colleges of Radiology and of Pathology have derived time-measured value units for their tests and examinations. Operating room, anesthesia, recovery room, and special care units are charged on the basis of either minutes of service or man-minutes. Such a conversion procedure must be considered in designing hospital accounting systems for the future.[10]

The allocation of routine charges (room and board) to diagnoses-related groups is a bit more complex. Preliminary studies seem to indicate that most of the variables in this cost category are in routine nursing services. We are now exploring characterizing the total stay of as many patients in these diagnostic groups as possible according to a standard patient classification system, originally applied to many patients on the intermediate care floors, in order to estimate the staffing required for each day. When these categories, i.e., intensive, intermediate, or minimal care, are fixed to a particular patient and that patient's total classification history during his stay is derived, a valid estimate of his— and consequently, his diagnostic group's— requirements for routine care can be approximated.

Resource Allocation Implications

The diagnostic-specific approach offers the unique characteristic of being expressed on a clinical case, thereby offering the opportunity of physician involvement in cost and price decisions in terms both acceptable and meaningful to the medical staff and hospital administrators.

The operation of a hospital can be described in terms of a complex resource supply system that is awaiting the demands of individual patients. These resource demands can then be viewed either as those required for the treatment of an individual patient or as an aggregate of the value of resources expended, which is subdivided into aggregates of various types of resources such as raw food costs, medical and surgical supplies, laboratory costs, etc. The problem is that, until now, resource data could not be aggregated by the medical problem the individual patient presented.

Although the physician is responsible for activating the utilization of resources for the individual patient, his major concern with these elements relates to their ability to satisfy patient-centered demands. Conflict arises when the physician's patient-centered demands clash with administrative and institutional responsibilities concerned with the availability of finite resources. Diagnostic-specific resource utilization data can illustrate these conflicts in a way easily understood by clinicians and related to his own clinical activity and those of his peers. Frequency distributions of the dollar value of these costs can, when compared with the previous data for the same diagnoses such as we have presented, give the physician a clearer idea of his own contribution to those costs—a view impossible if costs per undifferentiated patient stay or patient day are the only data available. The issue is not whether the physician should be involved in resource allocation—he already is the primary allocator within the hospital. The only question is at which level this involvement will come (solely at the patient level or at the institutional level as well), and whether or not he can use his clinical frame of reference in an informed manner at both levels. The diagnostic-specific patient stay costs may well assist in such an effort.

Reimbursement by Diagnostic-Specific Patient Stay

The central problem here is to select a reimbursement method for hospital inpatient services that will promote the effective use of this most expensive community resource and at the same time not adversely affect the availability of that resource or its quality.

This study has already demonstrated several drawbacks of the "reasonable cost" of a patient day as a basis for reimbursement for inpatient hospital care. There are indications that a pre-admission or concurrent length of stay will, through the utilization review process, be establishing one type of patient total treatment standard. The next logical extension of this approach is to reimburse hospitals based on this approved length of stay.

Such pre-admission or concurrent approvals will be granted for an established number of hospital days based on the admitting diagnosis and other factors weighted in the analysis of regional data. When coupled with average charges or cost data, such an approval could be expressed as a dollar amount for routine (bed and board) services. Such an approval merely requires a transformation from days to dollars in order to change the reimbursement target from patient days to patient stay. Third-party reimbursement policies could then be directed toward the use of the diagnostic-specific case cost as the method of paying for hospital services, rather than patient days.

It is the analysis of the special service costs as projected in this study that will complete the concept of diagnostic-specific case costs, which would, if used as the basis for reimbursement, result in coupling the financial and utilization factors into one rate and place the hospital in the position of co-insurer, or at least one who is negotiating for an exception of an established rate for the total cost of treating a case. Such a method of reimbursement would generate a real incentive for controlling both hospital costs and length of stay.

Conclusion

The generation of diagnostic-specific case costs based on demonstrated differential patterns of resource use seems to be a most promising approach in the development of more rational reimbursement for acute hospital care. Although the basic programs reported here are operational, more experience with application to hospitals in various settings and regions should be attempted. Diagnostic groupings must be extended to include a higher percentage of the patient population and refined by the direct use of the special services prices as the first dependent variable rather than as a second dependent variable to patient days as was carried out in group definition here. Serious consideration should be given to the use of these diagnostic-specific case costs as a basis for reimbursement for hospital services.

References and Notes

1 Lave, J. R. and Lave, L. B. "The Extent of Role Differentiation among Hospitals," *Health Services Research* 6:15 (Spring 1971).
2 Thompson, J. D.; Mross, C. D.; and Fetter, R. B. *Case Mix and Resource Use*, Yale University, Institution for Social and Policy Studies, Health Services Research Program, Working Paper No. 33, 1974.
3 Lave, J. R. and Lave, L. B. "Estimated Cost Functions for Pennsylvania Hospitals," *Inquiry* 7:3–14 (June 1970).
4 Feldstein, M. S. "Hospital Cost Variations and Case-Mix Differences," *Medical Care* 3:95–103 (April–June 1965).
5 Shuman, L. J.; Wolfe, H.; and Hardwick, C. P. "Predictive Hospital Reimbursement and Evaluation Model," *Inquiry* 9:17–33 (June 1972).
6 Babson, J. H. *Disease Costing* (Manchester, England: University of Manchester Press, 1973).
7 Mills, R. E.; Fetter, R. B.; and Carlisle, J. "Automated Grouping System," *Users Manual*, Yale University Institution for Social and Policy Studies, Health Services Research Program, 1973.
8 If the reader wishes to examine any or all of the basic tables, he is referred to Mross, C. D. *Diagnostic Mix and Cost Variation*, Essay presented to the Department of Epidemiology and Public Health, Yale University, 1973, University of Michigan Microfilm Service, Ann Arbor, MI 48106.
9 Fetter, R. B. and Thompson, J. D. "A Decision Model for the Design and Operation of a Progressive Patient Care Hospital," *Medical Care* 7:450–462 (November–December 1969).
10 *Connecticut Hospital Association Accounting Manual*, Connecticut Hospital Association, New Haven, CT, October 1, 1974.

Ralph E. Berry, Jr.

On Grouping Hospitals for Economic Analysis

Reprinted with permission of the Blue Cross Association, from *Inquiry:* Vol.X, No.4, pp.5-12. Copyright © 1973 by the Blue Cross Association.

Originally Published in December 1973

Economic analysis of hospital services has attracted considerable attention in recent years. The interest of many economists is undoubtedly due in part to the significance of the policy implications of hospital research, but it also derives in part from the nature of the theoretical and analytical challenges posed by the production and provision of hospital services.

The theoretical challenge revolves around the question of what motivates the behavior of nonprofit enterprises. A number of economists have contributed to the literature of what might be termed the theory of nonprofit hospital behavior.[1] For the most part, the concern has been with the nature and form of the objective function that nonprofit hospitals are engaged in maximizing. Among the maximands postulated to explain nonprofit hospital behavior have been the prestige of the institution, the quantity and quality of care provided, the net revenue of the hospital, and the income of the medical staff. In the main, the literature concerned with nonprofit behavior has been characterized mostly by theorizing. Little work has been done in testing the several theories against observed behavior of hospitals.

Perhaps the most significant analytical or empirical challenge in the context of hospital cost and production research is the problem of coping with product differences. The nature of the hospital industry is such

Ralph E. Berry, Jr., Ph.D. is Associate Professor of Economics, School of Public Health, Harvard University (55 Shattuck Street, Boston, Massachusetts 02115).
The analysis presented in this paper was supported in part by Grant #10-P-56002 from the Social Security Administration, DHEW.

that differences in the quality and the complexity of the scope of services provided are of signal importance. Whatever else may be characteristic of them, the units of production in the hospital industry certainly do not produce a homogeneous product.

The theoretical and the analytical challenges are related. In the context of the theory of nonprofit hospitals the question is what motivates and determines the specific quality and complexity of services that hospitals provide. In the context of empirical analysis the question is how are adjustments to be made for product heterogeneity among hospitals.

A number of researchers have dealt with the problem of product mix differences in a variety of ways with varying degrees of success. When case mix data have been available, for example, they have been used to some advantage in adjusting for product heterogeneity.[2] In many studies the facilities and services available in different hospitals have been used to some advantage as surrogates for product differences.[3]

Since hospitals should be viewed as multiproduct firms in the sense of both patient care-teaching-research and the complexity of each, considered attempts have been made to deal with the phenomenon of product differences. The available data representative of product mix differences in hospitals can be analyzed in order to ascertain whether or not the multidimensional character of hospital output can be rationalized. The results of such analysis can provide insight into the product mix phenomenon. In an earlier paper in this journal,[4] for example, the author outlined the results of a factor analysis of

Table 1. Distribution of short-term general hospitals by number of facilities and control

Number of facilities	All hospitals		Voluntary hospitals		Government hospitals		Proprietary hospitals	
	Number	Mean bed size	Number	Mean bed size	Number	Mean bed size	Number	Mean bed size
1	1	17.00	0	0.00	0	0.00	1	17.00
2	0	0.00	0	0.00	0	0.00	0	0.00
3	12	34.25	4	53.50	5	22.80	3	27.67
4	37	28.05	11	29.91	5	26.40	21	27.48
5	92	30.50	34	30.50	31	32.13	27	28.63
6	206	33.60	82	33.41	72	33.22	52	34.42
7	276	37.29	112	36.66	90	37.09	74	38.47
8	350	42.26	164	41.10	115	44.86	71	40.72
9	328	48.86	156	49.99	104	50.18	68	44.29
10	362	59.51	182	60.17	116	57.42	64	61.42
11	322	66.72	170	65.66	95	68.04	57	67.67
12	318	75.75	194	77.23	86	68.84	38	83.84
13	254	89.35	143	91.83	79	84.90	32	89.28
14	246	107.46	162	106.06	62	109.98	22	111.05
15	221	124.24	150	125.43	50	119.76	21	126.38
16	219	151.23	152	151.45	51	152.65	16	144.63
17	203	174.65	157	173.89	37	179.03	9	170.00
18	219	205.06	172	206.46	40	219.65	7	87.14
19	189	235.05	151	227.74	37	265.62	1	208.00
20	159	254.51	125	249.02	31	301.29	3	155.00
21	139	296.94	111	277.66	27	387.22	1	187.00
22	148	363.20	115	329.67	32	488.47	1	210.00
23	110	409.78	83	341.24	27	620.48	0	0.00
24	101	470.40	79	403.14	21	744.38	1	30.00
25	83	444.32	62	424.82	21	501.90	0	0.00
26	46	548.35	34	513.71	12	646.50	0	0.00
27	32	746.38	19	608.11	13	948.46	0	0.00
28	25	901.72	15	694.33	10	1,212.80	0	0.00
29	14	1,369.00	7	807.57	7	1,930.43	0	0.00
30	2	1,007.00	1	732.00	1	1,282.00	0	0.00

Source: Derived from data provided by the American Hospital Association.

some 40 variables which were related to product mix. Eight common factors were identified that explained approximately 60 percent of the variation in the variables used to represent product mix. Among the more important factors were medical education, basic services, complex services, length of stay, and outpatient activities. The factor analysis served to emphasize the relative importance of facilities and services among available data in explaining product mix.

At this point, a related question is raised as to whether or not there is a systematic pattern to the availability of facilities and services in short-term general hospitals. Further, if such a pattern prevails, what additional insight does it provide into the general nature of product mix and its im-

pact upon the production and provision of hospital services. The purpose of this paper is to explore the pattern of facilities and services in short-term general hospitals.

Facilities and Services in Short-Term General Hospitals

Table 1 contains a summary of the distribution of all short-term hospitals in the United States by number of facilities, mean bed size for a given number of facilities, and ownership. These have been derived from data provided by the American Hospital Association. A number of characteristics of short-term hospitals are evident from this distribution. There are relatively few hospitals with either very few or very many facilities and services. The majority of short-term hospitals have between 10 and 20 facilities and services. Proprietary hospitals as a group tend to have fewer facilities and services than voluntary and government hospitals; in fact, almost 90 percent of proprietary hospitals have 15 or fewer facilities and services. There is a less dramatic difference between voluntary and government hospitals; but, on balance, voluntary hospitals tend to have a somewhat greater number of facilities and services than government hospitals. Finally, there is the expected relationship between the number of facilities and hospital size. Hospital size increases with increased numbers of facilities and services. In fact, the increase in size is more than proportional.

The question to which we seek an answer is whether or not there is any pattern to the specific facilities and services that hospitals have when they have different numbers of facilities and services. Can hospitals be grouped according to the types of facilities and services they have? Further, if hospitals can be so grouped, do such groupings provide any insight into the product mix phenomenon?

The Pattern of Facilities and Services

A method of analysis was developed which allowed a determination of whether or not there is a systematic pattern to the specific facilities and services that hospitals tend to have. First a 30 by 30 element matrix was formed with the number of facilities and services forming the rows of the matrix and the 30 specific facilities and services forming the columns of the matrix. Thus, a given element of the matrix, a_{ij}, would indicate the number of i facility hospitals which had the jth facility. (For example, how many 10 facility hospitals have a blood bank?)

A similar matrix was then formed by dividing the 30 elements in each row of the original matrix by the sum of the elements in that row. Hence, a given element of the new matrix, b_{ij}, indicated the proportion of i facility hospitals which had the jth facility. (For example, what percentage of 10 facility hospitals have a blood bank?) By analyzing this matrix it was possible to determine the pattern of facilities and services.

Four sets of matrices were formed and analyzed—all short-term general hospitals, voluntary hospitals, proprietary hospitals, and government hospitals. A summary of the analysis of these matrices is presented in Table 2. The data in Table 2 actually reflect for each of the 30 specific facilities and services how many facilities and services hospitals have before the specific facility or service is common to at least 50 percent of the hospitals, or at least 75 percent of the hospitals, respectively.[5] Thus, for example, a clinical laboratory is present in at least 50 percent of all hospitals with four facilities and services; and it is present in at least 75 percent of all hospitals with five facilities and services. As a further example, a blood bank is present in 50 percent of all hospitals with 10 facilities and services, and present in 75 percent of all hospitals with 14 facilities and services. These data suggest that a very systematic pattern exists.

It should perhaps be emphasized that the form of Table 2 was suggested by the data rather than by any *a priori* expectations. Thus, the several categories of services were identified after the apparent clusterings implicit in the data outlined in the table were observed. The groupings were, in fact, suggested essentially by the discontinuities in the clusters of values in the body of the table.

There is a group of some five facilities and services that are basic—and there would seem to be such a thing as a basic service hospital. In fact, these five services seem to be added prior to any others. As the data in Table 2 indicate, the basic services become established very early. All five basic services are present in more than 50 percent of the hospitals by the time they have five facilities; and they are present in more than 75 percent of the hospitals no later than when they have six facilities. This pattern prevails for all hospitals regardless of the type of ownership.

After the basic services are established, hospitals apparently begin to add facilities and services that can be characterized as

Table 2. Summary of pattern of facilities and services

Type of services	Number of facilities when facility is							
	Present in 50 percent of hospitals				Present in 75 percent of hospitals			
	All	Volun-tary	Govern-ment	Propri-etary	All	Volun-tary	Govern-ment	Propri-etary
Basic								
Clinical laboratory	4	5	4	3	5	5	4	4
Emergency room	5	5	4	5	6	6	5	6
Operating room	3	3	3	3	3	6	5	6
Delivery room	3	3	3	4	5	5	3	6
X-ray, diagnostic	3	3	4	3	4	3	4	3
Quality-enhancing								
Blood bank	10	10	9	12	14	14	14	14
Pathology laboratory	12	12	13	11	14	14	15	15
Pharmacy with pharmacist	12	12	12	10	14	14	15	12
Premature nursery	10	11	9	11	15	16	14	17
Postoperative recovery unit	10	10	10	10	12	12	13	11
Complex								
Electroencephalography	19	19	21	15	22	22	22	18
Dental facilities	17	18	16	17	24	25	19	20
Physical therapy	13	13	13	11	16	15	16	16
Intensive care unit	19	19	19	15	22	22	24	20
X-ray, therapeutic	16	16	16	16	19	18	22	19*
Radioisotope therapy	17	17	19	17	19	19	20	17
Psychiatric inpatient unit	22	23	20	21	25	27	22	21*
Cobalt therapy	24	24	25	19	27	27	27	19*
Radium therapy	17	17	17	16	20	19	24	19*
Community								
Occupational therapy	23	24	21	18	26	26	23	24*
Outpatient department	19	19	19	17	22	23	20	20
Home care program	27	27	28	24*	29	29	29	24*
Social work department	22	22	19	....	23	23	21	19*
Rehabilitation unit	26	26	22	....	28	28	27	19*
Family planning service	27	27	27	....	29	29	29	22*
Special								
Hospital auxiliary	8	6	7	16	12	10	12	20
Chaplaincy	16	15	14	....	24	24	23	24*
Chapel	13	13	13	....	19	18	15	22*
Routine chest X-ray on admission	23	25	15	17	26	28	22	19*
Routine blood sugar on admission	28	26	28	16	30	30*	30*	19*

*One hospital only.
Source: Same as Table 1.

quality-enhancing. The quality-enhancing services are established (present in 50 percent of hospitals) when hospitals are 10 to 12 facility institutions; they are more firmly established (present in 75 percent of hospitals) when hospitals reach a size of 14 or 15 facilities. Again the pattern is consistent among hospitals of all ownership groups.

After the quality-enhancing services are

established, hospitals apparently add facilities and services that are perhaps best characterized as complexity-expanding services. At this stage of expansion, hospitals tend to expand the scope of services offered and add the capacity to treat a wider variety of ailments. Complexity-expanding services are established in hospitals of approximately 20 facilities; they are firmly established soon thereafter. As in basic services and quality-enhancing services, hospitals of each ownership group display a similar pattern in the case of complexity-expanding services. At this stage of the expansion process, short-term general hospitals are still essentially inpatient oriented institutions.

After hospitals add outpatient activities there is a tendency for certain of them to add a group of facilities and services that transform the institution from one concerned essentially with inpatient activities to one that evolves into a community medical care center. In effect, this group of services can be described as community services. These community services are present in only those hospitals that could be characterized as full-service institutions, in the sense that they tend to have virtually all facilities and services. In fact, community services are not established until hospitals reach the level of some 25 facilities and are not firmly established until the institution is essentially a full-service hospital. During this phase of the expansion process, the consistency of the pattern of expansion among ownership groups is broken. As the data in Table 2 show, proprietary hospitals never become community oriented institutions.

On balance, it would seem that there is a definite and systematic pattern to the expansion of facilities and services in short-term general hospitals. There is such a thing as a basic service hospital. As hospitals add facilities and services, there is a strong tendency to first add those that enhance the quality of basic services. Only after the services that enhance the quality of the basic services have been acquired do short-term general hospitals display a tendency to expand the complexity of the scope of services provided. The final stage of the expansion process for certain hospitals occurs when they add those facilities and services that essentially transform them from inpatient institutions to community medical centers.

Characteristics of Different Hospital Types
This analysis seems to be worth pursuing in a number of directions. It is of some interest, for example, to consider the size

implications of the implicit pattern of expansion. In order to do this, the mean bed size counterparts of the data in Table 2 were calculated and are presented in Table 3.

Basic service hospitals are exceedingly small; their average size is well below 50 beds. The addition of quality-enhancing services does imply some increase in average size, but these services are established in hospitals when they are still relatively small. The addition of complexity-expanding services does, however, imply a significant increase in average hospital size. For the most part, short-term general hospitals that provide a relatively complex scope of services are quite large. Finally, of course, those institutions that can be characterized by their provision of the community services are exceedingly large hospitals.

The basic grouping format seems reasonable and has an analytical appeal. In order to pursue the analysis, each hospital for which facilities and services data were available was assigned to one of the four groups: 1) basic service hospitals, 2) quality-enhancing service hospitals, 3) complex service hospitals, or 4) community service hospitals. The actual assignment was made by means of a simple algorithm and based on the availability of the specific facilities and services in each category.[6]

A summary of descriptive statistics for a variety of characteristics of interest for each of the four groups is presented in Table 4.

Since a substantial amount of information is presented in Table 4, it should suffice to outline a few of the salient characteristics. As previously noted, basic service hospitals are small, the mean size being only 43 beds. While the addition of quality-enhancing services increases the average size to 95 beds, these hospitals are still relatively small. It is with the addition of complexity-expanding services that there is a significant increase in average hospital size, the mean size now being 231 beds. For the very large community service hospitals, the mean size is 450 beds.

The effect of the average sizes of the

Table 3. Summary of expansion of facilities and services

Type of services	Mean bed size when facility is							
	Present in 50 percent of hospitals				Present in 75 percent of hospitals			
	All	Volun-tary	Govern-ment	Propri-etary	All	Volun-tary	Govern-ment	Propri-etary
Basic								
Clinical laboratory	30	30	24	32	29	30	24	29
Emergency room	29	29	28	29	32	34	29	31
Operating room	23	16	24	28	23	16	24	28
Delivery room	22	19	24	23	30	30	24	32
X-ray, diagnostic	21	16	31	28	25	16	31	28
Quality-enhancing								
Blood bank	60	57	52	89	107	107	107	108
Pathology laboratory	85	85	96	78	115	114	127	136
Pharmacy with pharmacist	85	86	76	76	113	111	129	92
Premature nursery	56	64	51	66	118	153	111	140
Postoperative recovery room	67	67	66	67	80	82	86	70
Complex								
Electroencephalography	244	240	438	158	371	332	521	96
Dental facilities	170	192	150	175	427	417	274	155
Physical therapy	91	96	98	63	152	130	156	144
Intensive care unit	245	238	275	119	366	339	764	155
X-ray, therapeutic	160	164	140	182	205	211	488	208*
Radioisotope therapy	190	186	273	204	242	236	290	204
Psychiatric unit	387	353	333	187*	577	640	519	187*
Cobalt therapy	449	414	681	208*	753	686	854	208*
Radium therapy	181	179	189	205	252	223	726	208*
Community								
Occupational therapy	457	417	455	89	554	517	665	30*
Outpatient department	230	224	252	111	374	349	323	155
Home care program	754	567	916	30*	**	842	**	30*
Social work department	380	328	313	208*	418	340	405	208*
Rehabilitation unit	548	510	575	208*	879	640	934	208*
Family planning service	767	645	951	210*	**	808	**	219*
Special								
Hospital auxiliary	40	30	34	78	73	57	68	155
Chaplaincy	145	123	180	30*	481	401	653	30*
Chapel	88	95	76	210*	238	207	119	210*
Routine chest X-ray	461	387	108	138	540	705	521	208*
Routine blood sugar	952	522	**	100	**	732*	***	208*

*One hospital only.
**Mean bed size over 999.
***One hospital only with mean bed size over 999.
Source: Same as Table 1.

different types of hospitals on the number of patients treated is reflected in the numbers of admissions and total patient days. The mean numbers of patients admitted to the four types of hospitals are: 1,578 to basic service hospitals; 3,706 to quality-enhancing service hospitals; 8,911 to complex service hospitals; and 11,486 to community service hospitals. Similarly, the mean number of patient days in each type is 10,301 in the basic service type; 25,502 in the quality-enhancing service type; 66,751 in the complex service type; and 135,400 in the community service type.

The average length of stay increases with the type of hospital: Mean stay is shortest for the basic service hospital and longest for the community service hospital.

Table 4. Summary of characteristics of four hospital groups

Characteristic	Basic services	Quality-enhancing services	Complex services	Community services
		Hospital type		
Number of hospitals	1,414	1,327	1,011	543
SMSA size[1]	3.9	10.2	17.0	24.0
Adult beds	43.1	95.4	230.8	450.4
Bassinets	8.2	15.3	31.2	37.3
Admissions	1,578	3,706	8,911	11,486
Inpatient days	10,301	25,502	66,751	135,400
Newborn days	672	2,020	5,359	7,429
Emergency outpatient visits	973	3,108	9,231	18,514
Total outpatient visits	3,803	8,515	24,763	74,628
Average daily census	28.2	69.9	182.9	371.0
Adjusted ADC[2]	30.3	74.5	196.4	411.9
Occupancy rate	63.3	71.3	77.8	80.8
Average length of stay	6.8	7.2	7.5	14.2
Full-time nurses	26.6	72.3	193.5	317.1
Part-time nurses	9.7	25.5	59.9	53.6
Total part-time personnel	15.7	40.9	103.4	116.6
Full-time-equivalent personnel	58.3	162.5	451.0	862.5
Student nurses	0.9	7.2	46.8	85.2
Interns and residents	0.04	0.60	6.20	48.10
Average cost per patient day	$34.58	$40.16	$43.93	$47.07
Average annual wage rate	$3,261	$3,655	$3,943	$5,001
Total expenditures	$337,960	$1,011,460	$2,940,770	$6,292,550
Assets per patient day	$55.47	$64.56	$74.11	$79.84
Capital/labor ratio[3]	$9,434	$10,056	$11,027	$12,086

[1]Standard Metropolitan Statistical Area size. The code for SMSA population size is:
  0 = non-SMSA
  11 = less than 100,000   22 =   600,000- 699,999
  12 = 100,000 - 199,999   23 =   700,000- 799,999
  13 = 200,000 - 299,999   24 =   800,000- 899,999
  14 = 300,000 - 399,999   25 =   900,000- 999,999
  15 = 400,000 - 499,999   31 = 1,000,000-1,999,999
  21 = 500,000 - 599,999   41 = 2,000,000 and over.
[2]Adjusted average daily census = ADC plus 20 percent of the average daily outpatient visits.
[3]Capital/labor ratio equals total assets per full-time-equivalent personnel.
Source: Same as Table 1.

The mean lengths of stay are: basic service hospitals — 6.8 days; quality-enhancing service hospitals—7.2 days; complex service hospitals—7.5 days; and community service hospitals—14.2 days.

Occupancy rates increase in a fashion similar to lengths of stay. Basic service hospitals as a group have a mean occupancy rate of only 63 percent. Quality-enhancing service hospitals as a group have a mean occupancy rate of 71 percent. Complex service hospitals have a mean occupancy rate of 78 percent. Finally, community service hospitals have the highest mean occupancy rate as a group, 81 percent.

There are also significant differences among the types of hospitals in terms of in-puts and input combinations. These differences are reflected in the numbers of personnel, the assets per patient day, and the capital/labor ratios. Thus, for example, community service hospitals not only employ more labor and more capital than any other type of hospital, but they also employ more capital per unit of labor. These differences in inputs and input combinations are consistent with product differences implicit in the groupings.

It would seem that the results of this analysis support the contention that there are significant differences among short-term general hospitals and indicate that it is possible to identify groups of similar hospitals. The groups of hospitals formed in the analysis are distinct, they cover the range of services provided, and they seem to have significant intuitive appeal. Further consideration of the phenomenon of groups of hospitals certainly seems to be indicated.

Conclusion and Implications

A final characteristic can be compared which perhaps best represents the potential value of the analysis. The range of services provided in hospitals extends from the most basic services provided in a small institution with exceedingly limited facilities, through a somewhat higher quality of essentially basic services, through the more complex services, to the services provided in a hospital that serves as a community medical center in addition to its role as an inpatient institution. Different patients presumably need different services. For some, the services of the basic service hospital would be quite appropriate. Others need higher quality basic services or more complex services. Still others can only be treated adequately in a community service hospital. This is related to the question of the appropriate mix of available capacity—what is the optimal mix of types of hospitals? The importance of this question is emphasized by the significant

differences in average cost per patient day among the four types of hospitals.

Basic service hospitals had a mean cost per day of $34.58. Quality-enhancing service hospitals cost $40.16 per patient per day. Complex service hospitals operated at an average cost per day of $43.93. Average daily treatment costs in community service hospitals were $47.07. The differences in dollar costs are paralleled by differences in real costs as reflected by labor and capital inputs. These data are from the period 1965 through 1967. Costs in each type of hospital have increased significantly since then and the relative differences imply an even greater absolute difference for the present and years to come. This is an important issue.

Clearly there is a relationship between the availability of facilities and services and the capacity of hospitals to provide specific services. There is undoubtedly a relationship between the provision of specific services and hospitals costs. Much hospital cost analysis has been preoccupied with the question of what is the optimal size of hospitals. A more fundamental question is what is the optimal mix of complexities of scope of services, or what is the optimal mix of types of hospitals?

References and Notes

1 See, for example: Davis, Karen. "Economic Theories of Behavior in Nonprofit Private Hospitals," *Economic and Business Bulletin* 24:1-13 (Winter 1972); Feldstein, Martin S. "Hospital Cost Inflation: A Study of Nonprofit Price Dynamics," *American Economic Review* 51:853-872 (December 1971); Lee, Maw Lin. "A Conspicuous Production Theory of Hospital Behavior," *Southern Economic Journal* 38:48-58 (July 1971); Newhouse, Joseph P. "Toward a Theory of Nonprofit Institutions: An Economic Model of a Hospital," *American Economic Review* 60:64-74 (March 1970); and Pauly, Mark and Redisch, Michael. "The Not-For-Profit Hospital as a Physicians' Cooperative," *American Economic Review* 63:87-100 (March 1973).

2 See, for example: Feldstein, Martin S. *Economic Analysis for Health Service Efficiency: Econometric Studies of the British National Health Service.* Volume 51 of *Contributions to Economic Analysis* (Amsterdam: North-Holland Publishing Co., 1967).

3 See, for example: Berry, Ralph E., Jr. "Product

Heterogeneity and Hospital Cost Analysis," *Inquiry* 7:67-75 (March 1970); and Carr, W. John and Feldstein, P. J. "The Relationship of Cost to Hospital Size," *Inquiry* 4:45-65 (June 1967).

4 Berry, *op. cit.*

5 The choice of 50 percent and 75 percent is arbitrary; they were simply chosen to provide reasonable base lines for comparison.

6 The specific algorithm was: Put a hospital in the Community Group if it has three or more of the community services; if not, put it in the Complex Group if it has four or more of the complex services; if not, put it in the Quality Group if it has three or more of the quality services; if not, put it in the Basic Group. This algorithm is, of course, arbitrary. A variety of algorithms could be employed and the final groupings are obviously a function of the specific algorithm used. In fact, the groupings that resulted from this particular algorithm were checked thoroughly and seem to represent unique clusters. They are certainly valid and useful for present purposes.

Part IV

Pricing and Efficiency

The theme that runs most insistently through this section is the need to introduce an incentive system for efficiency for suppliers and consumers. Indeed, this section presents what might be termed the central problem of health economics: how to have a workable price system for suppliers and consumers when the third-party payment method is the rule rather than the exception. Whatever method one may choose for containing health care costs, its success rests on devising the proper incentive system for efficiency—the same kind that a competitive market system offers. Without a proper system, no amount of regulation can achieve X-efficiency or allocative efficiency.

In the introductory piece in this section, Kong-Kyun Ro proposes marginal cost pricing as a method to promote provider and consumer efficiency. Ro envisions marginal cost pricing as enhancing both kinds of efficiency through interactions between consumer and provider in the right direction. Under marginal cost pricing, a consumer will be given incentive to be admitted on an off-peak day for a nonemergency case because the marginal cost of treating him on an off-peak day will be less than it would be for treating him on a peak day. If enough consumers respond to such an incentive, hospitals can arrange working hours for the staff on a staggered schedule to operate on a seven-day week basis. This will reduce overhead cost.

In the next paper, Mark Pauly presents a framework of analysis of various reimbursement schemes in relation to provider and consumer efficiency. He lists three kinds of reimbursement plants for hospitals and three kinds of pricing plans for consumers. Given the assumption of net income maximizing behavior for both hospitals and physicians, as well as minimizing payment for consumers, one should be able to predict various provider and consumer responses to various incentive schemes. Pauly avoids committing himself as to which scheme is best, but his thesis provides a basis for the reader to choose among them, given the reader's preferences.

Dowling's paper evaluates prospective reimbursement vis-a-vis cost reimbursement in terms of promoting provider efficiency. If a prospective reimbursement scheme uses the hospital budget, hospitals would be motivated to minimize cost in order to maximize residual income after costs. But if the prospective rate depends on the ex-post cost, minimizing cost in the current year means a lower rate for the next year. Thus, the incentive for efficiency is diluted. Any prospective reimbursement scheme that relies on past cost figures would have similar effects to that of the Cost Containment Act which sets a limit on the annual increment for reimbursement, regardless of the past cost differences among hospitals. There is a long way to go before it can come close to being a substitute for the market's system of survival of the fittest for efficiency.

189

Kong-Kyun Ro

Reprinted with permission of the Blue Cross Association, from *Inquiry:* Vol.VI, No.1, pp.28-36. Copyright © 1969 by the Blue Cross Association.

Incremental Pricing Would Increase Efficiency in Hospitals

Originally Published in March 1969

With the political controversy generated by rising hospital costs, hospitals have become increasingly aware of the efficiency issue. To achieve efficiency, many cost-saving devices have been recommended and adopted. These devices fall into two categories: those for shifting the production function of hospital services and those for changing the organizational structure of hospitals. Attempts to alter hospital pricing policy have been few.[1] This paper proposes incremental pricing in the hospital industry as a means of promoting social as well as private efficiency.

There appears to be a general agreement that the rate structure in the hospitals reflects a number of significant departures from the norm of competitive pricing. The majority of patients are not charged in proportion to the cost incurred on their behalf. However, the obvious and simple means of correction—an incremental pricing—has seldom been advocated because it is thought that introducing such a pricing system into the hospital industry is not feasible nor desirable.

Arguments against Incremental Pricing

There are several arguments against an incremental pricing of hospital services. The most common one is that marginal cost

Kong-Kyun Ro, Ph.D., is Assistant Professor of Economics, City College, City University of New York, and Research Associate, National Bureau of Economic Research, Inc., New York City. This paper was written during the summer of 1968 while visiting Chicago under a grant from the American Medical Association. The author wishes to thank Bruce E. Balfe, Russell H. Clark and Christ N. Theodore for valuable comments.

pricing exists only in a hypothetical world of textbooks, and that in actuality marginal cost and revenue calculations play no or a relatively small role in the price decisions of business practice. This argument is similar to that against the profit maximation principle which maintains that businessmen do not maximize profit— only those in the textbook do. Alchian's survival criterion refutes this line of argument.[2] Although management operates with unit costs and prices rather than with marginal calculations, in general those firms whose decisions conform closely to the line of action which would have been followed if marginal pricing were undertaken will survive while others fail. Thus, at any given time, the majority of ongoing business concerns practice an incremental pricing of one form or another, regardless of what businessmen themselves may call it.

The second argument against incremental pricing is that the accounting and operating data available in the hospitals are uniquely unadaptable to marginal cost and revenue calculations. But the hospitals do not enjoy such distinction. In considering the use of accounting costs as the basis for pricing, one must recognize the fact that in a large part of the business world nothing deserving the name of cost accounting exists. In all cases, some arbitrary standard of allocation is adopted to satisfy the requirements of a "cost accounting system." As matters stand, it is unlikely that one can know more than that practices differ widely among industries and among firms in the same industry. The extent to which such arbitrary accounting practices alone serve to shape pricing decisions is a problem shared by all industries.

To contend that such standards are "arbitrary" does not imply that they are useless or erroneous. They serve invaluable purposes as the data for decisions on internal cost control, pricing, and relative outputs of different products. The arbitrary cost data are never automatically translated into prices but are used as a basis for constant price modifications, as subsequent data filter in, to improve the profits position. The hospitals do not lack such crude data. What is at issue is the fact that the hospital industry has never established a price policy based on an equal-cost concept, on an equal-service concept, or on any other economic criterion.

Price Policy Based on
Economic Criterion

It has been argued that the price policy of the hospital industry should not be based on any economic criterion because it is essentially a nonprofit organization and, therefore, prices should not be designed to maximize profit. In the hospital industry, capital expenditures are usually financed from donation or taxation or both, whereas operating costs are covered by revenue from charges made to patients. This has created a tradition which distinguishes operating costs from capital expenditures, the latter sometimes treated as a free good.[3] Under the circumstances, prices designed for optimum utilization of capacity are unlikely to be sought.

If the concept of public services is accepted for the hospital industry and its objective is defined as that of making its services available to the widest population possible, a case can be made using prices as a device for income redistribution. In welfare economics, however, it has been demonstrated that where actions designed for private efficiency do not lead to social efficiency, an explicit system of subsidies or penalties is preferable to a covert one.[4]

In order to avoid confusion the hospital should distinguish its function as a production unit of health services from that as a public service agency. As a production unit of health care, a hospital should strive for economic efficiency using pricing as a means for this purpose as well as others. The public service function of a hospital should be pursued separately with awareness of the costs involved.

Instability of Occupancy and Incremental Pricing

There are two characteristics of the hospital industry that suggest incremental pricing as an appropriate means for increasing efficiency. First, the demand for hospital beds fluctuates considerably. Second, a substantial portion of hospital costs recurs daily regardless of occupancy, constituting the fixed component of total costs. If incremental pricing reduces the instability of occupancy by providing an economic incentive for hospital use during trough (or valley) periods, it can increase the overall economic efficiency of hospitals. In the short run, operating costs per patient will be cut through a reduction in the "stand-by" expenses during the low-occupancy period. In the long run, capital expenditures as well as operating expenses will be cut by reducing the capacity requirement for a given volume of demand.

There appears to be two reasons for instability of occupancy. First, the occurrence of illnesses requiring hospital care is often unpredictable and uneven. Second, patients, physicians, and hospital personnel prefer to avoid hospital confinement or work on weekends and holidays. Except for elective cases, the fluctuations in hospital use caused by the first reason are unavoidable. The systematic variations in hospital use caused by the second, however, can be reduced by incremental pricing.

Weekend and Holiday Occupancy

How much weekends and holidays affect occupancy is well documented by various studies. For example, a study of 14 hospitals during the four-month period from

Figure I. Relationship between occupancy and the percent deviation range of census by the day of week*

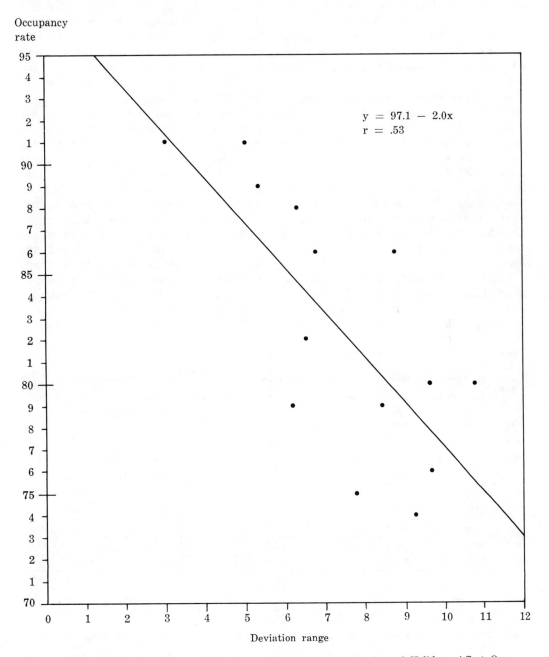

Occupancy
rate

$y = 97.1 - 2.0x$
$r = .53$

Deviation range

*Data are from London, Morris, and Sigmond, Robert. "How Weekends and Holidays Affect Occupancy," *The Modern Hospital*, Vol. 97, No. 2 (August, 1961), Table 1 on page 80.

November, 1959 to February, 1960 shows that a percent difference in daily census between the trough periods—Saturdays and Sundays—and the peak period was negatively correlated with occupancy rate, with a correlation coefficient of .54 (See Figure I). The same study also shows that on Christmas Day the total census for all 14 hospitals declined 40 percent below normal.[5]

What is more significant for its implication for an incremental pricing is the discovery of how the systematic variation in hospital use by the day of week is brought about. A study of about 4,000 patients admitted into six hospitals in the Pittsburgh area during the six-month period from July 1, 1964 to December 31, 1964 shows that weekends affect occupancy by influencing the timing of elective admissions and the timing of all categories of discharges.[6]

Table 1 shows that, except for admissions of emergency patients, there was a distinct pattern of statistical significance in timing of admissions and discharges by the day of week for all cases. The pattern reflects the desire on the part of patients and doctors to avoid weekends. Thus, admission tended to be heaviest on Sunday, lower on Monday through Thursday and declined to the lowest point on Friday and Saturday. The reverse was true for discharges. The day with the greatest number of discharges was Saturday and the smallest number of discharges was recorded for Monday.

Physicians wish to avoid weekends not only because of weekend family activities but also because hospital practices prevent them from providing normal patient care on weekends. It is interesting to note that most hospital personnel are on duty on weekends except those who provide "ancillary" services. For example, in a hospital in New Jersey,[7] 80 percent of the hospital personnel worked around the calendar and most of the remaining 20 percent who were absent on weekends worked in X-ray, heart station, laboratories, pharmacy and all special test areas.

Patients have reasons of their own to

Table 1. Daily admissions and discharges of all patients*

| Day | All cases combined | | | | Emergency patients | | | | Elective patients | | | |
| | Admissions | | Discharges | | Admissions | | Discharges | | Admissions | | Discharges | |
	Pa-tients	Per-cent	Pa-tients	Per-cent	Pa-tients	Per-cent	Pa-tients	Per-cent	Pa-tients	Per-cent	Pa-tients	Per-cent
Sun.	887	22.5	619	15.7	327	14.1	372	16.0	560	34.4	247	15.2
Mon.	517	13.1	350	8.9	333	14.4	206	8.9	184	11.3	144	8.9
Tue.	581	14.7	535	13.6	366	15.8	333	14.4	215	13.2	202	12.4
Wed.	555	14.1	648	16.4	346	14.9	400	17.3	209	12.8	248	15.2
Thu.	520	13.2	583	14.7	320	13.8	325	14.0	200	12.3	258	15.9
Fri.	446	11.3	516	13.1	325	14.0	284	12.3	121	7.4	232	14.3
Sat.	439	11.1	694	17.6	301	13.0	398	17.2	138	8.5	296	18.2
Total	3,945	100.0	3,945	100.0	2,318	100.0	2,318	100.1	1,627	99.9	1,627	100.1
E. =	564	14.3	564	14.3	331	14.3	331	14.3	232	14.3	232	14.3
$\chi^2 =$	245.37		135.25		7.64		87.02		572.79		59.90	
	SIG.		SIG.		NOT SIG.		SIG.		SIG.		SIG.	

Note: Throughout all the tables of this section of the study (A) the symbols should be interpreted as follows:

    SIG.   —Significant difference in the distribution at the .05 level and the .01 level;
    S/N   —Significant difference in the distribution at the .05 level but not at the .01 level; and
    NOT SIG.—No significant difference at the .05 level.

*Reproduced from Lew, Irving. "Day of the Week and Other Variables Affecting Hospital Admissions, Discharges, and Length of Stay for Patients in the Pittsburgh Area," Inquiry, Vol. 3, No. 1 (February, 1966), p. 8.

avoid weekend stays in hospitals. The public has become aware that not much is done for patients on Saturdays and Sundays and, therefore, weekend stays mean longer periods of hospital confinement and higher charges. In terms of costs to patients, even if the entire expenses of hospital services are covered by insurance or other arrangements, longer stays indicate higher costs of time. The more valuable is one's time, the greater incentive one has to choose "service-intensive" type of care over "time-consuming" type by avoiding weekend stays.

The five-day service has become the practice of most hospitals not because physicians and patients saw an intrinsic value in it but because the emergence of an increasing number of required new diagnostic and therapeutic procedures conducted by ancillary service personnel coincided with that of the 40-hour five-day week in America. Note that nurses have continued the practice of weekend work, although work hours per week have shortened. Incremental pricing, if applied to both hospital charges and the pay scale of hospital personnel, would provide incentive for patients to enter the hospital and for hospital personnel to work on weekends.

Pay Scale to Reflect Differences

The first action to take in this direction is to establish a pay scale which reflects differences in value of service rendered. Thus work-hours on weekends should be "rewarded" with compensation commensurate with the cost which more even occupancy saves the hospital. Then, reflecting individual hospital personnel's preference as shown in balancing the traditional aversion of weekend work against extra pay, a schedule of days-off or on-duty days should be established for each individual. This does not mean that any individual's work week is to be extended beyond 40 hours. In fact, if one preferred to work on weekends for extra pay, he would be able to shorten his working hours below 40 hours yet maintain the same weekly pay. What

is required is hiring personnel on a staggered week basis.[8]

Reflecting the changing relative requirements for services between weekdays and weekends and also the relative supply of services between the two, a pay schedule based on incremental pricing would obviously be continuously modified. This would, however, cause no more serious problems than those encountered in the operation of price system in competitive industries. What is required is the introduction of such competitive pricing, and subsequent mutual incremental adjustments would take care of any imbalances arising thereafter.[9]

Consumer to Have Choice

On the consumer side, incremental pricing of hospital services should be established which reward those admitted in trough periods, with a discount commensurate with the cost which he saves the hospital, and "punish" those admitted in peak periods with a higher charge. In view of increasing public criticism of hospital costs in recent years, it is somewhat surprising that the hospitals have never been held accountable for not giving the public a choice between off-peak and peak period admissions, with patients receiving a discount in off-peak periods or paying an additional fee for the cost of "rush" services in peak periods. An incremental pricing system which reflects differences in the value rendered the individual patients is already accepted as standard practice with the regulated monopolies.

Once the principle of incremental pricing is accepted by the hospital industry in pricing its product and the factors of production, the mutual adjustment mechanism of the competitive process would be set in motion. Individual hospital employees, in an effort to maximize their income for given effort, would assure an uninterrupted supply of services throughout the entire week as demanded. Except for emergency cases, the patients also, acting on the utility maximization principle subject to budget constraints, would choose to be admitted on off-peak periods. The end result would be an increase in efficiency through better utilization of facilities and better satisfaction of consumer and worker preferences.

The Sources of Payment and Hospital Price Policy

Hospital price policies are in general based on a full-cost or a cost-plus principle. However, the price differentials in the current rate structure by the sources of payment—Blue Cross, commercial insurance companies, governmental agencies, private patients and any combination thereof—contain many noneconomic considerations. The price differentials reflect in part cost differentials but are more influenced by the "public service" concept of the hospital industry and the relative political strength of the parties involved.

The substantial discounts given to Blue Cross patients are justified on the ground that there exists a difference in the costs incurred on behalf of Blue Cross patients and others for the same services provided. This is because the direct billing system and coordination between hospitals and Blue Cross result in savings in administration expenses, including those connected with bill collection. In other words, Blue Cross acts as an administrative agency of hospitals for billing and collection of hospital charges.

Another source of savings for Blue Cross patients is the fact that the standard rates for individual policies of Blue Cross are offered on the basis of the community ratings and full service benefits principles. This results in cost savings for hospitals in terms of the reduction in bad debts and in the number of patients in "free service" and "write-off" categories. These expenses are incurred because of the "public service" concept that a hospital, as a quasi-public agency, cannot refuse services to those who cannot afford to pay. Blue Cross, in this connection, plays the role of an agency who redistributes income from those whose actuarial rating would give them low premium to those whose actuarial rating would give them higher premium. If no discounts are given to Blue Cross patients, commercial insurance companies, whose rate structure reflects the actuarial rating of each individual, would put Blue Cross competitively in a disadvantageous position. Even with such discounts, it has been pointed out:

> Blue Cross faces the critical and difficult decision of whether to retain its philosophical ideals at the expense of competitive position or to rationalize away the social and humanitarian elements of its philosophy in an attempt to meet competitive pressures.[10]

Separation of Dual Functions

It is again suggested that a separation of the dual functions of the hospital industry —the production of health and the promotion of public services—would enhance its ability not only to perform the former function but also to pursue the latter goal. If such a separation is achieved in practice as well as in concept, incremental pricing could be adopted to promote efficiency in the production of health by the hospital industry. In providing public service, an explicit system of subsidies could prevent the distortion in resource allocation, and cost the minimum amount of public money.

As the first step in adopting an incremental pricing, Blue Cross should be paid for the administrative work done on the behalf of the hospitals. This would be a relatively easy transition because Blue Cross is already acting as an intermediary between the Federal government and hospitals in administering the Medicare program. Thus, there exists a basis for establishing the scale of compensation for the administrative work on a contractual basis within the framework of competitive bidding.

The public service performed by Blue Cross in enabling people to enroll on community rated individual policies should be compensated in a systematic way, not by hospitals but by a public agency. Then, Blue Cross would offer new individual policies based solely on actuarial ratings, thus enabling it to compete with insurance companies. Those who cannot afford to pay the premium due to their high-risk ratings or low income could be subsidized by the public agency. If the local government concerned is not willing to subsidize, the costs could be levied equally among all third parties involved and private patients.

Charges Based on Expenses Incurred

If the administrative work of bill collection and other bookkeeping activities of Blue Cross and the public service activities are undertaken separately and efficiently, hospitals could introduce an incremental pricing system charging everyone, regardless of who pays the bill, exactly the amount of expenses incurred on his behalf. Naturally, depending on the work load of a hospital at a given time and the type of room accommodation a patient chooses, hospital charges would differ among patients even if they receive the same hospital services.

A price policy based solely on economic considerations not only enhances the efficiency of hospitals but also consumer satisfaction. Individual patients can now have a wide choice. A consumer now can choose a hospital, through his doctor, on an economic basis: the greatest utility per dollar being sought. He can also choose the time of admission on the same basis.

Such consumer choices need not be restricted even if one has service benefit prepayment arrangements. Blue Cross can offer standard reimbursement to the hospital and the hospital can give a cash refund to those patients who have chosen a lower cost room accommodation or a lower cost time of admission. Conversely, those who wish to have deluxe accommodation or do not wish to wait for an off-peak period for hospitalization can pay the hospital the difference between what it costs and the standard reimbursement.

Patient Care and Training Activities of Hospitals

As hospitals have emerged as the nucleus of community health activities, training and research have increasingly become an integral part of the general operations of hospitals. Traditionally, hospitals have trained their employees in a more formal fashion than do other industries. Those who are formally trained in hospitals include interns, residents, student nurses, practical nurses, laboratory technicians, dieticians, and so forth. This training is usually conducted by larger hospitals.

In recent years, increasing attention has been given to expenses involved in these educational programs. Trainees, however, in most instances also provide services to hospitals. In fact, a school of nursing was considered to be a source of net income— rather than net cost—to its hospital up until the late 1940's.[11] Today it is generally agreed that nursing schools constitute sources of net financial cost.[12] This is in response to the accrediting agencies' efforts to upgrade the educational standard; nursing schools have reduced the amount of student service and increased the amount of classroom teaching.

The expenses involved in training interns and residents have also increased in terms of the gross outlays—stipends, maintenance, the salaries of full-time chiefs of clinical service, the cost of a broader range of tests conducted to establish the concept of "normal" results, etc.[13] Concurrently, it can be assumed that the value of services rendered to patients by the house staff, particularly by residents, has increased, not only because attending physicians' services have been priced higher than before, but because, contrary to nursing students, the house staff now spends more time with patients than before.[14] Therefore, the net cost to patients of medical education in hospitals is difficult to assess.[15]

Educational Programs Benefit All

It can be said that the net costs of operating a nursing school and medical educational program are the price of assuring a supply of graduate nurses and a house staff. However, the supply is for the health industry as a whole—not for the individual hospitals which undertake the training. Hospitals without these programs, which are for the most part smaller ones, benefit from the external economy. On the other hand, the external economy accruing to nontraining hospitals is essentially of an intra-industry nature. The net cost of the industry's investment in nursing and medical education might be more than adequately recouped by the benefit the industry receives through the increase in the supply of nurses and doctors and through the savings in payroll. For example, payroll costs of nurses must have been higher if student nurses themselves had financed the entire cost of nursing education.

Why should there be any concern about the external economy accruing to smaller hospitals when a certain number of larger hospitals undertake the training programs voluntarily? Does this not indicate that the direct and indirect benefits of training to those hospitals which undertake it are greater than its costs? Such a conclusion may be justified in a competitive industry, but in a nonprofit, public-oriented industry like hospitals one cannot rely on *a priori* reasoning of this nature without cost-benefit analysis.

Separate Two Activities

Under the circumstances, the efficiency of the hospital industry in both activities—providing patient care and training—can be increased by separating the two activities from one another and by introducing incremental pricing as the method of financing. For this purpose, although the cost accounting involved is difficult to develop to a satisfactory degree of accuracy, a cost allocation between the two activities should be initiated, based on the calculation of both the cost of education *per se* and the income from the services rendered by the trainees. Once a beginning is made, such cost allocation can be adjusted and improved continuously serving as the basis for decision making as to who should pay what cost. The principle of incremental pricing requires that the patients should be charged for expenses involved in providing patient care only and a systematic and equitable method should be developed to distribute the cost of training in hospitals to all those who benefit from it.

It is suggested that an institutional change will facilitate the development of such a system. An autonomous body within hospitals should be made responsible for running various training programs in coordination with the activities involved in providing patient care. As would two independent business enterprises, such a body should pay competitive prices for the use of the hospital facilities and charge to the hospital the value of the services the trainees provide at competitive prices. The difference between the amount of the outlays and incomes of the training body should then be financed through taxation or donation or both.

Concluding Remarks

Hospitals today face the difficult problem of how to pursue their social and humanitarian ideals with economic efficiency. Although efficiency has recently been emphasized, the rate structure and pricing policy of hospitals contain many noneconomic features which are now enshrined with all the virtue accorded to long-standing tradition. It is suggested that an incremental pricing based solely on economic criteria would not only increase efficiency in terms of cost savings but also enhance the ability of hospitals to carry out their traditional social commitment. What is required for an incremental pricing is functional differentiation of several activities of hospitals—patient care, training, research, public services, etc.—so that a price policy may be based on the equal-charge-for-equal-cost concept. Once the principle of incremental pricing is accepted, the difficulties involved in its implementation would not be insurmountable. Gradually, cost accounting could be improved and a systematic method of financing the public service and other nonself-paying functions of hospitals could be developed.

References and Notes

1 Two examples are: Feldstein, Paul. "A Note on the Pricing of Hospital Services," Appendix C, *An Empirical Investigation of the Marginal Cost of Hospital Services* (University of Chicago: Graduate Program in Hospital Administration, 1961), and Weisbrod, Burton. "Some Problems of Pricing and Resource Allocation in a Non-Profit Industry —The Hospitals," *Journal of Business,* Vol. 38, No. 1 (January, 1965).

2 Alchian, Arman A. "Uncertainty, Evolution and Economic Theory," *Journal of Political Economy,* Vol. 58, No. 3 (June, 1950), pp. 211-221.

3 Long, Millard F. "Efficient Use of Hospitals," *The Economics of Health and Medical Care* (Ann Arbor: University of Michigan, 1964), p. 213.

4 The rationale behind this argument is the same as that which, in order to avoid distortion in the allocation of resources, prefers income taxes to excise taxes and direct subsidies to farm price support program. See Hicks, J. R. *Value and Capital* (New York: Oxford University Press, 1946), p. 41.

5 London, Morris, and Sigmond, Robert M. "How Weekends and Holidays Affect Occupancy," *The Modern Hospital,* Vol. 97, No. 2 (August, 1961), pp. 80-81.

6 Lew, Irving. "Day of the Week and Other Variables Affecting Hospital Admissions, Discharges, and Length of Stay for Patients in the Pittsburgh Area," *Inquiry,* Vol. 3, No. 1 (February, 1966), pp. 3-39.

7 The hospital in question is Cooper Hospital at Camden, N.J. See Garrett, Robert Y., Jr. "Six-Day Service Makes Money and Sense," *The Modern Hospital,* Vol. 99, No. 6 (December, 1962), pp. 89-90.

8 A step-by-step method of implementing a gradual transition from five-day to seven-day hospital operation is outlined by Gluckman, Earl C., M.D., in "Operating a Hospital Seven Days a Week," *Resident Physician* (January, 1963), pp. 53-64.

9 Seven-day week operation has already been adopted with apparent successes by several hospitals. For a listing of literature on this subject, see Stenn, Frederick, M.D. "Seven-Day Utilization of the Hospitals," *Illinois Medical Journal,* Vol. 134, No. 55 (July, 1968), pp. 51 and 106.

10 Hedinger, Fredric R. "The Social Role of Blue Cross: Progress and Problems," *Inquiry,* Vol. 5, No. 2 (June, 1968), p. 11.

11 A study which the U.S. Public Health Service made in 1946 of a selected group of schools participating in the Cadet Nurse Corps showed that, although more than half of these schools did report expenses in excess of income, average income exceeded expenses by about 5 percent. See Block, Louis. "The Nursing School—Its Costs," *Hospital Progress* (September, 1947), p. 306.

12 A 1958 survey of 25 schools by the Illinois Hospital Association estimated the next cost per student at $1,620. No doubt the figure has increased since then. See Illinois Hospital Association, *Report on 1958 School of Nursing Cost Study,* Vol. 1 (Chicago, 1959), p. 33.

13 Until 1936, New York City, for example, did not pay any stipend to interns in municipal hospitals. Recently, hospitals with good teaching programs, that have no difficulty in recruiting house staff, have also substantially raised the stipend payment.

14 The Bane Report shows that residents, on the average, spend three-quarters of their working time on patient services, and the remaining one-quarter primarily on research and education. Bane, Frank, *et al. Physicians for a Growing America,* Report of the Surgeon General's Consultant Group on Medical Education, USPHS Pub. No. 709 (Washington, D.C.: GPO, 1959), p. 35.

15 A study of hospitals in Western Pennsylvania during 1953-1963 shows that whether a hospital has an approved internship or residency program does not significantly affect the cost per patient day of hospital care. See Ro, Kong-Kyun. *A Statistical Study of Factors Affecting the Unit Cost of Short-Term Hospital Care* (Ph.D. dissertation, Yale University, 1966), pp. 104 and 106.

Obviously, the cost to hospitals has certainly increased recently because hospital costs as recorded in hospital accounts are expenses incurred *by* the hospital, not *in* the hospital. Attending physicians practice in hospitals, but not for hospitals. Accordingly, the charges for their services do not enter into the hospital cost. Theoretically, if the house staff's services are not available, they can be supplied free of charge to hospitals by attending physicians. In terms of replacement cost, therefore, house staff's services are free.

Mark V. Pauly

Efficiency, Incentives and Reimbursement for Health Care

Reprinted with permission of the Blue Cross Association, from *Inquiry:* Vol.VII, No.1, pp.114-131. Copyright © 1970 by the Blue Cross Association.

Originally Published in March 1970

In this paper I wish to consider the relationships among the several sources of inefficiency that can arise in the provision of health care, the organizations or persons who provide or consume that care, and the incentive schemes implied by various ways—actually used or potentially usable—of paying for health care.

It is possible to distinguish a number of different requirements for efficiency in any economic system or subsystem:

1 Whatever combination of inputs is used must produce maximum feasible output. This is often termed "technical efficiency" or "X-efficiency" and describes being on, rather than within, the relevant isoquant.
2 The combination of inputs chosen should reflect the relative factor costs of those inputs. This choice of optimal proportions is usually represented by the tangency of an isoquant with an isocost line.
3 Given that inputs are combined in optimal proportions by each producer to produce maximum output, the size of each productive facility should be such as to minimize the cost of the total output produced by all producers. In simpler language, plants should be of optimal scale. Since we often define and measure scale by the amount of capital input, either in physical terms (e.g., number of beds) or in value terms, this

also relates to the efficiency of the capital allocation process.
4 The total quantity of output of each kind of good or service should be optimal. Generally, we represent this condition by equality between marginal rates of substitution and marginal rates of transformation (i.e., between marginal evaluation of benefits and marginal cost). However, I shall indicate that there are reasons why we might expect that equality not to hold for some kinds of medical care. There are really two problems here: the first, to achieve the optimal mix of the various kinds of services—hospital care, physician care, home care, etc.—which comprise what we call "health care"; and the second, to ensure the optimum production and consumption of "health care" relative to other goods and services on which the consumer can spend his budget.

These four conditions pretty well sum up the notion of economic efficiency for a static, world-of-certainty model. When uncertainty is present, we should add a fifth condition, which we can describe simply as:

5 Insurance should be provided optimally. This comprises both insurance in the sense of insurance policies and such insurance substitutes as preventive care.

Effect of Incentives

My intention is to show how incentives affect each of the three major components in the medical system—the hospital, the physician, and the consumer—with respect

Mark V. Pauly, Ph.D. is Assistant Professor of Economics, Northwestern University.

to those various sources of efficiency (or inefficiency).

Before proceeding with the analysis, we need to specify some kinds of incentives which will not be discussed. The first class involves incentives to make specific, precisely-defined changes in organization or methods of procedure. For instance, the government might give grants to hospitals which provide renal dialysis service or provide guaranteed low-interest loans to physicians starting up group practice arrangements. The goals of such incentives, and whether or not they will reduce costs, are debatable; but it does not seem useful to analyze the incentives as such.

The second and similar class to be omitted consists of situations in which acceptance of regulation, which will be particular to individual agents, is tied to reimbursement. For example, in the state of Indiana eligibility for Blue Cross reimbursement was tied to acceptance of the "advice" of areawide planning agencies on specific capital expansion projects.[1] Here again the major effects would be those of the regulation as such; and the incentives implied by reimbursement would be important only insofar as some hospitals rejected the regulation and, along with it, reimbursement.

Rather, I wish to consider what we might call "parametric" incentives in which a number of economic agents face given common sets of values for some variables, and have only to adjust to those common variables, not to engage in behavior specified for each different agent. The incentive to increase purchases of some good that a fall in its market price gives to utility-maximizing consumers is an example.

Incentives for Physicians

Incentives for Technical Inefficiency

We do not ordinarily suppose that physicians, in their private practices at least, behave in a technically inefficient manner. Income maximization, generally assumed implicitly if not explicitly, is usually thought to induce the physician to get the most out of the inputs that he uses, including his own labor.

The fee-for-service method by which physicians are usually paid also is relevant here. Since the physician's income depends upon how many units of service (here defined as office visits or procedures done, without regard to the efficiency or appropriateness of such procedures) he renders, there is an incentive to the physician to get the maximum number of units of service out of his inputs. This would explain, for instance, why most physicians no longer make house calls, and why, because of the telephone and the automobile, physician productivity increased significantly in the post-war period.

Mix of Inputs

It has been suggested that, in office and hospital alike, physicians use too much of their own labor relative to that of paramedical personnel such as retreaded military corpsmen or highly-trained nurses. Obviously, the immediate incentive for such behavior, if it occurs, is the fact that the use of such persons would often violate laws against practicing medicine without a license. But since physicians primarily determine the content and existence of such laws, this explanation cannot be pushed too far; and so we are left with a puzzle. If, indeed, the use of such persons does increase efficiency, there are potential income gains to physicians who employ them. Hence, the lack of widespread support among practicing physicians for such practices may indicate that the gains, and hence the incentives, are absent. It may be, however, that physicians oppose relaxation of licensing and the use of paramedical personnel because they fear that satisfactory performance by such persons might reduce the size of fees that physicians can charge for procedures. This would reduce monopoly gains arising from licensing, which prohibits anyone but a physician from treating patients.

Or, consider procedures done in the office. The physician must pay for non-physician labor and capital used, whereas if those procedures are done in the hospital, no charge is made to him. Two conflicting forces are felt here. On the one hand, if the procedure is done in his office, the physician may be able to obtain the profit from the use of other labor and capital that otherwise would have gone to the hospital, or would not have been extracted. On the other hand, he may prefer to let the hospital accumulate capital and other labor for his use, for which he does not have to pay directly. It is not strictly correct to think that the physician treats hospital labor and capital as though it were free. For self-pay patients at least, the patient is interested in the total cost to him of the procedure, not the physician's bill alone. *Ceteris paribus*, increased hospital charges reduce the amount the patient is willing to pay the physician.[2] But, in any case, the physician will be less conscious of the cost of hospital labor and capital than if it were employed in his own office. The incentive here arises from the separation of payment for all inputs in hospital-physician care.

Inefficiency Due to Non-Optimal Scale

One of the shibboleths of medical economics seems to be that solo practice is a less-than-optimal scale for the practice of medicine. The advantages of group practice, often in conjunction with prepayment and a hospital tie-in, are widely touted. Roemer[3] has defined group practice as an arrangement in which three or more physicians share common facilities and net income according to a prearranged scheme. The last condition appears unnecessary to obtain some economies of scale, since the physical sharing of equipment and facilities certainly could be accomplished under a variety of methods of paying for their use; and indeed, there is a fair amount of non-group practice sharing of such things. But for the free coordination envisioned by the usual discussion of group practice, income sharing is probably essential.

One would expect increased efficiency from such coordination, if present, to induce physicians to form medical groups, since by so doing they could see more patients and provide better service, thus increasing their incomes. But even though organized medicine has dropped its opposition to group practice, the relative growth of such practice in recent years has not been very great. The explanation for the failure of group practice to spread may be that there are no significant cost savings arising from economies of scale; and there is some empirical evidence of this.[4]

There is another disincentive to group practice that I can think of, and it involves the sharing scheme. We can envision the group practice as analogous to the firm, with the physicians as profit-receivers. But whereas stockholders contribute equity capital which is homogeneous, easily measured, and contributes service flows in a specific fashion so that sharing can be precisely defined, physicians contribute labor. Ideally, the physician's share of the profits should depend on the quantity and quality of labor he provides, but these are difficult to define in an acceptable manner ex post. If the sharing scheme is defined ex ante, each physician has an incentive to minimize his labor input, since if he does so he avoids the full disutility of labor but reduces his share of profits by only a fraction of the amount by which he reduces total profits. So, rather than be faced with the problems of haggling over profits and getting each member of a group to do his share of the dirty work, the physician may decide to remain in solo practice.

Incentives with Regard to Output

The output of physicians' services may be affected by the way in which the physician is paid for his services. Of course, the consumer makes the final decision whether to receive services; but since the physician not only renders those services but also provides information on which services to seek, the incentives faced by the physician may be expected to have some effect on the quantity of services the consumer ultimately takes.

There are three broad categories of ways in which a physician can be reimbursed: 1) fee-for-service—a piece-work basis; 2) a salary fixed for some time period; and 3) capitation—an amount per person "owned" or "assigned," fixed for some time period. There are many possible combinations of each of these methods with solo practice, group practice, physician-entrepreneurship, or physician employment. Each is also compatible with prepayment or point-of-service pricing.

Fee-for-Service Reimbursement

I have already mentioned that the fee-for-service reimbursement methods provide a strong productivity-increasing incentive, at least if the product is defined as patient visits or procedures performed. Since the physician does have some effect (like advertising) on the quantity of his services taken, and since the physician's income under such a system varies directly with the number of units of service rendered, one might expect the fee-for-service system to induce the physician to try to get patients to consume more units of service than they would have consumed under other kinds of reimbursement. (It is not possible to say whether patients get more doctoring than they need, since "need" is an imprecise and undefinable term.) The quantity-increasing influence of any one physician is somewhat circumscribed by potential loss of over-doctored patients to other physicians, although restrictions on the dissemination of information about fees and service by physicians—which is enforced by medical societies — mitigates the force of competition.

Capitation Payments

The reason why the physician has an incentive to maximize the number of procedures done under fee-for-service is because his income is directly affected by the number of units of service he renders. Under other schemes in which his income does not depend on the number of units, a different incentive will be present. Suppose, for example, instead of fee-for-service, each patient paid his physician a mutually agreeable lump-sum amount each year, in return for which the physician agreed to provide physician care. This is a kind of capitation scheme. Unless the agreement precisely specified the quantities of care to be provided in each situation, the physician, because he finds the provision of care laborious and costly in terms of the expenses he has to pay, would have an incentive to minimize the amount of care he renders and to prefer less laborious types of care. Since his gross money income is fixed by the capitation scheme, the physician would maximize his real net income by reducing the amount of service provided. (The patient, on the other hand, would be induced to maximize the amount of care he seeks because its marginal cost is zero.) In any case, we would expect the amount of care actually rendered to differ, depending on the way in which the physician is paid.

There is a second incentive under a capitation scheme for physicians which may be expected to mitigate, to some extent, the effect of the first. The physician's income under capitation schemes ultimately depends on the number of persons he can "enroll" or "obtain," and the price he receives from each one. (Of course, if the price is fixed and persons are assigned on an arbitrary basis, then only the first incentive discussed pertains.) Hence, the physician will try to maximize the number of high-profit patients he obtains. Competition among physicians would limit the amount any one physician could scrimp on services. Equilibrium under such a system is not easy to describe. It would appear to obtain when the going price for each kind of person (given his expected use of medical services) was such as to yield equal profits to physicians of equal "quality" and was the same for all persons with the same expected use of services.

But this might be obtained either by large numbers of low-use, low-cost individuals or by a small number of high-use individuals comprising the practice of various physicians. Note that capitation payments to physicians could also be combined with point-of-service pricing to consumers, although this would not be possible under the individual physician-entrepreneur arrangement. Finally, it should be noted that fixed capitation payments and fee-for-service reimbursement imply different risk-taking situations for the physician.

Under fee-for-service, the physician knows for certain his maximum loss—it is the amount of fixed costs he has to pay to remain open for business—but his maximum income is unlimited. Under capitation payment, the physician's maximum income is limited; it is the total of his capitation receipts less his fixed costs. But his maximum possible loss is unlimited, since if all of his patients became ill, he would have to render large volumes of service and purchase large quantities of medical inputs. If the physician is a risk-averter, he may prefer the fee-for-service scheme to a capitation scheme with the same or a higher expected income. Unless physicians can obtain insurance in some way against the high potential loss of capitation schemes, otherwise desirable capitation schemes may be rejected by physicians.

Salaried Practice

The use of a salary as the sole form of reimbursement necessarily rules out the physician-entrepreneur, either on an individual or group basis; but it is compatible with (physical) solo practice and either prepayment or point-of-service pricing. The incentive effects of salaried practice obviously depend upon the way in which salaries are determined. To take an extreme case, if salaries were based only on number of years of practice, the physician would have an incentive to minimize the amount of labor he performs, as under a capitation scheme, but with no offsetting incentive to seek additional enrollees by

giving good service. In general, if payment does not vary with the number of procedures performed, there will be an incentive to minimize the number of disutility-generating procedures performed. At the other extreme, if next year's salary depended directly on the number of procedures performed this year, the incentive effects of salaried practice would be almost identical with those of fee-for-service. Since we do not know how salaries are or might be determined, no further generalizations are possible.

Effect of Incentives on Locus of Patient Treatment

In the previous section we considered the effect of incentives on the output of total physician services. In this section we wish to analyze the effect of incentives on the locus of patient treatment, whether in the hospital as an inpatient or in some other capacity. Under the present arrangement, separate bills are submitted for hospital and physician services, even though to the patient they are joint consumption goods. If the patient paid in full for both kinds of care, he generally would consider the price of care to be the sum of the two bills. In such an arrangement, the physician would need to consider the size of the hospital bill, since, unless demand is perfectly inelastic, the amount he can get is reduced by increases in the hospital bill. As noted above, the fact that charges are made separately may provide less of an incentive to the physician to consider hospital costs than if a single bill were rendered, because he may not know precisely what hospital costs are. But, in general, the income-maximizing physician would consider hospital costs in determining whether or not to hospitalize a patient.

Effects of Insurance

Factually, however, insurance pays the hospital and physician bill for many persons for inpatient hospital care, but not otherwise. This has the obvious incentive for consumers to use inpatient care whenever possible, and the physician who wishes to maintain his practice will be induced to go along. The physician will have little incentive to consider the hospital bill. Although hospitalization of a patient who could be treated elsewhere will ultimately raise insurance premiums and may cause some people to cease buying insurance, from the viewpoint of the individual patient or physician this effect is so remote and diffuse that it is unlikely to affect the physician's decision. The fact that patients will get marginally better care in the hospital (even if the benefits, in some sense, fall short of the cost) and that the hospital may be a convenient, centralized location for the physician to see his patients (even though the costs of travel and disutility are less than the hospital costs) will induce the physician to put patients in the hospital even if patients were indifferent on financial grounds.

I wish to postpone discussion of the insurance incentives to consumers until later. It is sufficient here to note that no amount of reorganization of physician practice will remove incentives to hospitalization unless the insurance structure which provides incentives to consumers is also changed. Provision of insurance which covers both hospital and out-of-hospital care removes some of the incentives to hospitalization for patients, but has no particular effect on incentives for physicians. If such insurance leaves a patient indifferent as to the locus of treatment, there still will be the convenience incentives to physicians for "over-hospitalization."

One way to get around this problem has been suggested by Paul Feldstein.[5] Feldstein suggests providing insurance which covers both hospital and physician care, with the physicians (organized in groups) being paid on a capitation basis for both physician and hospital care. The usual capitation incentives would be present here, and in addition, it is argued, physician "overuse" of the hospital would be reduced because such overuse would reduce the profits going to physicians. Two

comments seem relevant here: 1) While there would be an incentive to reduce hospital use, it is not clear why provision of fewer services is necessarily desirable; and 2) if there are n physicians, a physician's decision to admit a patient to the hospital reduces his profit by $\frac{1}{n}$ times the cost of hospitalization, but provides him with the full benefits of centralized location, round-the-clock care of his patient, etc. The larger n is, the less is the disincentive to hospitalize that will be felt by each physician. So it seems unlikely to me that the incentive to the physician will have much effect, unless perhaps the physician's cut of the profits is made to vary inversely with the number of hospital days his patients generate.

Incentives Arising from Insurance

Let us first consider preventive care — which seems to be widely regarded as being underprovided in the current system —as it relates to the incentives facing physicians. In deciding how much preventive care to urge the patient to use in various situations, the income-maximizing physician will, under fee-for-service, compare his expected income under various combinations of preventive care and curative care.[6] While he generally gets more if the patient is ill, many office visits for checkups may yield more net income than the occasional big bill for therapeutic procedures that those checkups prevented. Thus, he will favor additional preventive care when the revenue from such care exceeds that of the curative care he would have given had the preventive care not been provided. Under a capitation scheme, on the other hand, the physician will choose additional preventive care if the cost of such care is less than the cost of the therapeutic care it prevents.

If we assume that price approximates cost under fee-for-service, we get exactly opposite incentives under the two arrangements. Since the optimal consumption of preventive care for a risk-neutral consumer if that amount at which the marginal cost of preventive care (including the bother of making the visit) just equals the mean expected benefits (in terms of curative costs avoided), it seems clear that the capitation method provides incentives in the right direction; whereas fee-for-service encourages both underuse of preventive care (when costs of curative care exceed costs of preventive care) and overuse of preventive care (when costs of curative care fall short of costs of preventive care).

Physician Payment and Insurance

The final theoretical consideration is concerned with the way in which physicians are customarily paid by insurance. In general, payment schemes are of three types: 1) a prearranged amount is paid directly to the physician (service benefits) ; 2) a prearranged amount is paid to the consumer, but the amount of the bill from the physician that the consumer pays can be greater or less than the insurance payment; 3) the insurance pays the charge the doctor levies, as long as it is his "usual and customary" fee for the procedure.

The first type of insurance is used for low-income patients under Blue Shield; the second (indemnity) approach for some middle-income Blue Shield subscribers and commercial insurance purchasers, and the last for Medicare recipients, until recently, and for some Blue Shield subscribers. The incentives under these plans are not complicated. Under all three approaches, there is an incentive to maximize the number of procedures. Under the last (Medicare) approach, a physician could increase his income by increasing his fees as long as the gain from these more than offset the loss of self-pay or indemnity-paid patients due to higher "usual and customary" fees. This incentive to raise fees under Medicare may have had an influence in the rise in physician fees. The service-benefit approach (for low-income Blue Shield subscribers) provides an incentive to the physician to minimize the input of services for each procedure, since

increases in effort on his part—even when they result in increases in "quality"—do not increase his income. (But, as compared to the alternative, in which no payment would be made by the poor, the physician may in fact render higher "quality" care.) The indemnity approach I shall discuss in more detail later on; it is sufficient here to note that it more closely approximates the no-insurance situation than either of the other two.

In an effort to hold down the costs of Medicare and Medicaid, the "usual and customary" approach has been altered by the Department of Health, Education, and Welfare, and it may be useful to speculate on the incentive effects of those changes. For his Medicaid patients, the physician will henceforth receive payments from a schedule based on the lowest prevailing Blue Shield payment for non-governmentally-provided medical care. For his Medicare patients, the physician's receipts per unit of service have been frozen until 1970. In both situations, the physician now receives a fixed price per unit of service. So, he will be motivated to reduce his input for each procedure as long as he receives only the fixed government payment for that procedure, since provision of "higher quality" care will not increase his net income. Presumably the higher-wealth Medicare patients and the higher-relative-income Medicaid patients might supplement the government payments with funds of their own, but the net effect of these changes will be to reinforce the physician's incentive to practice two-standard medicine, with low levels of service for the low-price, low-profit Medicare and Medicaid patients, and a higher standard for private-pay patients and those Medicare and Medicaid patient-recipients who make overt or covert supplementary payments.

Incentive Effects and
Organizational Effects

To conclude this section, I wish to point out the importance of distinguishing clearly between the incentive effects which arise from the way in which physicians, assumed to be income maximizers, are paid and the effects of various ways of organizing the provision of physician care. For example, in his discussion of group practice, Rashi Fein[7] expands at considerable length on the advantages of group practice, discussing considerations of specialization, of the optimal usage of various facilities, of economies of scale, and so on. But the evidence he cites to support these advantages is drawn wholly from studies of *prepaid* group practice in which physicians' incomes do not vary directly with the number of procedures they perform and in which patients pay a lump-sum annual fee for all physician and hospital care. The effect of such plans appears to be to reduce hospital usage in the neighborhood of 20 to 50 percent, without much increase in physician usage. As I have indicated, there is some reason to doubt whether this effect is necessarily beneficial for all persons. But the point I wish to emphasize here is that these effects do not follow necessarily from group practice as such. They may arise from the incentives that fixed salaries and hospital profit-sharing provide to physicians, and probably just as important, from the effects of comprehensive insurance on subscribers' demands. It is not correct to attribute them to group practice *per se.*

The experience of prepaid group practice has not been analyzed, from the economists' point of view, as well as it should. One major difficulty with analyses that compare two "similar" groups, one of which opts for prepaid group practice and the other chooses conventional forms of care, is the problem of self-selection. The fact that the two groups made different choices indicates in and of itself that they were *not* similar. Thus, their experiences are not strictly comparable. But even if the experience were analyzed properly, we would still be faced with the problem of distinguishing the effect of fixed payments on physicians from the effect of comprehensive insurance on consumers. Conceptually it is possible to separate the two influences by an arrangement in which physicians were paid salaries but in which consumers paid for each visit. Such an arrangement might be interesting empirically as well.

Incentives for Hospitals

The bulk of short-term care in the United States is given in so-called voluntary hospitals, which are private but not-for-profit corporations, with the rest of care given in hospitals operated by governments. Only a very small fraction of care is given in for-profit or proprietary hospitals. We have no acceptable behavioral model for analyzing either of the two major types of short-term hospitals. We do not know what they maximize, if anything; and there is almost no theory spelling out the differential consequences of various assumed maximands. The lack of a model has a very important consequence for the theoretical analysis of hospital behavior. It means that we cannot determine a priori what the hospital will do when confronted with various ways of paying it for care, because we do not know what the hospital is trying to achieve, or even whether it is meaningful to speak of "the hospital" as a single entity. Most discussions of hospital incentives, surprisingly enough, have implicitly used as a behavioral model that of hospital profit-maximization,[8, 9] although some have used variants of constrained sales or output maximization.[10, 11] But the absence of general agreement on the appropriate model will make most of the theoretical conjectures on the effects of various reimbursement schemes even more conjectural than usual.

Because the hospital does not explicitly maximize profits, it is widely believed that it is technically inefficient—that there is a lot of "slack" in its operations. Why this should be so is not immediately obvious. If the hospital were a constrained output-maximizer, for instance, or a profit-maximizer, it would use inputs in the technically most efficient way to produce the maximum feasible output. It might produce the "wrong" output, either quantitatively or qualitatively, but it would produce that output at least cost. Behind the discussion that hospitals are not-for-profit —and so "of course" are not subject to the same incentives for efficiency to which we like to think profit-maximizing firms, either competitive or monopolistic, are subject—lie two distinct models:

1 Hospitals are not maximizers but are satisficers, muddling through to meet some targets and generally trying to make things easy for themselves regardless of the kind of reimbursement scheme;
2 Hospitals are maximizers of something (of profit, even), but the way in which they are reimbursed provides them with an incentive (or at least no disincentive) for technically inefficient behavior.[12]

If model (1) is appropriate, improvement can only come—barring the substitution of different institutional arrangements— from interference with the technical process of the production of hospital output. This problem must be left to the technicians; if the economist is to analyze this model, he must postulate some maximand. Doing that would effectively convert model (1) to model (2), and so I shall analyze technical efficiency with the reimbursement scheme, rather than the model of the hospital, as the operative influence.

Technical Efficiency with the
Reimbursement Scheme

Most hospital bills are not paid directly by the person who receives the care. Instead, third parties (either an insurance firm, the Federal government, or local governments) pay the bill themselves or reimburse the patient for payments he has made. No precise figures are available, but it appears that approximately 80 percent of hospital revenue from patient services comes from third parties.

There are a number of ways in which reimbursement could be made, but the most common approach — used by Blue

Cross in many states and by the government in Medicare and Medicaid—is to pay hospitals the explicit costs of patient care, oftentimes with a "plus" either for cost not explicitly accounted for or for capital expansion purposes. This cost-pass-through method of reimbursement is alleged to lead to technically inefficient operations, since, it is argued, the hospital has no incentive to keep costs down or to anticipate unfavorable developments. "Cost-plus" contracts of this type provide a kind of insurance for the supplier since he is protected from loss. The "moral hazard" connected with this insurance is precisely the incentive just mentioned. (It is interesting to note that cost-plus plans should lead hospitals to take more risks, in terms of investment and other long-term commitments, than they would otherwise have done. But there does not seem to be much evidence of this.) The precise behavioral model of the hospital is not really too important here; the cost-expansion effect occurs in all models in which the thing being maximized is costly. Indeed, in cost-plus plans profit maximization suggests that the hospital will consciously try to push costs up and thus maximize the size of the plus.

The empirical basis for the existence of technical inefficiency or slack is less solid. In part it arises from the impressions of technical men that not all hospitals are operating as efficiently as they should, in terms of using new techniques. But the major evidence appears to be the wide range of unit costs, of output, and of the components of output experienced by hospitals which appear to be otherwise similar in terms of the input prices they face and the quality of output they produce.[13] It is argued that costs are $80 a day in one hospital and $40 a day in another because of slack.

It seems to me that this argument is not convincing since the presence of slack is neither a necessary nor a sufficient condition to explain variability in hospital unit costs. That it is not sufficient can be shown by considering the following: If hospitals, as personified either by their administrators, their medical staff or their boards of trustees, were provided an incentive for slack by the existence of cost-based reimbursement schemes, and if these hospitals were otherwise identical, we would expect them to maximize slack, in some sense, and so inflate costs. But we would expect *all* of them to do so; we would expect all hospitals to have the $80 costs. Slack is not sufficient to explain variability. There is, in short, no easy explanation of why people at the $40 hospital do not make things easier on themselves by letting costs go up to $80. Perhaps there is some random distribution of the propensity for slack or the propensity to tolerate slack.

That the presence of slack is not necessary to explain cost variation is a little more difficult to show. But let us suppose that, in every hospital, administrators and medical staff were working hard to get the maximum output of their inputs that they could. There are two reasons why we might still expect costs to differ even if there is no technical inefficiency. In the first place, costs at any point in time depend on both current and past behavior. If the hospital has made unwise or unlucky decisions in the past, with regard to investment, hiring, future demand, or organization, it may be experiencing high costs. But it may not be able to reverse those decisions immediately, no matter how hard today's administrators or medical staff try. The administrator saddled with an antiquated plant can hardly be faulted for having higher costs. Over time, these effects should be mitigated, but it will still be true that comparisons of costs at any point in time do not necessarily say anything about technical efficiency at that point in time.

Absence of Rents and Quasi-Rents

The second consideration is concerned with the absence of rents and quasi-rents in hospital cost. Suppose it were true that the head administrator determined, through his management skill, the level of hospital

costs. (I believe the medical staff may be more important overall, but that would complicate the example.) Suppose that these skills were distributed more or less randomly over the population of administrators, and that every administrator receives the same salary. Suppose finally that each administrator does the best job he can in managing his hospital. Then we could expect a variation in hospital costs, with the $40 hospital being the one with the best administrator, the $80 hospital being the one with the worst administrator, and so on.

If these were profit-maximizing firms in a competitive market, these ability differences would soon be reflected in salary differences. Competition for managers would bid up the salary of the best, and the equilibrium salary would be set at that level sufficient to attract the marginal manager. Rents would be earned by the infra-marginal administrators. Costs would tend toward equality, as the costs of formerly "low-cost" hospitals were bid up. But under a cost-based scheme, the $80 hospital has no incentive to offer higher wages to lure away the manager of the $40 hospital, nor does the $40 hospital have an incentive to raise his wages to induce him to stay.

We could substitute for "administrator" the medical staff, the board of trustees, or even the physical plant, and get the same results. In the latter case, the absence of competition probably results in a failure to alter the valuation of assets to reflect their productivity, so that the results of unwise investment, carried on the books at historical cost (or worse, replacement cost), bias cost figures. In sum, cost differences may be due to differences in the productivity of specialized resources, not to slack. The effect of cost-based reimbursement is simply to obviate the generation of rents and quasi-rents. (If factors are specialized, this also means that there is not necessarily a single "optimum" size of hospital.) We shall return to the question of incentives for slack after considering the related problem of optimal scale.

Very little other empirical evidence exists on whether or not slack exists. A study I did with David Drake[4] was designed to look at the effects of cost and charge-based reimbursement schemes on hospital costs. We compared the cost per patient day in all hospitals in four states, two of which use cost-based reimbursement and two of which used charge-based reimbursement. Our theory was that in cost-based states, hospitals would tend to inflate costs as indicated, but that in charge-based states, with charges given at any point in time, hospitals would try to keep their costs as low as possible in order to minimize losses or to maximize profits. But in hospitals in the two groups of states we found no statistically significant differences in costs which could be attributed to the reimbursement scheme. While there may have been variations in "slack" among the hospitals in each state, there were no consistent differences in hospital costs between pairs of states which were attributable to differences in reimbursement schemes.

Incentives for Reduction of Slack

A number of kinds of incentive schemes, which have as at least one of their goals the reduction of slack, have been suggested, and some are now being tried out on an experimental basis by HEW. The general form of these schemes is to select some target for costs, reward the hospital if its actual costs are less than the target, and penalize it or reward it less if they exceed it. The reward usually involves giving the hospital some or all of the difference between the target and actual unit cost; the penalty generally involves making the hospital bear some or all of the difference between the target and its cost.

In the absence of a model of the hospital, there is no basis for making any conjectures about the results of such "incentive" schemes. But if we make ad hoc behavioral assumptions, for instance, that hospitals dislike losses and like profits, then we might suppose that these schemes provide incentives to reduce slack.[15] Such

a conjecture would be strictly correct only if we assume that the hospital desires to maximize profits. It is within the realm of possibility that a hospital would respond to a target set above its costs, not by striving still harder to get its costs down, but by ballooning costs up to the level of the target.

One point to be noted is that, so far as incentives for reduction in slack are concerned, once the unit of output whose cost is to be the target is chosen, then a priori one fixed target is as good as another. The amount of the target determines the amount of the reward, positive or negative; but since we do not know whether there is any differential effect, there is no reason to prefer, say, average cost to last year's cost. Whether there is an asymmetric effect between profits and losses and whether an additional dollar of profit will have the same effect if profits are high as if they are low is a nice empirical question; but it is a question to which theory suggests no answers. There is, moreover, no basis for the common suggestion that setting as a target a given increase in costs will make things easier for high-cost hospitals, because high-cost hospitals do not necessarily have more slack.

Definition of Unit of Output

What does make a difference is the definition of the unit of output whose cost is to be the target. Suppose cost per patient day is chosen. Then the hospital which likes profit will have an incentive to maximize the number of low-cost patient days it produces. It can do this by keeping the hospital full at all times, by closing its outpatient department, by admitting easy-treatment patients, and by keeping patients in for long stays. On the other hand, if costs are based on the number of admissions or cases treated, stays will be shortened so that the number of cases can be increased. In both examples, the hospital will try to seek out low-cost cases and discourage the admission of high-cost ones.

This dilemma might be avoided by using not cost per case or cost per patient day, but by specifying the price to be paid for each type of case. A hospital which treated many low-cost cases, such as tonsillectomies, would not benefit unless its cost for performing a tonsillectomy were low. And a hospital that treated a costly, long-stay case could still gain if its cost for treating *that kind* of case were low. Lumping all patient days or all cases together ignores the possibility that some hospitals might be more efficient in treating some kinds of cases but less efficient in treating other kinds. This technique would also provide a strong incentive for hospitals to allocate their costs properly among departments.

The incentive experiments actually being tried in Connecticut define units of output as physical measures—number of meals, number of pounds of laundry, etc. There is no incentive here to affect length of stay; but there is clearly an incentive, for instance, to serve low-cost meals, which can be done both by lowering the "quality" of the meal and by discouraging the prescribing of more expensive meals for patients.

Competition with Non-Participating Hospitals

Finally, we should note that the effect of such schemes in a situation in which other competing hospitals in the area do not participate may not provide much information on what would happen if the same incentive schemes were made mandatory for all. This is so for two reasons:

1 What any hospital can do under the scheme is circumscribed by the possibility that patients may be lost to other hospitals. A hospital could not reduce the palatability of its meals too much so long as competing hospitals, operating on orthodox cost-based reimbursement, continue to provide costly but tasty meals. But if all hospitals were trying to maximize profits when faced with a target, the quality of meals in general might be reduced. This is a toy example, but it brings up an important point that might be emphasized here. In general, the performance of a particular kind of reimbursement scheme, for any of the vendors of care, will be very different in a situation in which it competes with other kinds of reimbursement schemes from that in which it alone exists. So one should be very cautious about concluding from the results of various isolated prepayment experiments that it would be a good thing if *all* payment for medical care were made in a particular way, and things would be better. People differ, physicians differ, and hospitals differ. My suspicion is that there is no single insurance scheme or reimbursement device which is the most efficient for all. Perhaps we should not be seeking the single best device, but devices which are viable when they compete with other devices.

2 Under the incentive schemes now being conducted, participation in them by hospitals is voluntary, although the administration has proposed that Congress give HEW the power to require participation of institutions. Hospitals will join only if they think participation will benefit them under the current scheme. This self-selection of the sample means that comparisons of the results for participants and nonparticipants is likely to be invalid, unless all nonparticipants would have been willing to participate, since the fact that some hospitals agreed to participate while others did not indicates that there is a systematic difference between the two groups.

Evaluating Results of Incentive Experiments

How can one evaluate the results of incentive experiments? There are many things which affect a hospital over time, in addition to the effort on the part of management to prevent slack. So, the result of any increase in that effort may be hidden by results of other things that change. It is usually suggested that results be evaluated by comparing the performance of the hospital or group of hospitals with that of a similar group which did not participate in the experiment.[16] If the effects of incentive reimbursement are large, they may come through in such a comparison. But if they are small, it will not be possible to control for all the other variables, some identified and others random, which affect hospital costs. If there is a reasonably comparable sample, it is likely to be too small to eliminate stochastic variation. In our paper, Drake and I tried to avoid this problem by the use of multiple regression. We tried to explain as much of the variance in costs as we could by variables which we suspected affected hospital costs, and then we determined whether addition of a dummy variable for the type of reimbursement explained any of the residual variance. This technique allows the use of a much larger sample than the "control group" approach.

Optimum Combination of Inputs

There is little to say on this topic, especially since we do not know what would constitute a suitable model of the hospital. We may reasonably conjecture that if reimbursement fails to pay for certain kinds of inputs, but will cover any costs "attributable" to other kinds of inputs, then the covered inputs would tend to be substituted for the uncovered inputs. If, for instance, insurance does not pay for depreciation, the hospital would not be induced to provide capital through borrowing. The incentive effects of failure to provide depreciation for capital built with donated funds or operating funds, or the failure to include a normal profit, are less clear. The main effect of such procedures would be to reduce the amount of investible funds that otherwise would be available; but we have no way of knowing whether hospitals will get and use the "optimal" amount of capital funds anyway. They presumably will use all the donated "free" funds they can get, but that amount may be limited by individuals' willingness to give and by the cost of solicitation. And the normal profit or im-

plicit interest is needed *only* if hospitals have a long-run alternative use for investible funds other than investment in hospital facilities. If they have no alternative, there is no opportunity cost of capital which must be paid to them.

The Optimal Scale: Hospitals

There are two problems in the optimal scale of hospitals which are related to the method of reimbursement. The first is concerned with duplication of specialized facilities. It has been alleged that voluntary hospitals tend to provide specialized facilities, such as heart-lung machines or surgical facilities, which are used at less than full capacity, and some hardly used at all. Excess capacity is not necessarily inefficient if demand is stochastic. Closed staffing policies of hospitals also may go a long way toward explaining "duplication." But certainly a large part of it can be traced directly to the cost-based method of reimbursement. Under such a method, the administrator has an incentive to push for a facility as long as it gives him prestige; the medical staff has a similar incentive as long as the facility makes some positive contribution to the staff's real incomes. This incentive would be present regardless of the institutional nature of the hospital, whether profit-seeking, not-for-profit, or governmental. Evidence for a particular influence of the voluntary form would have to be sought in cases of hospitals which have crowded general patient facilities, indicating excess demand, yet which spend uncommitted investible funds on rarely used but utility-increasing specialized facilities. A payment scheme which fixed the level of hospital receipts, such as a capitation scheme or a target price scheme, would provide a disincentive for these kinds of investments.

The second problem of optimal scale is concerned with the overall total size or capital stock of the hospital. Under cost-based reimbursement, the hospital, of course, has an incentive to invest as much as possible, so long as depreciation can be included in costs and the hospital can borrow funds. But the major way, apparently, in which it is thought that reimbursement affects hospital size and growth is by influencing the amount of "profits" earned.[17] The notion seems to be that hospitals which earn high profits will invest and grow. A reimbursement scheme which pays the average cost of a group of hospitals will cause the low-average-cost hospitals to be the ones which earn high profits. The low-cost hospitals, it is suggested, will grow; and this is desirable because this growth will cause cases treated in high-cost hospitals to become a smaller proportion of the total.

Reasons for Cost Differences
Among Hospitals

There are at least two reasons why one hospital may have lower costs than another: 1) It may have less slack in its operation; or 2) it may be experiencing economies or diseconomies of scale. If the latter reason is the only one operative, then the average-cost reimbursement scheme is not desirable. If we wish to produce a given output at least cost, output should be allocated on the basis not of average cost but of marginal cost. If we assume a U-shaped average-cost curve, we would wish hospitals with high average costs which are on the decreasing portion of the curve to grow, and hospitals with lower costs which are on the increasing portion of the curve to shrink. But payment on the basis of average costs will cause some too-large hospitals to grow and some too-small hospitals to shrink. If we admit the possibility of slack, so that some hospitals' long-run cost curves are everywhere above those of others, then the average-cost reimbursement scheme necessarily produces a desirable result only if costs are constant. If not, economies of scale may offset slack.

But even in the constant cost case, average-cost incentive schemes may not produce the desired effect. If "profits" from incentive schemes are specifically earmarked for capital expansion, then this facet of the scheme is only a capital allocation process, not an incentive as such. If funds are not earmarked, the conclusion follows only if it is assumed that high realized profits do induce investment by not-for-profit hospitals and that low or negative profits discourage it. Such an assumption could be based on an implicit model of profit maximization, in which past profits are used as a guide to future profitability of investment. But the discussion seems rather to suggest a liquidity or "bottomless pit" theory of hospital investment, in which the amount of investment varies positively with the funds available for it. There are some problems with such a model in this case. Profits are not necessarily available for capital investment; they may be used to raise the salaries of key personnel, for instance. More importantly, profits are not the only source of investible funds. The hospital with low profits can borrow and still make investment, even if it is high-cost. And the hospital with high profits does not necessarily have to *increase* investment; it may simply use profits as an offset against borrowing or donation solicitation which it would otherwise have done. Finally, there is no incentive for patients or physicians in this scheme to transfer cases to low-cost hospitals; and this is a serious defect.

The Optimal Quantity of Output: Hospitals

We already have investigated the problem of distribution of output between hospital and non-hospital facilities in connection with physician incentives. It is a little difficult to talk of hospital incentives in this area, or with regard to total output, unless we know what its goals are. But if the hospital likes profit, it generally will desire to avoid providing costly services if its revenues are fixed, as under a capitation plan. It is doubtful, however, that much discretion is available to "the hospital" as distinct from the attending physician; but it would be true that the profit-seeking hospital would try to move patients out faster and discourage them more from entering under a capitation plan as opposed to a cost-based plan. We already have discussed plans which fix costs per unit of output.

Incentives for Consumers

To complete our discussion of incentives, we need to consider the way in which consumers are reimbursed for medical care they purchase under insurance. Although it might be interesting to consider the consumer as a kind of firm producing "health care" by combining various medical inputs, I shall pass over that problem to consider the effects of various insurance devices on the total quantity and mix of medical care the consumer uses.

For our purposes, it is useful to distinguish three broad categories of insurance:

1 Those in which the payment depends upon the cost of the medical care obtained. This payment could be made either directly to providers of service (and in various ways—cost basis, fixed amount per unit, or capitation), as in service benefit schemes; or it may be made to the consumer to reimburse him;
2 Those in which the consumer receives a fixed indemnity for each kind of medical condition experienced. (An example might be a flat $75 payment for physician maternity benefits);
3 Those in which the consumer receives a fixed indemnity for each unit of service received. (Example: $50 for each day spent in the hospital, or $5 for each radiological procedure.)

Cost-Coverage Insurance

It may be useful to compare the incentives faced by consumers under insurance which covers the cost of care to the consumer, whatever the level of cost, and those faced by the vendors of care under different combinations of cost-coverage insurance and various ways of reimbursing producers. In every case, the consumer, once he has paid a premium, has an incentive to try to get care both in terms of quantity and quality up to the point at which a money measure of its marginal utility equals the price. The major effect of such insurance is identical to that of a price cut, since the insurance lowers the price to the user at the point of service, and the premium, once paid, has no additional effect on purchases. If demand is not perfectly inelastic, the consumer will respond to the price cut by increasing the quantity of care he demands, the amount of the increase varying directly with the elasticity of demand. This is called in the insurance literature "moral hazard," but it is very much an economic phenomenon. If only one of two substitute types of care are covered by insurance (e.g., inpatient hospital expenses but not care in the physician's office), the insurance will induce the consumer to substitute the covered service for the non-covered one. Extension of coverage to the previously uncovered service will remove this incentive, but only at the cost of substituting an incentive to increase consumption of previously uncovered kinds of service. As I have shown,[18] the final effect of such increased comprehensiveness may or may not be beneficial, depending on the strength of risk-aversion, the variability of expenses, and the elasticities of demand. It is not possible to say a priori whether increased comprehensiveness of coverage is efficiency-increasing or not.

If the vendor of care is paid on a cost-incurred basis, he also has quantity- and quality-increasing incentives. This combination, therefore, suggests a strong likelihood that care will be "overproduced" and "overused." If we combine price-coverage insurance with payment in a fixed or target price per unit basis to producers, the consumer still will want to increase the quantity and quality of care he receives. The profit-maximizing producer, on the other hand, still will wish to increase quantity; but he will wish to reduce cost per unit of output, which will probably mean some reduction in quality. We would expect him to try to get the consumer to substitute quantity for quality to some extent, but there will be a conflict of interest. Finally, if we combine price-coverage for consumers with capitation payments to producers, incentives go in exactly opposite directions. Consumers want to receive a lot of high-quality costly care; producers want to produce small amounts of cheap care. Conflict is increased, but so is the likelihood that "overuse" (meaning, I suppose, increased use) will be avoided. The quantity-increasing incentive of price-coverage insurance can be mitigated by charging some price at the point of service (coinsurance), and by other devices.

Indemnity Based on Illness

The second type of insurance (indemnity based on illness) is very attractive from the viewpoint of incentives to consumers. If we assume that the occurrence of illness is a random event, the consumer who receives a lump-sum indemnity faces the same incentives as the consumer without insurance, except for the probably minor income and insurance effects.[19] If he is charged a price per unit of service, then he will consume that good until his marginal rate of substitution between it and money equals its price per unit. Here there is an incentive to the consumer to keep down his consumption of the good both in a quantitative and qualitative sense, since additional consumption costs him additional money. If the vendor of care is paid on a fee-for-service basis, there will be conflict, but if the consumer pays on a fee-for-service basis while the vendor is paid through capitation, both groups will wish to hold down the quantity of care rendered. But this kind of insurance is probably infeasible in general, since it is impossible both to distinguish between the myriad types of "illness" and to determine whether or not a specific illness has occurred.

Indemnity per Unit of Service

The last type of insurance pays a fixed indemnity per unit of service. This is similar, insofar as the consumer is concerned, to the variable cost insurance suggested by Newhouse and Taylor.[20] For consumers, a quantity-increasing incentive would be provided, but not a quality or cost-per-unit increasing one. Consumers would have an incentive to take notice of differences in the prices (and the costs, if prices reflect costs) of the unit of service. An interesting result is obtained by combining this scheme for consumers with one in which the hospital is paid on a per-unit basis. Consumers would then have an incentive to seek out low-price, high-quality hospitals (at least as they judge quality), and to avoid high-price and/or low-quality hospitals. Hospitals which sell good services at low prices would prosper, and high-cost hospitals would have few patients. In effect, the plan fixes a price (the price the consumer is willing to pay) for each hospital, and the hospital must do the best it can, given that price. Here, as in other fixed-price plans, competition among hospitals is likely to prevent quality deterioration; but it does it even better here since the consumer is looking not just at quality but at quality for a price. This might provide an incentive to hospitals to reduce slack by introducing competition between hospitals on the basis of price.

There is one defect with this scheme. If the quality that a consumer will desire can vary with the type of illness, etc., this kind of insurance would not provide him with protection against the risk of quality variation. An interesting aspect of the scheme is that, on balance, even if it is most efficient, competition between it and a cost-coverage reimbursement plan for hospitals will not necessarily cause the indemnity approach to survive. This is because the incentive effect to hospitals will cause all patients to benefit, not just those on indemnity insurance. Since the prospective purchaser of indemnity insurance cannot capture all the benefits that his insurance brings, he may purchase only a small amount of it or may not purchase it at all. So in this particular case, competition between various insurance devices does not necessarily produce a desired result.

This insurance device does cause some problems — exposure to price-variation risk, quantity-increasing moral hazard (which may be exacerbated because the consumer can actually pocket money if he chooses a low-cost hospital)—but my feeling is that it deserves a try.

Summary and Conclusion

For any provider of service, his income depends on the price he gets per unit of output and the number of units of output he produces. If we assume that both physicians and hospitals are net income maximizers, this truism suggests the following threefold catalog of incentives for the vendor of care under various reimbursement plans:

1 If neither P nor Q is fixed (parametric) from the viewpoint of producer, the vendor will be induced to push up both P and Q. He will have an incentive to push up price directly if he is a physician paid on a usual and customary basis; and if the producer is a hospital paid on a cost-incurred basis, it will push up those costs through technically inefficient operation and additional investment in rarely used facilities. For either kind of producer, there will be an incentive to increase the output of high-priced units of output.

2 If P is fixed and Q is not, as in fee schedules for physicians or incentive plans for hospitals, there will be an incentive to push down the cost per unit of output by reducing slack, by reducing the "quality" of the output, and by producing only low-cost output. But net revenues can be increased by increasing the number of units of output.

3 If both P and Q are fixed, as under a capitation plan, there is an incentive both to reduce costs per unit output and to keep output down.

A similar classification is suggested for consumers by noting that the total price the consumer has to pay depends on the price per unit and the quantity of units purchased:

1 If variations in price and quantity both cause the total price paid by the consumer to vary, as when he buys on his own account or is reimbursed by a specific-illness indemnity, there is an incentive to seek out lowest priced units for the quality desired and to hold down the quantity purchased to that at which the marginal rate of substitution between medical care and money equals its price. Of course, the amount and type of information available to the consumer will influence this.

2 If price variations cause the total price to vary but quantity variations do not, there still will be an incentive to seek out the lowest price, but quantity will be increased beyond that indicated by the equality above. Indemity per unit schemes have this effect to some extent, since the quantity variations affect the total bill only when price differs from the indemnity price, but price variations affect the total bill directly.

3 If neither price nor quantity variations cause the total bill to vary, then the consumer will maximize both quantity and quality and pay no attention to price. Cost-coverage insurances for hospitalization and those which pay any physicians' bills over a wide range of usual and customary charges have these effects.

Numerous combinations of these devices are possible. Prepaid group practice, for instance, combines (3) for consumers with (3) for producers; and the typical Blue Cross plan combines (3) for consumers with (1) for producers. Some other combinations that might be of interest are (2) for consumers with (3) for producers, or (1) for consumers (when possible) with (2) for consumers.

I have deliberately avoided trying to make judgments about which scheme is "best" or "most efficient," both because, as can be seen, every method has incentives which potentially go in the wrong direction, and because there is no easy way to specify what constitutes "efficiency" in the provision of care. What we need is more information on the empirical strength of the various tendencies present in each of the schemes; and this information can be obtained either directly from experience or indirectly by the use of a model of the hospital (or the physician, for that matter) which has been empirically verified.

References and Notes

1 For a description of this situation, see Pauly, M. V., and Drake, D. F. "Effects of Blue Cross Reimbursement Plans." Paper given at the Conference on the Economics of Health, Baltimore, December, 1968.

2 For a description of a physician profit-maximization model of the not-for-profit hospital based on this notion, see Pauly, M. V. "Notes on a New Model of Non-Profit Hospital Behavior and Investment." July, 1969. Processed.

3 Roemer, M. I. "Group Practice: A Medical Care Spectrum." *The Journal of Medical Education* p. 1156 (December 1965)

4 Bailey, R. M. "Economies of Scale in Medical Practice." Paper presented at the Conference on the Economics of Health, Baltimore, December, 1968.

5 Feldstein, Paul J. "A Proposal for Capitation Reimbursement to Medical Groups for Total Medical Care." In *Reimbursement Incentives for Hospital and Medical Care.* (Washington, 1968)

6 It is obviously true that preventive care will be in disfavor among consumers, and hence to some extent among physicians, if insurance follows the practice of Medicare in not covering routine checkups.

7 Fein, Rashi. *The Doctor Shortage.* (Washington, D.C.: The Brookings Institution, 1967) ch. 4.

8 Feldstein, Paul J. "An Analysis of Reimbursement Plans." In *Reimbursement Incentives for Hospital and Medical Care.* (Washington, 1968)

9 National Advisory Commission on Health Manpower. *Report, Vols. I and II.* (Washington, D.C.: GPO, 1967)

10 Newhouse, J. P. *Toward a Theory of Non-Profit Institutions.* (Santa Monica: The Rand Corporation, P-4022, 1969) Processed.

11 Newhouse, J. P., and Taylor, V. *A New Approach to Hospital Insurance.* (Santa Monica: The Rand Corporation, P-4016, 1969) Processed.

12 A third model, which predicts technically inefficient behavior directly, includes some *input* characteristics in the utility function being maximized.

13 National Advisory Commission on Health Manpower. *Report.*

14 Pauly and Drake. "Effects of Blue Cross Reimbursement Plans."

15 If, however, cost differences were due to the absence of rents and quasi-rents, then competition for skilled administrators would simply raise their salaries, bringing all costs together by raising the costs of low-cost hospitals.

16 Waldman, S. "Average Increase in Costs: An Incentive Reimbursement Formula for Hospitals." In *Reimbursement Incentives for Hospital and Medical Care.* (Washington, 1968)

17 Feldstein. "An Analysis of Reimbursement Plans."

18 Pauly, Mark V. "The Welfare Cost of Health Insurance." *Health Services Research.* In press.

19 By "insurance effect" I refer to the possibility that the availability of insurance, by increasing the risk-averting consumer's real income though allowing him to avoid risk, may cause him to alter his consumption of medical care. By "income effect" I mean the net effect of the payment of the premium and the receipt of insurance benefits in the demand curve for care. This effect will be negative for those with below-average expenses and positive for those with above-average expenses.

20 Newhouse and Taylor. "A New Approach to Hospital Insurance."

William L. Dowling

Prospective Reimbursement of Hospitals

Originally Published in September 1974

The rapid increase in hospital costs during the 1960s and early 1970s can be attributed in part to the methods by which hospitals are paid. Cost reimbursement and charges reimbursement, the prevailing methods of third-party payment, are inherently inflationary in that they fail to provide incentives for cost containment. Recognizing this, government agencies and third-party payers are now investigating alternative approaches to reimbursement that incorporate such incentives.

Financial incentives can be directed at hospitals to encourage cost-containment practices, or they can be directed at physicians or patients to change their behavior with regard to hospital use. Because it appears that direct and separate reimbursement of hospitals will continue for the foreseeable future, this paper focuses on incentives that can be directed at hospitals via the methods by which they are reimbursed. Hospital incentive reimbursement schemes can focus on *process*, rewarding (penalizing) hospitals for initiating (not initiating) certain processes (e.g., improved budgeting techniques), or achieving (not achieving) certain goals (e.g., reduced length of stay) that are believed to

William L. Dowling, Ph.D. is Associate Professor and Director of the Graduate Program in Health Services Administration and Planning, Department of Health Services, School of Public Health and Community Medicine, University of Washington (Seattle 98195). At the time this paper was written, Dr. Dowling was Associate Professor and Associate Director of the Program in Hospital Administration, School of Public Health, University of Michigan.

The research leading to this paper was supported by the Division of Health Analysis, Office of the Secretary, Department of Health, Education and Welfare. The author wishes to thank Peter Fox and Joe Eichenholz for their valuable suggestions.

affect costs. Alternatively, incentive schemes can focus on *performance*, rewarding (penalizing) hospitals 1) if their costs are below (above) some ceiling or rate defined retrospectively—for example, by the average cost or average cost increase for comparable hospitals; or 2) if their costs are below (above) some amount or rate defined prospectively.[1] Because of the current interest in and apparent potential of prospective reimbursement, this paper examines the characteristics and possible impacts of this approach to paying hospitals.

The purposes of this paper are 1) to develop a framework for examining different approaches to prospective reimbursement that have been proposed or that are in use; 2) to identify areas of hospital performance that might be affected by prospective reimbursement; 3) to suggest, and where possible to support with evidence from existing reimbursement schemes, changes in hospital performance that might occur under different approaches to prospective reimbursement; and 4) to discuss alternative methods that can be used to set budgets or rates prospectively.

Definition

Prospective reimbursement—or more accurately, prospective budget- or rate-setting and reimbursement—is a method of paying hospitals in which 1) amounts or rates of payment are established in advance for the coming year; and 2) hospitals are paid these amounts or rates regardless of the costs they actually incur.

Prospective reimbursement clearly shifts some of the risk for costs from third-party payers to hospitals, in contrast to retrospective cost reimbursement where payers assume the

219

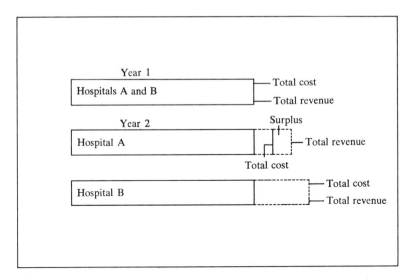

Figure I. Prospective versus cost reimbursement

risk for whatever hospitals spend. Incentives operate several ways. First, hospitals are motivated to anticipate and justify future expenditures and to establish the need for new facilities and services in attempting to gain recognition of the costs of their plans in their prospective rates. This could lead to greater cost-consciousness in capital and operations planning. Second, hospitals are motivated to identify and monitor the cost implications of the quantity, quality, and scope of services they provide to assure themselves that they can operate within their rates. This could lead to improved forecasting, budgeting, cost-finding, and cost-control techniques. Third, hospitals are motivated to keep their actual costs below their rates to avoid losses or to achieve surpluses. This could lead to more effective and efficient operations. An interesting question is whether hospitals are more responsive to the potential of losses (negative incentives) or surpluses (positive incentives). There is some evidence to suggest that rewards alone are not sufficient.[2]

Proponents of prospective reimbursement argue that inefficient hospitals would suffer losses and might be forced to curtail or cease operations. Hospitals that could contain costs might expand (perhaps using accrued surpluses). Thus, in the long run, there would be a shift from more costly to less costly hospitals. As will be discussed later, however, the changes

in hospital performance that might occur under prospective reimbursement depend on the design of the reimbursement scheme, and dysfunctional or unwanted changes can occur.

Lave *et al.* propose that an effective reimbursement system must meet two tests: 1) it must make hospitals viable (i.e., allow them to continue to serve patients in the long run); and 2) it must motivate hospitals to be efficient (i.e., to contain costs).[3] That a hospital, by containing its costs, can earn a surplus to provide the funds it needs to maintain its viability while at the same time receiving less revenue than it otherwise would receive is central to the concept of prospective reimbursement. In Figure I, hospitals A and B have the same total costs in year 1. Under cost reimbursement, their total revenues would equal their total costs. In year 2, hospital B's costs rise 15 percent as does its revenue under cost reimbursement. Suppose that, for hospital A, a prospective rate is set which generates 110 percent of its year 1 revenue, and that the hospital contains its cost increase to 5 percent. Hospital A would earn a surplus, although its revenue would be less than that of hospital B. Hospital B would be both more costly and less well off with regard to its surplus position. As Pauly has noted, however, in the absence of a behavioral model of nonprofit hospitals, it cannot be assumed that they would prefer spending less and earning a surplus under prospective reimbursement to spending more and earning no surplus under cost reimbursement, if participation in prospective reimbursement is voluntary.[4]

Payment Units

The impact on hospital performance of alternative prospective reimbursement schemes can most clearly be analyzed by identifying and evaluating separately the two components of reimbursement: 1) the payment unit and 2) the method of controlling or determining the amount to be paid per unit. Alternative payment units are discussed here and methods of rate-setting in a later section.

The bases of payment or payment units that could be used in prospective reimbursement include:

1 Total hospital budget
2 Departmental budgets
3 Family or person (capitation)
4 Episode of illness
5 Case or stay
6 Day
7 Specific services (departmental outputs)

As Table 1 indicates, all but one of these payment units has been used or is being considered in one or more prospective reimbursement schemes.

Areas of Performance

To evaluate the alternative payment units, it is first necessary to identify the changes in hospital performance likely to occur if each is used (i.e., its potential consequences, effects, or impacts).[5] The expected changes serve as criteria for choosing among the payment units. Judgments must be made as to the desirability of each change and its importance or significance weighed. A payment unit may cause some desirable and some undesirable changes; for example, an improvement in efficiency *and* a lowering of quality. No payment unit is without potential negative impacts of some kind, if only because the state of each area of performance differs from hospital to hospital. This suggests that additional controls or incentives might be needed to supplement the prospective reimbursement scheme itself.

Table 1. Prospective reimbursement schemes

Payment unit used
Hospital budget
Blue Cross Plans and Hospital Associations of Iowa and South Dakota
Blue Cross of Michigan
Departmental budgets
Connecticut Hospital Association (SSA)
Capitation
Colorado Blue Cross (1964)
Episode of illness
None
Case or stay
Blue Cross of Northeastern Pennsylvania
Day
Blue Cross of Alabama
Blue Cross of Northeast Ohio
Blue Cross of Western Pennsylvania
Connecticut Blue Cross – Connecticut Hospital Association
New Jersey Hospital Association
Blue Cross of Greater New York
Blue Cross of Rhode Island
Specific services
Blue Cross of Southwest Ohio
Blue Cross of Indiana
Kentucky Blue Cross
Montana Hospital Association
Nebraska Hospital Association
Blue Cross of Oklahoma
Virginia Hospital Association
Wisconsin Blue Cross

Prospective reimbursement can be considered from three perspectives—that of hospitals, the health system, or patients—and the three are interrelated. For example, prospective reimbursement might cause hospitals to reduce the average length of stay of patients, thereby shifting part of the burden of care to long-term care facilities and patients' homes. At the hospital level, costs might be reduced; at the system level, costs might also be reduced by more appropriate use of alternative facilities, but patients might suffer if they are not adequately covered by insurance for out-of-hospital care. This analysis focuses on hospital impacts, but system and patient impacts will also be considered.

The areas of hospital performance that might be affected by prospective reimbursement can be identified *a priori* by considering the factors that determine cost levels in hospitals. The following is proposed as a complete although general list of these cost-influencing variables.[6]

Table 2. Expected changes in hospital performance under alternative payment units

Payment unit	Cases treated	Length of stay[1]	Complexity of case-mix[2]	Intensity of service[1]	Scope of service	Amenity level	Quality level	Efficiency	Input prices	Investment in resources	Teaching programs
	Areas of performance (cost-influencing variables)										
Total hospital budget	↓	↓	↓	↓	↓	↓	↓	↑	↓	↓	↓
Departmental budgets	↓	↓	↓	↓	↓	↓	↓	↑	↓	↓	↓
Family or person (capitation)	↓	↓	↓	↓	↓	↓	↓	↑	↓	↓	↓
Episode of illness	↓	↓	↓	↓	↓	↓	↓	↑	↓	↓	↓
Case or stay	↑	↓	↓	↓	↓	↓	↓	↑	↓	↓	↓
Day	↑	↑	↓	↓	↓	↓	↓	↑	↓	↓	↓
Specific services	↑	↑[3]	↑	↑	↑	↓	↓	↑	↓	↓	↓
Cost reimbursement	↑	↑	↑	↑	↑	↑	↑	↓	↑	↑	↑

[1] It is assumed that intensity of service and length of stay are not substitutes (i.e., hospitals do not have to increase intensity in order to discharge patients sooner). Underlying this assumption is the belief that reductions in length of stay would come from the last few days of hospitalization, which are primarily convalescent.

[2] Admissions and case-mix are interrelated in that the case types that would be denied admission if admissions were reduced would be the least complex. Therefore, the case-mix of hospitalized patients that would result would include a higher proportion of more complex case types. At the same time, however, a hospital could attempt to select easier case types whenever possible.

[3] The direction of change in length of stay depends on the occupancy level. If a hospital is operating at high occupancy and has patients waiting for admission, payment on a per service basis should cause it to discharge patients sooner (reducing the average length of stay) in order to substitute patients requiring the more service-intensive first few days of hospitalization. Hospitals operating at low occupancy could both admit more patients and increase the length of stay to increase the quantity of services produced. The direction of change indicated is based on the observation that hospitals have extra or unfilled beds much of the time.

1 Cases treated
2 Case-mix
3 Length of stay
4 Intensity of service
5 Scope of service
6 Amenity level
7 Quality level
8 Efficiency
9 Input price levels
10 Investment in the maintenance and improvement of human and physical resources
11 Teaching programs

It is proposed that hospitals must act through these variables in attempting to keep their costs below their prospective rates. Further, given the form of a particular prospective reimbursement scheme (specifically, the payment unit used), the directions of changes in these variables that might be expected to occur can be hypothesized. It should be emphasized, however, that these hypotheses are based on the assumption that the prospective reimbursement scheme is the only constraint or incentive to which hospitals must respond. Clearly, other goals and pressures affect hospitals; therefore, the hypotheses proposed may not hold in any particular situation.

The matrix in Table 2 shows the directions of changes in the areas of hospital performance expected to occur under the different payment units. The payment units are ordered from the most aggregate to the most specific. It is important to note that hospital revenue under the first three payment units is only indirectly related to output, since once the amount to be paid is set for the coming year it does not vary with the quantity of services provided. Under the other four payment units, which are in effect different measures of output, hospital revenue is directly related to output. Retrospective cost reimbursement is listed last for comparison purposes.

The matrix does not include cost as an area of performance, despite the fact that cost containment is the central goal of prospective reimbursement. This is because the costs incurred by a hospital depend on the state of its performance with regard to the cost-influencing variables. The cost effect of prospective reimbursement results from changes in cases treated, length of stay, quality, efficiency, etc. In the absence of well-specified relationships between the areas of performance and costs, however, the exact cost effect of a given change cannot be predicted. Generally, it is just assumed that changes in the "right" direction in some area of performance (if not offset by changes in the "wrong" direction in others) will moderate cost increases. Three matters will be discussed in the following sections: 1) the expected directions of the changes, 2) the expected magnitudes of the changes, and 3) the desirability of the changes.

Expected Changes in Performance[7]

If a prospective reimbursement scheme uses the hospital budget, departmental budgets, or capitation as the basis of payment, hospitals would be motivated to contain increases in or reduce both the number of cases treated and the length of stay of hospitalized patients, since once the amounts to be paid under these payment units are set, they would not be affected by admissions or patient days of care provided. A hospital would simply receive, each month, the third-party payer's share of one-twelfth of the total amount agreed to for the year. Hospitals might attempt to admit more selectively and to discharge patients sooner to alternative facilities or to their homes. Depending on the adequacy of reimbursement for out-of-hospital services, hospitals might develop pre-admission testing, outpatient surgery, outpatient diagnostic and treatment services, and home care programs to prevent or shorten hospitalizations.

In addition to the incentive to reduce admissions and patient days, these payment units provide an incentive for hospitals to contain increases in costs by changing the composition of patients treated and by changing the nature of services provided them. Hospitals might admit fewer complex or serious case types (requiring costly services), thereby shifting toward a less costly case-mix. Hospitals might discontinue (or delay adding) costly programs and services, thereby reducing the scope of service they offer. These actions would tend to reinforce each other. Hospitals might also curtail the amenity level, quality level, and intensity of service they provide. All of these actions tend to moderate increases in expenditures for equipment, personnel, and supplies, and hence, act in the direction of keeping actual costs below prospective budget or aggregate capitation payment levels.

An incentive also exists for hospitals to improve efficiency, both by increasing input productivity and by shifting toward a less costly input mix. In addition, assuming that hospitals have some buying power, they might resist increases in input prices. An incentive also exists to reduce investments in the maintenance or improvement of human and physical resources. Cuts might be made in programs designed to improve employee morale and productivity over time and in programs designed to prevent deterioration of equipment and physical plant. These actions tend to moderate expenditures in the short run, although their impact on costs in the long run might be the opposite. Finally, an incentive exists to curtail teaching programs, both because of the direct expenditures involved, and because of the indirect impact of these programs on case-mix, intensity of service, and scope of service.

The overall effect of using any of these three payment units should be a reduction in both the quantity and cost per unit of hospital services, so that total hospital costs should be reduced. Total system costs should also be reduced with the substitution of alternatives to inpatient hospital care, if the cost of out-of-hospital services is less (for the quantities used) than the cost of hospital services that are eliminated. Whether or not patients would benefit from this shift would depend on the availability of alternative facilities and programs and on the adequacy of third-party coverage for them.

Evidence regarding the expected impacts of these three payment units is limited. The Michigan scheme has been in operation for only one year, and the Iowa–South Dakota scheme is in the planning stage. The Connecticut departmental budget scheme has been in operation for several years, and although the formal evaluation is not available yet, cost savings appear modest.[8] In this experiment, departmental budgets were not fixed, but were adjusted for actual volume. In addition, hospitals were reimbursed actual costs or adjusted budgets, whichever was higher. It may be that this no-penalty situation does not provide a strong enough cost-containment incentive. Evidence in support of the expected impact of capitation reimbursement is provided by the 1964 Colorado incentive reimbursement experiment with two hospitals in Yuma County.[9] Patient days per 1,000 Yuma County Blue Cross members dropped 7.5 percent during the year compared to a 3.5 percent rise in the use rate for Blue Cross members in the rest of the state. The 7.5 percent drop was achieved primarily by a reduction in the average length of stay, but the admission rate also dropped slightly.

One difference between the hospital budget and departmental budget payment units is that the latter focuses attention on departments where costs or productivity are out of line. In addition, departmental budgets could be used for departments over which the administrator has the most control, and cost or some other form of reimbursement used for the remaining departments. In the Connecticut experiment, only the administrative departments (representing about 28 percent of total hospital costs), were initially selected for target budget reimbursement.[10] Later, professional departments were added, under the assumption that administrators had gained more facility with budgeting and control techniques. Given the difficulty of identifying and measuring all of the relevant dimensions of hospital output (especially quality), a case can be made for using the departmental budget or specific services payment units for departments where output can be measured (or where quality is not a problem) and some other form of reimbursement for those where it can not.

Use of the episode of illness as the basis of payment, which would require that a hospital be associated with a medical group or health plan, would bring about the same responses as the three payment units just discussed. The problem of defining episodes of illness is substantial, however, and although included here for completeness, this payment unit has not been operationalized.

The case, the day, and the specific services payment units are all output related. In general, the use of any of these output measures as the basis of payment would motivate hospitals 1) to increase the quantity of that output (both to directly increase revenue and to spread fixed costs over more units of output to reduce the average cost per unit); and 2) to contain the amenity level, quality level, intensity, and scope of service provided per unit of output; to increase efficiency; and to contain input prices, investments in resources, and teaching programs, all of which act in the direction of reducing the cost per unit of output.

Specifically, payment of a fixed amount per case would motivate hospitals to admit more patients, but, if possible, to admit less complex case types, to shorten stays, and to reduce the intensity and scope of services provided. Concern that controls on per case reimbursement would adversely affect length of stay and intensity of service was expressed by the American Hospital Association in its opposition to the proposed Phase IV Economic Stabilization Program regulations.[11]

Evidence in support of the expected impact of per case reimbursement is provided by an experiment being conducted by Blue Cross of Northeast Pennsylvania with one hospital in Wilkes-Barre. Payment for the care of Blue Cross members is based on an average cost per case rate established by prospective budget negotiations. This rate is modified only if actual use is ± 8 percent of expected use, and therefore, it approximates a fixed rate. The difference between the hospital's actual cost and the fixed rate is shared 50-50. Preliminary evaluation based on the first six months of the experiment indicates a 1.1 day reduction in the average length of stay and a 12 percent reduction in the average cost per case.[12]

Admission selectivity (i.e., admitting less

costly case types) could be discouraged by establishing different rates for different case types. Hospitals treating less expensive case types would only be rewarded if their costs for such case types were low. Aggregating case types together and paying a single rate fails to recognize case-mix differences between hospitals and could lead to rewards or penalties that are not deserved.

Payment of a fixed amount per day would motivate hospitals to increase the days of care provided, by increasing admissions and/or lengths of stay, and to shift from more costly to less costly days by admitting less complex case types and by reducing the intensity and scope of services provided. Since the first few days of hospitalization are the most service-intensive (and, therefore, the most costly), hospitals might prefer not to admit more patients but to extend stays, if this would enable them to reach efficient occupancy levels. Where occupancy levels are high, hospitals might reach their desired output in this manner. Where occupancy levels are low, both admissions and lengths of stay might increase.

Payment of fixed amounts for specific services (e.g., nursing care, laboratory tests, surgical procedures, x-rays, etc.) would motivate hospitals to provide more services. Admissions and lengths of stay might be increased to increase the number of patients requiring services, if simply increasing the intensity of service provided hospitalized patients would not enable hospitals to reach the desired output levels of their departments. In contrast to the other payment units, hospitals might attempt to admit the more complex case types, since they need the most services.

All of the output related payment units provide an incentive for hospitals to increase the quantity of output, and this might be reinforced by long-run goals of growth and prestige. Of concern, of course, is whether inappropriate use would result. Again, no payment unit is without potential negative impacts. It would appear that controls over quality and utilization might assume more importance as cost-containment incentives are introduced. Another approach would be to attach additional financial incentives directly to performance; for example, by rewarding hospitals for reducing

their average length of stay. This has been tried by Blue Cross of Virginia.

The overall effect of using the case, the day, or specific services as the payment unit should be a reduction in the cost per unit of output but an increase in the number of units provided, so the net impact on hospital and system costs cannot be predicted. Pauly and Drake examined one specific services prospective reimbursement scheme, the Blue Cross of Indiana "controlled charges" program, in a comparative study of different methods of reimbursement. Hospital costs appear lower in Indiana than in states where cost reimbursement is used, although the differences are small.[13]

In summary, hospitals can attempt to contain costs in different ways. The actions hospitals actually take under prospective reimbursement will depend largely on the payment unit used. Selection of the payment unit, therefore, depends on how one wishes to change hospital performance. Hospitals could be left free to respond to prospective reimbursement as best fits their situation, or additional external controls could be applied to influence their responses. Hospital preferences for the different payment units would depend in part on their expectations about future use. If an increase in use is expected, the output related payment units would be preferred; if a decrease is expected, the budget or capitation payment units would be preferred.

Magnitudes of Changes in Performance

The magnitudes of the changes expected to occur under prospective reimbursement depend on several factors:

1 The tightness of the prospective rates. Obviously, if hospitals must take extreme measures to survive financially, changes would be greater than if the rates were more "reasonable."

2 The firmness of the prospective rates. If rates are adjusted for actual output or for changes in case-mix, input prices, etc., the influence of prospective reimbursement would be moderated.

3 The size of potential rewards or penalties. This depends on the proportion of any difference between actual costs and

prospective rates that is shared by hospitals and on the proportion of their patients covered by prospective reimbursement. Also, if hospitals are able to offset potential losses by increasing charges to direct pay patients, the influence of prospective reimbursement would be moderated.

4   The present state of hospital performance. Admissions or length of stay, for example, might decrease more under the appropriate payment units in hospitals where inappropriate use is substantial than in those where there is little overuse.

5   The physician's role in determining hospital performance. Admissions, case-mix, length of stay, etc., depend largely on decisions made by physicians; and therefore, changes in the medically-related areas of performance require their support.

In the Wilkes-Barre experiment, the Blue Cross per case reimbursement scheme is paralleled by a Pennsylvania Blue Shield program in which physicians are paid on a diagnosis-specific per case basis for the care of hospitalized patients. Examples of such complementary incentives, however, are rare. The financial incentives of hospital prospective reimbursement schemes have been directed at hospitals, not physicians; and hospitals have not attempted to pass on the rewards or penalties they incur. It is interesting to note that HR 13461, recently introduced by Representative Mills, would require hospitals to share any surpluses earned under prospective reimbursement with their employees and physicians.

The disposition of physicians toward cooperation with cost-containment efforts, especially where changes in patterns of practice are involved, is generally viewed as problematic. Certainly, differences exist from hospital to hospital. Nevertheless, most physicians will cooperate to some extent when the financial status of the institution is at stake. It may be that physician concern about hospital costs has not been more evident because hospitals themselves have given this goal low priority

under cost reimbursement. It may also be that administrators could gain physician support more readily if funds for adding services of interest to physicians depended on the ability of hospitals to earn surpluses. Hospital influence on physicians would be greater if all hospitals in an area were under a single prospective reimbursement scheme, and hence, sought to change patterns of practice in a similar manner, because this would reduce the possibility of physicians moving patients to less demanding hospitals.

Evidence regarding the cooperation to be expected of physicians is limited, although the Colorado experiment is pertinent. Capitation payments were made directly to the participating hospitals and covered only hospital services. There were no financial incentives for physicians. (It could be that physician income was decreased slightly by the shorter hospital stays.) Since reductions in admissions and length of stay occurred, it would appear that the hospitals were able to influence physician patterns of hospital use to further their own objectives. Blue Cross of Rhode Island claims to have achieved a $4.5-million reduction (from $144-million originally requested) in its negotiations with the 14 hospitals in the state over their FY 1970–1971 budgets. Much of this came from deletions of planned medical programs and services.[14] Again, it appears that hospitals were able to look to the medical side of their operations for cost savings. Rafferty apparently assumes that hospitals can influence physicians when he cautions that experimentation with incentive reimbursement should proceed slowly because of the danger of hospitals choosing easier case-mixes.[15]

Desirability of Changes in Performance

Judgments about the desirability of the changes expected to occur under prospective reimbursement depend on the present state of hospital performance. If, for example, inappropriate admissions are few in number, a reduction in admissions would be undesirable. If the reverse is true, a reduction would be desirable (assuming that unnecessary rather than necessary admissions would be the ones curtailed). The matrix in Table 3 contains the areas of

Table 3. Desirability of expected changes in hospital performance

Payment unit	Admissions	Length of stay	Complexity of case-mix	Intensity of service	Scope of service	Quality level	Efficiency
Hospital budget	+	+	?	?	?	−	+
Departmental budgets	+	+	?	?	?	−	+
Family or person (capitation)	+	+	?	?	?	−	+
Episode of illness	+	+	?	?	?	−	+
Case or stay	−	+	?	?	?	−	+
Day	−	−	?	?	?	−	+
Specific services	−	−	−	−	−	−	+
Cost reimbursement	−	−	−	−	−	+	−

performance most frequently discussed in relation to prospective reimbursement, with pluses and minuses indicating the author's judgments about the expected changes in performance. The assumptions underlying this matrix are discussed in this section.

Hospitals have been charged, in recent years, with abuses in every area of performance presented in the matrix. That community hospital utilization is 25 to 50 percent higher than experienced under prepaid group practice is often cited as evidence of overuse. Also, studies in which admissions and/or lengths of stay have been reviewed by panels of physicians consistently find inappropriate use, judged in terms of medical standards. It would appear from these studies that 10 to 20 percent of the patients in a "typical" community hospital on an "average" day do not need to be there. (Such a conclusion is warranted only if alternative facilities are available and covered by health insurance.) It is assumed here that there is some overuse of hospitals and that reductions in both admissions and length of stay would be desirable.

Less is known about the appropriateness of the intensity of service provided to hospitalized patients. Great increases have occurred in the per case and per day use of laboratory, x-ray,

etc., services over the last few years,[16] and this has caused much of the annual 3.8 percent increase (1955–1968) in labor and non-labor inputs used per patient day by hospitals.[17] Whether the increase in intensity is due to advances in medical technology; to changes in case-mix, improvements in quality, or shorter stays; or to the increasing threat of malpractice suits is unclear. Therefore, no judgment is offered about the desirability of reductions in intensity, although it is assumed that increases, especially if motivated by financial incentives, would be undesirable.

Evidence with regard to the appropriateness of the case-mix distribution across hospitals, which influences the scope of services they offer, is limited. Implicit in the charge of duplication of facilities and in the goal of rationalizing the delivery system is the assumption that some hospitals admit and treat case types that should be treated in referral hospitals. On the other hand, it is argued that if case-mix is too narrowly prescribed, some hospitals might not be able to maintain an adequate medical staff (since physicians prefer to locate most of their work in one hospital). It is also argued that hospitals must offer a reasonable scope of service to protect admitted patients. Not only may a patient's condition change, but the services required for treatment may not be known until the diagnostic work-up has been completed. Finally, frequent transfers, in addition to imposing social costs on patients and physicians, are medically undesirable. It is assumed that it would be dysfunctional for most hospitals to attempt to increase the proportion of complex case types treated or the scope of services offered. On the other hand, financial incentives should not motivate hospitals to admit only "easy" case types or to curtail substantially the scope of service they offer.

The findings of most studies of the quality of hospital care focus on the utilization aspects of quality, like unnecessary admissions, unnecessary surgery, or unnecessarily long stays. Few would argue that the remaining dimension of quality—the clinical or technical excellence with which diagnostic and treatment services are rendered—is too high. The level of training of medical and technical personnel is often

Table 4.   Classification of prospective reimbursement schemes by budget- or rate-setting organization and method

Organization	Budget- or rate-setting method[1]		
	Budget review and approval[2]	Formula	Negotiation
Federal agency		Economic Stabilization Program	
State agency	Arizona, California, Colorado, Connecticut, Massachusetts, New Jersey, New York, Washington		
Quasi-public special purpose agency	Maryland (HCAS)		
Third-party payer within the context of state regulation		Blue Cross of Greater New York[3]	
Hospital association within the context of state regulation	New Jersey Hospital Association		
Third-party payer	Blue Cross of Indiana Wisconsin Blue Cross	Blue Cross of Alabama[4] Blue Cross of Western Pennsylvania[5]	Blue Cross of Northeast Ohio, Blue Cross of Northeast Pennsylvania, Blue Cross of Western Pennsylvania, Blue Cross of Southwest Ohio, Kentucky Blue Cross, Blue Cross of Michigan, Blue Cross of Oklahoma, Blue Cross of Rhode Island
Hospital association	Connecticut Hospital Association (SSA), Nebraska Hospital Association, Virginia Hospital Association		
Joint third-party payer– hospital association	Connecticut Blue Cross– Connecticut Hospital Association, Iowa and South Dakota Blue Cross Plans and Hospital Associations		
Private special purpose agency	Montana Hospitals Rate Review Board		

[1] There are two additional methods of budget- or rate-setting that have not been tried:

Determination of reasonable costs of specific services
The National Advisory Committee on Health Manpower recommended that payment of hospitals be based on:
   . . . a small number of well-defined services or treatments. Those chosen should be well enough defined so that there would be reasonable assurance of meeting the criterion of equal payment for equal services, e.g., certain laboratory or radiology procedures, or the treatment of specified orthopedic or surgical cases. Careful studies would be made to determine the reasonable cost of providing each service. Evaluation would be made of the quality of each service in the participating hospitals. For each one, all hospitals in a locality would receive an equal base payment plus an increment that varied with the standard of service.

As noted, this method is not in use at the present time. See: National Advisory Commission on Health Manpower. *Report*, Vol. 1 (Washington, D.C.: GPO, 1967) p. 59.

Bidding
The bidding method of rate-setting might operate as follows: Hospitals would submit bids reflecting their expected costs of producing specific services (for which specifications would be developed), or their expected costs per day. For each service the average of the bids would be accepted as the reasonable cost. If a hospital's actual cost per unit of service was below its bid, it would be paid its actual cost plus a varying percent of the difference between its actual cost and its bid, the percent depending on how far the hospital's bid was below the average of all bids (to encourage hospitals to make low bids). Hospitals with actual costs above their bid or above the average of the bids would suffer losses. Again, this method is not in use at the present

used as a proxy for the quality of the services they perform, and it is possible to substitute less skilled personnel to perform certain functions without apparent harm. However, this is actually an improvement in efficiency, not a reduction in quality. Although it is possible for quality to be so high that the trade-off between quality and the availability of services or the ability to pay for them is unacceptable, it is assumed that a reduction in quality would be undesirable. Finally, it is assumed that improvements in efficiency would always be desirable.

Alternative Budget- or Rate-Setting Methods

It has been argued that the impact of prospective reimbursement (desirable or undesirable) on hospital performance depends largely on the payment unit used. Choice of the method used to control or determine the amount to be paid per unit should be based on an evaluation of how well alternative methods are able to establish fair but tight payment levels.

Table 4 classifies prospective reimbursement schemes in terms of the organization that sets the amount or rate to be paid and the method of budget- or rate-setting used. The budget- or rate-setting organization may be public, private, or a combination of the two. Various methods can be used to set budgets or rates—budget review and approval, formula, negotiation, determination of the reasonable costs of specific services, or bidding. The last two methods have not been tried, and so discussion about them is limited.

Uniform versus Individual Hospital Rates

The extent to which differences among hospitals should be taken into account in rate-setting is a basic issue in prospective reimbursement. The quantity and types of patients treated, facilities and services, teaching programs, input prices, and amenity, quality, and productivity levels differ greatly among hospitals. One point of view is that these differences should not be taken into account in

---

time. See: Hinderer, H. "Reimbursement: Past, Present, and Future." In: *Public Control and Hospital Operations*, Graduate Program in Hospital Administration, University of Chicago, 1972, pp. 4–9.

[2] Existing methods of reviewing and approving hospital *charges* (e.g., the Blue Cross of Indiana "controlled charges" system) review a hospital's past cost experience and its future plans presented in the form of capital and operating budgets. The hospital's proposed charge structure can only be justified in terms of projected costs that are judged to be reasonable. Therefore, no distinction is made here between budget review and approval and charges review and approval methods, although proponents of the approved charges method might argue otherwise.

[3] The formula of Blue Cross of Greater New York is as follows: A hospital's per diem cost for the past year $t-1$ is increased by the percent increase in its per diem cost from $t-1$ to the present year t and a further percent increase, reflecting expected increases in input prices, applied to determine its prospective per diem rate for the coming year $t+1$. A hospital's $t-1$ cost and $t-1$ to t cost increase rate are both subject to adjustment downward (upward) if they compare unfavorably (favorably) with the average for comparable hospitals.

[4] Blue Cross of Alabama is using the formula method of prospective rate-setting in an incentive reimbursement experiment being conducted with 10 hospitals. A projected per diem rate, equivalent to each hospital's previous year's cost increased by the average percent increase in costs of all Blue Cross of Alabama hospitals, is set for each hospital. If a hospital's actual cost + 5 percent (the regular Blue Cross reimbursement level) is less than the projected rate, it receives an incentive payment equal to 50 percent of the difference. If its actual cost + 5 percent is greater than the projected rate, it is penalized 50 percent of the difference up to the amount of the 5 percent plus factor.

[5] Blue Cross of Western Pennsylvania allows hospitals to choose between cost reimbursement and either of two formula methods for prospectively determining reimbursement. In the predicted cost method, the coefficients of a statistically estimated cost function (which includes case-mix, location, services, size, outpatient volume, and teaching status as independent variables) are used to predict a hospital's total cost for the upcoming years. During the year, the hospital is reimbursed at an interim per diem rate computed from the lesser of its budgeted or predicted cost. The final reimbursement settlement is based on actual cost but includes a reward (penalty) if the hospital's actual cost is below (above) its predicted cost. In the prospective cost method, a hospital's prospective per diem rate is computed from its budget for the coming year with the maximum budget increase for each category of expense limited to the average of an applicable input price index increase rate and the hospital's actual cost increase rate (both for that category of expense) during the current year. During the year, the hospital is reimbursed at the prospective rate. The final reimbursement settlement is based on actual cost, but if the hospital's actual per diem is above (below) its prospective rate, 50 percent of the difference is added to the prospective (actual) rate to determine the final reimbursement rate.

setting rates, because to do so would fix existing performance variations, moderate the cost-containment potential of prospective reimbursement, and slow the shift from more costly to less costly hospitals. This argues for a single community or regional rate or uniform rates for comparable groups of hospitals. Alternatively, it can be argued that a separate rate should be set for each hospital, allowing hospitals with justifiable or uncorrectable (at least in the short run) high costs higher rates than hospitals with high costs due to inefficiency or overuse.

Of the alternative budget- or rate-setting methods, review and approval of the budgets of individual hospitals most explicitly recognizes cost idiosyncracies among hospitals (assuming arbitrary decision rules are not used). Hospitals attempt to justify their performance and problems, and acceptable differences can be reflected in their rates.

One-to-one negotiations between hospitals and rate-setting organizations also enable differences among hospitals to be recognized, although in arms-length negotiations, bargaining power could play a more important role. For example, in an area with many hospitals, a bargainer might simply say, "I can get x service for y dollars from several other hospitals, so that's all I'm willing to pay you, regardless of why your costs are higher." Conversely, in an area with only one hospital, a bargainer might be less powerful. Nevertheless, both the budget review and approval and negotiation methods allow a hospital to attempt to gain recognition of its financial requirements, as it sees them; and rate-setters to attempt to pay less than requested for a hospital's costs, if these seem inappropriately high.

Formula methods that apply averages, ceilings, price indexes, or projections of past cost trends disregard some of the causes of cost differences among hospitals, and may not fully account for changes from year to year in case-mix, facilities and services, use levels, etc. More sensitive are formula methods that employ cost functions or point systems in which the characteristics of individual hospitals influence their rates. Rates based on a determination of the reasonable costs of producing specific services

explicitly disregard the cost idiosyncracies of individual hospitals.

Combinations of rate-setting methods are possible. The budget review and approval or negotiation methods may employ averages, ceilings, or projections as guidelines or parameters; negotiation may take place within budget review and approval; and any method may group hospitals to account for cost differences that are systematically related to characteristics such as size, ownership, location, teaching status, etc.

The grouping of hospitals has generated much discussion. Few would argue that grouping by the above characteristics achieves complete homogeneity within groups. More refined methods assign points for facilities and services offered or case types treated and group hospitals by point totals. Such a system was experimented with in Saskatchewan 20 years ago. Points were assigned for different services, and per diem rates adjusted for point totals. The system was rejected after it became apparent that the assignment of points failed to reflect variations in the quantity, quality, and sophistication of services, all of which influenced costs. In addition, this approach caused hospitals to add services, some of which were not needed.[18] Another difficulty with grouping hospitals for the purpose of basing reimbursement rates on group means is the absence of cost-containment incentives for hospitals with costs below their group mean. Lave *et al.* studied hospitals in Western Pennsylvania, where Blue Cross groups hospitals and reimburses actual costs up to 10 percent above each group's mean. They found that hospitals with costs below their group mean had greater than average cost increases and hospitals with costs above their group mean smaller, with the overall cost increase rate for all hospitals no different than that for Pennsylvania or the nation.[19]

Cooperative versus Competitive Processes

It is meaningful to distinguish between cooperative and competitive approaches to rate-setting. Cooperative approaches emphasize discussion of or negotiation over the proposed budgets of hospitals as a means of achieving agreement on changes in cost-influencing activities or plans (i.e., joint problem-solving). Competitive approaches emphasize the setting of tight rates by whatever means possible and imply more distant relationships. Cooperative approaches require expertise in analyzing budgets, performance, and problems, and persuasive or political skills to gain acceptance of findings and recommendations; but they make it possible to focus on specific areas of performance. Competitive approaches may relieve rate-setting organizations of some of this detailed involvement, but at some loss of influence over specifics. Competitive approaches, however, may make it possible to set tighter rates, since agreement by hospitals is not implied. Cooperative approaches are employed in most of the existing prospective reimbursement schemes, perhaps because participation is voluntary. This may change, as more states mandate participation in cost-control programs.

Prospective reimbursement provides an opportunity to question hospital decisions before they are implemented. The effectiveness of the budget review and approval method of rate-setting depends on the expertise of the rate-setting organization. Rigorous analysis requires detailed capital and operating budgets, information about the assumptions and plans that underlie them, and department-by-department or program-by-program review. Projected use levels must be examined, and the appropriateness of the quantities and types of resources budgeted to accommodate these use levels judged. Few third-party payers have the expertise to achieve analytical rigor at the present time, and therefore budget review and approval may fall short of its potential at least in the short run. Another problem is the poor budgeting practices of many hospitals.

Negotiations over budgets presented by hospitals combine cooperative and competitive pressures, since this approach does not assume complete agreement on the outcome. Effectiveness depends as much on the bargaining power and skill of the rate-setter as on expertise in budget analysis. When the third-party payer setting the rate covers a large portion of a hospital's patients, and when a number of hospitals are available to its members, a tough bargaining stance may be taken. In such situa-

tions, it is likely that the freedom inherent in negotiation gives this approach at least as much potential as budget review and approval for setting tight rates.

The formula method of rate-setting is probably the surest, if least equitable, way to set tight rates. Assuming hospitals are required to accept the formula-determined rates, they can be arbitrarily set as tight as desired. The Economic Stabilization Program Phase II and III regulations provide an excellent illustration. It is unlikely that even the strongest third-party payers could have achieved such results. However, if hospitals are not required to accept formula-determined rates—by federal or state regulation, for example—there is a good chance the formula method will lead to loose rates or be rejected. The setting of rates based on a determination of the reasonable costs of producing specific services is the most competition-oriented method. However, no rate-setting organization has undertaken the extensive cost studies that would be required.

Rate-setting organizations can be assisted by other organizations to overcome limitations in their authority, expertise, information, or political skill. In several states, organizations have been created fully or partially separate from third-party payers to provide them with information and recommendations related to rate-setting. In Rhode Island, hospitals submit their budgets to Peer Review Committees (sponsored by the State Hospital Association and comprised of administrators, controllers, and trustees) for critique and recommendations before submitting them to Blue Cross as a starting point for negotiations. Neither Blue Cross nor the hospitals are bound by the suggestions of the committees, although significant reductions have resulted from the reviews. Before the Rhode Island prospective reimbursement scheme was discontinued with the advent of Phase II, the Rhode Island Legislature passed a bill which would have had the effect of making the state through its Budget Office a party to hospital–Blue Cross negotiations. Although this was not implemented, it represents one possible form of state participation.

In the Social Security Administration supported Connecticut and Southern California incentive reimbursement experiments, third-party payers depended on another organization to determine the amount to be paid to hospitals. In Southern California, CASH (an independent, nonprofit, consulting organization founded by Blue Cross and the Hospital Council of Southern California) sets departmental labor budgets that determine the amounts hospitals are rewarded for productivity. In Connecticut, Budget Approval Boards (sponsored by the State Hospital Association and comprised of administrators, controllers, directors of nursing, and a trustee) review and approve departmental budgets submitted by hospitals, actually establishing the target budgets that serve as the basis of reimbursement. These Boards, in turn, depend on two private consulting firms to determine expected departmental staffing levels.

In Maryland, HCAS (an independent, nonprofit, quasi-public cost-analysis organization with six of 11 board members appointed by the Governor) examines departmental costs by means of comparative HAS data and in-hospital investigations, determines whether costs are reasonable, and makes recommendations to Blue Cross of Maryland and state agencies about limitations that should be imposed on reimbursement rates in cases where costs are too high. Another form of reliance on outside organizations is the use of planning agencies to make decisions regarding the appropriateness of additions to or expansions of facilities and services.

Sponsorship of organizations that assist third-party payers can range from hospitals themselves (peer review) to state government, and their role can range from advising hospitals on the appropriateness of their budgets to determining for rate-setters what the budgets or rates that form the basis of reimbursement should be. Such organizations may supplement the expertise of the rate-setter, making the rate-setting process more effective and the resulting rates fairer and tighter than would otherwise be possible. Some approaches, like peer review, also make the process more acceptable to hospitals.

Another form of back-up is federal or state regulation. A "voluntary" prospective reimbursement scheme can operate within a framework of public regulation. In both New Jersey

and New York, where hospital rate regulation laws are in effect, state officials are relying, at least in part and for the time being, on the New Jersey Hospital Association budget review program and the Blue Cross of Greater New York rate-setting formula. State back-up can take the form of 1) establishing ceilings or guidelines within which the determination of rates could be made by the methods under discussion; 2) mandating participation by hospitals; and 3) serving as the final appeal for hospitals and rate-setting organizations. In some states, public regulation has completely superseded voluntary incentive reimbursement efforts. It should be noted, however, that the rate-setting methods discussed here are as applicable to public agencies or commissions as to private organizations.

Delegation of Control or Responsibility by Government

At present, federal and state agencies, through Medicare and Medicaid regulations, have control over the means by which hospitals are paid, but because cost (or, more accurately, program beneficiaries share of allowable cost) reimbursement is used in these programs, they have little control over the actual amount paid. The Economic Stabilization Program regulations represented government control over the amounts paid to hospitals. Presumably, any prospective reimbursement scheme that might cover Medicare and Medicaid beneficiaries would be acceptable to federal and state agencies only if it provided some control and predictability regarding payment levels.

The budget review and approval and negotiation methods, conducted by third-party payers as intermediaries, would provide little control unless supplemented by ceilings, guidelines, or regulations. Determination of reimbursement rates would essentially be delegated. Strong third parties, negotiating at arms-length with hospitals, might succeed in setting tight rates, while others might not; and it would be difficult for federal or state agencies to monitor the process or outcome (although, as in Rhode Island, state officials could sit as a party to the rate-setting process). The lack of control implicit in these methods might be unacceptable to federal and state agencies given their responsibilities to taxpayers. Parenthetically, it should be noted that allowing intermediaries to establish budgets or rates that would apply to Medicare and Medicaid beneficiaries, as well as to their own members, might greatly strengthen their hand.

The formula approach offers more control and predictability. A formula is simple and visible. The impact of alternative formulas on payment levels can be calculated with reasonable accuracy, and acceptable formula levels specified. The Commissioner of Health of New York accepts the formula method of setting target rates as consistent with the state's cost control law. The formula method also offers the appearance of treating all hospitals equally, a traditional aspect of government policy in many fields. Rates based on a determination of the reasonable costs of producing specific services would also be fixed and visible. It should be recalled, however, that certain payment units provide an incentive for hospitals to increase the quantity of services they provide. Hence, even if rates are controlled, without controlling service volumes, future outlays may be somewhat unpredictable.

Any method could be made more predictable to federal or state agencies if they were directly involved in the process of rate-setting. Federally mandated ceilings (like the 106 percent rate increase limit) have been mentioned. State public utility type rate-setting commissions might set ceilings or procedural rules within which hospitals and external organizations would be free to set rates; or they might directly set rates (giving them absolute control, if the realities of politics are ignored).

Administrative Feasibility

Another factor to consider in evaluating alternative budget- or rate-setting methods is administrative feasibility. The costs of administering the program and the costs of the rewards paid to efficient hospitals must be less than the cost savings obtained. The magnitude of the task of conducting budget negotiations with each of 7,000 hospitals appears almost prohibitive, although reconciliation of differences between third-party payers and hospitals could

be facilitated by arbitration procedures; and guidelines, parameters, and standards could be developed to simplify the negotiation process. However, negotiations are unavoidably expensive and time-consuming. In Rhode Island, over 100 negotiating sessions, each backed up by hours of staff work, were consumed in establishing prospective budgets for 16 hospitals. Blue Cross of Western Pennsylvania dropped an experimental negotiated budget scheme because of the time involved. Budget review and approval is somewhat less taxing because guidelines and review procedures can more easily be applied, but again the expense and time required is substantial. The administrative costs of either of these methods could be reduced by employing parameters for a preliminary screening of budgets or rates. Detailed review or negotiations might be conducted only for hospitals that appear out of line. The cost studies required to determine rates under the reasonable cost of specific services method would be substantial. The formula approach appears to be the least costly to administer, although much time may be spent in negotiating the formula itself with hospital representatives.

Acceptability to Hospitals

The acceptability to hospitals of any budget- or rate-setting method, assuming participation is not mandated, probably depends more on the expected payment level, compared to existing reimbursement levels, than on the method used to determine rates. Third-party payers have found it difficult to get hospitals to volunteer for incentive reimbursement experiments, not because of the method to be used, but because hospitals saw nothing to gain from giving up cost reimbursement to risk a lesser level of reimbursement. Some hospitals have dropped out of the Connecticut incentive reimbursement experiment, apparently because the difficulties experienced in developing departmental budgets and justifying them in the review process were not seen as worth the possible rewards. However, hospitals have been willing to participate in other experiments in which they could receive rewards but could not receive less than prevailing reimbursement rates.

In addition to their concern over reimbursement levels, hospitals are not likely to accept willingly the shift of authority to rate-setting organizations implicit in rate-setting unless adequate safeguards are built into the process. Hospitals prefer voluntary rate review (especially if they are well represented) to a unilateral stance by external organizations. The mechanisms for appeals, arbitration, adjustments of established rates, etc., are also of concern.

Another concern of hospitals is the issue of reimbursement for past capital projects and future capital needs. Reimbursement by third parties has become their major source of capital funds. Therefore, hospitals can only be expected to accept prospective reimbursement if they believe that rates will be set high enough to assure the capital funds they believe they need. It seems imperative that, at some point, an explicit decision be made (by whom is an interesting question) as to whether third-party reimbursement is or is not to be the primary source of capital funds. Assuming that it is, the concern of hospitals might be stated as follows. Even if capital needs could initially be met by accrued surpluses gained by keeping actual costs below prospective rates (and hospitals are not too sure about this), where would capital funds come from in the long run after inefficiencies, and hence surpluses, have been eliminated? Two approaches to this dilemma have been suggested. First (under the assumption that only efficient hospitals should have their capital needs met through third-party reimbursement), a dual incentive structure could be designed in which a hospital could earn surpluses both for its individual performance in beating its own rate and for its relative performance in beating some target reflecting the cost performance of comparable hospitals (e.g., the average of the costs or cost increases of comparable hospitals). Under such an approach, a hospital that is efficient relative to comparable hospitals could earn surpluses to devote to new facilities or services, even if little slack remained between its own cost performance and its own rate.

Second, consideration of capital needs could be separated from consideration of operating efficiency and explicitly treated as a separate

item in rate-setting. Under this approach, a rate would be established for each hospital covering only direct patient care costs (about 85 percent of the total cost of a "typical" hospital). Questions of efficiency, case-mix, and use and comparisons of operating cost performance among hospitals would be pertinent here. Once set, the operating cost prospective rate would provide an incentive for efficient operations, but it would not be expected that any surpluses so obtained would fully meet capital needs. Past, present, and future capital needs would be considered separately. Presumably, planning agencies would be called on to rule on the appropriateness of proposed capital projects. Then, for projects judged to be necessary, a determination would be made of the funds required, and these funds would be explicitly figured into a hospital's rate or provided through lump sum payments over time. The American Hospital Association strongly favors separate consideration of non-direct patient care costs in establishing rates. A number of Blue Cross Plans presently separate the costs of teaching programs, depreciation and interest, bad debts and uncollectables, etc. from operating costs, and examine these items separately in their budget review and approval programs. One advantage of this approach is that hospital costs are more comparable, and inefficient hospitals more visible, when non-direct patient care costs are separated from their budgets.

Hospitals are also concerned about whether prospectively set rates can be adjusted for uncontrollable or unforeseen events such as unexpected volume, equipment breakdowns, union wage settlements, etc. It would seem unfair to penalize (reward) hospitals for cost increases (decreases) beyond their control, but it is not always clear whether certain events could have been controlled or predicted. If adjustments are made too readily, the incentive to contain costs is weakened. Of particular concern is volume. One way to handle this problem would be to develop variable prospective budgets or rates for different use levels, although such a system would have to be carefully designed so as not to eliminate the incentive for hospitals to curtail (presumably inappropriate or unnecessary) admissions, lengths of stay, and services. Few hospitals have the sophistication to identify and separate fixed and variable costs or to develop accurate variable budgets at the present time, but improved budgeting methods might evolve quite rapidly if adjustments for volume were not otherwise made. Other kinds of unexpected events would probably have to be accommodated by renegotiating rates, although adjustments for increases in the costs of personnel and supplies might be made by a means of price index. In the Connecticut experiment, hospitals can appeal the peer review panels for adjustments of their departmental target budgets. In Rhode Island, either the Blue Cross Plan or a hospital can ask for renegotiation of the hospital's budget if actual volume is ± 2 percent of the expected level, or if major unforeseen events occur. Most other prospective reimbursement schemes make some provision for adjusting rates.

The American Hospital Association in its "Policy on the Implementation of the Statement on the Financial Requirements of Health Care Institutions and Services" (November 18, 1970), endorsed the concept of prospectively determined rates as offering "very real opportunities for improvement in meeting the objectives of public accountability, predictability, and preservation of institutional autonomy, as well as other objectives of the *Statement on Financial Requirements*." In its "Guidelines

for Review and Approval of Rates for Health Care Institutions and Services by a State Commission" (February 9, 1972), the AHA proposes guidelines regarding the authority and responsibility of state rate-setting commissions, their organization and financing, their relationship with the planning process, the rate review process, the basis for reasonable rates, and the appeal mechanism.

It is clear from these statements that the acceptability of any prospective budget- or rate-setting method to the AHA depends on three key points. First, it must result in budgets or rates that meet the financial requirements of hospitals (as defined by the AHA *Statement on the Financial Requirements of Health Care Institutions and Services* (February 12, 1969)). Second, rates should apply equally to all patients and third-party payers (i.e., rates should "result in the apportionment of financial requirements without discrimination among all purchasers of care with equal charges for comparable services"). Third, the AHA is concerned about the rate-setting process itself, including mechanisms for full hearing of a hospital's budget justification based on established criteria and standards, automatic approval of rate proposals not acted on within 90 days, planning agency approval of proposed capital projects, "emergency" adjustments of rates, and appeal rights including judicial review.

References and Notes

1 For more complete discussions of the great variety of possible approaches to incentive reimbursement, see: Bauer, K. and Densen, P. *Some Issues in the Incentive Reimbursement Approach to Cost Containment: An Overview*, Health Care Policy Discussion Paper No. 7, Harvard Center for Community Health and Medical Care, Harvard University, 1973; Feldstein, P. "An Analysis of Reimbursement Plans." In: *Reimbursement Incentives for Hospital and Medical Care*, SSA Research Report No. 26 (Washington, D.C.: GPO, 1968); Goldstrom, B. *Prospective Payment to Hospitals: Methods of Rate Determination*, Occasional Papers in Hospital and Health Administration 2, Graduate Program in Hospital Administration, University of California, Berkeley, 1973; Hardwick, C.; Meyers, S.; and Woodruff, L. *Incentive Reimbursement: Prospects, Proposals, Plans, and Programs*, Research Series No. 6, Blue Cross of Western Pennsylvania, 1969; Pauly, M. "Efficiency, Incentives, and

Reimbursement for Health Care," *Inquiry* 7:14 (March 1970); and Sigmond, R. "The Notion of Hospital Incentives," *Hospital Progress* 50:63 (January 1969).

2 "Incentive Reimbursement: The Carrot Is There But The Hospitals Won't Bite," and May, D. "Connecticut: Reward System Doesn't Work," *Modern Hospital* 119:79 (October 1972).

3 Lave, J.; Lave, L.; and Silverman, L. "A Proposal for Incentive Reimbursement for Hospitals," *Medical Care* 11:79 (March–April 1972).

4 Pauly, "Efficiency, Incentives, and Reimbursement for Health Care," *op. cit.*

5 For the purpose of this discussion, it is assumed that the amounts to be paid per unit would be set tight enough to motivate hospitals to exert a deliberate effort to keep their actual costs below their prospective rates.

Carol McCarthy

Reprinted with permission of the Blue Cross Association, from *Inquiry:* Vol.XII, No.4, pp.320-329. Copyright © 1975 by the Blue Cross Association.

Incentive Reimbursement as an Impetus to Cost Containment

Originally Published in December 1975

Incentive reimbursement experiments have been and are being tried in an attempt to promote cost containment in the hospital industry. Against the backdrop of a general discussion of incentive programs, this paper focuses on a cross-section of those programs instituted in response to Public Law 90-248. Five experiments utilizing the industrial engineering, budgetary, or physician-expander approach are presented for purposes of clarification and comparison. In addition, a number of suggested methods for calculating incentive payments are outlined. With reference to these programs and proposed formulas, recommendations are made on ways to stimulate greater success through the incentive reimbursement approach.

Health Insurance and Cost Control

Health insurance is essentially a risk transfer mechanism. Directed primarily at defraying the cost of illness rather than maintaining health, it operates to reduce for the individual the uncertainty of economic losses resulting from a random event. The providers of health services also benefit—both institution and practitioner—for when the patient cannot pay for care, neither the physician nor the facility is reimbursed. Thus, to the extent of covered benefits, health insurance guarantees subscribers financial access to medical treatment and providers, a certain viability. Does it at the same time encourage cost control?

In 1950, the nation's outlay for health care

Carol McCarthy, M.S. is the Associate Director for Program Development and Evaluation, Nassau-Suffolk Regional Medical Program (1919 Middle Country Road, Centereach, NY 11720).

totaled $12-billion, or 4.6 percent of that year's Gross National Product. By 1974, that outlay had risen to $104-billion, or 7.7 percent of the GNP of $1.3-trillion,[1] with 97.2-billion going for personal health care services.[2] Moreover, in fiscal 1974, as in previous years, hospital care comprised the largest segment of the personal health care dollar, accounting for $40.9-billion, or 42 percent of the total. However, largely as a result of the growth of private health insurance and the impact of Medicare and Medicaid, out-of-pocket expenditures for hospital care decreased significantly in the period from 1950 to 1974. More specifically, in 1950, 16.5 percent of hospital charges were paid by private insurance carriers, 3.6 percent by philanthropy and industry, 45.7 percent by government and 34.2 percent by the patient receiving treatment. By 1974, the third-party share had risen to 90 percent—52.9 percent coming from government, 1.3 percent from philanthropy and industry, and 35.4 percent from private insurance carriers.[3]

Can a causal relationship be postulated between increased third-party coverage and increased hospital costs? Lave, Lave and Silverman, among others, believe that it can. They cite as evidence a 15 percent per year increase in hospital costs since the passage of Medicare.[4] However, even if one rejects a causal relationship, sufficient documentation exists to question whether present hospital reimbursement schemes provide incentives for efficient delivery of care. In this vein, Sigmond cites the conclusions reached in the Gorham Report to the President on Medical Care Prices, the 1967 report of the National Advisory Commission on Health Manpower, and the Barr Committee

Report on Hospital Effectiveness.[5] Why should the patient, covered by insurance or public assistance, be concerned about the direct costs of hospitalization? What reason has the physician, guaranteed reimbursement, to select a less costly alternative to what he considers a proper (but expensive) mode of hospital treatment? Finally, why should the hospital reduce operating expenses when three-fourths or more of its revenue is obtained from third parties who reimburse on the basis of costs?

Since reimbursement at less than cost would promote hospital bankruptcy, other alternatives must be sought that will foster cost-conscious management. At the heart of the issue is the notion of incentives—factors that motivate, stimulate or incite to action. The reimbursement experiments supported by Blue Cross Plans, as well as by the federal and state governments, attempt to supply such incentives by offering financial rewards for efficient operation leading to a reduction in overall program costs.

Incentive Reimbursement Experiments

Incentive reimbursement experiments are not new. As Wolkstein indicates, they have been conducted for years in Canada and in Blue Cross Plans across the United States.[6] However, new impetus was given to their undertaking with the passage of section 402 of Public Law 90-248, the 1967 amendments to the Social Security Act. This section authorized the Secretary of Health, Education and Welfare to experiment with reimbursement programs that incorporated incentives for economy and at the same time maintained or improved quality in the provision of health services connected with Medicare, Medicaid, and the Maternal and Child Health programs. Participating providers would be allowed to keep at least a part of any savings realized, while the government would accept responsibility for additional costs accruing to the Medicare, Medicaid, or Maternal and Child Health programs as a result of the experiments. Plans could be developed in conjunction with public and private third-party payers, planning agencies, professional associations, organizations of providers, hospitals and others, with priority being accorded to proposals designed to

achieve overall effectiveness.[7] By 1968 the Department of Health, Education and Welfare had been presented with over 500 proposals.[8]

The forms hospital incentive reimbursement experiments may take are manifold. The type of incentive employed, the aspect of program operation chosen for attention, the time focus utilized—all condition the nature of the experiment. Incentives, for example, can be positive (gains to be realized), or negative (punishments to be incurred). Although the latter are more powerful, they are more difficult to administer. In addition, they are likely to occasion greater side effects. For instance, by agreeing to pay the hospital a fixed dollar amount based on projected costs with the stipulation that meeting the objectives carries no reward but failure to do so entails a penalty, the third-party payer may promote a decrease in quality as well as in costs.[9]

Second, incentives may be directed at outcome or process. If outcome is emphasized, the focus will be on overall program costs. If process is highlighted, rewards will be paid or penalties exacted if certain programs believed to foster efficiency and economy are or are not operative—programs such as a sophisticated approach to budgeting, shared services, utilization review and the like. This has been the approach of the Joint Commission on Accreditation of Hospitals with regard to quality control. The danger here, however, is two-fold: 1) innovativeness may be discouraged; and 2) the presence of certain programs may be taken as evidence of an optimally operating system when in fact the programs are poor in quality and ineffective.[10]

Finally, incentives can be oriented toward future or past performance. With future-oriented incentives, rewards or penalties hinge on performance with regard to projected costs. With past-oriented incentives, a hospital is rewarded when its incurred costs compare favorably with those of other hospitals similar in size, location, and services offered.[11]

For the most part, the incentive reimbursement experiments undertaken in response to the 1967 legislation have been prospective, outcome-oriented and largely positive in emphasis. Although a wide variety are in operation, this discussion focuses upon those utilizing

Table 1. Annual savings of projects as a percent of departmental payroll costs*

Project	Department	Annual payroll costs	Project annual savings	Percentage reduction in payroll costs
Metropolitan community				
Laundry	Laundry	$ 98,952	$ 16,800	17.0
Sewing room	Sewing room	23,556	12,600	53.5
Nurse staffing	Nursing	2,260,572	84,700	3.8
Inpatient tray preparation and distribution	Dietary	356,940	32,500	9.1
Freight elevator	Elevator operation	7,900	7,900	100.0
Subtotal		$2,747,920	$154,500	5.6
University advanced teaching				
Maid service, supervision, overtime	Housekeeping	$ 561,000	$ 16,300	2.9
Engineering and maintenance	Engineering and maintenance	461,500	31,150	6.8
Pharmacy man-hours	Pharmacy	84,200	9,150	10.9
Inpatient tray distribution	Dietary	777,700	62,000	8.0
Subtotal		$1,884,400	$118,600	6.3
Non-metropolitan				
Engineering and maintenance	Engineering and maintenance	$ 151,700	$ 23,300	15.4
Accounts receivable	Accounting	179,500	34,750	19.3
Nurse staffing	Nursing	1,731,700	33,550	1.9
Payroll check service	Purchased service	7,555	1,230	16.3
Subtotal		$2,070,455	$ 92,830	4.5
Grand total		$7,702,775	$365,930	4.7

* This table is taken from: Hardwick, C. Patrick and Wolfe, Harvey. "Evaluation of an Incentive Reimbursement Experiment," *Medical Care* 10:113 (March–April 1972). Reprinted with permission.

one of three different approaches: 1) industrial engineering; 2) budgetary; and 3) the employment of physician-expanders in a prepaid group practice. The experiments conducted by Blue Cross of Western Pennsylvania, and the Blue Cross Plan, Medicare and Medi-Cal in Southern California fall into the first category; those supported by the Connecticut Hospital Association and Blue Cross of Rhode Island fall into the second category; and the programs undertaken by Medicare and the Health Insurance Plan of Greater New York are in the third category.

The Industrial Engineering Approach

In 1968, Blue Cross of Western Pennsylvania contracted with the Department of Health, Education and Welfare to pay hospitals a bonus for cost savings realized through the use of industrial engineering techniques. For a 12-month period, management analysts on the payroll of Blue Cross of Western Pennsylvania were assigned to operate in a staff capacity to the administration of a metropolitan community hospital, a university-affiliated advanced teaching hospital, and a non-metropolitan hospital. Engineering applications could entail changes in facilities, equipment, supplies, operating methods, transportation, materials handling, planning, scheduling and clerical assignments that would result in a reduction in labor required, a reduction in materials or supplies utilized, increased output per unit of labor, or decreased overtime. Reductions in departmental costs attributable to a one-time savings, cost avoidance measures, a fall in market prices, or a decrease in productivity would not be recognized in calculating incentive payments; nor would reductions in costs unaccompanied by any change in method or practice.[12]

The workload scheduling projects undertaken in the various hospitals are depicted in

Table 1, along with the projected annual savings as a percent of departmental payroll costs. Table 2 outlines the incentive formula and demonstrates how bonus payments were computed. Payments were made only when savings were verified and not upon program implementation.

In their evaluation of the project, Hardwick and Wolfe indicate that although savings were realized (largely as a result of a reduction in personnel), the effect of the incentive payments was minimal. The dollar value of bonuses paid was negligible in relation to total hospital income or expenditures because the Blue Cross Plan was the only reimbursement agency participating. Moreover, hospital employees did not directly benefit from the incentive payment. Indeed, they were unaware of its existence. The greatest incentive, according to Hardwick and Wolfe, was the free services for one year of the industrial engineer. Furthermore, the study report indicates that the effectiveness of the engineer varied directly with the degree of support he received from the hospital's top management personnel.[13]

Begun in the last quarter of 1971 and designed to run until October, 1974, the reimbursement experiment undertaken by Medicare, Medi-Cal and Blue Cross of Southern California also relied upon industrial engineering input. Here, however, labor alone was the focus of interest. Productivity indices established by the Commission for Administrative Services in Hospitals (CASH) were used to measure efficiency in a stratified sample of 25 of the area's hospitals. Under the experiment, each participating facility received a share of the cost savings realized in the current year of operations as compared to the previous year. The rate of labor cost improvement and level of productivity in the particular hospital determined that hospital's incentive payment, with the third party paying a portion of the total based on the ratio of its subscribers' patient days to the hospital's total patient days.[14]

According to one report, more than $600,000 was saved by the end of the first year of operation, with one hospital responsible for 40 percent of the total. At that time, $326,896 in bonuses from the Blue Cross Plan, Medi-Cal and the Social Security Administration were

Table 2. Incentive reimbursement formula*

The incentive formula is expressed as follows:
Hospital's incentive portion = (adjusted current cost − new cost) × (applicable Blue Cross patient days ratio) × (predetermined incentive sharing ratio).

Therefore:

Current annual cost was	$160,000

And we adjust for changes during this year:

Cost of direct labor increased	6,200
Cost of direct materials increased	540
Current anual adjusted cost is	$166,740

If this year's new cost is	141,740
The cost savings are	25,000
If the applicable Blue Cross patient days are	40%
The net savings would be	$ 10,000
If predetermined sharing ratio is	50%
The hospital's incentive portion	$ 5,000

The Blue Cross reimbursement and the incentive payment to the hospital would be:

$$.4 \times \$141,740 + \$5,000 = \$56,696 + \$5,000 = \$61,696$$
or
$$\$61,696/\$141,740 = 43.5\% \text{ of actual costs}$$

Under the current system, the total reimbursement would be $56,696 or $56,696/$141,40 = 40 percent of actual costs.

Such bonus calculations will be computed for all projects implemented during the term of the contract. Therefore, the actual dollar incentive will be much greater than the $5,000 shown in this particular example for a particular department.

* This table is taken from: Hardwick, C. Patrick and Wolfe, Harvey. "A Multifaceted Approach to Incentive Reimbursement," *Medical Care* 8:184 (May–June 1970). Reprinted with permission.

distributed among nine hospitals on the basis of their audited performances. CASH projected that 10 to 12 hospitals would receive reimbursement at the end of the second year and 16 to 18 at the end of the third. Robert Edgecumbe, executive vice-president of CASH, believes hospitals are learning the wisdom of matching staff to requirements, shutting down poorly utilized wings and discontinuing unnecessary services.[15]

Unfortunately, however, it may not be possible to properly evaluate the California experiment. About the time the program was launched, occupancy rates in area hospitals began to decline. Reluctant to lay off employees on the basis of reduced work volume, hospitals experienced a decline in productivity.[16] Since incentive payments are in part determined by productivity level, they, too, were affected. What would have happened had occupancy remained essentially stable is a matter for conjecture.

The Budgetary Approach

In the experiment undertaken by the Connecticut Hospital Association, expectancy levels for departmental productivity were again set by industrial engineers, but the emphasis here was on the development of departmental target budgets. At the outset of the program in May, 1969, 18 hospitals, divided into three groups by size, were participants. Each group was assigned a project coordinator who aided in budget preparation and served as a consultant on budgetary problems. Since a uniform accounting system and cost finding program had existed in all the hospitals for 20 years, and since standardized reporting procedures were employed in the experiment, the departmental budgets developed by each hospital could be reviewed by a Budget Advisory Board composed of administrators, controllers, directors of nursing and trustees from other hospitals in its group. Thus the element of peer review was introduced.[17]

In the first year of the experiment, budgets were prepared for housekeeping, laundry, medical records and certain nursing departments. Second year additions to the list included administration, dietary, plant maintenance and pharmacy. By the third year, budgets had been developed for the operating room, recovery room, X-ray department, laboratory and anesthesia department. At each year's end, target budgets were adjusted to reflect actual volume; then hospital performance was reviewed. Those hospitals whose actual departmental costs exceeded target amount were reimbursed at cost. Where costs fell below budget, hospitals were paid the budgeted amount. In addition, any hospital under budget—i.e., operating a department at 10 percent or more below the average costs of like units in peer hospitals—was given a bonus of up to 2 percent of the incurred costs of the department.[18]

Under-budget payments made by Blue Cross of Connecticut and Medicare at the end of the first year totaled $436,000. However, as the experiment continued, problems began to arise.

Administrative costs of responsible budget review were found to be high. In addition, the peer review portion of the program proved ineffective as hospitals, confronted with unknowns, found themselves forced into making arbitrary decisions. At the hospitals' request, the third-party payers assumed responsibility for budgetary decisions on new programs and services. Finally, reward-seeking varied inversely with hospital size. In the second year of operation, one of the large hospitals withdrew from the experiment. By the end of 1972, five additional ones had followed suit, questioning, among other things, the validity of the industrial engineering standards and retrospective adjustment of target budgets for volume.[19]

In an article in the March, 1973 issue of Inquiry *("SSA-Connecticut Hospital Incentive Reimbursement Experiment Cost Evaluation," 12:47–58), Elnicki outlines the final results of the Connecticut experiment. The cost experience of participating hospitals from 1960 through the second year of the experiment, 1971, is compared with that of non-participating hospitals in the Connecticut Hospital Association. The last year of the experiment is excluded to eliminate the possibility of contamination due to the federal government's Economic Stabilization Program. For each of the eight departments with target budgets set in the first two years of the experiment, two regression analyses are performed. Paid personnel hours and supply costs constitute, in turn, the dependent variable.*

As Elnicki indicates, evaluation results lend no support to peer review of department budgets as an effective cost control mechanism. While five of the 16 regressions indicate cost reductions associated with the experiment, in one instance only—paid personnel hours in the housekeeping department—is the negative coefficient significant. Elnicki offers three possible reasons for the experiment's outcome: 1) the absence of any penalty for exceeding budgeted amounts militates against concerted efforts to eliminate layers of slack costs; 2) monetary rewards are inadequate incentives for cost control; and 3) peer review that extends only to department budgets and not to general operating policies and procedures can-

not provide the "structure" needed for cost containment.

In contrast to the departmental budget approach undertaken in Connecticut, Rhode Island Hospital, in Providence, signed a contract with Rhode Island Blue Cross in 1970 for global budget review. Lawrence Hill, who was vice president of the hospital at that time, is quoted as reporting a savings of $950,000 at the end of the first year of the experiment, half due to the abandonment of plans for new or expanded programs, half to efficient operation. In the second year, when the state took part in budget negotiations and was empowered to approve rates, an additional savings of $5-million was realized, reducing annual hospital costs to their lowest level in five years.[20] It should be noted here, however, that, for Hill, "savings" is simply the difference between anticipated and actual spending, between what might have been spent and what was actually spent. Unlike Hardwick and Wolfe, Hill does not restrict his use of the term to a difference between the anticipated and the actual that is attributable only to greater and sustained efficiency of program operation.

The Prepayment Approach

Unlike the reimbursement experiments discussed up to this point, the one undertaken by the Health Insurance Plan of Greater New York (HIP) was truly comprehensive in scope. Begun January 1, 1970, the program had three primary objectives: 1) to develop an efficient arrangement for the provision of medical, institutional and home health services to Medicare recipients; 2) to utilize "nurse clinician coordinators" in innovative patient-centered activities in order to stabilize physician utilization and reduce hospital admissions and lengths of stay; and 3) to realize additional economies by centering reimbursement for all services in a single agency.[21]

The achievement of economical program operation depended to a large extent on the nurse clinician coordinator. One nurse was assigned to each of six medical groups participating in the experiment. Her patient population was Medicare recipients suffering from chronic conditions that were likely to entail frequent physician visits and possible hospitali-

zations. By educating the patient in the management of his or her illness, explaining the treatment regimen prescribed by the physician, and arranging for coordinated services from community health organizations where indicated, the nurse worked in the office setting and the patient's home to help the patient reach and maintain a level of functioning that would result in a decreased demand for medical and institutional services. In hospitals cooperating in the experiment, the nurse assumed the role of discharge planner. Here the objective was a reduced inpatient length of stay for the Medicare patient and the prevention of rehospitalization.[22]

The experience of HIP Medicare beneficiaries meeting study criteria for age, residence and coverage (with special attention to Medicare recipients in the six medical groups served by nurse clinicians) was to be considered against that of a matched sample of non-HIP Medicare beneficiaries from the same geographic area. Attention was to focus on medical and institutional utilization rates and per capita costs. The per capita rates of the non-HIP group would be taken as the norm, and any incentive payments made would be based on the favorable experience of the HIP group with regard to absolute costs and rate of change in costs over the three-year trial period. All HIP medical groups would share the incentive payment, along with hospitals, extended care facilities and home health agencies participating in the experiment. Payments to the six medical groups using nurse clinicians would reflect their extra efforts.[23]

As of this account, only limited data are available on program results. With regard to utilization and costs of services, an assessment of the first year of program operation shows the experiment to be a success. The decline in both hospital discharge rate and length of stay between 1969 (the year preceding the experiment) and 1970 was greater among HIP Medicare patients than among the control group. Indeed, the decrease in hospital utilization rates was sufficient in the HIP group to offset the inflationary effect on medical care costs in 1970. While reimbursed inpatient charges per non-HIP Medicare beneficiary increased from $270 in 1969 to $287 in 1970, charges per HIP beneficiary dropped from $266 to $260 the same year.[24] As a result, an interim incentive payment of approximately $750,000 was paid to participants at the conclusion of the first year of the experiment.[25]

Although studies published to date fail to show lower utilization and cost for Medicare beneficiaries in medical groups with nurse clinicians, Bauer does indicate general acceptance of the nurse by physicians and patients participating in the experiment. Most of the medical groups involved, she notes, have retained their nurse clinicians; patients have recognized a rightful role for the nurse in health maintenance and the coordination of care. To the extent that the nurse clinician program falls short of its objectives, Bauer would direct attention to: 1) the scarcity of appropriate area facilities for long-term care; 2) tightened SSA eligibility criteria for nursing home coverage; 3) the more favorable per diem rate attendant on the care of Medicaid rather than Medicare patients; and 4) the tendency of both patient and physician to view the nurse clinician in a supplementary rather than a primary role in the delivery of ambulatory services.[26]

Incentive Reimbursement Formulas

Wherever possible, the bases used in calculating incentive payments in the various reimbursement experiments has been indicated. In one instance, that of the Western Pennsylvania program, the payment formula was given—for there is a degree of concern among those in the health field about possible inequities in this area. Hardwick and Wolfe point to the importance of rewarding the hospital not only for the current year's achievement but for achievement over the years. The hospital that is given a lower target amount after the first year, on the basis of its more efficient operation, has little encouragement for further cost reduction. To eliminate this eventuality, the authors propose reimbursement according to the following formula:

$$R_j = C_j + \sum_{i=1}^{j} (P_j - C_j) \, \frac{j+1-i}{\phi}$$

where R_j in the formula is total reimburse-

ment for the current year; C_j is actual hospital costs for the current year; P_j is projected hospital costs for the current year; and ϕ is the incentive rate percent of cost savings to be returned in bonuses. Using this formula, the incentive payment is a function of the time since the savings were realized. In year one, reimbursement will equal actual costs plus the incentive rate times the amount saved. In year two, reimbursement will total the amount saved in year one multiplied by ϕ^2; in year three, the amount saved in year one multiplied by ϕ^3. If ϕ equals .5, a 100 percent bonus will eventually be paid for cost reductions.[27]

Rafferty, however, raises the issue of the effects of budgetary incentives on patient case mix. Citing as evidence the situation in proprietary hospitals, he holds that cost consciousness leads to decreased capital expenditures, which, in turn, result in facilities geared to handling less complex, less costly cases. Thus, to assure equitable reimbursement among hospitals participating in incentive experiments, he recommends periodic readjustment of target rates to reflect case mix changes.[28]

Lave, Lave and Silverman point to increasing inflationary costs attendant upon an upward shift in the complexity of case mix. When a hospital is undergoing such a shift and the formula used for reimbursement ignores caseload, unfair pressure is exerted upon the administrator. Indeed, according to these health economists, if quality care is to be delivered at low cost, payments to hospitals must be based upon size, occupancy rate, average length of stay, case mix, difficulty of surgery and extent of teaching programs. Moreover, the variables should be re-evaluated every three years. Table 3 indicates in detail the suggested approach. D-1 through D-5 in the table represent aggregations or clusters, based on similarity of estimated marginal costs, of 17 ICDA diagnosis classifications.

If case mix remains constant, in the first year of incentive plan operation, Lave, Lave and Silverman would give the hospital an increase of 10 percent over the previous year's reimbursement, a further increase of 8 percent in the second year, and 6 percent in the third. Subsequent increases would be tied to the Consumer Price Index. Should the hospital's in-

Table 3.   A suggested reimbursement formula*

Variable	Mean	Standard deviation	Regression coefficient	t-statistic
Constant term			374.380	3.03
Utilization	80.92	9.38	.564	−2.94
Size	248.04	144.85	−.139	−2.60
Average length of stay	9.47	1.62	26.252	5.74
Percent patients with easy surgery	46.51	6.05	−.452	−.55
Percent patients with very difficult surgery	1.56	1.30	21.513	3.42
Fraction of patients who had surgery	.52	.10	38.744	.28
Percent patients with common diagnosis	57.11	6.66	−4.012	−2.29
Percent non-surgical patients with common diagnosis	18.28	5.55	−4.181	−1.49
Advanced teaching program	.29	.46	32.617	2.23
Teaching program	.28	.44	−16.199	−1.34
Percent self-pay patients	5.05	3.05	−10.159	−5.77
Percent Blue Cross patients	39.93	10.34	.250	.48
Percent patients < 14	15.22	12.14	.534	.44
Percent patients > 65	19.03	4.60	−5.364	−3.30
Metropolitan area	.45	.50	29.547	2.63
Shift	.58	.50	39.202	5.13
D1	.11	.29	−84.107	−2.03
D2	.57	.31	22.249	1.02
D3		— — — excluded variable — — —		
D4	26.22	6.97	7.221	5.06
D5	7.03	2.16	21.728	5.56
Average cost/case	453.11	125.11		

$R^2 = .926$
Degrees of freedom = 91

* This table is taken from Lave, Judith R.; Lave, Lester B.; and Silverman, Lester B. "A Proposal for Incentive Reimbursement for Hospitals," *Medical Care* 11:87 (March–April 1973). Reprinted with permission.

curred costs be lower than those projected through use of the reimbursement formula, half of the difference would be returned to the hospital to use as it saw fit. If actual costs exceeded projected costs, the institution would again receive only half the difference. In the latter instance, the hospital would have to turn to philanthropy or other sources to cover the deficit.[29]

Finally, the one incentive reimbursement formula currently a part of a Blue Cross hospital contract not only takes note of hospital case mix, it relies upon data secured directly from the participating hospitals. In this manner, difficulties inherent in utilizing information that is not uniformly reported (i.e., information from such sources as the AHA guide, Medicare audit reports, and HAS), or which is less than all inclusive (i.e., HUP reports) are avoided. More specifically, the independent variables incorporated in the multiple regression model outlined by Shuman, Wolfe and Hardwick and utilized by Blue Cross of Western Pennsylvania include:

1 A dummy variable designating one of four locations: metropolitan, urban, non-urban or Pittsburgh (within city limits);

2 A dummy variable representing one of five size classifications based on average daily census—0–99, 100–199, 200–299, 300–449, 450 or more;

3 A service variable arrived at by summing the psychometric weights of inpatient services provided by the hospital and included among the 20 such procedures identified by hospital administrators, physicians, and controllers as significantly influencing both direct and indirect costs;

4 An index representing the summation of relative weights assigned by hospital administrators, physicians and controllers to educational undertakings impacting on hospital costs—resident, intern, nurse and technician training programs;

5 A case mix variable rooted in hospital medical staff attributes, namely, the number of Board-certified, Board-eligible and other staff physicians;

6 An indicator of outpatient activity based on the ratio of outpatient charges to total hospital charges.

The dependent variable is the total audited costs of the hospital.

The accuracy of the resultant non-linear model as a predictor of hospital costs was demonstrated when its developers estimated 1970 costs for 85 hospitals from data available in the three prior years. All but 3.6 percent of the variation in 1970 costs was explained.[30]

Present reimbursement procedures based on this model call for the establishment of "control bands" about predicted costs. Bonuses are paid when actual costs fall below the band that allows for standard error in the predictive model; penalties are assigned when costs are above the band. The size of the bonus or penalty varies with the size of the difference between actual and predicted costs, with the restriction that incentive payments may not exceed 12 percent of actual costs.[31]

Conclusion

In a memo circulated internally in the summer of 1972, officials of the Social Security Administration indicated their disappointment with the modest progress of the incentive reimbursement program. They attributed the slow advance to "the lack of research capacity in the health care field, misunderstandings of the basic concepts of incentive reimbursement and the requirement that participation be voluntary."[32] Perhaps the difficulties are even more fundamental.

Essentially, incentive reimbursement attempts to introduce elements of the competitive private marketplace into the voluntary, not-for-profit sector. There are certain weaknesses inherent in this approach. Community hospitals differ in their pricing, sources of revenue and philanthropic support; thus, they will react differently to cost incentives. Moreover, the quality of patient care, the pursuit of excellence and recognition, the satisfaction of the

medical staff—these and similar goals have traditionally been stronger motivators than profit among members of the voluntary hospital community. For the hospital not walking a fine line between solvency and insolvency, a change in priorities is necessary if cost containment is to become a primary and not a secondary objective. Full staff cooperation is needed, as well as, perhaps, organizational change. Hill suggests enlarging the role of the physician in institutional decision-making and elevating the administrator to the position of voting Board member to increase his "structural leverage." Physicians and managers, says Hill, must be given greater power if they are to assume greater responsibility for poor as well as good results.[33]

How can the third-party payer apply sufficient leverage to stimulate cost consciousness? There is certainly nothing wrong with attempting to identify cost waste areas through incentive reimbursement experiments. What can be questioned, however, is the form most of these experiments have taken. As the evaluators of the Western Pennsylvania experiment indicate, minimal financial bonuses have minimal motivational value. Thus, any attempt at incentive reimbursement should be a cooperative venture among all major third-party payers. Second, all incentives must be two-edged. Once realistic cost projections are set, rewards should follow achievement and punishment, failure. Admittedly, the threat of financial sanctions proves a deterrent to participation in experiments. However, rather than employ the rewards-only approach, participation should be made mandatory. When all major third parties are supporting an incentive program, delivering such a mandate is at least a possibility.

There is a valuable by-product to this approach, namely, improved reliability of experiment results. As Pauly indicates, at this point in time, participating hospitals are in competition with non-participating institutions. Moreover, as long as a program is voluntary, study groups are self-selected.[34] Both situations can contaminate study conclusions.

Finally, the instrument used to calculate reimbursement should be as comprehensive and individualized as that suggested by Lave, Lave and Silverman, and as sensitive to subjective assessment and uniform reporting procedures as that developed by Shuman, Hardwick and Wolfe. In addition, attention must be directed to performance over time if payments are to be just and equitable.

Properly administered, incentive reimbursement arrangements provide the hospital with a mechanism for achieving responsible self-control. In these days of rampant inflation, such arrangements may well constitute a means of salvation for the voluntary health system.

References and Notes

1 Worthington, Nancy L. "National Health Expenditures, 1929–74," *Social Security Bulletin* 38:5 (February 1975).
2 *Ibid.*, p. 9.
3 *Ibid.*, p. 18.
4 Lave, Judith R.; Lave, Lester B.; and Silverman, Lester B. "A Proposal for Incentive Reimbursement for Hospitals," *Medical Care* 11:79 (March–April 1973).
5 Sigmond, Robert M. "The Notion of Hospital Incentives," *Hospital Progress* 50:63 (January 1969).
6 Wolkstein, Irwin. "Incentive Reimbursement Plans Offer a Variety of Approaches to Cost Control," *Hospitals* 43:63 (June 16, 1969).
7 Sigmond, *op. cit.*, p. 68.
8 "Connecticut Gets Green Light on Medicare Incentive Pay Plan," *Modern Hospital* 111:88 (December 1968).
9 Hardwick, C. Patrick and Wolfe, Harvey. "Incentive Reimbursement," *Hospitals* 44:46 (September 16, 1970).
10 Hill, Lawrence A. "Financial Incentives: How They Could Reshape the Health Care System," *Hospitals* 43:62 (June 16, 1969).
11 Lave, Lave and Silverman, *op. cit.*, p. 80.
12 Hardwick, C. Patrick and Wolfe, Harvey. "A Multifaceted Approach to Incentive Reimbursement," *Medical Care* 8:173–188 (May–June 1970).
13 Hardwick, C. Patrick and Wolfe, Harvey. "Evaluation of an Incentive Reimbursement Experiment," *Medical Care* 10:114–115 (March–April 1972).
14 Martin, Glenn J. "Incentives for Economy," *Hospitals* 45:52–53 (October 1, 1971).
15 "California: Lesson in Belt-Tightening," *Modern Hospital* 119:85–86 (October 1972).
16 "Incentive Reimbursement: The Carrot Is There but the Hospitals Won't Bite," *Modern Hospital* 119:81 (October 1972).
17 May, Dennis P. "Connecticut: Reward System Doesn't Work," *Modern Hospital* 119:83–84 (October 1972).
18 "Incentive Reimbursement: The Carrot Is There," *op. cit.*, p. 80.
19 *Ibid.*, p. 81; May, *op. cit.*, p. 84.
20 "Incentive Reimbursement: The Carrot Is There," *op. cit.*, p. 82.
21 Martin, *op. cit.*, p. 53; Greenberg, Sidney M. and Galton, Robert. "Nurses Are Key in HIP Experiment to Cut Health Care Costs," *American Journal of Nursing* 72:272–273 (February 1972).
22 Greenberg and Galton, *op. cit.*, pp. 273–275.
23 Jones, Ellen W., *et al.* "HIP Incentive Reimbursement Experiment: Utilization and Costs of Medical Care, 1969 and 1970," *Social Security Bulletin* 37:5–8 (December 1974).
24 *Ibid.*, pp. 9–10.
25 Bauer, Katherine G. *Containing Costs of Health Services through Incentive Reimbursement* (Boston: Harvard Center for Community Health and Medical Care, 1973), p. 268.
26 *Ibid.*, pp. 279–280.
27 Hardwick and Wolfe, "Incentive Reimbursement," *op. cit.*, pp. 47–48.
28 Rafferty, John. "A Comment on Incentive Reimbursement," *Medical Care* 9:518–520 (November–December 1971).
29 Lave, Lave and Silverman, *op. cit.*, pp. 84–88.
30 Shuman, Larry J.; Wolfe, Harvey; and Hardwick, C. Patrick. "Predictive Hospital Reimbursement and Evaluation Model," *Inquiry* 9:18–27 (June 1972).
31 *Ibid.*, pp. 29–30. Information on 12 percent ceiling, personal communication from Harvey Wolfe, December 19, 1974.
32 "Incentive Reimbursement: The Carrot Is There," *op. cit.*, p. 80.
33 Hill, "Financial Incentives," *op. cit.*, pp. 61–62.
34 Pauly, Mark V. "Efficiency, Incentives and Reimbursement for Health Care," *Inquiry* 7:125 (March 1970).

Bernard Friedman

Reprinted with permission of the Blue Cross Association, from *Inquiry:* Vol.X, No.3, pp.31-35. Copyright © 1973 by the Blue Cross Association.

Consumer Response to Incentives under Alternative Health Insurance Programs

Originally Published in September 1973

Practical alternatives to current health insurance in the United States are being examined in the context of broader government intervention in the market for health services. A better insurance system would provide better protection for families against large monetary loss and offer less incentive to inefficient use of resources.

This paper will present some general discussion of the economics of an improved health insurance system. Special attention is given to an argument that the complete elimination of copayment formulae[1] in health insurance would yield social gains from earlier treatment of serious illness, and that these gains would outweigh the losses due to unwarranted utilization.

Ideal Insurance

As a standard or ideal form of insurance, an argument can be made for a system of indemnities—by which we mean lump-sum money transfers conditional on an objective state of illness in the absence of treatment.[2]

When health services consumed by an individual affect social welfare only via the individual's own utility evaluation, and when there are no externalities or increasing returns in production (placing obvious restriction on the illness conditions being considered), the following strong result ensues:[3] any *ex post* (after treatment of illness) social welfare opti-

Bernard Friedman, Ph.D. is Assistant Professor of Economics, Brown University (Providence, Rhode Island 02912).

mum can be accomplished by an appropriate *ex ante* distribution of general purchasing power together with the unfettered market behavior of perfect competition.

Indemnity insurance purchased in a competitive market may need to be supplemented by additional transfers to achieve the *ex post* welfare optimum.[4] But any other form of insurance that transfers purchasing power to an extent based on quantity of services purchased is not consistent with efficient allocation. Inefficient allocation associated with reimbursement insurance arises because the insured individual makes his decision on how much care to purchase based on a net price $k \cdot P$ (where k is a marginal rate of copayment), which is less than the social opportunity cost P that would prevail in the situation of no insurance. Impediments to perfect competition in the market for medical care present an argument for some government planning and/or self-regulation, but do not invalidate the indemnity form of insurance.

This kind of insurance has not been favored by voluntary market forces. A serious obstacle to pure indemnity policies would be the precise and stable specification of health events to be covered. Pauly[5] has discussed the feasibility of indemnity insurance, but he proposes a "compromise" which in fact is quite different. He suggests that for a particular *treatment* the lower of cost or a fixed limit be reimbursed. Expenditure above the limit would be only partially reimbursed. Such coverage would have very little advantage over the major current plans if it implied about the same average rate of copayment.[6]

Health Sector Peculiarities

Ideal assumptions are far from being appropriate in the health sector. This is primarily because most consumers cannot adequately judge the alternatives for preserving their health. In addition, there may be emotional obstacles to the making of careful decisions by a family when one member has a health problem. Arrow[7] discusses peculiarities of the market for medical care as a response to pervasive uncertainty. It is worth noting that Blue Cross Plans originally saw as their mission to serve as the collection arm of the hospitals. It can be inferred that hospitals sought an opportunity to provide their desired quality of care even though the value of this care would not be apparent to many of their customers. Such a development is consistent with the institutions and professional norms seen by Arrow as a natural response to consumer ignorance and uncertainty.

There are two additional considerations that permit policy planners to feel comfortable with some degree of specific subsidy to health care. First is the apparent positive value individuals place on the health of others. This interdependence justifies some stimulation of demand by subsidy. Second is a desire to preserve free choice of provider. This preference has supported reimbursement of providers on the basis of "reasonable and customary" charges.

For the foreseeable future, we can expect to remain with some system of health insurance involving a degree of distortion between net prices faced by consumers and the social costs of service. The size of this distortion and its effect under new plans will depend on the government response to pressures for more reduction of the risk to families of financial catastrophe due to illness.

Recent calculations by Feldstein[8] suggest that the distortions of the current system are so large that the public would be better off with a higher average coinsurance rate for hospital care. The basis for his conclusion, and the existence of some conflicting evidence are given in the next section.

Risk Reduction

It is more valuable to a risk averse family to receive a dollar of insurance benefit when its health expense is high than when it is low. This is a key result from the sensible assumption that consumers derive decreasing marginal utility per dollar of owned assets as the quantity of assets rises. The degree to which a consumer is risk averse with respect to uncertain monetary loss will depend on how steeply marginal utility decreases when assets rise and other variables are held constant. The premium for insurance against monetary loss that would be offered by the consumer for a given policy will be higher if he has a higher degree of risk aversion.

Suppose one consumer with an initial insurance policy purchases a new policy with more comprehensive benefits, the prices of health services remain constant, and his premium is raised by the difference in actuarial cost. This consumer is better off; the gain from risk reduction offsets a loss from expected increase in utilization.

However, when everyone obtains more comprehensive coverage, the prices of health services are observed to rise because of the pressure on supply which in the short run does not expand at constant unit cost.[9] This pure price rise indicates a loss in well-being to each consumer that serves to offset any potential gain due to risk reduction.

When quantitative assumptions about the degree of risk aversion and about demand and supply elasticities for hospital services are made, Feldstein calculates that there would be a net utility gain to consumers by changing to a higher average copayment in hospital insurance plans. Some evidence, however, suggests that consumers are more risk averse than he assumed.

An attempt to estimate quantitatively

the strength of risk aversion was recently made by this author.[10] Federal employees, who select health insurance coverage from a wide range of options, were assumed to make these choices based on the average expected utility that could be obtained under each option by persons of their own age and income. Estimated values of the implied strength of risk aversion for single employees were much greater than have been previously assumed.

Aside from the question of whether, on average, the rate of copayment is too high or low, the treatment of catastrophic versus small expenses requires further careful attention.

Catastrophic versus Small Expenses

There is no guarantee that consumers would be better off for long with a policy charging current premiums and eliminating large copayment losses. Anyone incurring the maximum copayment has no incentive to limit his claim on resources. When individual suppliers are paid only on the basis of actual or customary cost *per unit*, they also have no incentive to limit expense on behalf of their patient who will bear no added cost himself. It is to be expected that the ceiling and/or premiums would continually rise.

It is so far not possible to compare the persistent inflation associated with current insurance to the persistent inflation that would be associated with ceilings above which service is free to the consumer but returns actual cost to the supplier. Any plan that really protects against catastrophic loss is subject to this problem.

Feldstein[11] proposes insurance with protection against large losses combined with high deductibles to promote efficiency. He asserts that if most services were paid directly, the standard or customary charge would give a meaningful reference for covering expenses of persons who have already exceeded the catastrophic limit.

The catastrophic limit would need to be rather small so that most families would not be inclined to purchase additional insurance privately. Such a limit could

prove to be astoundingly low. The Feldstein argument also seems to confuse "customary charge per day" with "customary charge per case." In the catastrophic cases, the hospital has strong reasons to expand the quantity of care so long as they can receive the cost per unit of service.

It seems inevitable that expanded nonprice rationing of care will be required when moderate ceilings on copayment loss are instituted. Such control mechanisms would weaken the effect on demand of incentives to the consumer.

Early or Preventive Treatment

A somewhat extreme position might be taken that, regardless of the nature of copayment for moderate and high expenses, more of the financial obstacles to early or preventive care should be eliminated. It is doubtful that specific mass screening programs are an efficient substitute for routine office and clinic visits.[12] Even if health problems are discovered during screening, many copayment plans give an incentive to delay treatment until a more serious condition develops. Proponents of this view, therefore, recommend the complete elimination of copayment.

One reply to this position against copayment is that ignorance and stronger psychological phenomena are the chief obstacles to earlier treatment of disease.[13] Programs aimed at specific target populations may be a preferable alternative to general subsidies.

The results of Friedman, *et al.*,[14] do not support the view that eliminating the direct expense to consumers of medical care is a meaningful stimulus to the early diagnosis of breast cancer.

The female breast is the most common primary site of cancer and one of the most accessible to self-diagnosis. The disease is believed to spread from a single mass of cells. If treated before there is evidence of cells in other regional tissues or lymph nodes, the five-year relative survival rate[15] is esimated at 82 percent. When regional tissues are involved, the survival rate drops to 53 percent. Spread of the disease to distant organs makes a cure virtually hopeless. Despite the obvious gains from early diagnosis and public education efforts, the proportion of cases treated while still localized has remained less than 50 percent.

This study contains a multiple regression analysis of the determinants of early breast cancer diagnosis, seeking to isolate the independent effects of insurance coverage. Blue Cross members tend to be diagnosed significantly earlier in the course of disease than patients with no insurance. However, the complete coverage of medical costs under the Medicaid program does not seem to be an effective stimulus to early diagnosis.

Concluding Observations

This paper has considered possible innovations in health insurance for families at the high end of the expenditure distribution and at the low end.

For those families covered by the major health insurance plans today, important reductions of family financial risk can be achieved through a lower maximum copayment in the event of "catastrophic" losses. This change in coverage can be expected to generate inflationary pressures on costs of medical care which would require more formalized non-price rationing.

At the lower end of the expenditure distribution, the complete elimination of copayment does not seem to be the answer to shortening the delay between appearance of symptoms and treatment for serious illness. Insurance plans must then be supplemented by programs to meet this challenge.

References and Notes

1 The term copayment will be used for any direct, out-of-pocket cost to consumers of health care.
2 Not to be linked to the general use of this term in the health insurance policies of private insurance companies. These policies typically provide indemnities conditional on the amount of services consumed rather than conditional on the occurrence of illness. Some insurance companies have offered insurance with lump-sum transfers in the event of accidents (such as loss of an arm or leg) for over 100 years.
3 Since it is not our intention to advocate this form of insurance, we do not wish to distract the reader with a more rigorous exposition of social welfare maximization. The result has been recognized in: Arrow, K. J. "Uncertainty and the Welfare Economics of Medical Care," *American Economic Review* 53, No. 5 (1963); and Pauly, M. V. "Indemnity Insurance for Health Care Efficiency," *Economic and Business Bulletin* (Temple University, School of Business Administration) 24, No. 1 (1971).
4 Individual risk preference may be inconsistent with the way in which individual utility enters the social welfare function. The social welfare function, for example, may be symmetric in the utility of every individual, but individuals may have different degrees of risk aversion leading to nonoptimal indemnity transfers.
5 Pauly, "Indemnity Insurance for Health Care Efficiency," *op. cit.*
6 The gain from this scheme would be due to the consumer choosing an economical supplier. If the indemnities were large, misallocations among

treatments may remain since they tend to be accepted on physician advice, and the inducement to a more desired style of care could turn the limits into floors. High limits would mean larger coinsurance rates at the high end of expenditure, which implies utility loss due to risk aversion. Low limits of the first-dollar coverage would make the plan almost indistinguishable from current plans.
7 Arrow, "Uncertainty and the Welfare Economics of Medical Care," *op. cit.*
8 Feldstein, M. S. "The Welfare Loss of Excess Health Insurance," *Journal of Political Economy*, forthcoming.
9 Important references are, among others: Feldstein, M. S. "Hospital Cost Inflation: A Study in Non-profit Prices Dynamics," *American Economic Review* 61, No. 5 (1971); and Pauly, M. V. "The Economics of Moral Hazard," *American Economic Review* 58, No. 4 (1968).
10 Friedman, B. S. "A Study of Uncertainty and Health Insurance," unpublished Ph.D. dissertation, Massachusetts Institute of Technology, 1971. The relevant analysis is available in mimeograph from the author.
11 Feldstein, M. S. "A New Approach to National Health Insurance," *The Public Interest* 23 (Spring 1971).
12 In practice, a high proportion of persons entering voluntary screening programs have self-recognized symptoms. See: Goldsen, R. K. "Patient Delay in Seeking Cancer Diagnosis: Behavioral Aspects," *Journal of Chronic Disease* 16:431 (1963). The diagnostic importance and cost of patient histories favor continuity of routine care

Part V

National Health Insurance And Alternative Modes Of Delivery

This section examines the various forms of national health insurance and alternative modes of delivery. The first paper by Berki sets the economic framework within which national health insurance programs can be analyzed. Newhouse's paper offers an insight on how the demand for medical services varies with the price the consumer pays out-of-pocket for such services. Since various national insurance plans differ in the amount consumers are to pay out-of-pocket, Newhouse's paper should be helpful in estimating the demand under alternative plans. Barton and Smiley's paper offers a framework within which costs of various (national) health insurance plans may be estimated.

While the first three papers offer criteria and frameworks of analysis for evaluating various national health insurance plans, they should be followed up by actual evaluation of existing national health insurance proposals. What, for example, would be the demand under the Nixon–Ford plan versus the Ribicoff plan? How would the delivery system be altered under the American Hospital Association plan versus the Kennedy plan? Whose plan promises to minimize administrative costs? What are the distributions of costs among different income groups under different plans? These are some of the important questions to be asked in evaluating alternative national health insurance plans.

Many studies have been made that compare performance under prepaid group practice versus fee-for-service practice. Donabedian's paper reviews the literature on the subject. His review confirms the generally held belief that input-mix in the use of health resources under group practice approaches the optimum more than under fee-for-service practice. Donabedian also finds that, although there have been doubts about the level of "technical quality" of care under prepaid group practice, there are evidences to suggest that it has been maintained and safeguarded. He concludes that prepaid group practice will be more acceptable to consumers and providers as information on the relative merits becomes more readily available.

The last paper, by Coleman and Kaminsky, offers a computerized financial planning model (FPM) to improve financial planning and management practices of a Health Maintenance Organization. Simulations are presented showing the economic impact of different admission rates, costs, premium pricing strategies, and the rates of cost inflation. An increased input from industrial engineering and operations research are most welcome in the health field. Coleman and Kaminsky's model not only will acquaint health services administrators and policy-makers with a useful management tool but also will encourage more people in industrial engineering and operations research to become interested in the health field.

Sylvester E. Berki

Reprinted with permission of the Blue Cross Association, from *Inquiry:* Vol.VII, No.2, pp.37-55. Copyright © 1971 by the Blue Cross Association.

Economic Effects of National Health Insurance

Originally Published in June 1971

The nearly ubiquitous dissatisfaction with the state of affairs in medical care has permeated even the corporate ranks of business and management. In the introduction to a series of articles on "Our Ailing Medical System," *Fortune* magazine acknowledges that "American medicine, the pride of the nation for many years, stands now on the brink of chaos."[1] And the lead article in the series begins with this description of the system:

> Our present system of medical care is not a system at all. The majority of physicians, operating alone as private entrepreneurs, constitute an army of pushcart vendors in an age of supermarkets.[2]

Most major current proposals for the alleviation of "chaos" in health care rely on the institution of national health insurance. This paper presents the outlines of an analytic framework for the identification and analysis of the economic effects of such plans.[3]

The Framework of Analysis[4]

The characteristics distinguishing "national health insurance" from a "national health scheme" are organizational.[5, 6] National health insurance is basically a na-

Sylvester E. Berki, M.A. is Lecturer in the Department of Medical Care Organization, School of Public Health, University of Michigan.

This paper is a slightly abridged version of one presented to a Joint Session of the Medical Care Section, A.P.H.A., and the Conference on the Social and Behavioral Sciences in Health at the 98th annual meeting of the American Public Health Association, Houston, Texas, October 25, 1970.

tionally organized financial mechanism based on social risk-sharing: a public system for the collective financing of privately provided services. Its possible impact on the basic medical care variables of utilization, quality, clinical delivery systems, and outcomes is *indirect*, attained through a system of incentives, rewards, and regulations. National health schemes, on the other hand, are *direct* systems: in addition to the financing mechanism, both the organization of the health system as a whole, and of the individual personal care delivery units within it, are collectively determined; their objectives collectively established; their performance criteria set and enforced by legally constituted public bodies; and, often, the providers of service are salaried employees on the public payroll. Within it, the role of the private provider of care varies from the minimal to the marginal.

The collective provision of a financing mechanism for medical care within the framework of national health insurance, aside from ideological, sociological, and political considerations, finds its economic rationale in the presence of two basic conditions: private markets for the provision of the service either do not exist or, if they do, perform in an unsatisfactory manner;[7, 8, 9] and/or the service to be collectively provided is invested with the public interest.[10] In this sense, national health insurance is not basically different from rural electrification, T.V.A., or flood control. It is a public project writ large.

One appealing framework for evaluation of the economic effects of a large public project is cost-benefit analysis.[11]   A basic difficulty in attempting to investigate the economic effects of national health insurance, however, is that in previous scholarly discussions, as well as in the present political debate, "economic effects" have come to be identified with "cost effects." Reflected as increased budgetary expenditures, in increased utilization, or in increased administrative expense, costs presumably are hard-nosed facts—definable, identifiable, measurable.[12, 13]   Benefits, on the other hand, whether expressed in terms of increased levels of preventive care, in terms of reduced mortality and morbidity, or in terms of greater accessibility for major subsets of the population, are more difficult to measure.   They are less amenable to the application of refined analytic techniques, more "intangible" and hence tend not to be accorded the dignity of data. As a result, benefits are left out of the analysis.

This analytic asymmetry must continually be borne in mind when discussing the "economic effects" as in fact cost effects. The analysis of costs effects in the absence of measures of expected benefits will be useful if, by considering the likely effects of such a national payment system on the organizational and behavioral elements in medical care, it will permit predictions, at least at the level of orders of magnitude, of the differential cost implications of different values of policy variables.

In the short run the total direct and indirect private and social costs of any given national health insurance system will be determined by the interaction of its impact on utilization (satisfied effective demand) and the existing availability of resources (resource constraints).[4, 14, 15, 16] The effect on utilization, however, is itself a composite of population and benefit coverage, as well as provider attitudes, incentives, quality criteria, and present levels of pent-up demands, along with such policy parameters as the population's age, sex, income, and urban-rural distributions, not to mention its attitudes toward health, the sick role, and the system.[17, 18]   It appears to be a useful exercise, therefore, to attempt to disaggregate the possible effects and to order them within a framework capable of illuminating their interdependencies.

The Instrumentalities of Policy: Policy Variables

Consider as *policy variables* those elements of the system which are tractable to social policy decisions, and *policy parameters* those that are not.   Target population, for example, is a direct and, in most cases, crucial policy variable, while the resource constraints existing at a given time are parameters.   What is a variable and what is a parameter is partially determined by the time horizon chosen: elements which for purposes of policy-making must be considered parametric in the immediate period (say, five years) may be considered variables over a longer time span.   The objective of policy is to induce desired behavior through the interactions among the policy variables and those phenomena —economic, sociological, psychological, and institutional—which for the purposes of public policy-making must be considered parametric. The problem for the economic analysis of public policy—in this case national health insurance—arises from the multiplicity of interactions among the policy variables and parameters and their differential direct and indirect effects on costs.

Consider a simple schematic representation of the basic policy variables (Figure I) and what, for economic analysis, are the basic parameters: resource constraints. Prior to a somewhat more detailed discussion of the *dimensions* of the variables and of their direct and indirect effects (outlined in Table 1), it may be said that the list of available policy variables are:

A. Target Population
B. Target Benefit Coverage
C. Target Utilization
D. Payment Mechanisms
E. Incentive Mechanisms
F. Organizational Modalities

Figure I. Schematic representation of basic policy variables and parameters

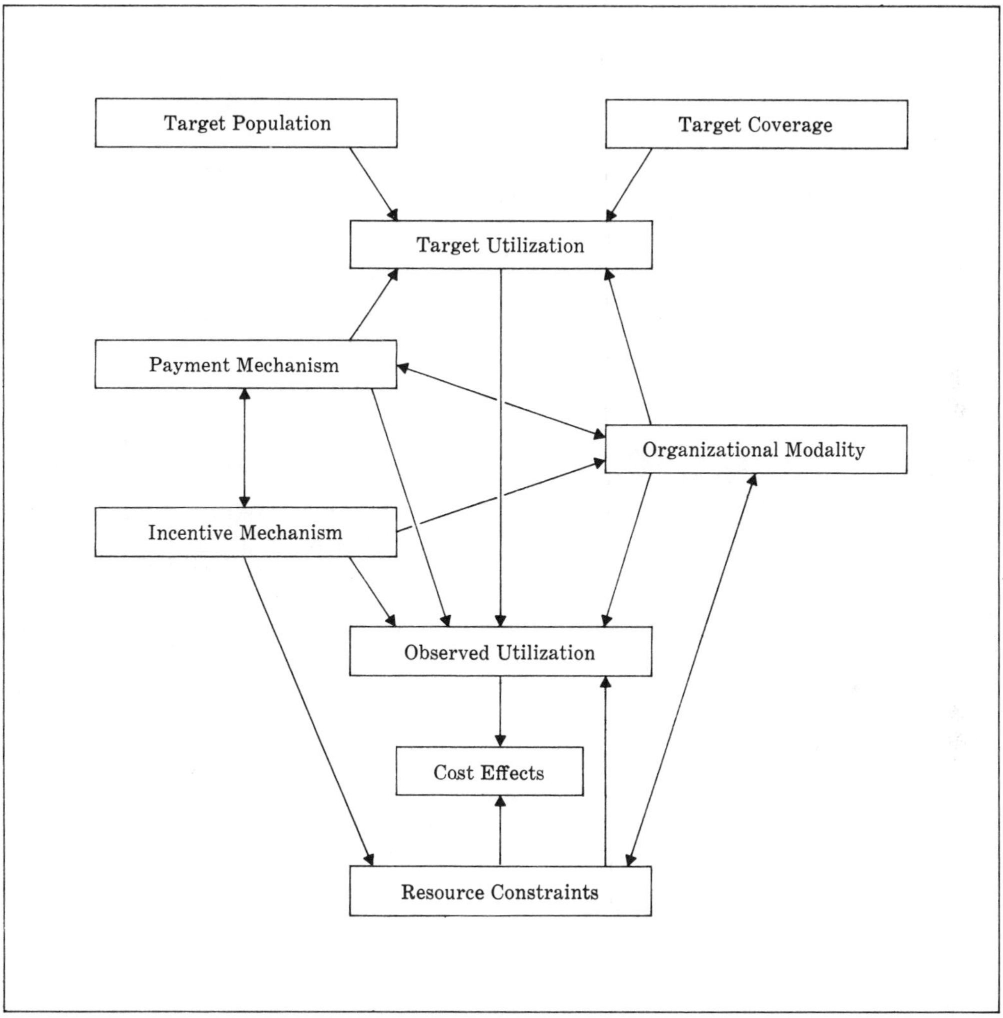

The dimensions of Target Population, in terms of the definition of the population groups to be the beneficiaries of the plan, and the dimensions of the Target Coverage, in terms of what services are to be covered, will jointly but not exclusively determine Target Utilization. Target Utilization may further be specified in terms of patterns of care along the dimensions of, say, comprehensiveness and quality criteria. It is, therefore, the combination of Target Population, Target Coverage, and Target Utilization — the interaction of three independently variable policy tools— that would appear to result in Observed Utilization.

The chosen Payment Mechanisms, Incentive Mechanisms, and Organizational Modalities will also have significant direct and indirect effects on Observed Utilization. Furthermore, Observed Utilization will be directly affected by Resource Constraints. The interaction of the direct and indirect effects of Target Population, Target Coverage, Target Utilization, Payment and Incentive Mechanisms, and Organizational Modalities of any given plan and the existing Resource Constraints determine

Table 1. Policy variables and effects

Policy variable	Dimensions	Direct effects	Indirect effects
A. Target Population	Who is to benefit	Increased accessibility	Effects on non-target current utilizers
	Methods of exclusion	Changes in perceptions of medical care phenomena	Effects on non-target current non-utilizers
	Methods of inclusion	Changes in attitudes toward medical care phenomena	Displacement of current categorical programs
B. Target Benefit Coverage	What is to be covered: definition of range of services	Impact on provider service orientation Prevention-diagnosis-treatment process effects	Innovational processes Supplemental private insurance effects
C. Target Utilization	Criteria for the intensity of use: comprehensiveness, continuity, accessibility	Differential utilization effects by population, by facility, by medical condition Allocative efficiency effects	Income effects on providers Income effects on users
	Medical criteria for acceptable processes	Regional allocative effects	Distributional effects Macroeconomic effects
D. Payment Mechanism	Methods of provider payment	Administrative cost effects	Current program effects: Federal, state, local, private
	Bases of provider payment	Budgetary expenditure effects, Federal, state, local	Non-health program effects Tax base effects Distributional effects
	Methods and bases of revenue collection	Private sector cost effects: carriers, individuals, providers, suppliers Budgetary revenue effects: Federal, state, local	Income effects Derived demand effects Tax base effects
E. Incentive Mechanisms	Nature and dimension of incentives: financial, professional, market competition	Allocation and distribution effects: utilization, costs Organizational modalities	Inter-systems effects Long run effects: market entry, supply functions
	Incentive, objectives: providers, patients		
	Impact of incentives: providers, patients		
F. Organization Modalities	Changes in existing delivery systems	Allocative efficiency effects	Observed utilization Regional effects
	Changes in relationships among existing delivery systems	Distributive efficiency effects	Quality effects
	New delivery systems		
	Acceptance of existing delivery systems and interactions		

the costs of that plan. We must be careful, as we shall show later, not to confuse "cost effects" with *net* cost effects: reductions in current levels of governmental expenditures for existing categorical programs as well as programmed reductions in current levels of private disbursements for services must be netted out to arrive at the *net additional costs* of the plan.

We indicate (by arrows) that Resource Constraints, in addition to determining Cost Effects conjointly with Observed Utilization, have direct effects on Observed Utilization itself, while at the same time they interact with Organizational Modalities. Resource Constraints, along with the policy variables, will be reflected in observed costs and prices; but, in addition, to the extent that the Payment and Incentive Mechanisms within the existing Organizational Modalities do not effectively ration existing resources among the demanders of services, alternative allocative mechanisms will evolve and in turn affect Observed Utilization over time. One such non-price allocative mechanism is the queue: waiting lists of office appointments, for elective admissions, for kidney machines. Interaction with Organizational Modalities and through it with Payment Mechanisms is designed to indicate that the nature and effectiveness of non-price allocative mechanisms to emerge are not independent of the given set of delivery systems and reimbursement mechanisms. That is, the rationing of services cannot be assumed to be independent of whether we are concerned with a group practice reimbursed by capitation, or a group or solo practice reimbursed by fee-for-service; nor yet of whether we have vendor payment, user prepayment, postpayment, or tax credit. Cost and Observed Utilization, therefore, are seen to be the resultants of a multiplicity of forces, many of which are subject to manipulation by policy tools and many of which are not.

We are attempting to specify a comprehensive set of variables and parameters and, by indicating their dimensions and interactions, to establish the bases for the development of quantitative models to predict the expected effects of any given plan. Not all of the policy variables need be incorporated in every plan for national health insurance: the argument here is that we can compare and evaluate alternative plans by considering which policy variables are operational along which dimensions. Neither the A.M.A.'s "Medicredit" proposal nor the Javits Bill directly incorporates as operational policy variables Organizational Modality. Under both of these proposals services would be rendered by existing delivery systems. Under the Javits Bill, however, changes in existing delivery systems would be encouraged indirectly via the formulation of Incentive and Payment Mechanism variables designed to foster the growth of comprehensive delivery systems. There are similar and greater differences among the proposals currently on the table in

terms of policy variables we have identified. The effects of each of the plans, it may be maintained, will be determined by the direct and indirect effects of the variables. Let us, therefore, consider them in greater detail.

Direct and Indirect Policy Effects

In Table 1 we list the policy variables and enumerate their dimensions as well as some of their direct and indirect effects.

The first dimension of policy variable A, Target Population, is obvious: the set of potential beneficiaries must be defined. The second and third dimensions are somewhat more problematical: a set of potential beneficiaries may be easily defined; but for all plans in which not all members of society are included there must be established mechanisms for inclusion and exclusion. If the excluded set is that comprised of "nonresident aliens" the mechanisms for exclusion are simple and obvious. When exclusion is based on family income, as in the 1970 Pettengill-Aetna proposal,[19] methods of exclusion to limit target coverage to the target population may be in conflict with other criteria: the undesirability of "demeaning" mechanisms for the establishment of eligibility, such as the means test.[20] In either case, Methods of Exclusion may be relatively more simple to devise than Methods of Inclusion.

For any defined dimension of the Target Population and for any increase in potential accessibility (a direct effect), the regional distribution of facilities, Payment and Incentive Mechanisms, Target Utilization criteria, patient perceptions of need and attitudes toward the medical care system, as well as the orientation of existing and to-be-designed delivery systems, together determine whether those who are eligible for services will in fact utilize them. That is to say, Observed Utilization and hence cost effects can not legitimately be directly and uniquely related to Target Populations: it is not who *may* use the services that counts, but who *shall*. One of the direct effects may well be changes in patient perceptions and attitudes, changes in social definitions of the "sick role."[18] Indirect effects of plans with less than universal population coverage on current utilizers *not* included in the Target Population may be difficult to predict but are nonetheless important. If the increased demands on existing facilities for providing services result in increased costs, such cost increases may have negative income effects on the excluded utilizers.

Policy variable B, Target Benefit Coverage, varies along several dimensions. The most important ones are: 1) ambulatory, inpatient, long-term; 2) physiological, mental; 3) preventive, diagnostic, therapeutic; and 4) inclusion or exclusion of dental, optometric, pharmaceutic, and rehabilitative services. The direct effects, in combination with the Payment and Incentives Mechanisms, can be expected to influence the service orientation of providers as well as currently practiced preventive and diagnostic patterns. While the distinction between prevention and early diagnosis is somewhat unclear, increased emphasis on both would tend to shift current relative demands for diagnostic and therapeutic facilities. Indirect effects may be manifest in a change of policy options offered by private carriers, either as supplementals for target populations, for services not covered, or as comprehensive coverage for excluded population groups. To the extent that generally high risk populations would be covered, the development of private plans for population subsets with lower risk would be enhanced. Indirect effects may also redirect the orientation of innovation toward the development of facilities, equipment, and processes, as well as manpower qualifications, for use in care patterns emphasized. The recent examples of multiphasic screening and the Papanicolau Test remind us of the impact of scientific and social orientation on innovative emphasis.

Utilization Criteria

Given the levels of Population and Benefit Coverage, it is useful to consider as a related yet separate variable the one we have called Target Utilization. While it is true that covered population at risk times covered services will more or less equal expected utilization, we should like to stress both the "more or less" and the desirability of explicitly considering utilization criteria. Such criteria, considered as dimensions of this policy variable, fit into two basic categories: Intensity of Use and Medical criteria. Whether any given plan explicitly considers comprehensiveness and continuity of care, they all generally, if implicitly, include medical criteria minimally in the requirements for certification standards to be met by vendors. We must also bear in mind the possibility of explicit inclusion of peer review mechanisms, organizational or other professional monitoring, or quality relevant information gathering and analysis systems such as MAP-PAS, to mention but a few readily available means designed to attain minimum acceptable standards of care. Implicitly or explicitly, criteria of appropriateness of care are imbedded in Payment and Incentive Mechanisms.[21, 22] Whether it is "Volkswagen" or "Cadillac" medicine that any given proposal is designed to deliver, the inevitable effects of the payment and Incentive Mechanisms introduced will have to be evaluated; and in fact, both Incentive and Payment Mechanisms should be designed with quality effects in mind.[23, 24]

From the points of view of analysis of the plans and evaluation of their effects on costs, there must exist some, even if vaguely defined, objective function. Since "economic effects" include benefits as well as costs, it is difficult if not impossible to analyze and to evaluate the costs of producing an undefined output. Quality of care is a basic dimension of medical care output, whether defined in terms of end results, processes, or services. If by "objective function" we mean the specification of the set of goals or objectives we wish to attain—or in economic terms, to optimize —the exclusion of quality standards means that the outputs we wish to optimize and whose costs we wish to evaluate are only partially defined. Further, while there may well exist trade-offs between quality and cost, we surely do not wish to pay "Cadillac" prices for "Edsel" quality—in fact we may not want "Edsels" at all.

Target Utilization criteria, whether specified or not, will in either case have significant resource allocation effects. Recall that Target Utilization, in addition to incorporating separable criteria, is the resultant of the composite effects of Population and Benefit Coverage. Its differential effects in terms of demands for services on segments of the health care delivery system (which while it may be a "many splintered thing" nevertheless exhibits significant interrelationships) may, for example, shift a significant proportion of investigative and diagnostic services now performed on an inpatient basis to ambulatory patterns. From the point of view of resource allocation the efficiency of such a shift cannot be evaluated unless we know which resources are the ones in relatively shorter supply. That is to say, the resource allocative effects of reduced rates of hospitalization together with increased office waiting lists and laboratory queues are not *obviously* in the direction of increased efficiency. Other resource allocation effects, also reflected in costs, may be more easily evaluated. The encouragement, by Target Utilization Criteria, Payment and Incentive Mechanisms, as well as by the Organizational Modality variable, of the development of progressive patient care acute and long-term facilities, including home care programs, imply the use of less capital intensive and more labor intensive processes, where part of the labor, as a matter of fact, is provided by the patient. The same three policy variables are also expected to have regional effects. The distribution of available facilities and manpower by geographic region, by political boundary, or by urban-rural-suburban divisions is by no means homogeneous. Thus the allocative effects can be expected to have very different regional effects—reflected in sig-

nificantly different regional cost effects, as well as in accessibility.

Prior to proceeding to the discussion of the other effects and variables, note that in the delineation of Target Utilization effects we have been continually forced to mention the interactions of the Payment and Incentive Mechanisms. As an aside to those who have a preference for tidy analyses of well delimited problems in terms of a small number of variables, consider that a system of national health insurance is just that: a *system* and *national*. In a nation where the population is heterogeneous along a multitude of dimensions, where the existing delivery units and facilities are a rich mix of private, public, nonprofit, proprietary, high quality, low quality, "pushcart vendors" *along with* supermarkets, the effects of a *national* system of financing and organizational improvement are not tractable by "partial equilibrium analysis." We cannot, that is, disaggregate the multitude of possible effects and then focus in on just one or two, assuming *ceteris paribus*. We are dealing with a system in many interacting variables, none of whose values can be determined in absence of the values of the others. One of the wonders is the purported ability of some "analysts" to produce "actuarial" estimates of costs of national health insurance plans without any specification of even the most obviously expectable effects. One set of such effects is listed under Indirect Effects of Target Utilization.

Any national health insurance plan—regardless of its specific Payment and Incentive Mechanisms — which to any extent alters utilization patterns will have at least indirect income effects on both providers and utilizers. Payment and Incentive Mechanisms may be designed to modulate such effects to attain desired objectives. But the income effects will be present. By income effects we mean that the incomes of both utilizers and providers will be affected. There is sufficient evidence of this—in a case more clear-cut and less controversial than that of physician incomes—in terms of Medicare effects on the net revenue position of hospitals.[25, 26] The introduction of Title XVIII was rapidly reflected in increased net revenues. Physician incomes were also affected minimally by the resulting higher collection ratios.[27, 28] While no studies of changes in incomes of the aged resulting from Medicare coverage are available, positive income effects can be deduced. Those previous utilizers whose out-of-pocket expenditures were reduced realized actual increases in their money incomes, now available for other consumption expenditures; and those previous non-utilizers who under Medicare *became* utilizers experienced an increase in their real income to the extent that they consider medical care services a desirable component of consumption. But income effects are even more pervasive. Expenditures by the non-aged for services for the aged, to the extent replaced by Medicare, represent increases in the income of the non-aged. The broader the population coverage and the more comprehensive the set of services covered, the greater the potential income effects will be and the more pervasive the potential distributional effects. By distributional effects we mean the differential income effect by income class. "Potential" must be emphasized, for the net resultant income distributional effect will be equally determined by the Payment and Incentive Mechanisms adopted. That is to say, whether beneficiaries in the lower income groups will receive relatively larger benefits than those in higher income groups will depend on what the Population and Benefit Coverages are, and, for any given set of these, on the Payment Mechanism. We shall return to these questions.

Consider also that one of the basic arguments for increased levels of medical care utilization, including prevention, rests on the nature of medical care as investment in human capital. Whether it is investment or maintenance, if increased levels of utilization result in lower mortality and morbidity rates among the working age population, the national manpower pool and its effectiveness will have been increased. This is one of the macroeconomic effects to consider. The other is that increased utilization resulting in the expansion of the health care sector implies the reallocation of resources from other sectors to this one, in a stable economy; or, in a growing economy, the redirection of some proportion of the increased productive capacity into the health sector. The consideration of these effects is not trivial relative to a sector which currently absorbs about 6.5 percent of the G.N.P., in the neighborhood of $70-billion.

Financing Mechanisms: Payment and Repayment

Much of the current discussion and many of the basic differences among the various proposals for national health insurance is in terms of the financing mechanisms to be employed. While the nature and extent of any given financial mechanism are directly intertwined with the intended and unintended incentive schemes embedded within it, we propose to consider separately at first the three major dimensions of the Payment Mechanism: Methods of Provider Payment, Bases of Provider Payment, and Methods and Bases of Revenue Collection — or what in public finance terms may be called "repayment."

The multidimensionality of Provider Payment Methods is indicated by the existing mix of reimbursement schemes. The possibilities may be outlined as in Table 2. Most of the entries in the cells are self-explanatory. Under the direct vendor prepayment method we may have capitation as the basis. But capitation payment may be limited to selected income groups, as has been done experimentally already.[29, 30, 31, 32] Postpaid cost of service user reimbursement may also be limited and/or graduated by income class. The current proposals include a variety of Bases and Methods of Payment listed in Table 2, with the exception of prepaid credit. A "credit card" system could technically be established: each member of the Target Population to be issued a "credit card"

Table 2. Methods and bases of payment

Methods of payment	Bases of payment		
	Prepayment	Postpayment	Mixture
Direct (Vendor payment)	Capitation Geographic Occupational Income class	Fee-for-service Customary Negotiated Limited Partial	X
Indirect (User payment)	Prepaid credit Prepaid premium	Cost of service Customary Negotiated Limited Partial Cost of Insurance Reimbursement Tax credit	X
Mixture	X	X	X

valid for the provision of Covered Services with or without specifying provider certification. The "credit card" could be sold to each covered individual at a price functionally related to a variety of consumer characteristics, such as age, family size, and income. Vendor payment could also be on a variety of bases, from capitation to fee-for-service. Under this plan, however, repayment methods and bases, or Revenue Collection, is one of the major determining forces. It is important to stress that the methods by which revenues to cover expenditures are to be collected, and the bases of such revenues, are separate and separable questions from the issues involved in the selection of Provider Payment Mechanisms.

The major income distributional effects on consumers will be determined by the choice of the repayment mechanism, together with Population and Benefit Coverage. Given a level of potential benefits in terms of coverage, if repayment is to be on a tax basis, then the choice of the base of the tax (payroll, income, employer-employee contributions, personal-business profit combination) and the nature of the tax (progressive, proportional, or regressive—although that is to some extent already determined by the choice of tax base) is at the heart of the question of equity. It will also at the same time have significant geographically differentiated Tax Base Effects on those state and local governments which currently use any of the tax bases for their own taxing purposes. That is to say, a program financed by payroll taxes will be more regressive than one financed by graduated income taxes, or income surtaxes in combination with non-personal taxes. But to the extent that local and state taxing authorities employ income as a tax base, their tax bases will shrink, generating a negative local tax effect. The net effect on state and local budgetary expenditures, however, will be determined by two other completely different issues: the proportion of state and local budgetary expenditures currently devoted to health care programs, and the extent to which such programs would be superseded by a national insurance plan. This question does not appear to have received previous attention. It is notable, however, that those states currently expending a significant proportion of their revenues on medical care, either under Title XIX or other categorical programs, would gain the most by those proposed plans that would obviate such existing programs.

Administrative Cost effects are related to methods of payment and repayment, as well as to the organizational variables in the provision of services. The extent of the use of third-party carriers (whether private or Blue Cross and Blue Shield), the method of vendor or user payment, the presence or absence of copayment, the degree of administrative centralization and coordination, all have to be considered prior to an estimation of the administrative cost attributes of any given plan. Needless to say, Private Sector Cost effects are the subject of the same set of variables, as are the Incentive Mechanisms to be employed.

The Carrot and the Stick: Incentive Effects

Incentive Mechanisms vary along three basic dimensions: objectives, nature, and impact. In terms of objectives we may consider rate of utilization, in which case the desired impact is on providers, potential utilizers, or both: the objective is to eliminate or to reduce medically unnecessary and economically inefficient patterns of care. The capitation system is said to have this effect on providers,[33, 34] although other proposals have been discussed.[35, 36, 37, 38, 39] Non-financial incentives, such as peer review, are also possibilities with yet different effects. The impact of incentives, or more generally disincentives, on users has been much discussed, mostly in terms of "moral hazard" or "high" price elasticity. But basically both hypotheses boil down to the same argument: if out-of-pocket costs are eliminated utilization will increase because a "free lunch" is free because its price is zero.[40, 41, 42, 43] The effects of incentives and disincentives on users is difficult to predict since previous analyses have assumed that the consumer is the sole decision-maker in choosing between more or less care, lower or higher rates of utilization. This may be correct in terms of the demand for initial physician contact, but certainly for that broad class of services where felt need or effective demand cannot be translated into utilization (satisfied demand) without physician legitimization, observed utilization is determined by patient *and* by provider

preferences. Thus the utilization of any service, or process, which requires a prescription, admission slip, or any other form of physician legitimization cannot be predicated on the bases of assumptions about consumer preferences or "morality." There are categories of demand for services that may be said to be *physician originated;* however, the total observed set of satisfied demands, or utilization, is a composite of patient-originated and provider-originated demands. The distribution of those demands among various care patterns is as much, or more, a function of organizational, financial, and incentive variables as of patient preferences.[44]

Recall that in Figure 1 we indicate a relationship between incentives, resources, and organizational arrangements. The reallocation of service functions in view of differential resource scarcities can be influenced by the appropriate system of incentives and will be influenced by any plan. One of the explanations for increased rates of hospitalization under insurance plans covering a wider variety of hospital than ambulatory services is that the price faced by the patient of covered services is lower than the price of uncovered services: when certain diagnostic procedures are reimbursed on an inpatient but not on an ambulatory basis, the patient naturally prefers, financially, the inpatient process. And so might the physician. The *less* comprehensive the insurance, the more selective in terms of services the national health insurance plan, the *more* built-in incentives for inefficiency obtain.

It must also be noted that less than comprehensive coverage would have long-run incentive effects as well. Service areas experiencing relatively higher rates of utilization would lead to relatively higher (derived) demands for inputs employed in the production of those services. To the extent that higher demands for inputs are reflected in their higher earnings, whether in terms of wages and salaries or returns on capital, those higher earnings can be expected to lead to increased entry of factors of production into those service areas. This does not imply that incentives with long-term effects may not be devised. One answer to the physician shortage, if it exists, is not only the expansion of medical school training capacities but subsidies to reduce the financial costs of training to students. The discussions of shortages and training needs tend unfortunately to assume a high degree of regional homogeneity: payment and incentive mechanisms must be analyzed with a view to their likely effects in bringing about a better regional allocation of facilities and providers. One of the ways of attaining the direction of new resources or the redirection of existing ones into areas of relatively greater unmet need is by the development of new Organizational Modalities jointly with Payment and Incentive Mechanisms designed to attain that objective.

The Organizational Modality aspects of national health insurance plans may vary all the way from emphasizing new delivery systems to the complete acceptance of prevailing ones. An obvious example of the latter is "Medicredit." Changes in existing systems may be along the lines of developing and instituting improved production processes, improved systems of increased accessibility such as "outreach" and neighborhood health centers, or simply increased emphasis on the development and expansion of outpatient departments. Changes in the relationships among existing systems would have to consider the nature and role of referral patterns, the role of community hospitals *vis à vis* community physicians, as well as the complete isolation of general medical practice, dental care, and optometric services into sealed off categories.

Questions of comprehensiveness, continuity, accessibility, and appropriateness of care relevant under the rubric of Target Utilization are equally relevant under Organizational Modalities. To whatever extent relationships between these dimensions of care and the organization of delivery systems exist they must be jointly considered. Questions of the differential

economic efficiencies of different delivery systems are equally important. Whether because of the existence of economies of scale or of the use of different technologies, varying resource combinations, or simply different attitudes regarding the importance of the use of resource-saving processes, where alternatives exist the organizational framework most likely to minimize the use of resources to attain specified objectives will result in the lowest attainable cost effects. That is the meaning of allocative efficiency. Questions of distributive efficiency are also involved, as well as those of regional and quality effects. "Mainstream" delivery systems designed to deliver "mainstream medicine" to the white middle-class insured suburban silent majority are the most likely to perpetuate the patterns of medical neglect of the poor, the rural, and the black. Note, therefore, that the envisaged Organizational Modalities must be evaluated by a variety of criteria: allocative and distributive efficiency, utilization criteria, regional effects, incentive and payment effects.

Analytic Conclusions

We have come full circle. We have started our discussion of the economic effects of national health insurance by emphasizing that they include not only costs but benefits as well; but benefits are hard to measure and hence usually get lost in the analysis. Partly they are hard to measure because the monetary values to be attached to "comprehensive, continuous, one-door, one-class, high-quality" care cannot be based on market signals. Market values, the prices observed in private transactions, are not accurate reflections of real scarcities in markets characterized by elements of monopoly, legal, traditional, professional, and economic restrictions, the prevalence of risk and uncertainty, and inefficient resource allocation indicated by duplication, fragmentation, and rigidity. Neither can prices be taken to reflect "consumer preferences" or value received in markets which, for them, are shrouded in secrecy, shot through with uncertainty and fear; and where demands, episodic in nature, are expressed in ignorance of alternatives or of consequences. Much work needs to be done to enable us to evaluate benefits even at that level of approximation at which we can estimate costs. It is with that in mind that perhaps the framework we have here outlined may be useful. It should enable us to list all relevant effects and to try to identify their complex interactions. As an example, let us briefly consider within this framework a proposed plan typical of national health insurance plans employing the tax credit mechanism: The Fannin Bill (S. 4419, September 30, 1970), a variation of "Medicredit."

An Application of the Analysis: The 1970 Fannin Bill

The 1970 Fannin Bill, like "Medicredit," had three separate parts: general health insurance, catastrophic illness insurance, and peer review procedures. Consider general health insurance first, Title I.

The Target Population is less than clearly defined as all U.S. citizens and those who must file a Federal income tax return, presumably including resident foreigners. This is, however, the *potential* Target Population: the mechanism of exclusion is generally simple, on the basis of the income tax return; but the mechanism for inclusion is not specified at all. The Bill establishes no direct procedure by means of which those eligible would necessarily be included in the covered population. This is, in fact, one of its claims: ". . . coverage should be extended without Government interference on a voluntary rather than compulsory basis." An indirect mechanism of inclusion may potentially be present in the use of existing private carriers: to the extent that insurance carriers, agents, and brokers should find it financially rewarding to extend their population coverage under this Bill, they may undertake advertising and other sales strategies and thereby increase the percentage of the potential Target Population that becomes actual. The effect of such competitive be-

havior, if any, on the relative position of private carriers and Blue Cross and Blue Shield is, for these purposes, irrelevant. Current categorical programs would not be replaced. The accessibility effects of the Bill are difficult to estimate, partly because the benefits are differentiated by income, partly because the Bill has nothing to say on vendor incentives or organizational modalities, and little on target utilization. Individuals who qualify under the eligibility standards for either of the two methods of payment the Bill specifies must apply to receive the benefits. Since the tax credit method is rather simple and tied to the already well known Federal income tax filing procedures, participation under this method is likely to be high. But participation under the "insurance premium certificate" method is likely to be rather low, if at all predictable, because its potential beneficiaries are members of socioeconomic groups of more limited information and lower accessibility to established carriers.

Whereas the "Medicredit" proposals presented by Dr. Russel B. Roth in November, 1969 specify Target Benefit Coverage by specifying the minimum service coverage of insurance plans "qualified" for tax credit along a number of dimensions, the Fannin Bill does not do so. For its purposes it defines as a "qualified medical care insurance policy" all existing insurance programs operating in accordance with state law except that they must be "without regard to any pre-existing health condition" and "guaranteed renewable." Part B of Title XVIII, the supplementary plan under Medicare, is included. The differences are both interesting and relevant since while under "Medicredit" supplementary benefit coverage may be written subject to deductible (usually 20 percent), there is no explicit limitation of service coverage under the Fannin Bill. That is, if private carriers wished to do so they could write whatever policy would be salable and meet state regulations. But existing restrictive state legislation, with respect to prescription drugs for example, and the persistent problems of adverse preselection would not be mitigated by the Fannin Bill or by "Medicredit." It is unlikely that changes in the currently privately available insurance plans would be induced, particularly regarding long-term, psychiatric and dental care, and prescribed drugs. Since there are no mechanisms present designed to alter the existing nature of insurance coverage, there are no direct or indirect effects to be expected. Thus the current emphasis on acute, episodic, fragmented care of variable quality would not be disturbed.

It may be argued that within the rubric of Target Utilization we may expect some such changes, particularly with respect to quality. Title III of the Bill established the "Peer Review Organization," or PRO. The envisaged function of the PRO is to "review the need for and quality of . . . medical and other health services" provided under Titles V, XVIII, and XIX of the Social Security Act. In each state, and where applicable at a lower political level, the state or local medical society, in agreement with the Secretary of Health, Education and Welfare, is to establish a "PRO Commission" to administer the unspecified program. Advisory panels composed of representatives of the professions, carriers, and the public are provided for. The plan for the PRO does not specify its functions along any of the dimensions we have considered under Target Utilization and appears, in fact, to be designed to invest state and local medical societies with an additional level of legal legitimacy. To the extent that medical societies have not been active in encouraging resource-saving care processes, organizational innovation, or system-wide integration of care at the local level, but rather have been, by and large, actively opposed to such developments, the Bill appears to assure that the current system of resource-wasting inefficiency will be maintained. The Payment Mechanism assures this.

There are two basic payment mechanisms in the Bill: tax credit and the "insurance premium certificate." The tax credit mechanism permits individuals fil-

Table 3. Schedule of allowable tax credits

Adjusted gross income	Individuals filing Federal income tax return	
	Single, no dependents; married, filing separate returns (percent)	Unmarried with dependents; joint returns (percent)
Not over $2,500	100	100
Over $2,500, not over $5,000	75	100
Over $5,000, not over $7,500	50	75
Over $7,500, not over $10,000	25	50
Over $10,000	25	25

ing a Federal income tax return to reduce their tax liability by a *percentage* of the *allowable* premiums they have paid to private carriers, and under Part B of Title XVIII, according to their income. The schedule as set forth in the Bill is shown in Table 3.

This appears to be rather progressive up to about $10,000 for a family. But there is no allowance for the number of wage earners in the family generating the income nor for the number of individuals within the family.

It can be argued that family size is already taken into account by the deduction for dependents. While that is correct, the specification of *maximum allowable* premiums paid during the year eliminates that degree of progressivity (Table 4). That is, a head of household filing a joint return specifying the adjusted gross income for the family for the year to have been $8,000 may deduct a maximum of $300 ($400 x .75) from his tax liability,

Table 4. Schedule of maximum allowable premiums

	Type of tax return		
	Single, no dependents	Married, separate returns	Unmarried with dependents; joint returns
Maximum allowable premium per year	$150	$200	$400

Table 5. Combined income effect of cash value of employer contribution and of tax credit

Adjusted gross income	Federal income tax (Schedule II, 1969)	"Tax credit"	Net after tax income	Net income after tax and premium
$7,200	$1,228	0	$5,972	$5,972
$7,500	$1,285	$225	$6,440	$6,140
				Net gain $ 168

if he paid at least $400 for insurance premiums during the year. This is regardless of how many dependents he has. Note that the deduction is based only on his own contributions and not on contributions by employers, which is subject to a different schedule. This raises several interesting problems. Generally individuals whose major or sole source of taxable income is wages and salaries have their taxes deducted during the earning period. The tax credit then becomes postpayment: it will be refunded and hence unavailable for consumption purposes during the period earned. At low levels of income this is a serious consideration. Further, employer "contribution" to premiums, from the point of view of economic analysis, is a form of income: a "fringe benefit" very much within the total earnings package which is the subject of negotiations within the framework of collective bargaining. But such income is not included in adjusted gross income.

The value to the employee of employer contribution would *decrease* with increasing income. Suppose an employer contributes $300 per year and one family's adjusted gross income is $7,200. Consider that, alternatively, the employee is to receive as cash income the $300 previously contributed by the employer (Table 5). The employee would stand to realize a *net gain* of $168 in cash or in tax refunds (deferred cash) and still have the same insurance. The cost of such a net gain to the individual would be a loss of $168 in Federal tax revenues, for a net social gain, on the assumption of no increases in tax rates, of 0. There could be few strong arguments then for maintaining one of the most

important organizational bases for providing care to the low-income population. It is unlikely that corporations would welcome this aspect of the Fannin Bill. The pattern of gains would diminish along the income distribution, reaching a net cash gain of $9 at adjusted gross income of $10,000. This aspect does not appear to have been considered in previous estimates of the cost of "tax credit" payment mechanisms even though it leads to some interesting possibilities.

Unions whose membership has gross income up to about $10,000 before dependent and other allowances would have an incentive to bargain for new arrangements: if employer contribution to health insurance premiums is $225 or more, the employee would be better off to receive the cash value of that contribution as income. The union could become the collection agency for premiums now deducted from the employee's pay check as his payment for the allowable insurance premium. The union, therefore, and not the employer could become the major consumer representative and bargaining agent *vis à vis* the carriers —a bargaining agent carrying the punch of cash. Further, as in our previous example, the employee could increase the amount he pays for premiums to the maximum allowable of $400 and still realize a net after tax, after premium payment, cash or tax refund benefit of $143. One need not push too far to argue that the union then could attempt to convince the membership to pay $400 a year in premiums at the gross income level of $10,000, and still have a net cash gain of at least $143. It is interesting to note that the cost of providing *complete* medical care per family, excluding dental but including total physician services in the home, office and hospital, 111 days per year per condition in the hospital, total laboratory and X-ray services as well as all prescription drugs, optometric and ambulance services, mental health clinic services, etc., has been estimated to cost $492 per year.[32] This is not to argue that the $492 figure is generally tenable. It is to suggest, however, that if employer payments can be converted to cash income, that—in combination with the Federal subsidy, which tax credit is—might be just the sufficient financial incentive and financial enabling factor to move unions and consumer groups, such as cooperatives, into the development of prepaid plans; or at the very least, into becoming the financially potent bargaining agents on behalf of their members with the carriers. In either case, this aspect of the Fannin Bill, unlikely to have been intended by its sponsors, should not be overlooked by those interested in attaining what the sponsors of the Bill were anxious to prevent: organizational change.

In the case of nonincorporated employers the situation is complicated by the potential for conflicting interests built into the Bill. Employers who are also taxpayers and file a Federal income tax return, such as solo physicians, may deduct 60 percent of their "contributions" toward their employees' premiums from their own tax liability. Consider that in the previous example the employer is a nonincorporated businessman, or professional. We have seen that the employee would prefer to receive the $300 "contribution" as cash income since he would stand to have a net gain of $168 and still have the same insurance. But the employer could now reduce his own tax liability by $180 ($300 x .6) ; hence the net cost of his "contribution" of $300 would be only $120. The employer, presumably, would prefer this arrangement. But note also that the gains to be realized are asymmetrical, always an indicator of economic inefficiency. The employer would tend to gain $180, the employee $168. If we value gains to each at

face value, the maintenance of the system of employer "contributions" entails a net loss of $12 per case ; in the case of only one million workers, a net economic loss of $12-million.

The conflict of interest and the inefficiency is somewhat more obvious if we consider an adjusted gross income of $10,000. Assuming the same $300 contribution, we have seen that the employee would stand to gain a net cash benefit of $9. But in this case the employer's gain of $180 is clearly much larger. We are in the weird and wonderful world of subsidies and taxes: it would be to the employer's benefit to maintain the "contribution" pattern and presumably he would be inclined to increase the cash income of his employee by anything up to $180 per year to maintain it. At the marginal tax rate of 22 percent, the employee would then gain about $140 in net after tax income. From the social cost point of view, not considering any other effects, this would be clearly desirable: the employee would gain $140, the employer at least $1 and tax revenue loss would be minimized at $140 (the $180 tax credit of the employer less the $40 increase in the employee's income tax). Among other things, *this is a demonstration that any arrangement of taxes and subsidies is an income redistribution scheme;* and further, that the impact and magnitude of the redistribution depends on institutional arrangements.

As if these arrangements were not yet complicated enough, the Fannin Bill also establishes the "Insurance Premium Certificate" for those whose income tax liability in a given tax year is less than $150 for single individuals without dependents, and less than $400 for heads of household. Such individuals may apply for the specified "Insurance Premium Certificate" which can be used solely for the purchase of qualified insurance coverage. This proviso, with the maintenance of Title XIX and other state welfare programs, would assure that the present multiclass system of service would be maintained.

It can be seen, then, under Direct Effects

of the Payment Mechanism, that the Administrative Costs of the plan would be high. To the current administrative costs of carriers and public agencies would be added another layer: the Federal bureaucracy to handle the "premium certificates" ("Federal Supplementary Medical Insurance Fund"); and yet another, under Title II, the "National Catastrophic Illness Insurance Fund" to handle reinsurance under that Title, which we shall discuss below. In addition would be the administrative costs of the PRO. The budgetary effects on the state and local level would be negligible, if anything, the complete cost being borne at the Federal level. As we have seen, the nature, magnitude, and impact of income distributional effects are unpredictable: they would depend on induced institutional changes, as would Federal budgetary costs. There would be no changes in existing methods of provider payments by carriers, hence all the present inefficiencies would be perpetuated. Neither would there be any regional reallocations, while the effects on current health care programs would be negligible.

The Incentive effects of the plan will be to reinforce the currently operating incentives for inefficiency, fragmentation, duplication, inappropriate patterns of care, high administrative and overhead costs, regional misallocation, and backdoor care for the poor. If the institutional changes in the form we have suggested above take place, changes in Organizational Modality would be encouraged by the plan.

The extent to which Title II of the Bill, entitled the "National Catastrophic Illness Protection Act of 1970" should be seriously discussed is debatable. It is introduced with the statement that:

It is therefore the policy of Congress and the purpose of this title to establish a national catastrophic illness insurance program under which the Federal Government, with the cooperation of the States and their insurance authorities and with the active participation of the private insurance industry, will encour-

age the issuance of private insurance policies which offer *adequate* health insurance protection on such terms and conditions as will guarantee that such protection is available to *all* Americans . . . (p. 13, emphasis added.)

The Target Benefit Coverage of Title II is exceptional: all services are covered, nothing is excluded. All services and products which are considered appropriate for purposes of computing the medical expenses deduction under I.R.S. regulations are included. The Target Population Coverage also appears to be exceptionally broad, if not universal: "Each statewide plan . . . shall be designed to make extended health insurance more readily available to all individuals in the State. . . ." (p. 16) The Payment Mechanism establishes the legitimacy of insurance pools for the purposes of offering high risk insurance as well as a Federally financed reinsurance scheme under a "National Catastrophic Illness Fund." Premium rates are to be established by state insurance authorities between the limits of actuarial estimates of what it would actually cost to make such insurance available on an actuarial basis on one hand, and what prospective beneficiaries would be willing to pay for it on the other. The mechanism is eminently fair, clear, and a reasonable extension of private procedures. Section 215 of the Bill establishes the deductibles.[45]

The deductible provisions of the Payment Mechanism modify somewhat "adequate" provision of catastrophic illness protection to "all" Americans: only *individuals* and *families* with *before tax* incomes of up to $2,000 per year are protected; and only individuals and families with incomes of $1,000 per year or less get complete coverage. A family with a $10,000 adjusted gross income before taxes and before medical deductions, and carrying coverage available under the subsidized plans, incurring uninsured costs of $6,000 would have a reduced taxable income of $4,000. This family would receive no benefits whatsoever. A family with the same costs and insurance but with an income before taxes and before medical deductions of $5,000 would now have a deductible of $3,500 and a benefit of $2,500. Note that a family in this situation with four dependents would have had an income not subject to tax of $2,400. Assuming no other exemptions or deductions, the family would have had a gross before tax income of $7,400. If it had paid its medical expenses incurred, it would have had $1,400 left over. With the benefit, paid *after* the tax year, it would have an income of $3,900.

Not only is this far less than "adequate" protection, this Bill accepts illness as the great social equalizer: 100 percent of all incomes, after exemptions and before deductions, in excess of $2,000 is to be used as the deductible. A family with $20,000 in gross income after exemptions and before deductions would have to incur uninsured medical expenses of *at least* $18,501 before it became eligible—then it would get a "benefit" of $1 as "adequate" coverage. If national health insurance is a form of socialism, this Bill surely supports leveling with a vengeance: let illness make paupers of us all. We have, of course, not taken into account the fact that this "insurance" would be sold at a premium, further reducing its net "benefits."

The catastrophic illness provisions of the Fannin Bill, then, offer protection to those who are already, by and large, covered under Title XIX. Those who are not covered under Title XIX, and depend for protection on the provisions of this Bill, will soon be.

Conclusion

We have argued that the "economic effects" of a national health insurance plan may be complex, pervasive, unintended, and in any case much more than its costs. Depending on its objectives, design, and mechanisms, a plan may alter the existing allocation and distribution of health care resources or it may rigidify them. It can bring about greater accessibility of better quality of care for all at a lower cost or it can solidify the existing system. Whatever estimates of costs are made, we must always ask: What are the benefits? The question of "What are you willing to pay?" is empty. We must ask: "What are you willing to pay for what, and what is it you want?"

> "Would you tell me please, which way I ought to go from here?"
> "That depends a good deal on where you want to get to," said the Cat.
> "I don't much care where—" said Alice.
> "Then it doesn't matter which way you go," said the Cat.
>
> LEWIS CARROLL

References and Notes

1 Anonymous. "It's Time to Operate," *Fortune* 81: 79 (January 1970).

2 Faltermayer, E. K. "Better Care At Less Cost Without Miracles," *Fortune* 81:80 (January 1970).

3 The economic implications of national health insurance have been discussed in some detail at least since 1936. See: Falk, I. S. *Security Against Sickness: A Study of Health Insurance* (New York: Doubleday and Doran, 1936). A more recent and more ideological discussion will be found in Campbell, R. R., and Campbell, W. G. "Compulsory Health Insurance: The Economic Issues," *The Quarterly Journal of Economics* 66: 1-24 (February 1952).

4 Since the time this paper was written in the summer of 1970 a number of new proposals have been introduced, especially the Kennedy Bill, S. 3, and the Fulton Bill, H.R. 4960, both 92d Congress,

1st Session. Although not done here, both are amenable to analysis by the framework outlined. The Fulton Bill is similar in principle and approach to the Fannin Bill, studied in detail.

5 Roemer, Milton I. *The Organisation of Medical Care Under Social Security*, (Geneva: International Labour Office, 1969) pp. 27-30.

6 Glaser, William A. *Paying the Doctor: Systems of Remuneration and Their Effects* (Baltimore 1970) pp. 6-24.

7 Arrow, K. J. "The Organization of Economic Activity: Issues Pertinent to the Choice of Market Versus Nonmarket Allocation." In Haveman, R. H. and Margolis, J. (eds.) *Public Expenditures and Policy Analysis* (1970) pp. 59-73.

8 Zeckhauser, R. "Uncertainty and the Need for Collective Action." In Haveman, R. H. and Margolis, J. (eds.) *Public Expenditures and Policy Analysis* (1970) pp. 96-116.

9 Akerlof, George A. "The Market for 'Lemons': Qualitative Uncertainty and the Market Mechanism," *The Quarterly Journal of Economics* 84:488-500 (August 1970).

10 Steiner, P. O. "The Public Sector and the Public Interest." In Haveman, R. H. and Margolis, J. (eds.) *Public Expenditures and Policy Analysis* (1970) pp. 21-58.

11 Grosse, R. N. "Problems of Resource Allocation in Health." In Haveman, R. H. and Margolis, J. (eds.) *Public Expenditures and Policy Analysis* (1970) pp. 518-548.

12 Waldman, S. "Tax Credits for Private Health Insurance: Estimates of Eligibility and Cost under Alternative Proposals." U.S. Department of Health, Education and Welfare, Social Security Administration, Office of Research and Statistics, Staff Paper No. 3 (October 1969).

13 Baird, C. W. "A Proposal for Financing the Purchase of Health Services," *The Journal of Human Resources* 5:89-105 (Winter 1970).

14 Falk, I. S. "The Economic Issues of Compulsory Health Insurance: Comment," *The Quarterly Journal of Economics* 66:572-591 (November 1952).

15 Campbell, R. R., and Campbell, W. G. "The Economic Issues of Compulsory Health Insurance: Reply," *The Quarterly Journal of Economics* 67:125-135 (February 1953).

16 Kemp, A. "Health Services and Political Economy," *Modern Age* 7:255-268 (Summer 1963).

17 Klarman, H. E.; Rice, D. P.; Cooper, B. S.; and Stettler, H. Louis III. "Sources of Increase in Selected Medical Care Expenditures, 1929-1969." U.S. Department of Health, Education and Welfare, Office of Research and Statistics, Staff Paper No. 4 (April 1970).

18 Coe, R. M.; Friedmann, E. A.; Peterson, W. A.; Sigler, J.; Saunders, H.; Marshall, D.; and Brehm, H. P. "The Impact of Medicare on the Utilization and Provision of Health Care Facilities: A Sociological Interpretation," *Inquiry* 4: 42-47 (December 1967).

19 For a summary see: Waldman, Saul and Peel, Evelyn. "National Health Insurance: A Comparison of Five Proposals." Division of Health Insurance Studies, *Research and Statistics Note No. 12*, Social Security Administration (Washington, D.C.; GPO, 1970).

20 Weisbrod, B. A. "Collective Action and the Distribution of Income: A Conceptual Approach." In Haveman, R. H. and Margolis, J. (eds.) *Public Expenditures and Policy Analysis* (1970) pp. 117-141.

21 Leveson, I. "Medical Care Cost Incentives: Some Questions and Approaches for Research," *Inquiry* 5:3-13 (December 1968).

22 Hill, L. A. "Financial Incentives—How They Could Reshape the Health Care System," *Hospitals* 43:58-62 (June 16, 1969).

23 Fuchs, V. R. "Let's Make Volkswagen Medicine Compulsory," *Medical Economics* 110-128 (November 10, 1969).

24 McGee, R. R. "Cadillac Medicine or Volkswagen Medicine?" *Medical Economics* 106-110 (November 10, 1969).

25 Feldstein, P. J. and Waldman, S. "Financial Position of Hospitals in the Early Medicare Period," *Social Security Bulletin* 18-23 (October 1968).

26 Feldstein, P. J. and Waldman, S. "The Financial Position of Hospitals in the First Two Years of Medicare," *Inquiry*, 6:19-27 (March 1969).

27 Donabedian, A. and Thorby, J. A. "The Systematic Impact of Medicare," *Medical Care Review* 26: 567-585 (June 1969).

28 Payne, Beverly C. "Medicare in Michigan." Reprinted from *Michigan Medicine*, 69:15-21 (January 1970).

29 West, Howard. "Group Practice Plans In Governmental Medical Care Programs: I. Group Practice Prepayment Plans in the Medicare Program," *American Journal of Public Health* 59:624-629 (April 1969).

30 Newman, Harold F. "Group Practice Plans In Governmental Medical Care Programs: II. The Impact of Medicare on Group Practice Prepayment Plans," *American Journal of Public Health* 59:629-634 (April 1969). .

31 Shapiro, Sam. "Group Practice Plans In Governmental Medical Care Programs: III. Serving Medicaid Eligibles," *American Journal of Public Health* 59:635-641 (April 1969).

32 Colombo, Theodore J.; Saward, Ernest W.; and Greenlick, Merwyn R. "Group Practice Plans In Governmental Medical Care Programs: IV. The Integration of an Old OEO Health Program Into a Prepaid Comprehensive Group Practice Plan," *American Journal of Public Health* 59:641-650 (April 1969).

33 Feldstein, P. J. "A Proposal for Capitation Reimbursement to Medical Groups for Total Medical Care." In *Reimbursement Incentives for Hospital and Medical Care*, U.S. Department of Health, Education and Welfare, Social Security Administration Research Report # 26 (1968) pp. 61-72.

34 Sigmond, R. M., "Capitation as a Method of Reimbursement to Hospitals in a Multihospital Area." In *Reimbursement Incentives for Hospital and Medical Care*. U.S. Department of Health, Education and Welfare, Social Security Administration, Research Report #26 (1968) pp. 49-60.

35 Ro, K., and Auster, R. "An Output Approach to Incentive Reimbursement for Hospitals," *Health Services Research* 177-187 (Fall 1969).

36 National Advisory Commission on Health Manpower. *Report, Vol. 1,* (Washington, D.C.; GPO, 1967) p. 147 ff.

37 Waldman, S. "Average Increase in Costs—An Incentive Reimbursement Formula For Hospitals." In *Reimbursement Incentives for Hospital and Medical Care*. U.S. Department of Health, Education and Welfare, Social Security Administration, Research Report #26 (1968) pp. 39-48.

38 Cross, J. G. "Incentive Pricing and Utility Regulation," *The Quarterly Journal of Economics* 84: 236-256 (May 1970).

39 Babnew, D., Jr. "Can the Profit-Motivated Center Stop the Medical Cost Spiral," *Hospital Management* 108:40-41 (August 1969).

40 Arrow, K. J. "Uncertainty and the Welfare Economics of Medical Care," *American Economic Review* 941-973 (December 1963).

41 Pauly, M. K. "The Economics of Moral Hazard: Comment," *American Economic Review* 531-537 (June 1968).

42 Arrow, K. J. "The Economics of Moral Hazard: Further Comment," *American Economic Review* 537-538 (June 1968).

43 Newhouse, Joseph P., and Taylor, Vincent. "The Economics of Moral Hazard: Further Comment," *Rand Reports* P-4080-1 (August 1969).

44 Bellin, S. S.; Geiger, H. J.; and Gibson, C. D. "Impact of Ambulatory-Health-Care Services on the Demand for Hospital Beds," *New England Journal of Medicine* 808-812 (April 10, 1969).

45 The first four paragraphs (pages 21-22) of Section 215 of the Fannin Bill are:

SEC. 215. (a) The total amount payable to or with respect to any eligible individual on account of costs of medical care paid or incurred in any year under an extended health insurance policy issued by an insurer or pool under a State plan approved under section 212 may be reduced by a deductible equal to so much of such costs, actually paid or incurred by such individual, as does not exceed the amount determined under subsection (b).

(b) The deductible for any individual or family for purpose of subsection (a), with respect to costs of medical care paid or incurred in any year, shall be—

(1) 50 per centum of the amount by which the adjusted income of such individual or family for such year exceeds $1,000 but does not exceed $2,000, plus

(2) 100 per centum of the amount by which the adjusted income of such individual or family for such year exceeds $2,000.

No deductible may be imposed in the case of an individual or family whose adjusted income does not exceed $1,000.

(c) Notwithstanding any other provision of law, the deductible applicable with respect to any individual or family for any year under this section shall be reduced by the amount of any payments made toward the costs of medical care of such individual or the members of such family under title XVIII or XIX of the Social Security Act or under any other public or private health insurance policy covering such medical care.

(d) As used in this section with respect to any individual or family for any year, the term "adjusted income" means the gross income of such individual or family for purposes of chapter 1 of the Internal Revenue Code of 1954, reduced by the aggregate amount of the personal exemptions allowed such individual or the members of such family for such year under section 151 of such Code.

Joseph P. Newhouse

A Design for a Health Insurance Experiment

Reprinted with permission of the Blue Cross Association, from *Inquiry:* Vol.XI, No.1, pp.5-27. Copyright © 1974 by the Blue Cross Association.

Originally Published in March 1974

This paper discusses the design of the experimental portion of the Health Insurance Study. The broad aim of the study is to improve the formulation of public policy in health care financing. To do this, several research objectives are being pursued, including measuring the effect of various financing provisions on the demand for medical services, establishing the effect of financing provisions on health status, and exploring administrative procedures concerning health insurance. We believe that this information will be useful to public decision-makers in considering legislation pertaining to health financing. The information should also be useful to those making decisions on financing health care in the private sector. Our methods are to analyze existing data and conduct an experiment to generate improved data. This

Joseph P. Newhouse, Ph.D. is Senior Staff Economist and Deputy Program Manager for Health and Biosciences, the Rand Corporation (1700 Main Street, Santa Monica, California 90406).

The research reported here was performed pursuant to a grant from the Office of Economic Opportunity to the Rand Corporation. The opinions and conclusions expressed here are solely those of the author and should not be construed as representing the opinions or policy of any agency of the United States Government, or of the Rand Corporation. The Health Insurance Study is now under the administrative auspices of the Department of Health, Education and Welfare, Office of the Assistant Secretary for Planning and Evaluation. Mathematica, Inc., Princeton, New Jersey, has contracted with Rand to perform field operations, administer claims, and assist with design and analysis.

While the author is indebted to well over 100 persons for their help in bringing the Health Insurance Study to the point of realization, he would especially like to acknowledge the contributions of Larry L. Orr. The original impetus to conduct an experiment was his, and he has provided many of the ideas used in the design.

paper considers the experimental portion of the work; the non-experimental portion has been discussed elsewhere.[1-11]

In the following section the objectives of the experiment are considered in detail and placed in the context of existing knowledge about health care financing. Alternative means of attaining those objectives are also considered. The next section summarizes our methods of procedure. We conclude with brief remarks about the significance of the work. Table 5 at the end of the paper summarizes the dimensions of the experiment.

Objectives

Effect of Price on Demand for Medical Services

A primary objective of the experiment is to measure how the demand for medical services varies with the price the consumer pays for medical services. We focus on price as a key variable for three reasons:

1 Since insurance operates to change the price, and since public policy can legislate the terms of insurance, public policy can exert considerable influence over price. Indeed, the ability of government to influence the terms of insurance is probably its most powerful available instrument for affecting the demand for medical services.

2 A well-established economic theory exists concerning the effect of price.[12] This theory gives us some confidence in our ability to understand the phenomena we are measuring.

3 Price may be a common denominator for measuring the effect of many variations in the details of insurance policies. For example, deductibles may be per person or per family, per quarter or per year.[13] To attempt to ascertain the effect of variation in detailed clauses of this kind —by observing actual variation with all else held constant—would require vast resources. One may be able, however, to approximate a particular variation as a variation in price; knowing something about the effect of a variation in price, one may then be able to estimate the effect of the particular provision.

We therefore assign participants randomly to insurance plans that systematically vary the price they face.

Measurement of the effect of price on demand can be refined in several ways. For example, we may wish to know whether the effect of price varies with income and total expenditure. Do poor families respond more readily to price than affluent ones? If so, they will benefit differentially from a generous health insurance plan. Do families with major illnesses respond differently from those with minor illnesses? If so, estimates of the effect of catastrophic health insurance must be based on data from only those with such illnesses.

The effect of price cannot be measured straightforwardly if the price changes with total expenditure. This would be the case if, as has been proposed,[14] the federal government were to provide a health insurance plan that paid the entire bill after the family had spent a certain amount in a given year. The problem this poses for analysis may be grasped intuitively by noting that if a person expected to spend less than the amount at which the plan takes over, he would act differently from the case where he expected to spend more than that amount. The "price" he faces is therefore not obvious. We will return to this problem in greater detail later.

The effect of the price of particular medical services on the demand for other medical services should also be examined.

For example, it is often alleged that the present, relatively generous coverage of inpatient services shifts utilization from the office to the hospital. We have therefore covered all services uniformly, hoping by comparison with a control group (many of whom will have the present kind of coverage) to determine the effect of the relatively scanty coverage of ambulatory services on the use of hospital services.

Another consequence of the relatively scanty coverage of ambulatory services, it is often alleged, is a neglect of preventive medicine, leading to increased utilization later. To provide maximum incentive for the use of preventive services, we have included a set of plans in which all outpatient care is free but inpatient care is subject to coinsurance. This will permit inferences about the effect of financial incentives in inducing the consumption of preventive services.[15]

We will also seek to measure the effect of price on demand for services other than typical hospital and physician services. It is generally agreed that hospital and most physician services should be included as part of a health insurance plan, but there is less general agreement on the inclusion of prescription drugs and vision and hearing, chiropractic, dental, and psychiatric and psychological services. Because little is known at present regarding the effect on demand of covering such services, most of them have been included in the scope of coverage.

Effect on Demand of Changes in Coverage

While a major objective of the experiment is to improve estimates of the responsiveness of demand to price, we are ultimately interested in the demand for medical services under any particular insurance plan. This will be determined not only by the responsiveness of demand, but also by the change in the amount of coverage that any particular plan will bring about. To compute this change, one must know the current coverage of the population; unfortunately, detailed information on this subject is rare. National Health Survey estimates can be used to determine the percentage of the population with no coverage, but they are not helpful if one wants to determine the improvement that would be caused by any particular plan—say, a full-coverage plan—among persons who now have partial coverage (as most do). The experiment will augment and update the existing scarce data on this subject (primarily the 1970 survey of the Center for Health Administration Studies).

The change in coverage that any legislation causes will also be partly determined by the degree to which consumers will purchase additional insurance to supplement a government policy, if the government plan stops short of full coverage (as, for example, it did with Medicare). Supplementation is an especially important issue in plans with large deductibles, which could leave the consumer bearing considerable risk. We will offer the participant the chance to supplement his experimental insurance in the final year of the experiment, and so will be able to generate evidence on the degree to which consumers would purchase additional insurance if a national health insurance plan were passed that did not provide full coverage.

How much additional insurance the consumer decides to purchase, if any, may well be a function of the tax treatment of insurance. Currently, the tax system provides a considerable subsidy to the purchase of insurance, since employer paid premiums are not taxable income, and individually paid premiums are 50 percent deductible (up to $150). This subsidy exists to stimulate the purchase of private insurance; but if a national plan were available, the rationale for the subsidy could disappear. As a result, some have proposed changing the tax treatment of insurance.[16] By altering the terms at which supplementary insurance is offered, we can determine the effect of various tax treatments of insurance premiums.

Effect of Insurance on Health Status

Estimating the response of demand to insurance is necessary (although not nec-

essarily sufficient) for estimating the *costs* of alternative financing legislation, or the resources that the nation would devote to health care. To determine the *benefits* of alternative legislation, one would like to know something about the effect of a change in utilization on the health status of individuals. This issue is often described as "necessary" versus "unnecessary" care; and the problem is to define how much additional health care of each kind is induced by more generous insurance. Improving the state of knowledge regarding this issue is a principal objective of the experiment, but will not be discussed further in this paper, since it is considered in a following paper by Arnold I. Kisch and Paul R. Torrens.

Administrative Aspects of Health Insurance

Another objective of the experiment is to contribute information on the administrative feasibility of various aspects of national health insurance. Obviously, the scale of the experiment will not permit replication of how a large organization, private or public, might administer a national plan, but it will permit some testing of various technical details. For example, the accounting period and the accounting unit must be determined for those plans that use deductibles or coinsurance which is eliminated after a certain amount of expenditure.[17] Although we shall use a uniform set of definitions, we hope that the data we collect can be used to simulate the consequences of alternative definitions. We also expect to contribute information on details of claims processing. If, for example, a large deductible applies to the family, what claims volume might be expected? What information can be obtained from claims forms that will permit ongoing evaluation of the insurance plan? While some information of this kind now exists among fiscal intermediaries, it is generally relevant to other types of plans than those we are considering in the experiment.

HMOs and Quality of Care

We wish to address certain issues related to health maintenance organizations (HMOs). In recent years HMOs have been advocated as an important reform for the delivery system. While HMOs encompass a wide variety of arrangements, a distinguishing feature is the prepayment of the physician or group of physicians for his (their) services. Thus, the method of reimbursement of the physician differs from the fee-for-service system. There is a growing volume of evidence that this change in the method of paying the physician considerably reduces the amount of utilization.[18] However, there is very little evidence on the effect of such a reduction on health status. We therefore plan to assign certain of our enrollees to such organizations in order to measure the effects of HMOs on both utilization and health status.

We also wish to address certain issues related to the quality of medical care. The principal instrument currently envisioned for improving the quality of care is some kind of peer review. There are those who doubt that peer review can be effective. By choosing sites where the extent of peer review varies, we hope to generate some evidence on relative effects. Note also that the experiment should provide data from before and after implementation of Professional Standards Review Organizations.

Interest in the quality of care is related to the debate over HMOs. It is feared that if physicians are given a fixed amount of money to care for their patients, they will be motivated to stint on services, thereby jeopardizing the quality of care. Considerable emphasis is therefore being placed on the development of measures of quality. Since one of the objectives of the experiment is to assess the effect of prepayment, it will be necessary to address the issue of quality-of-care measurement within the experiment. It is hoped that this effort will contribute to the growing amount of methodological work on the issue.

Effects in Different Communities of Varying Physician Workloads

A final objective relates to measuring the effects of the varying workloads of physicians in different communities. The type of services delivered by physicians when they are busy may differ from the type delivered when they are not. For example, waiting time for an appointment, waiting time at the office, time spent per patient, revisit rate, and profile of medical problems seen may all change as the physician becomes more or less busy.[19] This in turn may affect who gets what kind of medical services for what kinds of medical problems. A number of financing proposals would increase the demand for ambulatory physician services significantly, so that understanding the effect of a physician's being more or less busy is an important issue in the debate over financing; it is also important in formulating health manpower policy.

The experiment can contribute to understanding these issues, since physicians are considerably busier in some part of the United States than in others. For example, the best endowed of the four Census regions has around half again as many physicians per person as the least endowed. Yet the best endowed region has only 10 to 20 percent more physician visits.[20] This suggests that physicians in areas of the country where there are few physicians per person are likely to be 30 percent or more busier than their colleagues in well-endowed areas. By selecting sites with varying degrees of physician workload, the effects of physician workload will be measurable.

Research Strategy of Non-experimental Data

Advantages and Disadvantages

The use of existing, non-experimental data has certain advantages over conducting an experiment. A question can therefore be raised as to whether an experiment is a sensible research strategy.

The principal advantages of existing non-experimental data are that the analysis is faster and that it is cheaper than with experimental data. Both are significant. If it could promise the same kind of results, the analysis of existing data would be preferred. In addition, both existing and prospective non-experimental data avoid two difficulties found with experimental data, the Hawthorne Effect and the transitory problem. According to the Hawthorne Effect, individuals behave differently when they are being observed (in an experiment) from when they are not being observed. The transitory problem is analogous to the Hawthorne Effect; individual behavior in an experiment of limited duration differs from behavior in a national program that the participant expects to last indefinitely. However, as discussed in the next section, these two problems have solutions; so the important issues are speed and cost relative to the quality of results.

To achieve the objectives we have described, both experimental and non-experimental research should be pursued. But existing non-experimental data—from surveys and claim files—simply cannot provide answers to many of the questions posed. Where the data can provide some answers, the precision is likely to be low, because non-experimental data have a variety of weaknesses:

1 They generally provide little or no information on the health status of individuals. As a result, it becomes impossible to measure the consequences of more or less utilization. It is reasonable to believe that more rapid progress will be possible on this issue with a project of the scope described here.

2 Survey data rely on the ability of individuals to recall details of their utilization from memory. There are obvious possibilities for error here, the more so if utilization farther in the past must be recalled.[21] (The National Health survey estimates physician visit rates using data from the past two weeks because of the magnitude of recall error.)

Administrators of survey data either rely upon the respondent for details of his insurance policy or attempt to obtain the policy from an independent source. Such data are essential if the effect of changing the terms of the policy is to be measured. Yet so few respondents know the details of their policy that the National Health Survey has stopped asking such questions. Only two national probability sample surveys are known to us which have tried to obtain the policy from an independent source: the 1963 and 1970 surveys of the Center for Health Administration Studies. Two surveys represent relatively little data.

Existing data are by definition limited to the range of insurance policies currently in effect. Such policies seldom have deductibles greater than $100 per person and coinsurance rates greater than 25 percent. The effect on demand of a plan containing a large income-related deductible or coinsurance rate is therefore very hard to assess. Also, as has been pointed out, existing policies may vary along numerous dimensions. One policy may pay up to $60 per day for a hospital room, another may pay the full cost of a semi-private room, and still another may pay 80 percent of whatever the room charge is. Attempting to measure the effects of such policies is difficult. Finally, existing policies typically do not cover some medical services, such as psychiatric services; it is therefore difficult to learn much about the consequences of such coverage.

3 Data from the claim files of existing insurance plans are, of course, restricted to existing kinds of plans and therefore have the weaknesses just described. In addition, claim files typically contain little detailed information on the patient beyond age and sex. Without data on income, such data cannot be used to answer questions relating to the effect of insurance on different economic groups. In addition, if there is a deductible or upper limit in the policy, there will be no information on services consumed below the deductible or above

the limit. Thus, total demand may not be well measured. Finally, the necessary data in many claim files are not in machine-readable form. To reduce the data to this form is an expensive and time-consuming operation, tending to defeat the advantage of non-experimental data.

4 Consumers have by and large self-selected their insurance. Since there is evidence that those in poorer health have better insurance,[22] use of existing data may overstate the responsiveness of demand if insurance were extended to the entire population. While the overstatement can be corrected with enough data and appropriate estimation techniques, the cost of obtaining accurate estimates from non-experimental data is raised.

Another alternative to an experimental strategy would be to gather new, richer data from either insurance claims or survey data. To adapt such a strategy, however, is to give up most of the speed and cost advantages of non-experimental data. In addition, certain inherent weaknesses of existing data, as noted, keep the value of this strategy relatively low. The weaknesses were quite apparent to the Social Security Administration, when it responded to a 1971 Congressional request to analyze the cost of various national health insurance plans. In providing estimates, SSA commented: "The [percentage increases in demand] were chosen after a review of past experience, but no claim is made that any of [them] are based on solid empirical foundations."[23]

Methods of Procedure

Plan of Analysis of Demand for Services

We plan to estimate three different models of demand for medical services. The simplest, the easiest to estimate, and the least informative is an analysis of a covariance model. Essentially, this model estimates the mean annual cost of each plan, adjusting for measurable differences in demographic characteristics among individuals

assigned to different plans. Thus, the model to be estimated is

$$(1) \quad Y_i = \sum_k \delta_k D_{ik} + \sum_j \beta_j Z_{ij} + \epsilon_i$$

where Y_i is a general response variable (such as annual expenditure on medical services of the ith person); D_{ik} is a set of dummy variables, which take the value unity if the ith person is enrolled in the kth plan and the value zero otherwise; and Z_{ij} is a vector of demographic characteristics for the ith person (such as age or income). If no Z_{ij} are included, the estimated δ_k are simply the mean level of expenditures in each plan.

Demographic variables such as age and income are probably best entered in dummy-variable interval form to allow for non-linearities. To predict the cost of any particular plan when such variables are included, one must obtain the predicted cost for each demographic group and then weight such costs by the proportion of the total population that the demographic group represents.

The model specified in Equation (1) does not allow for interactions between the demographic variables and the insurance plans. Tests will be performed for the existence of interactions of interest (such as whether the effect of a particular plan differs by income group). If such interactions prove to be significant, they will be included.

There is no doubt that such a model can be estimated and that the results will be of interest. The results of estimating Equation (1), however, are not so useful as the results of estimating two other kinds of models, for two reasons. First, no theory underlies the model specified in Equation (1) that would afford an insight into the effect of health insurance on demand. And, second, the model specified in Equation (1) estimates discrete points on a response surface. It provides no basis for interpolating between points and, as a result, cannot readily be used to predict what would happen if the underlying plans were changed.

The second model is a traditional model of demand based on economic theory. An example might be of the form:

$$(2) \quad Y_i = \alpha + \sum_j \beta_j Z_{ij} + \delta_1 P_{iI} + \delta_2 P_{i0} + \epsilon_i$$

where variables are defined as before except that Y_i is expenditure for a specific service rather than total expenditure, P_{iI} is the price facing the ith individual for inpatient services, and P_{i0} is the price for outpatient services. P_{iI} and P_{i0} are functions of the insurance plan. The estimated values of the δ_1 and δ_2 can then be used to derive own-price and cross-price elasticities of demand for that service. Again, no interactions have been specified in Equation (2), but we will test for their presence. Specification of a linear form is not meant to be restrictive; logarithmic, polynomial, and other non-linear functions of P can readily be estimated.

Y_i must be disaggregated by service to prevent bias in δ.[24] Further disaggregation of expenditure into variation in quantity (physical units) and price (or style) may also be informative.[25]

As with the first model, there is little doubt that this model can be estimated, since a similar one has been estimated using existing survey data.[26] The model specified in Equation (2) is not much more difficult to estimate than that in Equation (1), and meets the two objections to that model. Since there is a well-articulated economic theory of the effect of price on demand, some explanation of the underlying phenomena is possible. Moreover, the model is embedded in a functional form, so that interpolation to other prices is possible.

The estimated coefficients of the Z vector (β) in Equation (2) will also be of interest. The Z vector will include a dummy variable that takes the value unity for those assigned to a prepaid (or HMO-type) plan, while the P variable for such individuals takes the value zero. The estimated coefficient of the dummy variable will then show the effects of prepayment, conditional upon zero price. We do not expect to assign individuals to prepaid plans that contain fees; if there is any interaction between price and prepayment, our design will not measure it.

The Z vector will also include estimates of community demand and supply, and their interaction with price. It is hoped that such estimates will show how services are rationed as community demand increases relative to supply, and therefore will indicate what might happen if national legislation were to change either element. Obviously, our estimates will be reliable only over the range of variation in community demand and supply observed in the sample. By deliberately selecting sites with extreme values and by taking account of seasonal changes in demand, we hope to observe considerable variation; but national legislation representing particularly marked change from the status quo may well raise community demand beyond any level we will be able to observe. In this case, prediction on the basis of our data will be hazardous.

Variables measuring the individual's price of time and its effect on demand will also be included in the Z vector. National legislation that reduces the money price and thereby increases demand may well increase queuing and thereby the amount of time required for medical services; this in turn would decrease the demand for services. Demand could be expected to decrease most among persons who set high prices on their time. The sensitivity of particular groups to changes in the time price could have a considerable effect on how a given supply of services is distributed in the population.[27]

Measures of health status will also be included as part of the Z vector. Such measures have been found to be among the most important ones in explaining variation in demand in cross-sectional studies.[28-30] For the purpose of estimating Equation (2), a general measure of health stock seems appropriate. This could be subjective ("Would you rate your health as excellent, good, fair, or poor?"), as well as objective (derived from physical examination of the individual). Inclusion of such variables will make the measurement of price effects more precise.

While the model specified in Equation (2) represents an improvement over that in Equation (1), two broad difficulties remain concerning the definition of price. The first arises most prominently with hospital services, where the relevant price variable for using the service at all may differ from the relevant price variable for decisions on how much of the service to use. The decision on whether to use hospital services at all has an all-or-nothing character about it and should therefore be estimated with a dichotomous dependent variable (with an appropriate estimation technique such as logit or probit) and a price variable that measures the price facing the individual for his total stay in the hospital. Decisions on how much of the service to use (once having decided to use it) may be more appropriately taken to be a function of the cost of remaining an extra day in the hospital.

These two prices are not necessarily proportional, since out-of-pocket costs become zero after a certain level of expenditure. As a result, hospital expenditure variation should be disaggregated into variation along several dimensions, each of which should be analyzed separately: 1) admissions, with total price as an explanatory variable; 2) length of stay, conditional on admission, with the cost of an additional day (marginal price) as an explanatory variable; 3) room and board price per day, with the coinsurance rate for an additional day as an explanatory variable; and 4) ancillary services expenditure per day, again using the coinsurance rate as an explanatory variable.[31] A similar disaggregation into quantity and price can be carried out for many different services (e.g., physician visits, drugs). However, the disaggregation of quantity into separate decisions on use or no use, and then on quantity conditional on use, is probably not necessary for services other than hospital, since the total price and the marginal price are probably approximately proportional. In sum, this difficulty can largely be handled within the context of Equation (2).

The second difficulty is more fundamental. The theory underlying the model given in Equation (2) is essentially an application of standard economic theory.[32, 33] Unfortunately, standard theory makes an assumption known not to hold in the Health Insurance Study; that is, price per unit is assumed to be a constant. Since plans for the study limit out-of-pocket expenditures to a fraction of income (because of policy interest in this type of plan), the price falls to zero after a certain amount of expenditure and the assumption of constancy does not hold. There is little or no prior work in modeling demand in this type of situation. Heuristically, the problem occurs because the consumer may take account of the expenditure limit in deciding how many services to consume, and therefore may act as if he faces a price other than the one he pays for any particular service.

Because of this problem, we are working on the development of a third model which differs from the first two by analyzing expenditure by episode. It views the consumer as incurring an illness episode, then making a decision on whether to seek care. (Chronic illness is treated as an episode that continues throughout the accounting period.) If the consumer does seek care, he or his physician then makes a decision on how much care by taking into account the probability that the consumer will exceed the expenditure limit at some time during the accounting period —and the value of the services consumed if he does so. The probability that the consumer will exceed the expenditure limit will depend on how far he is from the limit, the length of time remaining in the accounting period, his underlying health status, the severity of his current problem, and the probability distribution of expenditures for others in his family unit. The operational implication of this model is that expenditures must be classified by episode, and the data collection system is

Table 1. Coinsurance and maximum dollar expenditure variation in experimental insurance plans

Insurance plan	Inpatient coinsurance percentage	Outpatient coinsurance percentage	Maximum dollar expenditure (percentage of income)
1	0	0	NA
2	25	25	5
3	25	25	15
4	50	50	5
5	50	50	15
6	100	100	5
7	100	100	15
8	100	100	D
9	25	0	5
10	25	0	15
11	50	0	5
12	50	0	15
13	100	0	5
14	100	0	15
15	100	0	D
16	0	0	HMO

NA = Not applicable
D = $150 per person deductible, $450 per family maximum
HMO = health maintenance organization

set up to do so. This model is described elsewhere in more detail.[34]

Dimensions of Experimentation

In order to estimate these three models, we have structured the 16 insurance plans shown in Table 1. These plans are of three basic types. The first, represented by Plans 1 through 8, consists of plans in which the fraction of the bill that the consumer must pay (or coinsurance) varies between zero in Plan 1 and 100 percent in Plans 6, 7, and 8. In Plans 2 through 7, the maximum amount that the family can spend on medical care in a year is limited to 5 or 15 percent of its income; in Plan 8, the limit is $150 per person or $450 per family. The variation in utilization and health status observed across these plans will be the primary means of inferring the general effect of price.

The second basic type of plan (Plans 9 through 15) differs from the first in that all outpatient care is free, while inpatient care is subject to coinsurance or deductibles. Comparison of individuals enrolled in these plans with those enrolled in Plans 2 through 8 will permit statements about the possibilities for and consequences of shifting the place of care from an inpatient to an outpatient basis by using insurance. In addition, comparison of individuals in Plans 9 through 15 and Plan 1 with individuals in plans with positive coinsurance rates for all services (especially Plans 6, 7, and 8) should provide evidence on whether insurance affects demand for preventive services; and if it does, whether preventive services affect health status.

The third type of plan is Plan 16, the HMO plan. Ideally, a variety of HMOs would be included in the study, ranging from well-established prepaid group practices, such as Kaiser-Permanente, to medical foundations and new HMOs. However, difficulties in finding sites with HMOs and establishing data collection systems within HMOs that provide data comparable to those of the fee-for-service system will probably force limitation to one or two HMOs. Because no site for the experiment that contains an HMO has as yet been selected, we cannot at present be more specific about our procedures in this area.

In the remainder of this section we discuss, first, our choice of particular fraction-of-income limits, deductibles, and coinsurance rates, then the role of the control group, the period of participation, and the question of supplementary insurance.

Income Limits, Deductibles, and Coinsurance

Speaking formally, our choice of fraction-of-income limits of 5 and 15 percent and coinsurance rates of 0, 25, 50, and 100 percent means that we have constrained the design so that no families can be allocated to any other design point. Some such constraint is necessary for computational reasons. Our first task, therefore, was to decide how many design points we wished to have—that is, how many points we wished not to constrain to be zero. The answer to this question depends upon the functional relationship between the experimental "treatment" (in this case, coinsurance rates and expenditure limits) and the response (in this case, demand or health status). If, for example, the relationship were linear, maximum efficiency would be achieved by allocating all of the sample to the two extremes of the range of interest. If some of the sample were to be allocated to intermediate points, efficiency would be lost. If, by contrast, the relationship were non-linear, an optimal design would include some intermediate points, the exact number depending upon the non-linearity. If the functional relationship were in fact non-linear, but the sample was allocated wholly to extreme points, the non-linearity could not be measured. In either event, however, extremes of the range one is interested in would be included. Thus, plans calling for zero coinsurance and for 100 percent coinsurance were included. There is no reliable evidence as to what the functional form actually is. Because it was felt that the zero to 25 percent range might be of greater interest than higher ranges of coinsurance, a plan with 25 percent coinsurance was also included. Finally, a plan with 50 percent coinsurance was included to give some notion about possible non-linearities in the zero to 100 percent range.

Only two fraction-of-income limits were included, to permit relatively good estimates of the effect of any given plan. To have included a larger number of limits would have greatly increased the number of plans and would have had the practical effect of making the estimation of the model specified in Equation (1) meaningless, since precision in any particular plan would become low. It was felt that the speed and ease of estimating Equation (1), together with its heuristic value, meant that an effort should be made to keep the number of plans relatively small.[35] Five percent of income was chosen as the lower limit, because it was thought unlikely that a national plan would have a substantially lower value, unless all care were free (Plan 1). Fifteen percent of income was chosen as the upper limit, because 1) there was some evidence that

few families would reach the limit (especially in plans with 25 and 50 percent coinsurance), and so the variation in price would be preserved; 2) it seemed unlikely that a national plan would have a significantly higher expenditure limit; and 3) inclusion of a higher limit would be more expensive, because of the experimental reimbursement method described in a later section. Both limits have been modified to be the lesser of the appropriate percent of income and an absolute dollar amount. The effect of this "truncation" is to eliminate price variation in high expenditure ranges. There would be few observations in these ranges and the cost of each observation would be large if the truncation were not included.[36]

Plans with a $150-per-person deductible were included because it was thought that such a deductible could possibly be included in a national plan. The effect of expenditure limits related to income is to introduce a rather large family deductible. We believe that it would be difficult to estimate the effects of a per-person deductible if it were not included explicitly. The deductible was set at $150 because it seemed unlikely that a national plan with deductibles unrelated to income would have a significantly higher figure. A $450 out-of-pocket limit on family expenditures was included to save costs (given the nature of payments to families, as described below) and because such a limit could well be part of a national plan.

Role of Control Group

The experimental design includes a control group whose purposes are five-fold. The first is to provide a basis for measuring the Hawthorne Effect, the effect of observation of the families on their utilization. The method for doing this is to vary the frequency of interviewing in the control group. If greater involvement with the families has any effect on utilization, there will be differences in behavior among families who are interviewed with varying frequency. If the null hypothesis of no difference cannot be rejected (and the power of the test is reasonable, as it should be), one can be reasonably sure that the Hawthorne Effect is not large.[37]

The second purpose of the control group is to provide a basis for measuring transitory demand in the experimental group. Transitory demand occurs when consumers "take advantage of a sale"—that is, purchase at a different rate from their rate in the steady state. (In the high-deductible plans there can be negative transitory demand.) The problem occurs with services that produce a steady stream of benefits in the future and whose consumption is affected by the money price. Treatment of a self-limiting illness, for example, would not exhibit transitory demand, since the treatment does not produce benefits beyond the period of the experiment. Similarly, if the consumer would not purchase eyeglasses at any price, there is no transitory demand. But suppose that his purchase of eyeglasses is affected by their price, and that if they are not covered by insurance he would replace eyeglasses only infrequently. Then, if he is assigned to a generous plan, his rate of purchase would be expected to increase during the period of the experiment relative to what it would otherwise have been. But because the eyeglasses will continue to produce benefits after the experiment ends, his rate of purchase may exceed what it would have been in the steady state with generous insurance. The problem of transitory demand seems important for benefits relating to vision and hearing, dentistry, psychiatry, and elective surgery.

One method for assessing the degree to which transitory demand leads to an overstatement of price elasticities is to include a control group whose members continue coverage under their existing insurance.[38] To the extent that variation exists within existing insurance for these kinds of services, one has some assistance in estimating the amount of overstatement of the elasticities. Such estimates will not be very precise, in view of the difficulties of measuring the effects of existing insurance

described above; but they should provide some information.

Third, the control group will help in measuring the effect of specific exclusions in existing policies, a type of price variation not included among the experimental "treatments" because of the need to minimize the number of treatments. The effects of two exclusions common to existing policies are of interest. Psychiatric services are frequently not covered. It is sometimes alleged that this exclusion has the effect of raising the demand for other medical services. The implication is that the additional cost from covering psychiatric services is smaller than it might seem, because fewer services would be demanded from other physicians if they were covered. This hypothesis can be tested at sites where psychiatric coverage is quite rare; then the use of medical services in the control group (who by assumption do not have psychiatric coverage) can be compared with the use in the experimental group. Rarity of psychiatric coverage at a site is necessary to guard against adverse selection in the group without psychiatric coverage. (That is, those with psychiatric problems may seek employment where there is coverage, leaving a non-representative group without coverage.)

Preventive services (physical examinations, inoculations, and so forth) are also frequently not covered. It is sometimes alleged that this exclusion prevents early discovery of pathology and leads ultimately to poorer health and higher costs. Since the experimental "treatments" cover all services of physicians, comparison with the control group can establish the effect of covering only curative services rather than both curative and preventive services.[39]

Fourth, the control group will help measure the effect of covering inpatient services but not outpatient services. The experimental "treatments" include equal coverage of both services, and favorable treatment of outpatient services. We rely on the control group to help measure favorable treatment of inpatient services, since that kind of coverage is conventional in the population.

Fifth, unlike the administrators of a national plan, we will not have detailed fee profiles on all providers and therefore may be charged higher prices than would be charged under a national plan. While efforts will be made to eliminate this possibility, it is unreasonable to expect that they can be entirely successful. Moreover, the incidence of abnormally high prices is likely to be greater in the more generous plans—implying that the estimated price elasticities are overstated. The control group can provide some evidence on the degree to which this has taken place. Since the claims filed by the control group are paid by existing intermediaries, comparisons of prices for specific procedures charged to the control group with those charged to the experimental group (controlling for generosity of insurance) will throw light on any differences in charges between our methods and those of existing intermediaries.

Period of Participation

Those persons enrolled in the experimental group will participate for either three years or five years. The purpose of varying the participation time is to acquire better evidence than the control group is expected to provide on the extent of transitory demand at the end of the experiment. By comparing the behavior in the third year of those enrolled for three years with that of those enrolled for five years, the degree to which individuals "crowded in" or postponed services in the terminal year should be apparent.

The minimum length of participation is three years because this is the least period of time which can provide what we regard as a reasonable amount of steady-state data. We anticipate transitory demand at both the beginning and the end of the experiment; based on available data,[40, 41] we estimate that this demand will occur primarily in the first and last six months. Therefore, we will have about two years

of steady-state data from the three-year group. Five years was chosen as the period of participation for the other group for two reasons. On the one hand, it was sufficiently long to provide a good baseline against which to measure transitory demand in the three-year group. On the other hand, to have chosen a longer period would have reduced the number of individuals participating (given a fixed budget), and therefore the amount of information at any point during the project.

We expect about 52 percent of the sample to be enrolled for five years and the remainder for three years. This division is statistically optimal if the first six months of data are not useful because of catch-up demand and if the last six months of data are not useful because of transitory demand.

In the final year of the experiment those enrolled in plans with coinsurance and deductibles (that is, Plans 2 through 15) will be permitted to supplement their experimental insurance at rates that simulate varying tax treatment of insurance premiums. This will provide evidence on the amount of additional insurance that families might purchase if a national plan requiring out-of-pocket payments were enacted. After two years we will have a reasonably good estimate of the actuarial value of the plans, and so will know what premium to charge for supplemental insurance. Permitting supplementation will introduce adverse selection into the data; however, this can be controlled for by using simultaneous-equation estimators. In any event, the data from the last year may not be very useful for estimation purposes because of the problem of transitory demand. The issue of measuring demand for supplementary insurance is discussed at greater length elsewhere.[42]

Statistical Experimental Design

In this section we discuss methods of selecting families and allocating them to insurance plans, problems of refusal and attrition, and the expected precision of our estimates at the end of the experiment.

These issues are also discussed in greater detail elsewhere.[43-45]

The choice of families will proceed as follows. Four sites will be chosen for the experiment. From each, a clustered random sample of roughly 6,000 families will be chosen. These families will be given a screening interview in order to define the family unit, determine eligibility, and gather information on income, education, age, sex, race, and self-perceived health status. Using this information, we will choose a subset of 2,000 families to receive a lengthy baseline interview. These families will be chosen in accordance with the Finite Selection Model developed by Morris.[46]

Given a fixed budget and an equation or a set of equations to estimate, the model chooses families that yield the optimal variation in explanatory variables in order to estimate the equation(s). The baseline interview verifies the information from the screening interview (going into considerably more detail on such variables as income and self-perceived health status), and asks questions about prior utilization and insurance. These data are important for selecting families and will also be a source of non-experimental data for analysis (analogous to the 1963 and 1970 surveys of the Center for Health Administration). From the 2,000 families given baseline interviews in each site, approximately 500 will be chosen for enrollment in the experimental plans and 300 assigned to the control group. Thus, with four sites, there will be some 2,000 experimental families and 1,200 control-group families in all.

The number of families assigned to any one plan will be determined by the Conlisk-Watts model.[47] This model determines the number assigned to any plan so as to optimally estimate an equation or set of equations. It is similar to the Finite Selection Model except that variables related to particular insurance plans, rather than demographic characteristics of families, are used in the optimization process.

The families selected for enrollment will be allocated "randomly" to plans.[48] While the Finite Selection Model can, in principle, select optimal family-plan combinations (given a model to be estimated), random allocation offers some protection against latent variables. (That is, one can be reasonably sure that any such variable will be balanced among the treatment groups.) By allocating randomly, one pays a price in efficiency of estimation (if there are no latent variables). The price paid can be kept small if random allocation is made subject to a constraint of near balance among the treatment groups.[49]

In enrolling families, we make them an offer which ensures that they will be better off financially under any circumstances. As a result, we expect any refusals to participate to be random. This may not be correct, however; in addition, refusals to participate in screening and baseline interviews may also not be random. To test this, a larger payment will be offered by way of persuasion to a sample of those who refuse (at each stage). Analysis of data from these individuals should show whether there was any significant selection bias, and if so, should provide corrections for it. Attrition differs from initial refusals; since we will have some data on these people, we do not plan to re-enroll anyone who drops out.

Expected Precision of Results

What precision might be expected from data on 2,000 experimental families, 52 percent of whom are enrolled for five years and the remainder for three years? Because of uncertainties in estimating precision, we have defined "pessimistic" and "more likely" expected standard errors. In explaining this method of estimating precision, we shall discuss our ability to predict total expenditures; and at the end of this section we shall give expected precisions for particular medical services.

Two major factors affect our definition of "pessimistic" and "more likely" estimates. The first is the coefficient of variation. In the 1963 Center for Health Administration Studies Survey, the coefficient

Table 2. Estimated coefficients of variation for total health expenditure using experimental families

Estimate	Coefficient of variation of predicted expenditure
"Pessimistic" estimate Assumes model specified in Equation (1) and population coefficient of variation equal to 1.34	0.060
"More likely" estimate Assumes price represented by four parameters and population coefficient of variation equal to 1.00	0.022

of variation across 2,376 families for total expenditure was 1.34. We have used this figure to obtain a "pessimistic" estimate. However, the experimental expenditure data may have less measurement error, the data will be site-specific, and some of the variation will be explained. All of these factors will tend to reduce the residual coefficient of variation, the appropriate figure. As a "more likely" estimate, we have chosen 1.00, recognizing that even this may be high.

The second factor concerns the model we wish to estimate. Our "pessimistic" estimate uses the model described in Equation (1). A "more likely" model would assume that price can be represented by four parameters (rather than the 16 in Equation (1)), in which case standard errors would be halved. Using these two definitions, Table 2 shows the estimated precision at the end of the experiment. With the 0.022 figure, a 95 percent confidence interval around expenditure in an "average" plan would be less than plus-or-minus 5 percent of mean expenditures in that plan.

We next attempt to give some idea of the expected effect of other factors that could affect precision. While their net effect is unknown, it is reasonable to believe that on balance they leave the above estimates approximately unchanged.

There are four reasons why these standard errors might be too low. First, some attrition may occur, so that the final sample will be less than 2,000 families. If the attrition occurs early, additional families can be enrolled; later in the experiment, control of attrition may be better and much of the data will already be included. If there is a 10 percent (net) loss of family years, standard errors would rise by 5 percent. Second, although these calculations have assumed that family years are independent, there is likely to be considerable serial correlation in health expenditures for families. If the correlation from year to year is 0.3, as might be expected,[50] standard errors would increase by 10 percent. Third, the data from the beginning of the experiment may be useless because the steady state is not achieved or because of the Hawthorne Effect. If the first year's data are useless, standard errors will rise by 15 percent. There will also be some problem at the end because of transitory effects and because families will be able to supplement. However, the three- and five-year variation should permit measurement of the transitory demand, and the use of simultaneous-equation methods when families have chosen their insurance should mean relatively little degradation. As a result, precision should fall by substantially less than it would if the data were useless (15 percent). Finally, a number of parameters other than price will be estimated, which will cause a loss of degrees of freedom; estimation of 400 nuisance parameters (which seems high) will cause standard errors to rise by 2 percent.

A number of factors also operate to reduce the standard errors below those reported. First, the standard errors as reported assume a strictly random choice of families and an equal number in each plan. Based on Monte Carlo results, use of the Finite Selection Model and the Conlisk-Watts Model should reduce standard errors by at least 25 percent. Second, we plan to use Empirical Bayes methods in the analysis, particularly for site-specific parameters. A conservative estimate is that such methods could reduce standard

Table 3. Increase factors for the standard deviation of estimates

Service	Increase factor
Hospital non-obstetric days	2.5
Physician office visits	1.2
Surgeon in-hospital expenditures	3.2
Prescription drugs	1.3

errors by 10 percent.[51] Empirical Bayes methods may be particularly useful for coping with the problem of within-family correlation of utilization. Third, the control group and the baseline interview will provide additional data, although how much is unknown. Finally, part of the general philosophy of the experimental design is sequential implementation. While this can provide no improvement per se in the estimates given above, it forms the basis for altering the design if the assumptions on which it was based prove to be inaccurate. For example, if it should appear that standard errors had been underestimated based on data from the first site, eliminating half the plans in the last three sites would reduce standard errors in Equation (1) by 24 percent.

As might be expected, the coefficients of variation for expenditure on specific services are higher than the coefficients for total expenditure. Table 3 shows the factors by which standard errors must be increased, if one is interested in expenditure on a specific service. These factors are the ratio of the coefficient of variation for the specific service to the coefficient of variation for total expenditure (1.34) in the 1963 Center for Health Administration Studies Survey. Of course, since dollar expenditure on such services is smaller than total expenditure, in most cases the absolute errors (in dollars) will be smaller than those for total expenditure.

Breadth of Benefits

The following criteria were used in making decisions about which medical services should be covered: 1) The more likely that a service would be covered under a national plan, the more likely that the experiment would cover it; 2) the less the transitory or catch-up demand for a service, the more likely that the experiment would cover it; and 3) the less the cost of the service, the more likely that the experiment would cover it.

The rationale for our decisions will be explained in detail elsewhere.[52] In general, most services are covered, since it was felt that those making decisions about coverage as part of a national plan would value information on the effect of insuring many kinds of services. The way to generate such information is to include them in the scope of coverage.

There were some exceptions, however. It was felt that drugs not prescribed by a physician would never be covered in a national plan, so such drugs are excluded. (Prescribed drugs that could be obtained without a prescription are tentatively included.) While dental services for children are treated like any other service (except orthodontia, which is excluded on the basis of all three criteria), a compromise was reached on dental services for adults. Such services may not be included in a national plan, are subject to catch-up demand and do significantly affect cost; however, it was felt that some evidence on the responsiveness to price of dental services for adults would nevertheless be useful. Therefore, some or all of the families in Plan 1 (the free-care plan) will receive dental coverage for adults (again excluding orthodontia) ; the exact number will be chosen later. In addition, some families in Plans 4 and 5, the 50 percent coinsurance plans, may receive dental coverage, although in this case their out-of pocket expenditures will not count toward the Maximum Dollar Expenditure (to preserve comparability with the other plans). Since the remainder of the sample will typically not have dental coverage, comparison of the utilization of those with experimental coverage with the utilization of the remainder of the sample will provide evidence at a relatively low cost on the responsiveness of demand for dental services to insurance.[53]

Intensive psychoanalysis was excluded by limiting the coverage of outpatient psychiatric services to 52 visits per year; this was done on the basis of all three criteria. Those who use psychiatric services intensively (even for fewer than 52 visits) can be expected to satisfy their expenditure limit, which would mean that they face zero price for all other services. As a result, it was decided not to count expenditures on psychiatric services toward the expenditure limit, although they are covered at the coinsurance rate specified in the policy.

Selection of Sites

There are two problems in site selection: determining the optimal number of sites, and then choosing the actual sites. The optimal number of sites can be determined from an extension of the Conlisk-Watts model.[54, 55] The number of sites is chosen that minimizes the sum of between-site and within-site variances, subject to a budget constraint and a cost function of the form

$$(3) \quad C_s = C_f + \sum_{i=1}^{n} c_i$$

where C_s is total cost per site, C_f is the fixed cost per site, and c_i is the expected cost of an additional observation in any site. For estimated values of between- and within-site variances in the experiment and estimated costs, the optimal number of sites appears to be about four.

Given that we wish four sites, we have elected not to choose them randomly.[56] With only four sites to be chosen, a strictly random selection could result in quite bad estimates of national parameters. In addition, purely random selection is impractical, because the cooperation of state and local officials and local providers is essential if the experiment is to succeed. Sites are therefore chosen purposively. The desirability of potential sites will be assessed by using the Finite Selection Model. Site-dependent variables will be entered, and costs per site will be made proportional to a medical-care price index

for the site. Two variables are of interest. One is the capacity utilization of the local ambulatory care system. This is being measured by a telephone survey of physicians asking about workloads, scheduling of patients, and waiting times for appointments. The other is the presence of an HMO, Experimental Medical Care Review Organization, and medical foundation. The inclusion of the latter two institutions is to test for the possible effects of peer review upon utilization outcomes.

In addition, there are certain constraints on the choice of sites. Since there is evidence of regional disparities in the utilization of health services as well as in capacity utilization, regional diversity will be sought in the sites selected. As noted, the cooperation of state and local officials (including the Governor, the Insurance Commissioner, the Mayor, and the local Community Action Program) and local providers is a precondition in the choice of any site.

The first site chosen for the experiment is Dayton, Ohio; the other sites remain to be selected, but one is to be in the West and one in the South.

Rules of Operation

One of the major advantages of conducting an experiment over analyzing non-experimental data is that one is forced to consider a great many detailed rules of operation which are generally not considered in the non-experimental analysis, but which may in fact be significant determinants of demand. While there are too many such issues for full discussion here, a few are of sufficient importance to warrant brief mention. (A fuller discussion of the reasoning behind the actual rules of operation will be contained in a report now in preparation.[57])

In any plan containing income-related clauses, the family unit whose income is pooled, and the income itself, must be defined. Our definition of the family unit is based on the notion of an economic unit; persons who share income and expenditures are treated as one unit, since this was felt to be the relevant decision-making unit for medical expenditures. Thus, we consider a self-defined head and his or her spouse to be the nucleus of a unit. In general, persons dependent upon the head or spouse and residing with them are treated as part of the same unit, their income and expenditures being pooled for purposes of the expenditure limit.

Rules must also be defined to handle changes in family units through departures or additions. Because it simplifies analysis, we will recognize departures of non-heads only at the beginning of a new accounting period. At that time, those who have left the unit will be placed in a new unit and kept in the study. A departure of a head will lead to the formation of a new unit at once. Coverage will in general not be extended to additions to units because observations for a short period of time are not as useful (the problem of transitory demand), although newborn or adopted children and new spouses of heads will be covered.[58]

Income is defined quite comprehensively to reflect the resources available to a family unit for contingencies. Measurement of a number of components of income will permit us to simulate the consequences of using alternative definitions.

In any plan that includes a deductible (or, more generally, that makes price a function of total expenditure), the accounting period for expenditures must be defined. We will use a fixed 12-month period to minimize the effect of seasonality and concentration of discretionary expenditure. The accounting period is fixed and not a moving average, because a moving average is difficult to analyze. We have rejected the notion of a carry-over of unreimbursed expenses near the end of one accounting period to another because of the difficulties it creates for analysis.

These are the issues that an income-related national plan would have to resolve. But many other issues are peculiar to the experiment and would not be relevant to a national plan. Of these, two deserve discussion here, since they bear on the usefulness of the results and the ethics of the experiment. For both scientific and ethical reasons, families will be paid an amount of money sufficient to ensure that they will never be worse off financially from participating. This money will be independent of the family's utilization of medical care. It will therefore not alter the price of services and should be treated like other income by the family. The formula for calculating this amount to be paid is

$$(4) \quad P = B + \underset{E}{\text{maximum}} \ (0, \text{maximum} \ (I(E) - X(E) - R) \ )$$

where P is the sum paid to the family, B is the amount paid for interviewing fees and returning monthly forms, I is the amount paid by the family's existing insurance plan(s) conditional on expenditures E, X is the amount paid by the experimental plan, and R is the family's out-of-pocket insurance premium.

This formula may be explained as follows. The family heads are each paid $5 per interview (interviews are anticipated to be quarterly) and $10 per month for returning forms indicating family composition changes, job changes, or insurance changes. These payments are represented by B. To guarantee that the family will never be worse off from participating, the largest possible difference between what it would receive under its old policy and what it would receive under its new policy is computed. This is $I(E) - X(E)$ in the formula. For example, if a family has hospitalization insurance at present covering the first 30 days at a semi-private room rate, and we were to assign it to a plan with a 25 percent coinsurance rate subject to a maximum out-of-pocket payment of $1,000, we would pay the family $1,000. We would assume that a member of the family could spend 30 days in the hospital, and could incur total expenditures of $4,000 or more. In this case the family would have to pay $1,000 with its experimental coverage; but because the bill might have been paid in full under its old plan, the family exposes itself to a potential $1,000 loss. From this "worst case" payment is deducted any out-of-pocket premium payments that the family would have made on its old policy, since it will no longer have to make these payments.

If the family were not protected against its worst case, families who expected high expenditures would differentially refuse plans requiring large out-of-pocket payments. This would have the effect of overstating the responsiveness of demand to insurance when comparing results across plans. In addition, if worst case payments were not made, the family would be in effect participating in a lottery in which it could, under some circumstances, lose. Some consider it unethical for the government to make such a lottery available.

In addition to the payment P, we will reimburse the family's out-of-pocket premiums if it keeps its prior insurance in force, for two reasons. First, doing so guarantees that no family will become uninsurable by participating in the experiment. If the policy were not kept in force, a person who became sick might find that he could not obtain insurance afterwards. Second, keeping the policy in force guarantees that the family can withdraw from the experiment, if it chooses, and not be uncovered for a period of time.

In return for paying the family an amount equal to the most it could "lose" and reimbursing the family's out-of-pocket premiums, the families are asked to assign the benefits of their existing policies to us for services that we cover.[59] There are two reasons for this. By obtaining an assignment, we can be certain that the families are not being double-covered, thereby changing the price of medical care and defeating the purpose of the experiment. Second, by reclaiming against the family's old policy, it will be possible to recoup a portion of the funds paid to maintain the family's insurance in force.[60]

Payments to the family for participating will, in general, be made monthly. This is done to maximize the possibility

that the family will treat the money paid it as it would any other income, and therefore, when making decisions on medical care, will act as if it faced the price specified in the policy.[61] Although unlikely, if the money were paid at the beginning of the accounting period, the family might "put it in a cookie jar," use it for medical care, and treat its medical care as free. In this case, the family's behavior would differ from its behavior under a national plan, where it would receive no payments. However, if the family does not put the money in a cookie jar, a different problem may arise. The family might spend its payment, then be hospitalized and not be able to meet its bills. In this case, the family will be referred to local lending institutions. (Note that over the succeeding 12 months the family will be paid an amount equal to its largest possible bill.) During the course of the experiment, we will attempt to find out how families finance their medical care expenditures. If plans that call for substantial out-of-pocket payments cause the families financing difficulties, legislation that envisions such payments must give some attention to the financing question.

The monthly payment scheme will be changed in the final year; the money will be held in an escrow account for the family. The family may draw down its escrow account to finance medical expenditures, and any balance in the account at the end of the year will be paid to the family. The purpose of the escrow account is to prevent a situation where it is not in the family's interest to continue in the experiment, one that could occur if payments continued to be made monthly. For example, if an illness occurred in the middle of the last accounting period, a payment of $500 might be required from the family, but continued participation in the experiment might net the family only $250 (if $250 had already been paid), while dropping out of the experiment and returning to its old insurance might save the family the entire $500. Since this would tend to decrease reported expendi-

Table 4. Cumulative number of family years by site, by fiscal year

End of fiscal year	Dayton	Site 2	Site 3	Site 4	All sites	Multiple of final coefficient of variation
FY 1975	417	125	....	....	542	3.86
FY 1976	917	625	375	250	2167	1.92
FY 1977	1417	1125	875	750	4167	1.39
FY 1978	1717	1565	1375	1250	5907	1.17
FY 1979	1977	1825	1695	1630	7127	1.06
FY 1980	2020	2020	1955	1890	7885	1.01
December 31, 1980	2020	2020	2020	2020	8080	1.00

Assume enrollment complete in Dayton August 31, 1974; Site 2, March 31, 1975; Site 3, September 30, 1975; Site 4, December 31, 1975. Assume 500 families per site. The multiple of the final coefficient of variation is $(8080/x)^{1/2}$, where x is the cumulative number of family years at that time.

tures in plans with high coinsurance rates, it would lead to overstated responsiveness of demand.

A second issue peculiar to the experiment is the definition of eligibility. Those over 65 were deemed ineligible, since a national insurance program could well leave the Medicare program intact and since the different kinds of health problems among the aged would require a larger sample. Those with incomes greater than $25,000 were also eliminated. A relatively high income eligibility figure was chosen to permit generalization to most of the population. An income limit of $25,000 includes over 90 percent of the population, while it avoids the problem of using tax money to make large payments to very high-income families. Those with access to the military medical care system were also excluded, because it was felt that they might continue to use this system—making observations of their behavior not comparable to the other observations. Foster children were excluded, on the assumption that the state would continue to pay for their medical care in full, even if a national plan were enacted.

Schedule and Costs

In late November and early December, 1973, 50 families were enrolled as a pilot sample. Fifty-five offers were made and there were five refusals. The purpose of the pilot sample is primarily to test the operating systems to eliminate flaws be-

fore enrollment of the regular sample. These 50 families will continue in the experiment for three years and will serve as a group upon which interview instruments can be pretested. The pilot sample also permitted the testing of enrollment techniques.

The regular sample of 500 families will be enrolled in Dayton in late summer 1974; enrollment of 500 additional families in the second site will take place around March, 1975; enrollment is scheduled in the third and fourth sites in September and December, 1975, respectively.[62] Table 4 shows the cumulative number of family years by site by fiscal year if this schedule is followed. The last column of the table gives the multiple of the final coefficient of variation through time. The calculation of the coefficient of variation assumes that data from the first year are usable and that observations across time are independent.[63]

As might be anticipated, precision improves rapidly at the beginning of the experiment. By the end of fiscal year 1977, confidence intervals are only about 40 percent as large as they will be at the end of the experiment. Thus, useful data should be available relatively early.

The total projected cost of the experiment (1973 dollars) is $32-million. Of this figure, $12-million will be paid to families either as claims payments or as worst case payments. (This assumes that on the average about $1,550 per year will be paid to families and that $250 per year can be reclaimed from existing insurance.) Some $6-million will be paid in local field costs, primarily for interviewers and quality control operations. About $9-million of the cost is for design, analysis, and administration (exclusive of data processing), and $5-million for data processing. Administrative and data processing costs are high because of the volume of data being collected and the need to collect it in ways that make it amenable to different types of analysis. For example, one may wish to look at a subset of families over time or all families at one point in time. Similarly, we wish to analyze the data both by illness episode and by annual expenditure. Also, one must be able to identify individuals with family units, which may change through the course of the experiment.

Although they have been thoroughly reviewed, the uncertainty of the cost estimates must be emphasized. The better one is able to predict claims payments, the less compelling the rationale for doing the experiment. In addition, many aspects of the project are novel, making the prediction of cost hazardous. Because of uncertainties with regard to both cost and feasibility, the Department of Health, Education and Welfare has, to date, authorized enrollment only in Dayton. A review of progress will be made before enrollment takes place in each remaining site. If the project is not fulfilling its objectives, it will be curtailed.

Significance of the Results

The experiment must be appraised in the context of the debate over health care financing. In this debate, neither the costs nor the benefits of proposed legislation can be well predicted. One factor in estimating cost is the responsiveness of demand to insurance (price elasticity); yet existing estimates both in the popular press and in technical journals vary widely. For example, estimates of the effect of price on demand made in the economics literature

Table 5. Summary of the experiment's principal dimensions

Four sites (projected)

2,000 experimental families, each randomly assigned to one of the 16 plans

Families nearly evenly divided between three-year and five-year periods of participation

1,200 control-group families

Plans vary coinsurance rate from zero to 100 percent

All plans requiring out-of-pocket payments limit such payments to 5 or 15 percent of family income

Some families assigned to a health maintenance organization

Opportunity for purchase of additional insurance in the final year

differ by more than an order of magnitude from those made by the Social Security Administration.[64-67] Answers to more specific questions concerning the effect of price—such as how large a deductible would affect the demand for ambulatory services, or how much supplementation of a plan requiring out-of-pocket payments would occur—are much less certain. Reliable estimates of the effect of tax law changes are virtually impossible to make.

The benefits of insurance are even less well understood than the costs. The evidence suggests that additional medical care consumption has little effect on measured indices of health status.[68] Many observers find this statement counter-intuitive and suspect that if different aspects of health status were measured, significant results would be found. By obtaining objective and subjective measures of health status over time, the experiment should make a considerable advance in the data available to examine the question of the effect of insurance on health status.

Some have commented that the experiment is likely to be too late—that it would be valuable if we had the information now, but that by the time the experiment ends, a national plan will have been enacted. However, reasonably precise results will be available early on; within two years, confidence intervals will be about double their final level, and in four years, confidence intervals will be only 20 percent higher than their final level (see Table 4).

Furthermore, whatever plan is adopted is unlikely to remain immutable; the recent debates over altering the Medicaid and Medicare programs attests to that. Moreover, assuming a plan is adopted in the near future, the control group will provide data from before and after its implementation, thereby facilitating evaluation.

The principal dimensions of the Health Insurance Study are briefly summarized in Table 5.

While the experiment has been designed to provide better answers to some of the principal questions in the present debate over health care financing, it is also a basic research project concerning health care financing. The project should generate not only results of immediate usefulness and policy relevance, but also a data base that should be a valuable asset for health service researchers for decades to come.

References and Notes

1 Acton, J. P. *Demand for Health Care When Time Prices Vary More Than Money Prices* (Santa Monica: The Rand Corporation, 1973) R-1189-OEO/NYC.

2 Acton, J. P. *The Demand for Health Care Among the Urban Poor With Special Emphasis on the Role of Time* (Santa Monica: The Rand Corporation, 1973) R-1151-OEO/NYC.

3 Arrow, Kenneth J. *Optimal Insurance and Generalized Deductibles* (Santa Monica: The Rand Corporation, 1973) R-1131-OEO.

4 Arrow, Kenneth J. *Welfare Analysis of Changes in Health Coinsurance Rates* (Santa Monica: The Rand Corporation, December 1973) R-1281-OEO.

5 Mitchell, Bridger M. and Vogel, Ronald J. *Health and Taxes: An Assersment of the Medical Deduction* (Santa Monica: The Rand Corporation, August 1973) R-1222-OEO.

6 Newhouse, Joseph P. and Phelps, C. E. *Price and Income Elasticities for Medical Care Services.* Paper presented to a Conference of the International Economic Association, Tokyo, April 1973; to be published in the *Proceedings* of the Conference.

7 Newhouse, Joseph P. and Phelps, C. E. *On Having Your Cake and Eating It Too: An Analysis of Estimated Effects of Insurance on Demand for Medical Care* (Santa Monica: The Rand Corporation) R-1149-NC, forthcoming.

8 Phelps, Charles E. *The Demand for Health Insurance: A Theoretical and Empirical Investigation* (Santa Monica: The Rand Corporation, July 1973) R-1054-OEO.

9 Phelps, Charles E. and Newhouse, Joseph P. *The Effects of Coinsurance on Demand for Physician Services* (Santa Monica: The Rand Corporation, June 1972) R-976-OEO.

10 Phelps, Charles E. and Newhouse, Joseph P. *Coinsurance and the Demand for Medical Services* (Santa Monica: The Rand Corporation, 1973) R-964-OEO/NC. An abridged version, "Coinsurance: The Price of Time, and the Demand for Medical Services," is forthcoming in *Review of Economics and Statistics.*

11 Sloan, Frank A. *Supply Responses of Young Physicians* (Santa Monica: The Rand Corporation, 1973) R-1131-OEO.

12 Grossman, Michael. *The Demand for Health* (New York: Columbia University Press, 1972); and Phelps, Charles E. and Newhouse, Joseph P. *Coinsurance and the Demand for Medical Services, op. cit.*

13 Another example of a policy detail is limits on specific services: some hospital policies may reimburse for a semi-private room; others may have a specific dollar maximum; some may have a dollar limit for ancillary services; others may not have such a limit; still other policies may not cover such services at all.

14 Weinberger, Caspar W., to be Secretary of Health, Education and Welfare, "Hearings Before the Senate Committee on Labor and Public Welfare," 93rd Congress, 1st Session (1973) Part 2, Appendix.

15 The limited duration of the experiment (five years) creates obvious difficulties for estimating the magnitude of the effect of any preventive services on the later consumption of medical services, but any immediate effect should be noticeable.

16 Feldstein, Martin S. and Allison, Elizabeth. "Tax Subsidies of Private Health Insurance: Distribution, Revenue Loss, and Effects," Discussion Paper No. 237 (Cambridge: Harvard Institute of Economic Research, April 1972); and Mitchell and Vogel, *op. cit.*

17 The accounting period defines whether the deductible is annual, quarterly, or tied to some other period, whether the period is a moving average, and so forth. The accounting unit defines whether the deductible applies to the family or to the individual, and if it applies to the family, how the family unit is defined.

18 Donabedian, Avedis. "An Evaluation of Prepaid Group Practice," *Inquiry* 6:3-27 (September 1969).

19 Enterline, Philip E., *et al.* "The Distribution of Medical Services Before and After 'Free' Medical Care—The Quebec Experience," *New England Journal of Medicine* 289:1174-1178 (November 29, 1973).

20 National Center for Health Statistics. "Volume of

Physician Visits," *Vital and Health Statistics*, Series 10, No. 49 (Washington, D.C.: GPO, 1968) Tables 3 and 21; and American Medical Association. *Distribution of Physicians, Hospitals, and Hospital Beds in the U.S.* (Chicago: AMA, 1966).

21 Balamuth, Eve. "Health Interview Responses Compared with Medical Records," National Center for Health Statistics, Series 2, No. 7 (Washington D.C.: GPO, 1965); and National Center for Health Statistics, *op. cit.*

22 Phelps, *op. cit.*

23 Social Security Administration. *Analysis of Health Insurance Proposals Introduced in the 92nd Congress.* Printed for the use of the Committee on Ways and Means, 92nd Congress, 1st Session (Washington D.C.: GPO, 1971) p. 83, n. 1.

24 Newhouse and Phelps, *On Having Your Cake and Eating It Too, op. cit.*

25 Newhouse and Phelps, *Price and Income Elasticities for Medical Care Services, op. cit.*

26 *Ibid.*

27 While the experiment can measure the responsiveness of demand to changes in the time price, the amount by which any plan will affect the time price must also be estimated if the information is to be useful. This amount can be assessed to a limited degree in the study by observing the time price across communities with varying amounts of insurance coverage and varying supply. The experiment is not well suited, however, to measuring what would happen to time price if large changes in demand were to occur and supply could not be expanded; in this case one might wish to predict the level of demand using several different assumptions about the level of time price. See Enterline, *et al., op. cit.*

28 Andersen, Ronald, and Benham, Lee. "Factors Affecting the Relationship Between Family Income and Medical Care Consumption." In: Klarman, H. E. (ed.) *Empirical Studies in Health Economics* (Baltimore: Johns Hopkins Press, 1970).

29 Grossman, *op. cit.*

30 Newhouse and Phelps, *Price and Income Elasticities for Medical Care Services, op. cit.*

31 *Ibid.* The product of the first two dimensions represents the rate of patient days in the population; the sum of the third and fourth dimensions represents price per day. The product of the patient-day rate and price per day represents expenditures.

32 *Ibid.*

33 Newhouse and Phelps, *Coinsurance and the Demand for Medical Services, op. cit.*, Appendix A.

34 Newhouse, Joseph P. "Issues in the Analysis and Design of the Experimental Portion of the Health Insurance Study," *Proceedings of the Social Statistics Section*, American Statistical Association, 1974, forthcoming.

35 *Ibid.*

36 *Ibid.* Initially, this "truncation factor" has been set at $1,000. Work is now in progress to determine an optimal truncation factor by plan, being higher in the high-coinsurance plans.

37 If the null hypothesis is rejected, the next step is to determine whether there is any interaction between frequency of interviewing and generosity of insurance. To do this, the control group will be stratified in such a way as to guarantee vari-ation of insurance coverage within classes of frequency of interview. If the null hypothesis of no interaction is not rejected (that is, if there is no significant interaction), then the effect of interviewing would only be to change the intercept in our various models. If the null hypothesis is rejected, estimates will have to be made of the interaction (from control-group data) and appropriate adjustments of price elasticities made.

38 Since the present coverage is not randomly distributed, it will be necessary to treat existing insurance as endogenous when analyzing data from the control group.

39 If almost all members of the control group do not have coverage for either psychiatric or preventive services, comparisons of total utilization between the experimental and control groups will not, strictly speaking, help in identifying which exclusion is responsible for the results. In this case, comparisons must be made for those services thought likely to be affected by one exclusion or the other.

40 Sparer, Gerald, and Anderson, Arne. "Utilization and Cost Experience of Low-Income Families in Four Prepaid Group-Practice Plans," *New England Journal of Medicine* 289:67-72 (July 12, 1973).

41 Strauss, Mark A. and Sparer, Gerald. "Basic Utilization of OEO Comprehensive Health Services Projects," *Inquiry* 8:36-49 (December 1971).

42 Newhouse, *op. cit.*

43 *Ibid.*

44 Morris, Carl. *Determination of the Number of Sites in the Housing Allowance Demand Experiment* (Santa Monica: The Rand Corporation, R-1082-HUD) forthcoming.

45 Morris, Carl *A Finite Selection Model for Experimental Design* (Santa Monica: The Rand Corporation) forthcoming.

46 *Ibid.*

47 Conlisk, John, and Watts, Harold. "A Model for Optimizing Experimental Designs for Estimating Response Surfaces," *Proceedings of the Social Statistics Section*, American Statistical Association, 1969, pp. 150-156.

48 The idea contained in this paragraph was suggested by Bradley Efron.

49 Stated formally, the constraint is that there is near orthogonality between the demographic and plan variables.

50 In the Palo Alto data described in Phelps and Newhouse (see note 9), the correlation between physician expenditures in 1966 and 1968 was 0.15, while the correlation for the number of visits was 0.3.

51 Efron, Bradley, and Morris, Carl. "Limiting the Risk of Bayes and Empirical Bayes Estimators— Part II: The Empirical Bayes Case," *Journal of the American Statistical Association*, 67:130-139 (March 1972).

52 Clasquin, Lorraine. *Coverage of Services in the Health Insurance Study* (Santa Monica: The Rand Corporation) forthcoming.

53 The possibility of adverse selection in the choice of dental insurance (those who expect to use more services having better insurance) seems unlikely because such insurance is relatively rare, but will be tested by using a simultaneous-estimator.

54 Newhouse, *op. cit.*

55 Morris, Carl. *Statistical Design for the Health Insurance Study* (Santa Monica: The Rand Corporation) forthcoming.

56 Morris, *Determination of the Number of Sites, op. cit.*

57 Clasquin, Lorraine. *The Rules of Operation of the Health Insurance Study* (Santa Monica: California: The Rand Corporation) forthcoming.

58 Permitting additions other than these also raises the possibility of adverse selection, sick individuals becoming members of units with generous plans. Incentives for such additions in the experiment (which covers only a small fraction of the population) are much greater than the incentives would be in a national plan with universal coverage.

59 If we do not cover a service—such as dental services for adults in some plans—and the family's existing insurance covers such a service, the family will continue to be covered at the terms of its existing policy.

60 Note that if there were no reclaiming, there would be a windfall to insurance companies, since they would be collecting premiums on a policy that would not be used.

61 To test whether the family treated its payments as other income, we will enter the amount of the payment as an explanatory variable. There will be some variation independent of income and plan because of the truncation factor and variation in out-of-pocket premiums on pre-existing coverage; additional variation, created by paying something extra to a few families, is being considered.

62 About one year is required from the date of beginning operations in a site to the date of completing enrollment. This allows time for randomly choosing areas of the city, listing dwelling units in those areas, conducting screening and baseline interviews, verifying insurance coverage of those in the sample, contacting local providers, and enrolling the families.

63 If there is substantial serial correlation within families across time, these multiples are too large.

64 Social Security Administration, *op. cit.* (see note 23). The order of magnitude figure is derived by comparing the projected dollar cost of various plans and computing the implied elasticities.

65 Feldstein, M. S., "Hospital Cost Inflation: A Study of Nonprofit Price Dynamics," *American Economic Review* 61:853-872 (December 1971).

66 Rosett, R. N. and Huang, L. F. "The Effect of Health Insurance on the Demand for Medical Care," *The Journal of Political Economy* (March/April 1973).

67 Davis, K. and Russell, L. B. "The Substitution of Hospital Outpatient Care for Inpatient Care," *Review of Economics and Statistics* 54:109-120 (May 1972).

68 Haggerty, Robert J. "The Boundaries of Health Care," *The Pharos*, July 1972, pp. 106-110.

David M. Barton
Robert H. Smiley

Estimating the Cost of Health Insurance Programs

Reprinted with permission of the Blue Cross Association, from *Inquiry:* Vol.XIV, No.1, pp.51-62. Copyright © 1977 by the Blue Cross Association.

Originally Published in March 1977

Despite the obvious importance of program costs in choosing between competing proposals, the current debate over national health insurance has proceeded without reference to a methodological framework for estimating such costs (with but one exception which will be noted later). In this paper we present such a framework and use it to estimate the cost, in 1975, of a modified version of the Catastrophic Insurance Protection Plan (CIPP), a health insurance plan proposed for New York State.[1] Costs to the state include claims expense, administrative costs, and changes in state tax revenues directly attributable to the CIPP program. The costs of raising the revenues required to finance the program are not included.

While the cost estimates presented here apply to a specific proposal and are for a state rather than the nation, the methodology is applicable to various national health insurance schemes currently being considered since some features of the CIPP plan are shared by nearly all bills, including the Ford Administration's bill for catastrophic coverage of the elderly. In addition, the income and family size related private expense limit is common to CIPP and

David M. Barton, Ph.D. is Assistant Professor of Economics and Public Finance and **Robert H. Smiley, Ph.D.** is Assistant Professor of Business Economics, Graduate School of Business and Public Administration, Cornell University (Ithaca, NY 14853).

The authors wish to acknowledge the assistance of George Harris, Pamela Hornett, Bridger Mitchell, John McCann, John McClain, Gordon Trapnell and Robert Uris. Financial assistance was provided by the Regional Medical Program Service, Public Health Service, DHEW, and the Central New York Regional Medical Program. The views expressed are the authors' and not those of the sponsoring organizations.

the Ulman and Fannon bills. Finally, the CIPP plan is similar to the National Association of Insurance Commissioners' model bill in that coverage can be for family expenses, coinsurance is a feature of both bills, and the private expense limit is income related.

The only formal cost analysis of a national health insurance plan so far completed is one prepared by Arthur D. Little, Inc., (ADL) under contract with the Health Resources Administration.[2] The purpose of the ADL study was to estimate the cost of covering the entire U.S. population with several variants of the Aetna plan available to Federal employees enrolled in the Federal Employees Health Benefits Program (FEHBP). In addition to apparently being the only available study to provide both cost estimates and a clear description of the methodology used, the ADL effort also produced a valuable data base. A major preliminary effort involved assembling the claims expense records of a 20 percent sample of enrollees in the Aetna FEHBP. This data base is currently being used by the Social Security Administration National Health Insurance Modeling Group and was also used in making the cost estimates for CIPP.

Despite the contribution provided by the ADL study, the methodology is not directly applicable to estimating the costs of most national health insurance proposals. The reason for this is that the benefit structure of the Aetna plan differs from that envisioned by most national health insurance schemes in two respects: 1) the Aetna plan provides benefits based on expenses incurred by enrollees taken individually, and 2) the benefits do not vary with the income of the insured. In contrast, a number of national health insurance proposals have benefits that are based on total family expenses and vary according to family size and income. The importance of these differences can be seen by considering, for example, a simple type of health insurance plan with a benefit structure described solely by a deductible and a coinsurance rate. The cost of an insurance plan that covers each member separately in a family of four for 80 percent of all medical expenses after a deductible of $100 is met, will not be equal to the cost of a plan that covers a *family* of four for 80 percent of all medical expenses after a deductible of $400 is met. Second, the variation of benefits by family income requires the cost of the plan for a family of four to be computed for various levels of the expense limit corresponding to different family income levels.

In what follows, we describe the procedure used to estimate the costs of CIPP to New York State utilizing the data base provided by ADL. For our purposes, the important features of this bill are that benefits such as deductibles and expense limits are related to total family expenses and vary according to family income and size. In these respects it is similar to many national health insurance proposals. The fact that the word "catastrophic" appears in the title of this plan is of no real significance. By varying the parameters describing the coverage, the costs of a more comprehensive version could be estimated using the same approach.

It will be helpful to begin by presenting an overview of the estimation procedure. This will serve to describe the general framework and to divide the analysis into its component parts, which will be dealt with in subsequent sections.

Overview

In brief, the provisions of CIPP are as follows: After the family pays a deductible related to income and family size, CIPP begins paying for 80 percent of medical expenses. Once the family's portion of expenses in excess of the deductible equals an income related expense limit, CIPP pays 100 percent of all additional expenses. Only family-borne out-of-pocket expenses count toward meeting the deductible and expense limit, and the deductible is reduced

by the amount of any premiums paid for private health insurance.

Data supplied by ADL on expenses of individuals enrolled in the Aetna FEHBP form the basis of our cost estimates. However, these data were not directly usable since we required estimates of the expenses of families rather than individuals.

Our procedure was to begin with the observed sample frequency distributions of total annual medical expenses for individuals; find a probability density function (*pdf*) that provided a good approximation to the observed frequency distribution of expenses for individuals and then used these *pdf*'s to derive the *pdf*'s of expenses for a family. For example, assume that the observed frequency distribution of total annual medical expenses for a married male between the ages of 25 and 45, X_i, and those for a married female in the same age interval, X_j, can be approximated by:

$$g_i(x_i); x_i > 0$$

and

$$g_j(x_j); x_j > 0.$$

The joint distribution of expenses for these two individuals (assuming X_i and X_j to be independent) is the product of the individual *pdf*'s. From the joint distribution, the *pdf* of the sum of expenses,

$$X_{ij}(= X_i + X_j)$$

for a family composed of these two individuals can then be found. Denote the latter by

$$g_{ij}(x_{ij}); x_{ij} > 0.$$

Following the same procedure, the *pdf* of the total annual expenses for a family composed of any number of individuals can be derived.

Since these *pdf*'s apply only to the case for which some expenses were incurred, the probability, P, that the family will have some expense is also required; i.e., the probability that the relevant *pdf* will be applicable. Each *pdf* will, therefore, be associated with a particular value of P. Let this probability be denoted by P_{ij} for our hypothetical two-member family.

Given the *pdf* and the corresponding value of P, the expected annual cost per family, E, for this family with income k (and no private health insurance) would be calculated from the following expected cost function:

$$EC_{2,k,i,j} = P_{ij} \left(.8 \int_{D(2,k)}^{XL(k)} x_{ij}\, g\,(x_{ij})\, dx \right.$$
$$\left. + \int_{XL(k)}^{\infty} x_{ij}\, g\,(x_{ij})\, dx \right)$$

where D is the value of the deductible, related to family size (2) and income (k), above which CIPP pays for 80 percent of expenses until the expense limit is met; $XL(k)$ is the amount of out-of-pocket medical expense (income related) that would cause the family expense limit to be met. For medical expense in excess of XL, CIPP pays 100 percent of medical expenses.

The calculation of the cost of CIPP for the target population—that projected for New York State in 1975—requires that the calculation of EC be made for a large number of family-type/income-level combinations (henceforth, these will be referred to as "cells"). Therefore, data on the target population is required to determine the number of families within each cell. Once this is accomplished, the value of EC for each cell is multiplied by the number, n, of families in that cell. Summing $n \times EC$ over all cells gives the estimate of total annual cost for the target population.

This overview neglects various complexities specific to CIPP, such as its interaction with Medicaid and private health insurance and its effect on tax revenues. These will be dealt with in the following sections.

Since our interest is methodological, we have attempted to be clear in pointing out data limitations and our use of simplifying assumptions. As in all such endeavors, an implicit tradeoff had to be made between the costs of making additional refinements and the expected improvement in accuracy. It was often necessary to choose between reasonable alternative assumptions regarding, for example, an unknown value of some parameter. As a rule of thumb, the choice in such cases was made in favor of the alternative that would tend to overstate rather than understate costs.

Provisions of CIPP

CIPP is a state-provided insurance plan covering a broad range of medical assistance. The purpose of the plan is to provide umbrella protection for all residents of New York State. The salient features of the plan for the purpose of the cost estimates are:

1 A family size and family income related deductible (exclusion) with a minimum of $25. This is the portion of the family's medical expenses that must be paid by the family (not private health insurance), before the plan is effective. Table 1 shows the amount of the deductible by income and family size.

2 Once the deductible is met, a 20 percent coinsurance (cost-sharing) rate is effective. The family pays 20 percent of the expenses for which it is responsible.

3 The income related expense limit is given in the last column of Table 1. After the family pays this, in addition to the deductible, CIPP pays all expenses for which the family is responsible (i.e., expenses not paid for by private health insurance or Medicaid).

4 The deductible given in Table 1 is reduced by the amount of the family's annual premium for private health insurance, whether paid for by family or on its behalf by another party.[3]

ADL-Aetna Data Base

The cost estimates in this report are based on data provided to the authors by Arthur D. Little, Inc. The data come from a 20 percent (approximately) sample of individuals who submitted insurance claims to the Aetna FEHBP for the year 1970. These data have two characteristics that make them particularly useful.

First, the data can be used to construct frequency distributions of claimants and total annual expense by expense interval. The availability of expense data in the form of distributions is essential for estimating costs of an insurance plan with variable deductibles and expense limits. This is a crucial feature that distinguishes the ADL-Aetna data from expense data available from private insurance companies. As an example of the data on claims expense used in this study, consider males between the ages of 19 and 44 falling into the Aetna claimant category entitled "Active Male Employees" with self-only (non-

Table 1.   Characteristics of CIPP

Total family income	Annual family income exclusion (deductible) by family size												Expense limit
	1	2	3	4	5	6	7	8	9	10	11	12	
$1,000	$25	$25	$25	$25	$25	$25	$25	$25	$25	$25	$25	$25	$60
2,000	153	67	25	25	25	25	25	25	25	25	25	25	120
3,000	275	172	76	25	25	25	25	25	25	25	25	25	180
4,000	405	283	156	25	25	25	25	25	25	25	25	25	240
5,000	540	398	241	122	43	25	25	25	25	25	25	25	300
6,000	695	526	331	180	71	25	25	25	25	25	25	25	420
7,000	943	829	715	603	501	402	306	200	105	25	25	25	560
8,000	1,114	1,000	886	772	658	552	450	354	245	140	42	25	720
9,000	1,285	1,171	1,057	943	829	715	603	510	402	290	185	84	900
10,000	1,468	1,342	1,228	1,114	1,000	886	772	658	552	450	338	230	1,100
12,000	1,864	1,732	1,600	1,468	1,342	1,228	1,114	1,000	886	772	658	552	1,560
15,000	2,485	2,335	2,194	2,064	1,930	1,798	1,666	1,534	1,402	1,285	1,171	1,057	2,400
17,000	2,935	2,785	2,635	2,485	2,335	2,194	2,064	1,930	1,798	1,666	1,534	1,402	3,000
20,000	3,652	3,484	3,316	3,160	3,010	2,860	2,710	2,560	2,410	2,260	2,128	1,996	4,000
22,000	4,156	3,988	3,820	3,652	3,484	3,316	3,160	3,010	2,860	2,710	2,560	2,410	4,900
25,000	4,988	4,796	4,604	4,410	4,240	4,072	3,904	3,766	3,566	3,400	3,235	3,085	6,250
30,000	6,524	6,308	6,094	5,876	5,660	5,468	5,276	5,084	4,892	4,700	4,508	4,352	9,000
35,000	8,231	7,997	7,763	7,529	7,295	7,064	6,848	6,632	6,416	6,200	5,984	5,768	12,600
40,000	10,088	9,836	9,584	9,332	9,080	8,828	8,582	8,348	8,114	7,880	7,646	7,412	16,800
45,000	12,095	11,825	11,555	11,285	11,015	10,745	10,475	10,214	9,962	9,710	9,458	9,206	22,050
50,000	14,260	13,964	13,676	13,338	13,100	12,812	12,524	12,236	11,960	11,690	11,420	11,150	28,000

family) coverage. The experience of a 20 percent sample of such claimants in 1970 is given in Table 2.

Second, the Aetna plan provides very extensive coverage, with 20 percent cost-sharing after a $50 deductible for all expenses other than the first $1,000 in-hospital room and board expense, which is covered in full. As such, it represents a fully operational health insurance program with a benefit structure similar to that of CIPP. In particular, the coinsurance rate (cost-sharing rate) facing Aetna claimants who have met the deductible is the same as that faced by CIPP claimants for expenses between the CIPP deductible and expense limit. The similarity of the two programs over the range of expense containing

Table 2.   Distribution of claimants and total claims expense for a sample of active male employees, 19–44 years of age with self-only coverage

Expense interval	Number of claimants	Annual total claims expense
$1–1,000	427	$139,089
1,001–3,000	51	88,233
3,001–5,000	10	39,145
5,001–10,000	5	36,256
10,001 and over	1	11,624

the bulk of total expenditure is a particularly fortunate circumstance; the difficulties that one would otherwise face in estimating expenditure at one coinsurance rate based on the experience under a different coinsurance rate are largely avoided.[4]

A limitation of the data, at least for estimating the cost of CIPP, is that approximately two-thirds of the Federal employees in the 65-and-over age group covered by Aetna were not covered by Medicare. Since CIPP is concerned with expenses net of payments by any other health plan, only the distribution of expenses net of Medicare payments would be of interest. Using available data it is not possible to separate the Aetna claimants with Medicare coverage from those without such coverage. As a result, it is not possible to construct sample distributions of claims expense net of Medicare for the 65-and-over age group. The choice was, therefore, to either use a sample distribution of claims expense that would vastly overstate the expense relevant for CIPP, or to estimate the costs of the portion of the population under 65, as we have done in this paper.

A second, and more general, limitation of the data stems from the fact that the Federal employees insured under the Aetna-FEHBP are not a representative sample of the population. Being a predominantly white-collar group, their health experience is likely to be better than that for a cross-section of the general population (i.e., the Federal employees are likely to have lower annual claims expense than an average U.S. citizen insured under the same program). Our method of dealing with this problem is described at the end of the next section.

Lastly, the sample data could not be broken down by income categories. This, in effect, requires that we ignore the income elasticity of demand for medical services. In practice, however, this is most likely to lead to over- rather than underestimates of the cost. The average income of the Federal employees is greater than that of the general population. Therefore, medical services being a normal good, we would expect an average Federal employee covered under the FEHBP to have a greater demand for medical services than an average individual of the same age, sex, and marital status covered under a similar insurance plan.

From the ADL sample data, frequency distributions of claimants and total annual expense, such as that given in Table 2, were available for 10 claimant categories used by Aetna for its own record-keeping purposes and four age intervals (excluding individuals 65 and over) used by ADL in compiling the data. As Census classifications were used to stratify the population into cells for the cost estimates, supplementary information provided by ADL was used to recombine the 10 Aetna claimant categories into the six categories corresponding to those used by the Census. Age interval differed slightly in the case of the two youngest age intervals; we treated the 0–18 and 19–44 age intervals used by ADL as though they corresponded to the 0–24 and 24–44 age intervals used by the Census. The end result was a set of frequency distributions for the combinations designated by a star in Table 3.

Note that sample frequency distributions are not available for the youngest age group in the first five individual categories. The reason for this being that few, if any, employees covered by the Aetna FEHBP were less than 18 years old and those between the ages of 18 and 44

Table 3. Individual groups stratified by Census classifications for which sample frequency distributions were constructed

Individual	0–24	25–44	45–54	55–64
		Age		
Unrelated males		*	*	*
Unrelated females		*	*	*
Male heads of families		*	*	*
Female heads of families		*	*	*
Wives		*	*	*
Children	*			

we placed in the 25–44 age interval. For these we used the data for the next oldest group. This will introduce an upward bias in our cost estimates since we use the experience of an older group to estimate the expenses of a younger group.

The Expected Cost Functions

Having constructed frequency distributions of claimants and total annual expense corresponding to Census individual classifications, we now turn to the *pdf*'s used to approximate those frequency distributions; the derivation of *pdf*'s for family types made up of two or more individuals; and estimating the probability (P) that a family type will have some medical expense. Using the *pdf*'s and associated values of P, we can then construct expected cost functions for population cells.

In choosing a *pdf* to approximate the observed frequency distributions, two conflicting objectives had to be weighed. First, the *pdf* should be able to reproduce the observed frequency distributions with reasonable accuracy. Second, the variability of the limits of integration (because of the many family type and income levels considered) dictated that the resulting *pdf*'s for each family type have closed analytic forms in order to keep the computations managable.

Individual Frequency Distributions

Given these considerations, the *pdf* chosen to approximate the individual frequency distributions was the exponential that has a single parameter u, which can readily be estimated

$$1/u \; e^{-x/u}; \; x > 0$$

Table 4. Comparison of actual and estimated expense within claims expense interval (in $ thousands)

$ (000)		Actual	Estimated
Unrelated males			
25–44	$0–1	$138.9	$159.9
	1–3	87.3	78.5
	3–5	41.4	37.7
	5–10	33.6	26.0
	10+	13.2	12.3
45–54	0–1	162.1	208.2
	1–3	171.1	160.2
	3–5	77.1	73.6
	5–10	102.0	81.3
	10+	39.3	31.6
55–64	0–1	299.5	381.6
	1–3	337.6	316.1
	3–5	129.7	120.4
	5–10	136.1	116.5
	10+	52.9	46.8
Unrelated females			
25–44	0–1	156.2	186.0
	1–3	105.2	107.8
	3–5	56.0	55.3
	5–10	65.1	56.6
	10+	0.0	10.6
45–54	0–1	300.1	374.4
	1–3	296.7	266.5
	3–5	100.8	88.4
	5–10	50.7	40.5
	10+	9.3	7.6
55–64	0–1	360.6	503.1
	1–3	383.3	345.6
	3–5	142.0	131.7
	5–10	118.4	96.6
	10+	27.1	21.4
Male heads of families			
25–44	0–1	531.4	719.1
	1–3	327.3	305.0
	3–5	126.9	114.7
	5–10	113.2	79.9
	10+	11.3	10.9
45–54	0–1	871.2	1,194.4
	1–3	826.0	760.2
	3–5	328.7	305.8
	5–10	307.3	246.2
	10+	160.8	133.3
55–64	0–1	958.2	1,333.4
	1–3	973.6	886.9
	3–5	512.4	483.7
	5–10	314.4	256.0
	10+	250.2	143.9
Female heads of families			
25–44	0–1	187.4	213.1
	1–3	141.5	145.7
	3–5	7.9	8.9
	5–10	79.5	60.7
	10+	31.7	24.1

Table 4. (Continued)

$ (000)		Actual	Estimated
45–54	0–1	194.8	249.9
	1–3	207.9	204.1
	3–5	59.0	53.6
	5–10	34.9	29.4
	10+	50.9	26.8
55–64	0–1	192.9	263.5
	1–3	173.2	160.2
	3–5	65.7	66.4
	5–10	98.4	86.8
	10+	33.9	26.8
Wives			
25–44	0–1	1,498.9	1,661.3
	1–3	1,240.4	1,210.6
	3–5	268.0	266.2
	5–10	280.1	238.2
	10+	79.9	66.8
45–54	0–1	1,145.8	1,518.3
	1–3	1,177.9	1,094.3
	3–5	439.6	412.4
	5–10	407.8	344.0
	10+	158.3	98.8
55–64	0–1	917.0	1,242.2
	1–3	862.1	808.6
	3–5	499.3	468.6
	5–10	356.2	314.2
	10+	50.2	41.2
Children			
0–24	0–1	1,692.7	2,302.1
	1–3	652.4	557.2
	3–5	295.9	267.1
	5–10	179.9	141.9
	10+	176.7	111.1

using the sample data. For each individual type, the estimate of *u* is given by dividing the total claims expense by the total number of claimants.

In order to see how well the exponential distribution performed in approximating the observed sample frequency distributions we did the following: For each of the Census-type/age-group combinations marked by a star in Table 3, the exponential distribution (using the appropriate estimate of *u*) was used to estimate the total claims expense in five intervals (corresponding to the expense intervals used for tabulating the frequency distributions of the sample data). The estimated expense for each interval was then compared with the actual expense. The actual and estimated expense, by expense interval, are given in Table 4. These expenses are, of course, only for those families that actually had expenses.

As can be seen by comparing the actual with estimated expense,[5] the exponential distribution provides a reasonably good approximation to the observed distribution of expenses. The exception is the $0–$1,000 interval. For this interval the estimate using the exponential significantly overstates the actual expense.[6]

Family Frequency Distribution

The *pdf* of expense for a combination of individuals composing a family is derived from the *pdf*'s of expense applicable to its constituent members. In a trivial case—a single-member family—the *pdf* of expense is given by:

(1) $1/u_i \, e^{-x_i/u_i}; \; x_i > 0$

where the subscript refers to a particular Census-type and age-group combination, i.e., one of the applicable elements of Table 3. For a family with two more members, the *pdf* of sum of expenses is found by combining the *pdf*'s associated with the individuals composing the family. In order to do this, we assume that the individual *pdf*'s are independent. For a family with exactly two members, i and j, the joint *pdf* is therefore given by:

(2) $1/u_i \, 1/u_j \, e^{-x_i/u_i - x_j/u_j}; \; x_i, x_j > 0.$

Employing the change of variable technique,[7] the *pdf* of

$X_{ij} \, (= X_i + X_j)$

is given by:

(3) $1/(u_j - u_i) \, (e^{-x_{ij}/u_i} - e^{-x_{ij}/u_j}); \; x_{ij} > 0.$

The procedure just described can be extended to the case of families with three or more members.[8]

Since the *pdf* of total expense for a family is applicable only to families that have expenses, we require an estimate of the probability that total annual expenses will be greater than zero. Because the Aetna deductible is relatively small, only members with very small expenses are likely not to file claims. As a result the proportion of insured individuals becoming claimants under Aetna will be a good estimate of the proportion of insured individuals having any expenses at all. The probability of becoming a

claimant was used as the estimate of the probability of having some annual expenses, P. P is estimated by dividing the number of claimants by the applicable number of "exposures," i.e., the number of insured individuals.

For a family of more than one individual, the relevant P is the probability that one or more members of this family will have some expense that is equal to one minus the probability that none of the family members will have expenses.[9]

Having described the derivation of the *pdf*'s and P's, the expected cost function for a population cell can now be formed. A population cell refers to a particular family type (a particular combination of Census-type individuals) in a given income class. From this point on, it will be convenient to use subscripts to refer to a family type rather than individual types. The total annual cost to CIPP for a family of type j in income class k would take the following form (assuming that CIPP is the only health insurance in force):

$$EC_{jk} = P_j \left\{ .8 \int_{D(j,k)}^{L(k)} x_j g_j(x_j) dx_j + \int_{L(k)}^{\infty} x_j g_j(x_j) dx_j \right\}$$

where:

$P_j =$ the probability that one or more members of a family of type j will have medical expenses in a given year.

$x_j =$ the total dollar amount of family expenses (= the sum of expenses for individual family members).

$g_j(x_j) =$ the *pdf* of x_j.

$D(j, k) =$ the deductible. (This is written as a function of j and k because the deductible is a function of family size—one of attributes of a family type—and family income.)

$L(k) =$ the dollar value of medical expenses necessary to cause the expense limit of the family to be met. (A function of family income only.)

Multiplying EC by the number of families in that cell, n_{jk}, and summing over all population cells would give the estimated cost of CIPP to the target population assuming that CIPP was the only health insurance program covering the target population. The form of the expected cost function will be changed if a family is covered under another health insurance program. Our attempt to deal with this complication is described later.

Recall that the *pdf* used in the calculation of EC_{jk} is a function of the mean expense for each individual in family type j. The values of the u_j's used in the calculation of expected cost were those calculated from the sample data and then adjusted as follows:

1 Since the ADL sample data for each individual type is weighted to reflect the experience of a representative U.S. citizen of that type, some adjustment had to be made to reflect the cost of medical care in New York State relative to the national average. The adjustment made was to inflate each mean by a factor of 40 percent. This is the same as saying that in 1970 an average claimant living in New York State would have claims expenses that were 140 percent of those incurred by the average U.S. claimant, due to higher medical costs.[10]

2 Since the CIPP cost estimates are made for 1975, the means were also adjusted to account for inflation in medical prices from 1970 through 1972 (the last year for which medical care prices index figures were available when the cost estimates were made) plus that projected for 1973 through 1975.[11]

3 In addition to the above two adjustments made to all means, the mean was increased by 10 percent for adult members of blue-collar families. Each population cell was therefore divided according to the estimated number of blue-collar families in that cell. This adjustment is intended to reflect the (on average) higher expense incurred by adults who would be classified as belonging to blue-collar occupations.[12]

Estimate of the Population Distribution in 1975

This section describes the method used to estimate the distribution of families and unrelated individuals in New York State in 1975. The estimated 1975 distribution consists of numbers of families and unrelated individuals stratified by family type (e.g., husband-wife families), number of family members, age of head, and family income. In this study each stratum is called a cell.

The starting point for this estimate was the 1970 Census of the Population. The Census provides the distribution of families and unrelated individuals by family type, age of head, and family income. This three way stratification is then combined with a second stratification which breaks down (age, family-type) cells by size of family, to estimate the four way stratification needed for the cost estimate.[13]

Since the cost estimates in this study are for 1975, a distribution of families and unrelated individuals for 1975 is needed. The simplest possible method of predicting the 1975 distribution of families and unrelated individuals would be to take the 1970 distribution and increase each cell by the overall expected population growth. This procedure would ignore two major trends: inflation, which causes people's nominal income to increase—thus shifting their income class upward; and real income growth, which also causes individuals to shift classes, irrespective of the rate of inflation.

These trends can be taken into account using a projection made by the Data and Systems Bureau of the New York State Office of Planning Services (OPS). OPS projects the 1975 income distribution for families and unrelated individuals in 1970 dollars. The procedure followed was to adjust this 1975 projection for estimated inflation so that the projected distribution was in 1975 dollars. This along with the 1970 OPS population distribution and the 1970 Census estimates, was used to estimate the 1975 population distribution by the four-day stratification given above.

Interaction of CIPP with Medicaid, and State Tax Revenues

This section describes our procedure for estimating the effect of Medicaid on the cost of CIPP and the effect of CIPP on state tax revenues.

Even if the CIPP plan were in existence, it would clearly be to the advantage of some families to remain on Medicaid. This will certainly be the case if the family pays no expenses under Medicaid. A family qualifies for complete coverage under Medicaid if it meets the public assistance standard (has annual income less than a stated amount for its family size).

Annual income is defined as total annual income less income taxes, cost of health insurance premiums and payments for support of dependents made by court order. It has been assumed that a family will remain on Medicaid (and not shift to CIPP) if its income falls below the defined public assistance standard.

Families that do not meet this standard may still remain on Medicaid. If the public assistance standard is not met, however, the family may be required to meet an assets or allowable resources test (depending on its income) and may pay some portion of its own medical expenses through a cost-sharing provision. Cost-sharing is required for outpatient care for all families with income above the standard. Inpatient care is subject to cost-sharing only if the family's income is above the medical assistance standard.

The approach chosen to deal with the question of which families would remain on Medicaid and which would opt for CIPP coverage was based on conversations with several state officials who suggested that, were CIPP in existence, relatively few individuals would choose to spend down (thus reducing their assets) for Medicaid coverage. Unless families were already under the public assistance standard, most would choose CIPP coverage. This assumption has been operationalized in the following manner. Families are assumed to choose CIPP unless their income is low enough to qualify for public assistance or is one income class (usually $1,000) above the public assistance level. The assumed Medicaid cutoff is thus slightly higher than the public assistance level.

The CIPP plan would result in an increase in tax revenues to the state, irrespective of how the program was financed. Since the purpose of this report is to estimate the net cost to the state of CIPP, an attempt was made to assess this impact.

To understand the reasons for the tax revenue increase, consider an individual with a medical expense of a certain magnitude, with and without the CIPP plan in force. Without CIPP, if the individual itemizes deductions on his tax return, and his medical bills are sufficiently large to qualify, a deduction will be taken and the individual's tax liability decreased.

If, however, the CIPP plan was in force, and the individual qualified for assistance, the individual would not claim as a tax deduction the portion of the expense that the CIPP plan paid. His tax liability (and the state's tax revenues) would be higher with CIPP in force than without it. The amount of the increase would be the portion of the expense paid by the CIPP plan, multiplied by the individual's marginal state income tax rate.[14]

The expected increase in state income taxes for each cell is the product of three factors; the probability that a family in the cell would claim a medical deduction if CIPP were not in force; the expected marginal state income tax rate for the cell; the CIPP claims expense for the cell. The estimation procedure for the first two factors is described elsewhere.[15]

Private Health Insurance Coverage

The CIPP cost estimates depend crucially on the assumptions regarding the private health insurance coverage of the state population. Clearly, the passage of CIPP would have a major impact on the distribution and amount of such coverage. Many individuals and families, particularly those with low incomes, will have little incentive to purchase any private health insurance. For those that continue to purchase insurance, the existence of CIPP will provide incentives to change the form of coverage. Any change in private health insurance coverage designed to take advantage of CIPP will have the effect of raising the cost of CIPP to the state.

In preparing the cost estimates for CIPP, we were instructed to estimate the cost of CIPP on the rather unrealistic assumption that the present structure of private health insurance in force remains unaffected. Private health insurance policies vary enormously in detail; for example, some pay a simple proportion of expenses with or without a deductible; others pay stated dollar amounts or give benefits in terms of services covered rather than· dollar figures. In addition, policies vary according to the types of expense excluded from coverage and the maximum benefits that the plan pays.

Faced with such complexity, we were forced to make some rather drastic simplifying assumptions since there exist no studies describing (in sufficient detail to be useful) the policies carried by different segments of the population. These assumptions concerned the "representative" private policy, the number of people in the state covered by such a policy, and the premiums paid by the covered individuals (or by others such as employers). The policy is assumed to pay 75 percent of all costs after a deductible. The deductible is $25 for single individuals and $25 per person up to a maximum of $75 for families with three or more individuals. The maximum benefit paid by the plan is $10,000 for single individuals and $10,000 per person up to maximum of $30,000 for a family of three or more individuals. The annual premium cost (which reduces the CIPP deductible) is $240 for a single individual, $300 for a family of two, and $360 for a family of three or more individuals. The proportion of the population covered under the representative insurance policy is assumed to vary by income only and to be equal to the proportion of that income class with hospital insurance according to National Health Survey data for 1968.[16]

The representative policy is thus characterized by four parameters:

☐ PIC—Percent of expense paid by the insured individual or family
☐ PID—The deductible
☐ PIPREM—The annual premium
☐ PIMAX—The maximum amount of dollar benefits paid by the insurance plan.

Since CIPP payments are based on family expenses net of any other insurance payments, the value of gross medical expenses necessary to cause the CIPP deductible and/or expense limit to be met will never be less than, and in general will be greater than what they would be in the absence of private insurance.

The order in which the CIPP deductible (D), the private insurance deductible (PID), CIPP expense limit (L) and private insurance maximum payment ($PIMAX$) will come into play will depend on the value of the CIPP deductible and expense limit of the family. Let the value of gross expense, X, at which each of these four provisions becomes effective be denoted as XD, $XPID$, XL, $XPIMAX$, respectively. With four

values there are 24 possible orderings; however, it was necessary to consider only five.

To avoid reproducing a great deal of cumbersome algebra let us consider only one of these five cases and suppose that for a particular family we have determined the four critical values of X and they have the following order: $XPID$, XD, $XPIMAX$, XL.

The expected value of costs to CIPP in this case is given by the following expected value function:

$$EC_{j,k} = P_j \left(.8 \int_{XD_{jk}}^{XPIMAX} .25\, x_j g_j(x_j)dx + .8 \int_{XPIMAX}^{XL_K} X_j g_j(x_j)dx + \int_{XL_k}^{\infty} X_j g_j(x_j)dx \right).$$

For gross expenses less than XD there will be no cost chargeable to CIPP since it is only when gross expenses total XD that the out-of-pocket expenses of the family equal D. For gross expenses in excess of XD the CIPP pays 80 percent of the 25 percent of expenses not paid by the private insurance policy. When gross expenses total $XPIMAX$, the private insurance benefits are exhausted (the private insurance policy has paid an amount equal to $PIMAX$), and CIPP begins paying 80 percent. When gross expenses total XL, the out-of-pocket expenditure of the family has reached the CIPP expense limit, L, and any additional expenses will be borne entirely by CIPP.

For each population cell the values of XD, $XPID$, $XPIMAX$, and XL were determined and then, depending on the order of these values, one of five expected value functions was used to calculate the expected cost to CIPP.

Results and Concluding Comments

In the preceding sections we have outlined the methodology followed to estimate the cost to New York State of the CIPP plan. These costs incorporate claims expense, administrative expense, and changes in the state's tax revenues due to the plan. The results presented in this section separate out these costs effects and show the total costs to the state based on three different assumptions concerning the extent of private health insurance, and two different assumptions concerning the size of administrative costs based on Medicare and Medicaid experience.[17]

Table 5. Cost to New York State of CIPP plan (in $ millions)

	Private health insurance coverage		
	Existing coverage	**50% of existing coverage**	**No coverage**
1 Claims expense	$452	$2,034	$3,616
2 Tax savings	15	104	198
3 Costs before administrative costs (1 – 2)	437	1,930	3,418
4 Administrative costs at 5% of claims expense	23	102	181
5 Net costs to state with 5% administrative costs (3 + 4)	$460	$2,032	$3,599
6 Administrative costs at 10% of claims expense	45	204	362
7 Net cost to state at 10% of claims expense (3 + 6)	$482	$2,134	$3,780

Table 5 is a summary of the basic results. If the extent of private health insurance is unchanged under the CIPP plan, we estimate the total cost to New York State in 1975 to lie between $460-million and $482-million, depending on the amount of administrative costs. If, however, half the people currently carrying private health insurance drop their coverage, we estimate the cost to New York State in 1975 to lie between $2.032-billion and $2.134-billion. Finally, if everyone drops private health insurance following the enactment of the CIPP plan, the estimated cost lies between $3.599-billion and $3.780-billion.

The estimated costs are strongly influenced by effect of CIPP on the level of private health insurance coverage. The figures given for 50 percent of existing coverage give only a guide to the magnitude of the impact. This is due to the fact that our representative policy is a simplification and to the fact that merely dropping that coverage is an oversimplification of the response to a government imposed health insurance program.

In reality, two things will happen. Some people will drop their private coverage entirely, and perhaps more importantly, the benefit structures of private health insurance will change in order to take maximum advantage of coverage under CIPP. In both cases, however, the effect will be to raise the cost of CIPP above the cost if the present level of private health insurance were unaffected. We suspect that the higher figure—nearly $4-billion—is more likely to be in the neighborhood of the true cost.

Lastly, it should be pointed out that the estimates represent steady state costs of the program. There are a number of individuals who, but for financial reasons, would seek medical attention for existing but not debilitating ailments. Were the CIPP plan to become effective, some proportion of these individuals would begin treatments, have surgery, etc. This phenomenon would produce a surge in demand for medical care in the early years of the program, which would abate as the individuals with ailments existing at the time of passage of the bill were accommodated. While the magnitude of additional cost caused by this pent-up demand is interesting, we felt that the long-run steady state costs were of greater importance. Thus, the cost estimate for 1975 treats the demand in 1975 as if the program had been in effect for a sufficient period to allow the pent-up demand, existing at the time of enactment of the bill, to have been satisfied.

References and Notes

1 New York State, Senate Bill 5226-A (1973–74). The modification consists of assuming that CIPP does not cover persons over 65. As discussed in the text, data limitations precluded the possibility of reliable cost estimates for this age group.

2 Arthur D. Little, Inc., *Deep Coverage in Health Insurance and Treatment of Catastrophic Illness*, Preliminary Report to DHEW, Contract #HSM 110-71-197.

3 The purpose of this provision is to provide an incentive for families to retain private health insurance.

4 Where the benefit structures of the two programs differ, we have, in effect, assumed that the demand for health care is completely inelastic with respect to price.

5 Note that the observed frequency distributions referred to here are those that result from the recombination of Aetna claimant categories into those corresponding to census classifications.

6 For this reason the exponential distribution will not pass the X^2 test at conventional levels of significance (except in a few cases). An alternative would be to derive the distributions empirically. Better fitting distributions than the exponential might be found this way, but the computational effort required was beyond the scope of this study.

7 See, for example: Hogg, Robert V. and Craig, Allen T. *Introduction to Mathematical Statistics*, 3rd edition (New York: MacMillan Company, 1970) Chapter 4, especially pages 125–152.

8 For the purposes of making the calculations, an approximation to the theoretically correct distribution was actually employed. Barton, David M. and Smiley, Robert H. *An Economic Analysis of the Projected Cost to New York State of Proposed Senate Bill 5226-A*, Final Report to the New York State Senate Health Committee, 1974.

9 Consider a family of two adults, i and j, and n children. The P applicable in this case would be calculated as:

$$P_{i,j,nc} = 1 - (1 - P_i)(1 - P_j)(1 - P_c)^n.$$

10 This factor was derived by taking the ratio of the average daily service charge in New York Hospital, $59.02, to that of the nation as a whole, $42.42 [American Hospital Association. *Survey of Hospital Charges as of January 1, 1972* (Chicago: AHA, 1972) p. 140 ff, Table B2]. The average daily service charge includes room accommodation, food service, routine nursing care, and minor medical and surgical supplies.

11 The rate of inflation in the medical care component of the Consumer Price Index (CPI) between December, 1970 and December, 1972 was 8.2 percent or a little over 4 percent a year. Since the rate of overall inflation has risen in the past year, a rate of 6 percent was used as the projected rate of inflation from 1972 to 1975.

12 This factor was arrived at by asking an Aetna actuary to give his "best guess" regarding the increased cost of insuring a blue-collar population with benefits identical to those available under coverage by Aetna.

13 U.S. Department of Commerce, Bureau of the Census. *Census of the Population, 1970, Detailed Characteristics—New York*, Volume 34, Table 198 and 156.

14 There may be a related decrease in tax receipts, depending on how CIPP is financed. If, for example, CIPP were to be financed by employer contributions, employees' taxable income would decrease, and thus state corporation income taxes would decrease. However, since our analysis did not deal with the method used to finance the plan, this issue could not be addressed.

15 Barton and Smiley, *op. cit.* In the original report, we also discuss how state tax revenues will vary with the amount of private health insurance purchased, and how we account for this variation.

16 National Center for Health Statistics. *Hospital and Surgical Insurance Coverage, United States—1968*, Vital and Health Statistics, Series 10, No. 66 (DHEW Publication No. (HSM) 72-1033, January 1972) Table 3, p. 19.

17 Administrative costs for Medicaid and Medicare coverage between 5 and 10 percent of total claims for most states. See: *Medicare and Medicaid, Problems, Issues and Alternatives*, Report of the Staff to the Committee on Finance, United States, Senate, February 9, 1970, 35-7190, pp. 314–316.

Avedis Donabedian

An Evaluation of Prepaid Group Practice

Reprinted with permission of the Blue Cross Association, from *Inquiry:* Vol.VI, No.3, pp.3-27. Copyright © 1969 by the Blue Cross Association.

Originally Published in September 1969

Much has been written for and against group practice in general, and prepaid group practice in particular. This report will not deal with this controversy, nor with the theoretical advantages of one form of organizing medical care over another. It will restrict itself to a review of what is generally known about the *actual performance* of prepaid group practice plans as compared with alternative modes of organized financing for medical care. The review will be based almost entirely on published information. Moreover, it will include only those studies which permit fairly valid comparisons to be made. The following aspects of performance will be examined: choice of plan and satisfaction with the plan on the part of subscribers; the opinions of participating physicians concerning prepaid group practice and concerning subscribers to these plans; utilization of ambulatory and hospital services and costs incurred by comparable population groups served by a variety of insurance plans, including

prepaid group practice; productivity; and the quality of care provided by prepaid group practice and alternative plans. It is hoped that after these various features have been examined a clearer picture will emerge of what prepaid group practice has achieved so far and what it may have to offer in the future.

Limitations of space will not permit full documentation of the information and opinions offered in this paper. A more complete report including extensive documentation has been published as a separate monograph.[1] This paper summarizes information included in the monograph and adds the findings of more recent studies. Since the older studies are covered more fully in the monograph, this review devotes somewhat more space to the more recent studies than their relative importance might warrant.

The Subscribers

The first question that will concern us in evaluating the performance of prepaid group practice plans is the extent to which they meet the expectations of consumers and potential consumers of medical care. Three kinds of information have a bearing on this question. These are: 1) the frequency with which persons who are offered alternative choices elect prepaid group practice, the characteristics of those who choose a group practice plan, and the reasons given for election or rejection of the plans offered; 2) opinions expressed by

Avedis Donabedian, M.D. is Professor of Medical Care Organization, Department of Medical Care Organization, School of Public Health, University of Michigan. Valuable assistance in the preparation of this review was received from several colleagues in the Department of Medical Care Organization. The author is especially indebted to Professors S. J. Axelrod, C. A. Metzner and R. L. Bashshur and to Mr. S. E. Berki.

Financial support for part of the work on which this review is based was provided by a grant from the American Motors Corporation and the General Research Support grant (NIH-1-SO1-FR-05447-02) from the Public Health Service.

participants in prepaid group practice plans; and 3) the frequency with which plan subscribers use services outside the plan in preference to those available to them within the plan. These last two may be taken to provide subjective and objective evidence of consumer satisfaction.

Choice of Plan

It has become customary for employees to be offered at least two alternative health insurance plans from which to choose. The proportion of employees who select a prepaid group practice plan under these so-called "dual choice" provisions is one indicator of public acceptance. Data from several published studies suggest that, in different employee groups, anywhere from 20 to 60 percent of persons choose in favor of prepaid group practice.[2-4] There are also instances in which as few as 2 to 5 percent of employees initially give up coverage under a standard Blue Cross-Blue Shield plan in favor of prepaid group practice, even though the latter generally provides more benefits for an equivalent premium. On the other hand, in some small groups with special characteristics, prepaid group practice may be preferred by 80 percent or more of the members. Under the Federal Employees Health Benefits Program, employees are given a choice of a number of insurance plans including prepaid group practice where this is available in a given locality. The record shows that in 10 localities across the U.S. where such a choice is possible, the percent of Federal employees who choose prepaid group practice ranges from 2.5 percent in the St. Paul metropolitan area to 44.8 percent in the Los Angeles metropolitan area.[5] There appears to be a geographic factor probably related to plan characteristics. On the West Coast, in localities where the Kaiser-Permanente plans are in operation, more than 30 percent of employees select such a plan. In most other areas, group practice plans are chosen by less than 6 percent of employees. Henderson, who has reported these data, believes that the major reasons why employees do not select a group prac-

tice are 1) limitation of the geographic area within which the plans operate; 2) limitations on free choice of physician and, sometimes, of hospital; 3) ideological opposition to what is regarded as "socialized medicine"; and 4) gaps in coverage as compared with the two government-wide plans.

More systematic examination of the factors that influence choice should give some understanding of what aspects of prepaid group practice attract or repel prospective clients, and what the potential for further growth might be. The factors influencing choice have been studied by Wolfman,[2] Anderson and Sheatsley[6] and, most systematically, by Metzner and Bashshur.[7-10]

Metzner and Bashshur studied a sample of members of the United Automobile Workers Union (UAW) who were offered a choice between Blue Cross-Blue Shield and a hospital-based, union-sponsored prepaid group practice plan, the Community Health Association (CHA) of Detroit. They conclude that, in this population, general values and ideology were not significant elements in choice. Blue Cross-Blue Shield and CHA members were essentially similar with respect to general attitudes and values concerning progress, innovation, financial security, individualism and role of government. CHA members did, however, express somewhat greater approval of union involvement in medical care arrangements for workers and were, themselves, more involved in union activities.

More important in choice, according to Metzner and Bashshur, is a pragmatic evaluation of the specific attributes of the rival plans. According to their model, the choice between plans depends on 1) knowledge that a choice is available, 2) knowledge concerning specific health care plan attributes and their ascription to one, or other, or both of the plans, and 3) the degree of importance of, or valuation placed upon, each attribute. The application of such a model to their data, which included 26 plan attributes, has enabled a correct prediction of 88 percent of actual choices in a dual choice situation. This represents about 50 percent improvement over the prediction possible simply by knowing the percentage of those who chose each plan.

Knowledge for Choice

Data on the degree of knowledge necessary for choice confirm the difficulty with which new ideas permeate among members of the society, at least among the working class. In Detroit, 32 percent of the sample of UAW members who had selected Blue Cross-Blue Shield did not know that an alternative choice was available. Furthermore, among those who knew they had a choice, there was a large proportion who had little information, or were misinformed about the group practice plan.[7]

The predisposition to receive, and act upon, information may be related to the needs and interests of the potential recipient. In this connection, Bashshur and Metzner advance the notion of "vulnerability."[8, 9] This appears to depend on a subjective estimate partly of the probability of illness and the magnitude of expenditures for care and, partly, of the disruptive effect that illness and costs might have on an established, and relatively secure, style of life. In addition to bringing about receptivity to relevant information, vulnerability would also result in placing a much higher valuation on the greater protection against unforeseen expenditures attributed to prepaid group practice. Accordingly, knowledge concerning prepaid group practice, and the predisposition to choose it are greater among persons who are older, married, have a larger number of children, do not belong to the lowest income group, and own their homes (Table 1).

The importance of information becomes even more critical in the light of the finding, by Metzner and Bashshur, that of those who chose Blue Cross-Blue Shield, a majority considered as "very important" certain features of medical care that prepaid group practice tends to emphasize. These include the availability of certain

Table 1. Selected characteristics of members of the United Automobile Workers Union, by health insurance plan chosen, selected area in Detroit, Spring, 1964

	Plan chosen (percent)	
	CHA	BC-BS
Demographic characteristics		
Under 30	8	21
Married with children	75	66
Of those married, percent who have four or more children under 18	19	14
Family income under $4000	2	9
Opinions concerning importance of selected plan attributes[a]		
Coverage for home and office care	79 (96)	67 (89)
Family doctors and specialists work together in groups	68 (83)	46 (62)
Provision of shots and checkups	74 (94)	64 (86)
To have a family doctor or one to go to regularly	70 (90)	81 (94)
Seeing the same doctor most of the time	64 (91)	70 (89)
Picking the doctor to go to	61 (87)	79 (94)
Availability of specialists	62 (79)	51 (65)
Having a say in how the plan is run	46 (64)	30 (53)
Having the union arrange for medical care	64 (77)	46 (60)
Reasons given for choice[b]		
Financial reasons: lower expense, more coverage, etc.	51 (23)	
Complaints about Blue Cross-Blue Shield: mainly costs	16 (5)	
Incumbency: has BC-BS; parents had BC-BS; plan reputable, established, more dependable		38 (5)
Can choose own doctor or hospital		20 (16)
Did not know about choice or did not know enough about CHA	16	(4)
CHA too localized, not national	6	(2)

[a]Figures not in parentheses are percent of those in each plan who thought each specified attribute was "very important." Figures in parentheses are the sums of the percentages of those who thought the attribute was "very important" and those who thought it was "somewhat important." [b]Figures not in parentheses are percent of first mentions by respondents in each plan, and figures in parentheses are percent of second mentions. The few salient reasons are given in the table. Other reasons were very infrequently mentioned. Source: References 7, 8 and 10.

preventive services, the establishment of a stable relationship with a physician and the availability of specialists. Perhaps more to the point, 67 percent of respondents in Blue Cross-Blue Shield said that it was very important to be covered for doctor's home and office services, and 46 percent said that it was very important "that family doctors and specialists work together in the same place as a group." It was found, however, that those who chose prepaid group practice put, in general, a somewhat higher valuation on these features. The difference was most marked with respect to the desirability of having family doctors and specialists work together in the same place as a group. Sixty-eight percent of the sample of CHA enrollees thought this was very important, as compared to 46 percent of the sample of Blue Cross-Blue Shield enrollees (Table 1).

Persons who choose prepaid group practice most often say that they do so because of the greater security that these plans offer against the costs of illness. Those who select the alternative plan say that it offers them greater freedom to choose a physician. Wolfman[2] compared a sample of automobile workers who had selected Kaiser-Permanente. Of the 100 families who selected Blue Cross-Blue Shield, 37 had rejected the Kaiser plan outright without considering relative economic merit, because of hostility to this kind of service. It is a moot point whether ideology underlies this hostility. The remaining 63 families had given thought to economic factors but selected Blue Cross-Blue Shield nevertheless. Free choice seemed to be a more potent factor among the more educated and higher income families. According to Wolfman, "Some of these families seemed to regard freedom of choice in medical care, like owning a car, as a goal to which they aspired regardless of its economic merits. To be able to afford the opportunity of free choice appeared to be a symbol of economic and social independence—possibly a step upward from their previous circumstances."[2]

The findings of Metzner and Bashshur support these earlier findings to some extent (Table 1). Of automobile workers in Detroit who chose CHA, 51 percent mentioned in first place financial reasons including lower expenses, especially for larger families, and more protection re-

sulting from a larger range of benefits. An additional 23 percent mentioned financial reasons in second place. Of those who chose Blue Cross-Blue Shield, 20 percent gave as a first reason, and 16 percent as a second reason, the ability to choose a physician or a hospital. The emphasis on choice of hospital is especially interesting, but may have been more than ordinarily salient because of the historical associations of the prepaid group practice hospital in this particular plan.

Relationship with Doctor

Previous medical experience in general, and the prior establishment of a relationship with a regular doctor in particular, may be an important factor in which one of two plans is chosen. In addition to emphasizing lower cost and better coverage, many of those who had chosen Kaiser-Permanente, in preference to Blue Cross-Blue Shield, mentioned unfavorable reactions or experiences regarding the latter plan.[2] In Detroit, 16 percent of persons who had chosen CHA mentioned as a first reason complaints about rates, cost, coverage and service under Blue Cross-Blue Shield. An additional 5 percent gave similar complaints as a second reason. In another study, persons who joined the Health Insurance Plan of Greater New York (HIP), a prepaid group practice plan, had had a regular doctor and had received private medical care less frequently than those who joined Group Health Insurance (GHI), a plan that provides comparable benefits but permits virtual free choice of physician. HIP subscribers had used more clinic care and more often had been satisfied with such care.[6]

However, contrary to expectation, respondents in Detroit, although they emphasized freedom of choice and the desirability of having a stable relationship with a physician, very rarely mentioned existing ties with a doctor or hospital as a factor in selecting the plan to which they belonged. By contrast, pre-existing ties to the older insurance plan was the most frequent reason given by those who had not chosen the newer prepaid group practice plan. About 38 percent of those who had chosen Blue Cross-Blue Shield gave as the most important reason for doing so factors relating to incumbency: that the respondent or his parents had Blue Cross-Blue Shield, sometimes for long periods of time, and that this plan was established, reputable and dependable. This is in keeping with the experience of the Kaiser Foundation Health Plans which indicates that in employee groups that start with a dual choice program there is approximately equal enrollment in the two plans offered. But when dual choice is introduced to a group which already belongs to a prepayment plan, the established plan has a decided advantage.[11] As already pointed out, in addition to representing established and familiar ties, the existing form of organization is the beneficiary of the difficulty with which information about new plans is disseminated and acquired.

Finally, factors related to location and distance may be important in choice. The Detroit study strongly suggests that a disproportionately large share of the clients of the prepaid group practice plan were drawn from the vicinity of the central facility and its satellite clinics. Further study to establish more clearly the influence of distance is in progress. In the meanwhile it is reasonable to assume that an insurance plan that can tap a wide range of community resources and is not restricted to a relatively few sources of care would appear to enjoy a significant advantage.

It is difficult, on the basis of the studies reviewed, to arrive at a simple statement concerning the acceptability of prepaid group practice to people in general. It appears, however, that at least some segments of the population have acquired sufficient sophistication to appreciate many features of the organization of care that prepaid group practice tends to emphasize. What may be lacking is accurate information and the opportunity (real or perceived) for choice. Given information and opportunity, potential clients tend to choose not on the basis of general ideological factors, but on the grounds of which plan best meets their needs as they see them. Under these circumstances, expectations of greater protection against medical care expenditures, at worst without injury to quality, appear to be the strongest selling points for prepaid group practice. The greatest obstacle they face is the existence of reasonably satisfactory ties with an already established system. There may, of course, be other obstacles, such as opposition by the medical profession, which have not figured in the studies reviewed in this paper.

Subscriber Opinion

A question of central importance is whether persons who receive service in prepaid group practice plans have a favorable opinion of the care received, of the physicians who provide care, and of the conditions under which care is provided. A review of several studies suggests that the great majority of subscribers are satisfied with whatever plan they belong to in spite of substantial differences in the features of the plans compared.[6, 12-14] Although the majority of subscribers express satisfaction, there appears to be a small "hard core" of dissatisfied persons, roughly about 10 percent of all subscribers, who hold decidedly negative views of almost all aspects of the plan to which they belong. It appears that these intensely dissatisfied individuals are not likely to change their views and that to protect the plan, if nothing else, an alternative choice must be made available to them.

Those subscribers who complain, do so about a large variety of things: there is a certain impersonality about the care received; physicians are not interested and rush the patient out of the office, do not give him an opportunity to explain his trouble exactly, and do not tell him enough about his illness; there is the atmosphere of a clinic and of charity medical care; obtaining medical care is inconvenient; one waits too long to see the doctor; it is difficult to get a home visit. Less frequently there are complaints about the quality of care. Restriction of free choice of physician is seldom mentioned explicitly. Presumably those who make an issue of free choice have already ruled themselves out of the plan.

It is reasonable to assume, as some studies suggest, that an appreciable proportion of complaints made by subscribers to prepaid group practice plans apply to medical care everywhere.[13, 14] There are, however, certain features of organized group practice that appear to evoke fairly characteristic responses in their subscribers. Freidson[14] points out that prepaid group practice is thought by patients to promote the technical quality of care but to hamper the establishment of a satisfactory personal relationship with the physician. Subscribers seem to think that good quality occurs not because of the superiority of individual physicians in the plan, but through the use of the technical, diagnostic and consultative resources which the plan can muster. Furthermore, subscribers appreciate the absence of financial incentives in the use of these services. Data from the Labor Health Institute of St. Louis[13] indicate that subscribers tend to accept perceived limitations in care, so long as the quality of care is thought to be superior.

In contrast to its enhancing effect on the perception of quality, group practice by its very mode of organization is thought not to be conducive to personal interest and concern on the part of the plan and its physicians. According to Freidson, several factors are responsible for this. The first is alteration in the method of payment from fee-for-service to prepayment. The patient thinks this weakens the physician's incentive to care for him. There are, in addition, the many rules and regulations that govern practice and appear to render it less responsive to patient need. The complexity of the physical set-up and the larger number of persons intervening between the patient and the physician add to this feeling. High turnover in medical staff and interchange-ability of physicians make it even more difficult to develop a personal relationship. In fact as many as 35 percent of subscribers to the Labor Health Institute, and 38 percent of subscribers to one HIP group, did not consider the plan physician to be their "family" or "regular" doctor. In the Labor Health Institute, "although about 90 percent of the respondents who used medical and dental services felt that the doctors take the proper amount of professional interest in them, treat them as private patients, and provide them with good quality care, only 65 percent of these people feel that the physicians are their family doctors. . . . The accolade of family doctor is not easily won."[13]

A more recent study of consumer opinion in one prepaid group practice plan revealed an even higher level of satisfaction than reported in previous studies.[15] Seventy-eight percent of respondents said that they liked the plan very much. Furthermore, there was no evidence of a significant hard core of dissatisfied members. Dual choice and selective withdrawal from the plan may have helped to bring about this favorable situation. The study also reports some additional interesting findings. As many as 52 percent of members had joined the plan without strongly partisan feelings, seemingly to give it a try. About 70 percent of these, after approximately three years of experience with the plan, reported that they now liked the plan very much. By contrast, very few members (6 percent) had developed a less favorable opinion of the plan than they originally held. Further to the credit of the plan, there is evidence that need for service and use of service contributed to the acquisition of favorable opinions.

The study also inquired into whether the respondent had complaints or knew of someone who did. Although this form of questioning invites multiple counting, about 60 percent of respondents answered in the negative. Furthermore, the authors contend that complaints do not necessarily signify dissatisfaction with the plan but may represent concern for improving still further a plan which members fundamentally approve. This is supported by the observation that complaints were very specific in nature and that about 33 percent of persons who liked the plan very much had, or knew of, some complaint. It remains true, however, that complaints were reported twice as frequently by respondents who did not express strong satisfaction with the plan.

Use of Services Outside the Plan

One important indicator of consumer satisfaction might be the extent to which subscribers to prepaid group practice plans continue to use services outside the plans in preference to the corresponding services available to them within the plans. It is fairly well established that an appreciable proportion of subscribers continue to do so.[12-16] Outside physicians are used for 37 percent of surgical operations in the Health Insurance Plan of Greater New York, 14 percent of all paid physicians' services and 33 percent of home calls in Kaiser-Permanente, and 23 percent of physicians' and dentists' services in the Labor Health Institute of St. Louis. During a period of approximately three years, 39 percent of the members of the Community Health Association (CHA) of Detroit had used physicians outside the plan.

The use of outside services appears to be related to the nature of the service, the characteristics of the subscriber, the opinions of the subscriber about the plan, and the existence and nature of a prior patient-physician relationship. Freidson found in one HIP group that 41 percent of the outside use of surgical and obstetrical services was for childbirth and 26 percent was for gynecological operations. In 61 percent of instances a physician formerly known by the subscriber was used. Persons who use outside services were more likely to be of higher education and occupational attainments, more critical and selective in seeking medical care, more quick to take offense with real or fancied slights, more resentful of the "clinic" atmosphere and,

in many ways more negative in their opinions of the plan and its physicians.

These findings are partly supported by the CHA study in Detroit; but in this population group the responsibility of the wife for use of outside physicians was not so markedly dominant. Of the total number of reports that one or more family members had used a physician outside the plan, 35 percent represented use by the wife alone, 29 percent by the husband alone, 53 percent by the wife alone or in combination with some other member of the family, and 39 percent by the husband alone or in combination with another member of the family. In 31 percent of cases where only the husband or wife had gone to an outside physician one or more times, a specialist was consulted. In the case of the wife, the specialist was an obstetrician or gynecologist in 38 percent of reports. Respondents who reported use of an outside physician were less likely to have a favorable view of the plan and more likely to have complaints. Such attitudes may not, however, fully account for the use of outside physicians. As many as 68 percent of respondents who reported the use of outside physicians said that they liked the plan very much, as compared to 84 percent of respondents who had not used outside physicians; and the frequency with which complaints were reported by those who used outside physicians was only 42 percent as compared to 36 percent for those who had not used outside physicians.[10, 15]

Experience in both the Labor Health Institute and the HIP-Montefiore Group shows that subscribers who had a "family" or "regular" physician prior to joining the plan are much more likely to use outside services. But this does not hold if the subscriber was not satisfied with his "regular" physician.

Convenience is an additional factor that often leads to the use of services outside the plan. In the CHA study the occurrence of an emergency was cited as a reason by 12 percent of respondents who reported use of an outside physician.

In summary, it may be said that the use

of outside services is significant in group practice. It occurs partly because of dissatisfaction with services offered in the plan. Partly it is the expression of previously established relationships with an outside doctor and of the greater convenience, under certain circumstances, of obtaining care outside the plan.

At this point it may be useful to recapitulate some points, already made, which physicians need to ponder. Persons who have a regular physician with whom they are satisfied are less likely to choose prepaid group practice when an alternative plan that permits free choice of physician is offered. Should they join a prepaid group practice plan they are less likely to be satisfied with services offered by the plan and more likely to get outside care, often from the physician they knew before they joined. To some extent consumer acceptance of prepaid group practice plans is an expression of the absence of a prior patient-physician relationship or of a breakdown in such relationships.

The Physicians

Little is known about the kind of physician who chooses prepaid group practice in preference to the more prevalent and professionally acceptable ways of conducting practice. Even less is known about how these physicians view themselves, their practice and their patients. One published study on this subject deals with a nonrandom selection of groups in the Health Insurance Plan of Greater New York and of physicians within each of these groups.[17] Consequently, the findings cannot be accepted as representative of prepaid group practice in general. They are, nevertheless, sufficiently interesting to warrant mention.

About two-thirds of physicians felt that prepaid group practice was preferable to the traditional form and permitted them to practice, in association with their colleagues, the kind of medicine carried out at a teaching hospital. But a quarter to a third of physicians were also aware of certain adverse effects that they attributed

to this form of organization. They felt that by becoming associated with this type of practice they had lost status in the eyes of medical colleagues as well as of the patients they served. They felt that they did not have time to do a good job. They felt that their patients were demanding, made excessive use of services, complained too much and were lacking in loyalty. For an appreciable number of physicians then, prepaid group practice was seen as having an adverse effect on the patient-physician relationship and a hampering effect on their own careers especially in matters that involved the medical community in general. It is interesting that the viewpoint of these physicians reinforces the perceptions that some patients have of the strain that group practice imposes on the patient-physician relationship.

Utilization of Service

Concern over rising costs of medical and hospital care have intensified the search for more efficient methods of organizing medical care. This has directed a great deal of attention to utilization rates, especially of hospital services, in prepaid group practice as compared with other forms of health insurance. Utilization data are fairly easy to assemble and compare but very difficult to interpret. In the first instance, utilization of service depends on the occurrence of a condition which must be recognized by the patient, or by those responsible for him, to require medical attention. Once care is initiated by the patient, further use of service is largely determined by the manner in which the physician manages the case, subject, of course, to continuing cooperation by the patient.

The organization of service and of financing can affect this process of seeking and receiving care at various junctures and in different ways, some desirable and some not. Utilization might be increased appropriately through an eductional program that helps subscribers to recognize need for care, a program of detection through regular physical examination and screening procedures, more thorough clinical investigation at each patient visit, and removing barriers (financial and administrative) to seeking care and continuing care in accordance with medical recommendations. Utilization might be increased inappropriately through the absence of checks on excessive patient demands, the absence of checks on over-investigation and over-treatment by the physician, and the presence of incentives (of financial rewards, convenience, etc.) to over-treatment, excessive surgery, over-consultation or over-hospitalization.

Utilization might be decreased appropriately through early detection and prevention of illness, the effective management of illness, and the use of less expensive alternative services (of the clinic instead of the hospital, for example). It might be decreased inappropriately through neglecting patient education, erecting financial or administrative barriers to access to the doctor, erecting barriers to continuing care, and providing less than needed care. The key question is not what is the level of utilization that is associated with any system of organizing care but what precisely happens to utilization and why. In the following sections the available data on levels of utilization will be described. But the answer to the key question: "In what ways is utilization affected?" will remain largely a matter for speculation.

Use of Ambulatory Services

The use of ambulatory services has not been studied as thoroughly as has hospital utilization. From a review of three comparative studies that include a prepaid group practice plan[6, 12, 16] and some that do not[18, 19] one might safely say that the provision of ambulatory services as a benefit tends to increase the use of these services to a modest degree. But it is not possible, from the available evidence, to reach any conclusions about the comparative frequency of ambulatory services in a prepaid group practice plan and another plan that provides ambulatory care benefits but permits free choice of physicians.[6] In the three comparative studies reviewed (Studies 6, 12 and 16), roughly similar proportions of persons make one yearly visit only or 10 visits a year or more. This suggests that there is no remarkable abuse of the prepaid group practice plan, even when it provides broader benefits, either through use for trivial complaints or through repeated or excessive use. That insurance coverage for ambulatory service is not associated with conspicuous abuse is confirmed by other experience, notably in Windsor, Ontario.[20] In fact, even when most financial barriers are removed, about 25 to 30 percent of persons entitled to service make no visits at all during the year.

A more recent study[21] compares the utilization experience of Old Age Assistance recipients who obtained medical care through the traditional welfare system in New York City with another group who obtained care through an arrangement with a prepaid group practice (HIP). Although the two groups were selected on the basis of residence, rather than by a randomizing process, they were roughly comparable except that the clients of the group practice had a larger proportion who were from Puerto Rico or Latin America, and a smaller proportion from Eastern Europe. The aggregate use of physician services in the two groups was comparable both before and after the introduction of the program. There was, however, a change in the manner in which services were distributed and used. Under the prepaid program a) a larger proportion obtained at least some ambulatory care; b) previously low utilizers increased their use of service and those who previously were high utilizers decreased their use of service to some extent; c) home visits were strikingly fewer; and d) the use of ancillary services and supplies was greater. These findings are consistent with efforts made to reduce barriers to care (including provision of transportation), to adjust care to need, and to provide a wider range of services under group practice.

Hospital Utilization

There is much evidence, which will not be reviewed here, that the provision of insurance for hospital services, under any form, is associated with an increase in hospital use. It is generally believed that some of this increase in hospital use is justified and desirable; but that some is unjustified and excessive. Does prepaid group practice, first through the removal of financial incentives to the physician, and secondly through the operation of professional restraints within the group, offer one means of controlling unnecessary utilization? Table 2 assembles data from the major comparative studies that have attempted to answer this question. In the first of these (Study 16) a comparison is made between a sample that represents the subscribers of a prepaid group practice plan (HIP) and a sample representative of the New York City population (NYC). The excess in HIP admissions might seem at first sight to be due to the fact that about half of the NYC sample had no medical care insurance. But when the NYC utilization is determined for the insured and uninsured, the hospital rates are higher for the uninsured than the insured. This extraordinary finding has not been adequately explained but may be due in part to the ready availability of free care in New York City.

In the second study (Study 22) the comparisons are between HIP enrollees who are employees of New York City and a sample of workers in comparable employments covered by Blue Cross-Blue Shield (BC-BS). The Blue Cross-Blue Shield plan differs in at least two ways from HIP: it does not cover physician services outside the hospital and has few mechanisms for controlling the practice of individual physicians. Under these circumstances HIP appears to exert the greater control over utilization.

The circumstances are somewhat different in the third and fourth comparisons (Studies 6 and 3) between HIP and Group Health Insurance (GHI). The populations

Table 2. Hospital utilization by subscribers to specified medical care insurance plans[a]

Hospital utilization[b]	Study 16		Study 22		Study 6[c]		Study 3[d]		Study 4[d]		Study 12[e]			Study 23[f]		
	HIP	NYC	HIP	BC-BS	HIP	GHI	HIP	GHI	HIP	UP	K-P	MM	BC-BS	K-P	CWO	BC-BS
Hospital admission rate	81	74	81[d]	94[d]	63	110	70	88	64	64	79	71	76	62	104	96
Patient-day rate	859	858	588	688	410	870	744	955	535	534	610	610	580	607	810	756
Average length of stay (days)	10.6	11.6	7.6	7.2	6.5	8.0	10.4	10.8	8.3	8.4	7.7	8.6	7.6	6.3	7.8	7.9
Hospitalized surgical procedure rate	40	32	41	50	43	76	49	62	...	...	58	36	55	...	...	...
Tonsillectomy rate	3.4	4.9	4.7[d]	9.4[d]	...	...	0.5[g]	1.0[g]	18[h]	26[h]	9[h]	24[h]	27[h]	...	...	...
One day hospital stays as percent of all stays	10	10	14	14	...	...	6	6	12	14	29	31	27	...	...	...

[a]See text for explanation of column headings. The study numbers indicate the source references.
[b]All rates are per 1000 persons per year.
[c]Data are for matched samples. They permit comparison but not generalization.
[d]Standardized for age and sex.
[e]Non-obstetrical stays in short-term hospitals.
[f]Active employees only. Not adjusted for age or sex.
[g]Adult females.
[h]Children only.

See original sources or detailed monograph[1] for further qualifications on data.

are again comparable, but so are the benefits. Both plans cover the services of a physician in the home, office and hospital, and provide hospital coverage through Blue Cross. Presumably the only difference is in the organization of care: HIP is based on prepaid group practice and GHI permits free choice of physician. Under these conditions HIP again shows clear advantage in controlling utilization. This is so, even though the data include services received from physicians outside the plan.

In the fifth study (Study 4), comparisons are made between members of one union who have chosen either HIP or an alternative union plan (UP) that permits free choice of physician. Although one would expect the HIP rates to be lower, the results show that the utilization rates are almost identical. In attempting to explain this finding (so different from previous studies) the authors point out the exceptionally low utilization rate for both plans. They also find that the plan membership and the physicians participating in the union-sponsored plan are constantly alerted by the union to the proper use of the plan. In other words, although the union-sponsored plan permits free choice of physician it is able to exert controls of sufficient effectiveness to keep utilization in check.

The sixth study (Study 12) compares hospital utilization by blue-collar workers under the Kaiser-Permamente plan (K-P), a commercial major medical insurance plan (MM) and a generous Blue Cross-Blue Shield Plan (BC-BS). Unfortunately, the populations studied live in different parts of the country: West, Midwest and East respectively. Regional differences in hospital utilization rates make these comparisons very hazardous.

Geographic differences do not play a major role in the last study in the Table (Study 23) which compares hospital utilization by California state employees under several health insurance plans made available to them by a contributory state program. Among the three major plans compared, the lowest utilization rates occur under Kaiser-Permanente (K-P), the prepaid group practice plan, and the highest rates under the California Western States-Occidental plan (CWO), a cash indemnity plan, with intermediate utilization rates under Blue Cross-Blue Shield (BC-BS).

A recent study, not shown in Table 1, reports that hospital use by recipients of Old Age Assistance who obtain ambulatory care from a prepaid group practice is somewhat lower than hospital use by a roughly comparable group of OAA recipients who obtain care under the traditional welfare system: 6.0 days per person per year as compared to 6.9 days.[21] However, during the year of observation, hospital care for both groups of clients was provided in similar manner through municipal hospitals. A more decisive test of the effect of prepaid group practice on hospital use by a welfare population will become possible under the more recent Medicaid program which has permitted consolidation of ambulatory and hospital care under the prepaid group practice plan.[24]

The findings of these selected comparative studies reinforce the impressions gained from many other reports. For example, analysis of data reported by various plans under the Federal Employees Health Benefits Program has consistently shown a markedly lower rate of hospital use by those employees who have selected prepaid group practice. This difference persists when the data are grouped by state, level of benefits (high or low options) or by age.[25]

Hospital Utilization by Diagnosis

It was said above that the key question in evaluating the performance of a plan is not whether utilization rates are low or high but whether utilization is appropriate. Overall utilization rates give very little direct insight into this matter. Utilization by diagnosis might be more revealing. There are, of course, many pitfalls in the study of utilization by diagnosis. The medical usage of the various diagnostic labels

Table 3. Hospital admission rates per 100,000 for specified diagnostic categories likely to involve surgery, by type of medical care insurance plan[a]

Diagnostic category	Study 16[b]		Study 22 HIP compared with BC-BS[c]				Study 3 HIP compared with GHI[c]				Study 4	
			Males		Females		Males		Females			
	HIP	NYC	HIP	BC-BS	HIP	BC-BS	HIP	GHI	HIP	GHI	HIP	UP
Benign unspecified neoplasm	....	....	382	348	1148	1079	729	462	1439	1893*	584	500
Varicose veins	70	40	59	61	88	102	....	....	31	75	73	83
Hemorrhoids	200	130	132	230*	88	129	35	319*	221	310	185[d]	194[d]
Tonsillectomy and adenoidectomy	340	490	503	1018*	445	856*	....	....	48[e]	104[e]	1800[f]	2600[f]
Appendicitis	360	320	244	337	217	331*	....	....	169	154	113	243
Hernia	310	160	397	389	116	103	470	680	141	108	149	194
Diseases of the gallbladder	160	110	85	126	270	206	339	371	482	656	109	125
Diseases of the prostate	....	....	99	164*	....	....	693	331	....	....	....	....
Diseases of the female genital tract	780	550	....	....	803	544*	....	....	539	830*	....	

*Statistically significant differences: chances are less than 1 in 20 that the difference between rates is due to random factors. No significance test results are reported for the first and last studies tabulated.
[a]The study numbers and column headings in this table correspond to those in Table 2.
[b]Data in this study are for actual operations.
[c]Data adjusted for age.
[d]"Rectal disorders."
[e]Almost all are adults.
[f]"E.N.T." disorders in children under 15.
See original sources or detailed monograph[1] for further qualifications on data.

differs by physician and medical care institution. Reporting and coding vary in accuracy by procedure. The data presented in this section must be interpreted with these reservations in mind.

The one thread that runs with absolute uniformity throughout all the comparisons given in Table 2 is the tonsillectomy rate, which is always lower in prepaid group practice. This, plus the observation that surgical hospitalization rates are lower in the three major HIP studies (Studies 22, 6 and 3), would lead one to believe that unjustified surgery tends to be less frequent in prepaid group practice. Further evidence is offered in Table 3 which shows hospital admission rates for conditions that often require surgery as reported in several comparative studies which involve comparisons of HIP with an alternative plan. The first of these studies (Study 16) differs from the rest because about half the NYC sample had no insurance of any kind. In this case, the rates are higher in the HIP for all operations except tonsillectomy. In the other

three studies (Studies 22, 3 and 4), the pattern is reversed. The rates for HIP are significantly less for 8 entries in the Table, less in 17 entries, more in 10 entries and significantly more in only 1 entry.

Experience in the Federal Employees Health Benefits Program has also shown consistently a markedly lower rate for surgical procedures under group practice plans. The rate of all procedures under group practice is only 42 percent that under Blue Shield; it is 73 percent for cholecystectomy, 51 percent for female surgery, 50 percent for appendectomy and 23 percent for tonsillectomy and/or adenoidectomy.[27] These comparisons do not include adjustments for the possible performance of surgery outside the plan or for demographic and regional differences in the populations covered by the respective plans.

The study of comparative utilization for broader diagnostic categories including hospital admissions for medical conditions is, if anything, more speculative than the

Table 4. Disease categories by nature of differences in hospital admission rates in two studies that compare female subscribers to the Health Insurance Plan of Greater New York (HIP) with female subscribers to either Blue Cross-Blue Shield or Group Health Insurance (GHI), New York

Nature of difference	Disease categories
HIP rates significantly* lower in both studies	Diseases of the circulatory system Diseases of respiratory system Influenza, pneumonia, bronchitis
HIP rates lower in both studies; only one of the differences is significant*	Other diseases of heart Acute upper respiratory infection Tonsillectomy and adenoidectomy Other diseases of respiratory system Infections of kidney Diseases of bones and organs of movement Other diseases of musculo-skeletal system Accidental injuries
HIP rate lower in one study, higher in other. Lower rate significantly* different	Neoplasms: benign and unspecific Appendicitis Diseases of genitourinary system Symptomatic complaints
HIP rate lower in one study, higher in other. Higher rate significantly* different	Vascular lesions central nervous system
HIP rate lower in one study, higher in other. Both differences significant*	Diseases of uterus and female genital organs

*Statistically significant: chances are less than 1 out of 20 that the difference between the admission rate for any one diagnostic category in HIP and the rate for the same condition in the alternative plan is due to random factors.
Source: References 3 and 22.

surgical comparisons described above. Only two studies (Studies 3 and 22) in which the study design was good and the diagnostic coding comparable, will be described and discussed. One of these studies compares HIP with GHI (Study 3) and the other compares HIP with Blue Cross-Blue Shield (Study 22). Furthermore, only those categories in which a significant difference was recorded in one or other of the two studies will be considered. A few purely surgical categories will be included. Because there were very few male subscribers in one of the studies, only the data for females will be presented. The data selected as indicated above are shown in Table 4. For 16 out of 17 diagnostic categories, the HIP rate is significantly lower than that for the alternative plan in one or both of the comparisons made. In one comparison (vascular lesions of the central nervous system) the rate for HIP is significantly higher. In another condition (diseases of uterus, and female genital organs) the HIP rate is significantly higher in one comparison (HIP, BC-BS) and sig-

nificantly lower in the other (HIP, GHI). The findings are consistent with the conclusion that the alternative plans over-hospitalize for the common respiratory conditions and the more minor surgical conditions such as benign neoplasms, tonsillectomies and accidental injuries. Some critics have pointed out the fact that some HIP physicians have difficulty in admitting patients to hospitals and attributed lower utilization rates in HIP to this factor rather than the exercise of professional control. Further study has shown that when HIP groups are divided into those who have ready access to hospital and those who do not, there remains a large element of reduced utilization that cannot be attributed to difficulty of access to hospital beds.[26] The selective nature of reduced utilization, as demonstrated in the data reviewed above, also suggests that professional controls do play a role.

Summary on Hospital Utilization

The available data on hospital utilization are consistent with the notion that prepaid

Table 5. Yearly family expenditures for medical care by type of medical care insurance plan[a]

Expenditures	Study 6		Study 2		Study 12[d]			Study 23[c]		
	HIP[b]	GHI	K-P	BC-BS	K-P	MM	BC-BS	K-P	CWO	BC-BS
Premiums	....	....	$109	$ 99	$122	$110-120	$110	$284	$227	$285
Total costs: all services	$139	$154	$255	$312	$224	$247-257	$259	$373	$416	$485
Out-of-pocket expenditures	....	....	$147	$213	$102	$137	$149	$ 89	$189	$200
Percent of total expenditures paid by plan:										
All services	35	34	43[e]	32[e]	54[e]	45-47[e]	42[e]	76[e]	55[e]	59[e]
Hospital services	88	78	....	....	....	....	....	....	....	....
Physicians' services	80	59	....	....	....	....	....	....	....	....

[a]See text for explanation of column headings. The study numbers indicate the source references.
[b]See original reference for methods used in allocating HIP costs.
[c]Estimated annual cost of health services for typical family of one employee and three dependents. Medical costs limited essentially to physician services, prescription drugs and hospitalization. They do not include dental care, eye glasses or non-prescription drugs.
[d]Adjusted for regional medical care price differences.
[e]Premium as percent of total cost.

group practice through changing the nature of the incentives to the physician and introducing professional controls lowers the hospital utilization rates for many surgical and nonsurgical conditions. This effect seems fairly clear in relation to the common respiratory infections and the less severe surgical conditions in which there would seem to be a larger element of discretion. Confirmation of this provisional statement is possible only through further detailed studies in which the appropriateness of each admission and procedure is individually determined using accepted criteria of good medical care. For many reasons, including the fact that the criteria of good care are often not very precise, this would be a formidable undertaking.

Expenditures for Care

The data on medical care expenditures from four studies (Studies 6, 2, 12 and 23) are summarized in Table 5. Unfortunately, comparable data are not available from all of these studies and many specific questions about expenditures must remain unanswered.

The first two plans compared (HIP and GHI) are similar in benefits. They are also comparable in the proportion of total consumer medical care expenditures which they cover (35 and 34 percent respectively). But HIP has a moderate advantage with respect to physicians' services with 80 percent of such expenditures covered. This is because HIP physicians are permitted to make very few additional charges. Physicians who participate in GHI also undertake to accept scheduled fees. Nevertheless only about 60 percent of expenditures for physicians' service made to GHI families is covered. It is not known what part of this difference is due to the use of non-participant physicians and what proportion to lack of control on charges made by participant physicians.

The second study (Study 2) compares expenditures of families from one union who chose either Kaiser-Permanente (K-P) or Blue Cross-Blue Shield (BC-BS) under dual choice arrangements. Although Kaiser subscribers, by and large, seem to have received more service, their out-of-pocket expenditures were less.

The third study (Study 12) concerns expenditures incurred by blue-collar workers under three different plans (Kaiser-Permanente, a commercial major medical plan and Blue Cross-Blue Shield) in three geographic areas of the country (West, Midwest and East, respectively). The fourth study (Study 23) reports estimated expenditures for hospital and physicians' services and prescribed drugs incurred by a "typical family" of four persons. The subscribers are employees of the State of California who have a choice of several plans under a state contributory program. The Table gives data on three major plans: Kaiser-Permanente (K-P), a commercial cash idemnity plan (CWO), and Blue Cross-Blue Shield (BC-BS). In both Studies 12 and 23 the prepaid group practice plan (K-P) emerges with an advantage in terms of total expenditures and of percent of total expenditures that are covered by the plan. Moreover, the Kaiser plan has a smaller proportion of families who incur large expenditures each year.

It appears that prepaid group practice provides greater protection against the unforeseen costs of medical care by meeting a somewhat greater proportion of total medical expenditures and may even reduce the total level of expenditures for medical care. It should be noted, however, that all plans, even the most generous, cover a relatively small part of all medical expenditures. There is need for further extension of benefits in all plans, even those that are euphemistically referred to as "comprehensive."

Productivity

It is not clear what factors are responsible for the apparent ability of prepaid group practice to provide similar or more service at lower cost. One reason may be the rather clearly demonstrated capacity of prepaid group practice to reduce hospital use. Another may be the greater productivity attributed to group practice in general, and prepaid group practice in particular.

Fein[28] and Boan[29], among others, have discussed the theoretical reasons for expecting an increase in productivity, up to a limit, as the provision of medical care is organized into larger groupings of individual providers. These "economies of scale," as they are called, are thought to result partly from the division of labor which brings about the development of greater

skill in the performance of a smaller range of tasks by each employee, as well as more precise matching of skills to task requirements so that highly skilled and scarce personnel (for example, physicians) are not wasted on relatively low-order activities. Large scale organization also makes possible the greater use of machinery and equipment to help perform tasks at lower cost. Furthermore, since each item of equipment and each professional person is "indivisible," the chances that equipment and personnel do not stand idle, but are utilized to capacity, is expected to be greater as the organization becomes larger in scale.

While these theoretical expectations are reasonable, there is little direct information concerning physician productivity in prepaid group practice. One reason may be the conceptual and empirical problems of defining and measuring productivity in a manner suitable for comparison among different forms and scales of organization. The physician visit, which has been the usual unit used, is subject to great variability in duration, content and quality, and, therefore, in its ability to produce health. Surrogate measures of physician activity, such as income, add even further difficulties in interpretation.[28, 30, 31]

Boan has assembled some evidence (Table 6) that suggests greater physician productivity for group practice (not necessarily prepaid) as compared to solo practice in Canada.[29] A survey of Canadian physicians performed by the Royal Commission on Health Services has shown that, on a per physician basis, physicians in group practice employ more nurses, technicians, and clerical personnel than do physicians in solo practice. The same survey has shown that the average group practice has more medical and office equipment than the average solo practitioner. However, the value of such equipment per physician is less in group practice than it is in solo practice. The same is true for the cost of "paramedical" personnel per physician. On the other hand, the income of physicians in group practice is somewhat

Table 6. Number and cost per physician of specified personnel, value of capital assets and annual income, by type of practice, Canada, 1960

Specified items	Group practice	Solo practice	
		General	Specialist
Number of persons employed per physician[a]			
Nurses	0.5	0.3	0.3
Technical staff	0.4	0.05	0.07
Clerical and other	1.0	0.4	0.5
Average annual cost per physician[a]			
Nurses	$1,740	$2,470	$2,610
Technical staff	1,520	1,850	2,260
Clerical and other	2,540	1,580	1,970
Average depreciated value of capital assets per physician	$4,460	$8,840	$6,160
Average annual total net income[b]	$19,420	$13,820	$18,730

[a]Because of variably incomplete responses to the questionnaire by physicians in solo practice, each of the items under the headings "Number of persons employed per physician" and "Average annual cost per physician" may relate to a different number of physicians. Hence it is not possible to derive average cost per employee from the data cited. (Communication with author)
[b]Average annual total net income from medical practice and salaried appointment of active civilian physicians in Canada during 1960.
Source: Reference 29. Based on reports in a questionnaire on the economics of medical practice administered by the Royal Commission on Health Services to all physicians and surgeons in Canada, March 1962.

larger than that of specialists and considerably larger than that of generalists in solo practice.

This constellation of findings, summarized in Table 6, is interpreted by Boan (and by Fein) to support the theoretical expectation that the physician in group practice is more productive than his counterpart in solo practice, irrespective of the additional feature of prepayment.

Bailey, on the other hand, has criticized such indirect evidence of increased productivity.[30] His major argument is that "the medical firm" produces a range of products rather than only one product (a concept presented by Codman in his analysis of the product of a teaching hospital published over 50 years ago[32]). The increased revenue to group practice is postulated to be attributable not to greater physician productivity but to a different product mix that includes relatively more low cost, high price services such as X-rays and other diagnostic tests. This hypothesis is supported, according to Bailey, by his own empirical studies in the San Francisco Bay Area (Table 7).

These studies show that although physicians in larger partnerships and groups are supplemented to a greater extent by the services of other personnel, their productivity in terms of office visits is not increased. What is increased is income, and the proportion of revenue derived from ancillary services which require little clinician input. In the process of arriving at this conclusion, Bailey makes some correction for differences in type of visit made by size of firm. However, his study is based on a very small number of firms and does not fully assure comparability of product. Other study findings suggest that the lack of difference in office visits by size of firm is not brought about by compensatory differences in hospital visits.

Yett[33] used a sample from the A.M.A. list of self-employed physicians under age 65 to study the relationship between yearly "tax deductible professional expenses" per physician and patient visits per year per physician. The method of analysis was to postulate certain mathematical models of the relationship between professional expenses and patient visits and, using multivariate analysis, to determine which of the models best fit the data. Corrections were made for field of specialization, group versus solo practice, geographic

Table 7. Measures of input and of production, by size of firm, sample of internists, San Francisco Bay Area, April 1967

Measures of input and output	Firm size				
	Solo (N = 12)	2-man (N = 4)	3-man (N = 6)	4 to 5-man (N = 5)	Clinics (N = 4)
Input measures					
Average hours per physician	218	222	197	200	197
Average paramedical hours per physician	187	181	225	271	499
Average technical hours per physician	7	11	9	44	122
Average paramedical hours per physician hour	0.858	0.817	1.142	1.353	2.531
Average technical hours per physician hour	0.032	0.050	0.046	0.220	0.619
Output (production) measures					
Office visits per physician[a]	286	278	291	243	286
Office visits per physician time with patient[a]	3.4	3.0	3.5	3.1	2.9
Gross monthly income per physician	$4,777	....	$6,107	....	$6,725
Average percent of revenues earned by sale of ancillary products	15	....	34	....	48

[a]Office visits are weighted by assigning to the major categories of regular office visits, annual examinations, and complete histories and physical examinations, weights based upon the amount of time the physician normally devotes to each service output.

Source: Reference 30.

region and price differences as signified by salary figures for nurses, office aides and technicians. The author concludes that the data are consistent with the hypothesis that there are economies of scale. It also appears that at every level of output (patient visits) tax deductible professional expenses are lower in group practice than in solo practice, suggesting greater productivity in the former. However, as Yett himself recognized, these findings need further confirmation. The response rate to the questionnaire on which this study is based was only 41 percent and, due to additional depletion for other reasons, the final analysis is based on a mere 15 percent of the original sample. Three strikingly different mathematical models of the hypothesized relationship between expenses and visits fit the data about equally and all three models leave a considerable amount of variation unexplained (R^2 equals about 0.5).

Closer to the narrower concerns of this review is a report by McCaffree and Newman[34] that in a prepaid group practice plan the cost of prescribed drugs is 45 percent lower than the national average. This figure is reduced to 28 percent when corrections are made for the estimated purchase of drugs by group plan enrollees from outside pharmacies and for the fact that community pharmacies are subject to taxes, must make a profit and, in addition, often perform certain special services that add to the convenience of the purchaser (see Table 8). According to the authors, several factors related to organization and to size are responsible for the savings in drug costs. These include reduction of inventory and purchase of lower priced generic drugs brought about by the institution of a drug formulary, large volume purchasing, the manufacture of some pharmaceuticals on the premises, precounting and prepackaging of certain medications, and the use of pharmacy clerks in lieu of additional licensed pharmacists. The study makes a fairly good case for greater efficiency of the prepaid drug program partly due to increased productivity of the pharmacist. The case would have been stronger if the comparability of the service provided had been established, the costs under the prepaid program had been compared with costs for a similar population in the same community using identical sources of information, and if the quantitative effects of the

Table 8. Cost of prescribed drugs to the purchaser in a prepaid group practice plan as compared to average national figures, including specified elements of cost, 1966

Items	Prepaid group practice	United States	Difference as percent of U.S. gross average annual cost
Gross per capita annual cost	$8.80	$16.00	45
Decrement from U.S. cost attributed to profit and taxes	....	1.28	8
Increment of 15 percent to prepaid plan cost attributed to purchase of drugs outside the plan	1.32	....	8
Decrement from U.S. cost attributed to special services (credit, delivery, etc.) provided by community pharmacies	....	0.16	1
Total adjusted per capita annual cost	$10.12	$14.66	28

Source: Reference 34.

several cost reducing factors had been assessed.

From the studies reviewed one may conclude that prepaid group practice has the potential to increase physician productivity. The extent to which this potential has been realized has not been clearly established. The conceptual issues of measuring the physician's product remain unresolved. In addition, all the studies reviewed suffer from such deficiencies in design and measurement that their findings must be viewed with caution.

Quality of Medical Care

The quality of medical care is difficult to define and even more difficult to measure. There is no room in this paper to review the varieties of meaning which "quality" may have or the many approaches that may be made to its assessment.[35] For our purposes quality will be defined by the aggregate of items which will be described below. Before these items are described it might be well to summarize present knowledge and opinion concerning the quality of medical care without taking time to provide the necessary documentation. There is much evidence to indicate that the quality of care available under many circumstances falls far below acceptable levels. Furthermore, the patient is generally unable to assess the technical aspects of the quality of care he receives.

It is, therefore, necessary to incorporate into the practice of medicine professional and organizational safeguards to maintain and promote quality.[36, 37] It is the contention of those who favor prepaid group practice that this form of organization provides the framework for precisely that. Our task is to examine the evidence that pertains to this contention.

Effective Use of Service

Do subscribers to prepaid group practice plans make more effective use of medical care services as compared to the manner in which they used services prior to joining such plans, or as compared with subscribers in other plans? A number of studies provide partial answers to this question. These studies concern the subscribers' own perceptions of change in how they use medical care service subsequent to joining the plan, the establishment of a relationship with a personal or family physician, the use of preventive services, whether care is sought in the presence of illness, and delay in seeking care. The major findings will be briefly reviewed below.

When subscribers to "comprehensive" health insurance plans, including prepaid group practice, are asked whether being in the plan has affected their use of medical care services, relatively few (15 to 30 percent) say that it has.[6, 13] The changes reported include seeing the doctor more readily, reporting sooner for minor things, and more use of specialists, checkups and tests. To what extent these changes mean better quality is, of course, a matter for some debate. More generally accepted as conducive to quality is the establishment of a stable patient-physician relationship. Many prepaid group practice plans emphasize that one of their basic policies is to help subcribers choose a personal or family physician who is responsible for the management of their health care. We have already presented evidence to show that in about a third of cases they fail in making the subscriber feel that he has a personal or family physician. The available evidence indicates that prepaid group practice enjoys no superiority in the establishment of a *perceived* relationship between patient and physician. This does not mean that in actual operative terms the care of the group practice subscriber is not more centralized and integrated. A striking example of what happens where unlimited free choice is available comes from the three-plan study repeatedly referred to in this review.[12] The families in the Blue Shield and the major medical insurance samples were asked to report the name of every physician who had seen any member of the family during the survey year. They mentioned about 80 physicians for every 100 family members, or more than 3500 for the two samples together.

One avowed objective of prepaid group practice is to encourage the use of preventive services by their subscribers. There are some data from New York City[16, 38] comparing the use of preventive services by HIP subscribers to the use of such services by non-subscribers. It appears that HIP subscribers are more likely to use general checkups and prenatal and postnatal care than are persons in the general New York City sample. Moreover, HIP enrollment is associated with a greater increment of prenatal care to the usually underprivileged segments of the population (nonwhite and Puerto Rican). But when prenatal care by HIP enrollees is com-pared with the sample of New York City mothers who receive care from private physicians, the differences noted above are eliminated for white mothers and considerably reduced for nonwhite and Puerto Rican mothers. A report from California indicates that both white and nonwhite subscribers to Kaiser-Permanente are much more likely than persons enrolled in other health insurance plans to have a cervical cytology examination, almost always because the examination was recommended by a physician.[39]

The readiness with which patients seek care when illness strikes is another indicator of adequate medical care. Data from one study suggest that persons who have prepaid group health insurance are somewhat more likely to seek care in the presence of either acute or chronic illness than are persons in a general population sample, some of whom have and some of whom do not have the usual types of health insurance coverage. Delay in seeking care is reduced as indicated by the somewhat larger proportion of cases who seek care less than one day after the onset of a set of specified illnesses and injuries.[16]

A measure that has been proposed to test the effectiveness of a system for the delivery of personal health services is the extent to which it reduces the disparity between high and low socioeconomic groups in the use of such services.[40] We have already referred to several studies in which this disparity is shown to have been substantially reduced for persons in prepaid group practice. This includes the use of prenatal care by ethnic group in New York City[38], the use of cervical cytology by "native whites" as compared to "all others" in Alameda County, California[39], and the use of physician services by Old Age Assistance recipients in New York City who were born in Puerto Rico or Latin America as compared to those born in the continental United States or Eastern Europe.[21] A more recent study describes the experience of an indigent population whose care was undertaken by the Kaiser Foundation Health Plan in Portland,

Table 9. Qualifications of physicians and surgeons and accreditation status of hospitals used for specified purposes by type of medical care insurance plan[a]

Qualifications of physicians and hospital accreditation status	Study 16		Study 43		Study 44			Study 12		
	HIP	NYC	HIP	NYC	HIP	GHI	BC-BS	K-P	MM	BC-BS
Percent of families who use "special doctor for children":										
For children under 4	72	44								
For children under 1	90	50								
Percent of deliveries attended by:										
Diplomates of specialty boards			72	24						
Other specialists			28	15						
Not specialists			0	22						
Hospital ward physician			0	39						
Qualifications of physicians and hospitals:										
Use of qualified physicians					83[b]	57[b]	62[b]	....[c]	33[c]	33[c]
Use of accredited hospitals					64	71	79	98	98	95
Physician-hospital combinations:										
Qualified, accredited					56	46	54			
Qualified, not accredited					27	10	8			
Other, accredited					7	25	26			
Other, not accredited					9	18	13			

[a]See text for explanation of column headings. The study numbers indicate the source references.
[b]In this column, percent of operations performed by surgeons of given qualifications in specified types of hospitals.
[c]In this column, percent of all physicians used, including ambulatory care, and percent of all hospital stays.

Oregon, through an arrangement with the Office of Economic Opportunity.[41] It describes the extent to which levels of use by an indigent population can be made comparable to use by the general membership of the prepaid group practice plan, if a special effort is made to encourage use. In almost all studies, however, significant differences in the levels of use persist. Furthermore, there remain some interesting differences in the manner in which services are used. In Portland, Oregon, the OEO population used a greater proportion of emergency room services and a greater proportion of services after hours. Similar differences were reported by Nolan et al. for the use of pediatric services in the Kaiser Health Plan at Oakland, California.[42] For example, for Negroes, as compared to whites, a smaller number of visits were for health supervison, visits were less likely to be made by appointment, visits to the drop-in clinic were less likely to be made by prior arrangement with a particular doctor, and a smaller proportion of families named a Kaiser pediatrician as

their child's regular doctor. One may conclude that while prepaid group practice can significantly reduce the socioeconomic gap in use of services, the differential is not fully erased.

Kinds of Physicians and Hospitals Used

Prepaid group practice plans claim to exercise control over the qualifications of the physicians they employ and the type of hospital they use for providing care. It can be assumed that the use of qualified physicians and accredited hospitals contributes to the technical quality of the care provided. Table 9 summarizes some relevant data.

Data from New York City indicate that subscribers to HIP are more likely to use specialists to care for children and attend to childbirth than is the general population (Studies 16 and 43). Surgical operations are more likely to be performed by qualified surgeons (diplomate or equivalent) for HIP subscribers than for members of GHI or Blue Cross-Blue Shield

(Study 44). But accredited hospitals are least likely to be used by HIP surgeons. This means that a proportion of HIP surgery is performed by qualified surgeons in non-accredited hospitals, possibly because of difficulty in obtaining privileges for HIP physicians at some accredited hospitals.

Data from another study (Study 12) suggest that the frequency of use of accredited hospitals, and probably of qualified physicians as well, is similar for the three plans studied (Kaiser-Permanente, Major Medical and Blue Cross-Blue Shield). This is probably a reflection of the availability of accredited hospitals and of qualified physicians in the regions where the several plans operate.

Performance of Physicians

Data on how physicians perform in the actual management of cases are very hard to come by. The following information is extremely fragmentary but should be mentioned in order to round out the picture.

The evidence concerning the possible occurrence of unjustified surgery in various plans has been presented. Prepaid group practice appears to exert some control in reducing such surgery and, to that extent, contributes to the quality of care.

The Health Insurance Plan of Greater New York has sponsored and conducted several studies of the quality of care offered by physicians associated with its affiliated groups.[45-47] These studies have been significant contributions to methodology and have added to our knowledge of factors related to the quality of performance. But they do not give any direct indication of comparative levels of quality since there are no comparisons of HIP with non-HIP physicians. They do, however, suggest certain pertinent observations. The most important of these is that the manner in which a group is organized, staffed and equipped appears to be fairly closely related to the quality of physician performance as judged by a review of case records supplemented by interviews with the managing physicians. This means that

the groups can, and do influence quality by the manner in which they are set up. There are, however, aberrant cases in which well organized groups do less well on quality ratings, and less well organized groups do better. All the factors that influence physician performance are not as yet well understood. With greater understanding, the ability of organized medical care systems to assure higher levels of quality is expected to improve.

Effects on Health

The ultimate test on whether any form of medical practice is more or less successful than a competing form, is the health and well-being of the people it serves as compared with the population served by its competitors.[48] But health and well-being result not only from the use of medical services but from the operation of many biological, psychological, social and economic factors as well. Under ordinary circumstances it is difficult to isolate the effect of medical care from among the many interacting factors that affect health. This task is even more difficult when we wish to detect the effect of a medical care plan which most people join in their adult years and in which they have remained for relatively short periods of time.

There are three studies, all involving HIP, which have attempted to answer the seemingly simple question: "Are HIP subscribers more healthy?" The first is the comparison between representative samples of HIP and New York City populations which has been the source of so many data in this report.[16] The method used was to ask people about the diseases and disabilities they had during a given period of time. The results are inconclusive. "Although most specific conditions were reported with about the same frequency in the two samples, the kinds of conditions for which the HIP rate was higher are generally thought by the public as run of the mill, whereas those for which the New York City rate was higher are generally considered to be serious." With this method, it is not clear whether the differences noted are due to actual differences in health or due to different expectations or to different concepts of health and illness held by the respondents.

The second study[38, 43] is more sharply focused. It attempts to determine the rates of premature births and of deaths of infants at birth or during the first weeks of life (perinatal mortality). The study is well conceived and carefully designed and executed. The data are analyzed with due regard to differences in population composition. The results, shown in Table 10, are unequivocally in favor of HIP. The HIP population, compared to the New York City sample under the care of private physicians, experiences fewer premature births and fewer newborn deaths. This is true for whites and nonwhites. Belonging to HIP does not wipe out the differences between whites and nonwhites, but there is a suggestion that these are reduced. The rates quoted above have been adjusted for differences in age of mother. The differences shown to exist between the HIP and NYC samples are statistically significant. They could have occurred by chance with a frequency ranging from 6 times per 100 (differences in prematurity rates for whites) to less than once per 1,000 (differences in prematurity rates for nonwhites and newborn deaths for whites).

The third study[21] attempts to assess differential effects at the other extreme of the life span. A group of Old Age Assistance recipients who obtained care under prepaid group practice (HIP) were compared with a roughly similar group of OAA recipients who received care under the traditional welfare system. Mortality in the two groups was measured beginning six months after the initiation of the program. During the first year of observation mortality (adjusted for age, sex and country of origin) was roughly comparable: 7.8 per 100 for those in HIP and 7.9 per 100 for those who were not. Thereafter the mortality rates diverged significantly so that during the following 18 months the yearly mortality rate was 7.8 per 100 for the HIP

Table 10. Prematurity and perinatal mortality rates, by race, enrollees in the Health Insurance Plan of Greater New York (HIP) and private patients from a New York City sample, 1955-1957

| Prematurity and perinatal mortality rates | Study 43[a] | |
	HIP[b]	NYC sample: Private patients
Prematurity rate per 100 live births		
White	5.5	6.0
Nonwhite	8.8	10.8
Perinatal mortality rate per 1000 live births and fetal deaths		
White	22.7	27.3
Nonwhite	33.7	43.8

[a]The study number indicates the source reference.
[b]Adjusted to age of mother and ethnic distribution of NYC deliveries.

group and 8.8 for others—a difference of 14 percent. Data were also available, for the first year of observation only, on two groups of nursing home patients. Although the patients in HIP had a lower rate (19.9 per 100 compared with 21.8), the difference could have been due to chance.

The last two studies cited describe circumstances in which life itself is shown to be related to the precise way in which the provision of medical care is organized. Should these findings prove to be more generally true, their implications would be shattering.

Conclusion

Prepaid group practice represents the confluence of two powerful currents that are reshaping medical care today: health insurance and the greater organizational complexity demanded by the explosive growth of medical science and technology. As an important social innovation in its own right, it has attracted much criticism, and sometimes outright opposition. In this review an attempt has been made to summarize and evaluate what is known about the performance of prepaid group practice so that discussion and further research can be carried out on a more informed basis.

Least open to doubt are the capability of prepaid group practice to achieve a more rational pattern in the use of medical resources, its ability to control costs and the greater protection it generally offers against the unpredictable financial ravages of illness. Less is known about the levels of quality attained, but there is little to suggest that technical quality suffers and much to suggest that it is maintained and safeguarded. Although prepaid group practice has appealed to enough people to ensure a slow but steady growth, its acceptability to broad segments of potential recipients and providers of care remains in considerable doubt. Attachments to the traditional, and more familiar, forms of medical care run deep. But they can be strained or ruptured. There is much to suggest that prepaid group practice becomes acceptable to consumers to the extent that they become alienated from traditional practice. But the future growth of group practice need not depend merely on dissatisfaction with what now exists. There is evidence that consumers are able to judge rival plans on the grounds of their relative merits and to select what best meets their own needs as they see them. Insufficient information, rather than rejection, may be the major obstacle.

The great majority of subscribers and physicians in prepaid group practice are satisfied by what they have. Nevertheless, there are two problems that have not been fully solved: how to promote the full flowering of the professional spirit and how to nurture the sensitive personal relationships between professionals and their clients in complex bureaucracies that are governed by impersonal exigencies of their own. These are, of course, problems not not only of prepaid group practice but of medical care in all organized settings. They are, moreover, problems that face our society in many spheres in addition to the medical[49], and that need to be solved on a much broader front.

Other Reviews

The attention of the reader is called to two reviews that have also attempted to assemble and evaluate information concerning prepaid group practice. These are: 1) Klarman, H. E., "Effect of Prepaid Group Practice on Hospital Use." *Public Health Reports* 78:955-965. (November 1963), and 2) Weinerman, E. R., "Patients' Perception of Group Medical Care: A Review and Analysis of Studies on Choice and Utilization of Prepaid Group Practice Plans." *American Journal of Public Health* 54:880-889. (June 1964)

The present review was made without reference to the work cited above and, therefore, constitutes an independent evaluation.

References

1 Donabedian, A. *A Review of Some Experiences with Prepaid Group Practice.* Research Series no. 11. (Ann Arbor: Bureau of Public Health Economics, School of Public Health, University of Michigan, 1965) 74 pp.

2 Wolfman, B. "Medical Expenses and Choice of Plan: A Case Study." *Monthly Labor Review* 84: 1186-1190. (November 1961)

3 Densen, P. M., Jones, E. W., Balamuth, E. and Shapiro, S. "Prepaid Medical Care and Hospital Utilization in a Dual Choice Situation." *American Journal of Public Health* 50:1710-1726. (November 1960)

4 Densen, P. M., Shapiro, S., Jones, E. W. and Baldinger, I. "Prepaid Medical Care and Hospital Utilization." *Hospitals* 36:63-68 and 138. (November 16, 1962)

5 Henderson, M. B. "Federal Employees Health Benefits Program, II: Role of the Group Practice Prepayment Plans." *American Journal of Public Health* 56:54-57. (January 1966)

6 Anderson, O. W. and Sheatsley, P. B. *Comprehensive Medical Insurance: A Study of Costs, Use and Attitudes Under Two Plans.* Research Series no. 9. (New York: Health Information Foundation, 1959)

7 Metzner, C. A. and Bashshur, R. L. "Factors Associated with Choice of Health Care Plans." *Journal of Health and Social Behavior* 8:291-299. (December 1967)

8 Bashshur, R. L. and Metzner, C. A. "Patterns of Social Differentiation Between Community Health Association and Blue Cross-Blue Shield." *Inquiry* 4:23-44. (June 1967)

9 Bashshur, R. L. and Metzner, C. A. "The Relation of Vulnerability to the Spread of Health Care Information." Unpublished paper. 28 pp.

10 Metzner, C. A., Bashshur, R. L. and Worden, C. *Choice of Health Care Plans. A Survey of Auto Workers' Selection of Blue Cross-Blue Shield or Community Health Association: Basic Tables.* (Ann Arbor: Bureau of Public Health Economics, School of Public Health, University of Michigan, January 1965) 135 pp.

11 Yedidia, A. "Dual Choice Program." *American Journal of Public Health* 49:1475-1480. (November 1959)

12 *Family Medical Care Under Three Types of Health Insurance.* School of Public Health and Administrative Medicine, Columbia University. (New York: Foundation on Employee Health, Medical Care and Welfare, Inc., 1962)

13 Simon, N. M. and Rabushka, S. E. *A Trade Union and Its Medical Service Plan.* (St. Louis: Labor Health Institute, 1954)

14 Freidson, E. *Patients' Views of Medical Practice.* (New York: Russell Sage Foundation, 1961)

15 Bashshur, R. L., Metzner, C. A. and Worden, C. "Consumer Satisfaction with Group Practice, the CHA Case." *American Journal of Public Health* 57:1991-1999. (November 1967)

16 Committee for the Special Research Project in the Health Insurance Plan of Greater New York. *Health and Medical Care in New York City.* (Cambridge: Harvard University Press, 1957)

17 McElrath, D. C. "Perspectives and Participation of Physicians in Prepaid Group Practice." *American Sociological Review* 26:596-607. (August 1961) A more complete account in McElrath, D. C. "Prepaid Group Medical Practice: A Comparative Analysis of Organizations and Perspectives." Unpublished Ph.D. dissertation, Yale University, 1958.

18 Darsky, B. J., Sinai, N. and Axelrod, S. J. *Comprehensive Medical Services Under Voluntary Health Insurance.* (Cambridge: Harvard University Press, 1958)

19 Shipman, G. A., Lampman, R. J. and Miyamoto, S. F. *Medical Service Corporations in the State of Washington.* (Cambridge: Harvard University Press, 1962)

20 Darsky, B. J., Sinai, N. and Axelrod, S. J. "Problems in Voluntary Insurance: Some Answers from the Windsor Experience." *American Journal of Public Health* 48:971-978. (August 1958)

21 Shapiro, S., Williams, J. J., Yerby, A. S., Densen, P. M. and Rosner, H. "Patterns of Medical Use by the Indigent Aged under Two Systems of Medical Care." *American Journal of Public Health* 57:784-790. (May 1967)

22 Densen, P. M., Balamuth, E. and Shapiro, S. *Prepaid Medical Care and Hospital Utilization.* Hospital Monograph Series, no. 3. (Chicago: American Hospital Association, 1958)

23 Dozier, D., Krupp, M., Melinkoff, S., Schwarberg, C. and Watts, M. *Report of the Medical and Hospital Advisory Council to the Board of Administration of the California State Employees' Retirement System.* (Sacramento, 1964)

24 Shapiro, S. and Brindle, J. "Group Practice Plans in Governmental Medical Care Programs, III. Serving Medicaid Eligibles." *American Journal of Public Health* 59:635-641. (April 1969)

25 Perrott, G. S. "Federal Employees Health Benefits Program, III. Utilization of Hospital Services." *American Journal of Public Health* 57:57-64. (January 1966) Also see annual reports by Mr. Perrott in *Group Health and Welfare News.*

26 Densen, P. M. and Shapiro, S. "Hospital Use Under Varying Forms of Medical Organization." *Conference on Research in Hospital Use.* PHS publication # 930-E-2. (Washington, D.C.: Division of Hospital and Medical Facilities, 1963) p. 15.

27 Perrott, G. S. and Chase, J. C. "The Federal Employees Health Benefits Program: Sixth Term Coverage and Utilization." *Group Health and Welfare News* special supplement. (October 1968) 8 pp.

28 Fein, Rashi, *The Doctor Shortage, An Economic Diagnosis.* Brookings Studies in Social Economics, The Brookings Institution. (Washington, D.C.: May 1967) 199 pp. See chapter IV, pp. 90-129.

29 Boan, J. A. *Group Practice.* Royal Commission on Health Service, Queen's Printer. (Ottawa, 1966) 79 pp. See pp. 23-31.

30 Bailey, R. M. "Economies of Scale in Medical Practice." Paper presented at the Second Conference on the Economics of Health, Baltimore, Maryland, December 5-7, 1968. Processed, 28 pp.

31 Klarman, H. E. *The Economics of Health.* (New York: Columbia University Press, 1965) 200 pp. See pp. 149-157.

32 Codman, E. A. "The Product of a Hospital." *Surgery, Gynecology and Obstetrics* 18:491-496. (January-June 1914)

33 Yett, D. E. "An Evaluation of Alternative Methods of Estimating Physicians' Expenses Relative to Output." *Inquiry* 4:3-27. (March 1967)

34 McCaffree, K. M. and Newman, H. F. "Prepayment of Drug Costs Under a Group Practice Prepayment Plan." *American Journal of Public Health* 58:1212-1218. (July 1968)

35 Donabedian, A. "Evaluating the Quality of Medical Care." *The Milbank Memorial Fund Quarterly* 44:166-203, part 2. (July 1966)

36 Donabedian, A. "Promoting Quality Through Evaluating the Process of Patient Care." *Medical Care* 6:181-202. (May-June 1968)

37 Donabedian, A. *A Guide to Medical Care Administration, Volume II: Medical Care Appraisal—Quality and Utilization.* American Public Health Association. (New York, 1969) In press.

38 Shapiro, S., Weiner, L. and Densen, P. "Comparison of Prematurity and Perinatal Mortality in a General Population and in the Population of a Prepaid Group Practice, Medical Care Plan." *American Journal of Public Health* 48:170-185. (February 1958)

39 Breslow, L. and Hochstim, J. R. "Sociocultural Aspects of Cervical Cytology in Alameda County, California." *Public Health Reports* 79:107-112. (February 1964)

40 Rosenfeld, L. S., Donabedian, A. and Katz, J. "Unmet Need for Medical Care." *New England Journal of Medicine* 258:369-376. (February 20, 1958)

41 Colombo, T. J., Saward, E. W. and Greenlick, M. R. "Group Practice Plans in Governmental Medical Care Programs, IV. The Integration of an OEO Health Program into a Prepaid Comprehensive Group Practice Plan." *American Journal of Public Health* 59:641-650. (April 1969)

42 Nolan, R. L., Schwartz, J. L. and Simonian, K. "Social Class Differences in Utilization of Pediatric Services in a Prepaid Direct Service Medical Care Program." *American Journal of Public Health* 57:34-47. (January 1969)

43 Shapiro, S., Jacobziner, H., Densen, P. M. and

Weiner, L. "Further Observations on Prematurity and Perinatal Mortality in a General Population and in the Population of a Prepaid Group Practice Medical Care Plan." *American Journal of Public Health* 50:1304-1317. (September 1960)

44 Columbia University, School of Public Health and Administrative Medicine. *Prepayment of Medical and Dental Care in New York State.* (New York: Commissioner of Health and the Superintendent of Insurance, 1962)

45 Makover, H. B. "Quality of Medical Care: Methodology of Survey of the Medical Groups Associated with the Health Insurance Plan of New York." *American Journal of Public Health* 41: 824-832. (July 1951)

46 Daily, E. F. and Morehead, M. A. "A Method of Evaluating and Improving the Quality of Medical Care." *American Journal of Public Health* 46: 848-854. (July 1956)

47 Morehead, M. A. "The Medical Audit as An Operational Tool." *American Journal of Public Health* 57:1643-1656. (September 1967)

48 Shapiro, S. "End Result Measurement of Quality of Medical Care." *Milbank Memorial Fund Quarterly* 45:7-30, Part 1. (April 1967)

49 Solomon, D. N. "Professional Persons in Bureaucratic Organizations." *Symposium on Preventive and Social Psychiatry.* (Washington, D.C.: Walter Reed Army Institute of Research, April 15-17, 1957) pp. 253-266.

John R. Coleman
Frank C. Kaminsky

Reprinted with permission of the Blue Cross Association, from *Inquiry:* Vol.XIV, No.2, pp.176-188. Copyright © 1977 by the Blue Cross Association.

A Financial Planning Model for Evaluating the Economic Viability of Health Maintenance Organizations

Originally published in June 1977

With enactment of federal legislation (PL 93-222)[1] and subsequent funding to support the development of 300 to 500 Health Maintenance Organizations (HMOs) throughout the country by 1980,[2] HMOs are being proposed and developed at a rapid rate. The extensive operating deficits that usually occur during the first five years in the life cycle of an HMO, together with the consequences of dissolving one once it has become operational, make it absolutely essential that sound financial planning methodologies guide the growth of HMOs. To assure prudent planning, a computerized Financial Planning Model (FPM) is available that can be used by planning organizations involved in the development of a new HMO. In addition, the financial planning model also can be used by decision makers who are interested in examining alternative policies for the operation of existing HMOs. The planning model described in this paper is designed not only to help to guide the growth of financially sound HMOs, but also to fill a gap that exists in the state-of-the-art of financial planning for the health industry.

John R. Coleman, Ph.D., is Assistant Professor, Department of Public Administration, University of New Haven (West Haven, CT 06516).

Frank C. Kaminsky, Ph.D., is Associate Professor, Department of Industrial Engineering and Operations Research, University of Massachusetts (Amherst, MA 01002).

This research was supported in part by HS-00709 from the National Center for Health Services Research and Development.

Relative to other established industries, financial planning in the health industry has not achieved a comparable state-of-the-art. Before 1973, few financial planning methodologies were reported in the literature. These methodologies,[3-8] were concerned primarily with financial planning in hospitals and do not apply to HMOs. After 1973, financial planning methodologies and models for HMOs started to appear.[9-15] To anyone interested or involved in financial planning for HMOs, two shortcomings are apparent in an examination of recent planning models: The models are either conceptual and presented as incentive for future development, or they are models that have been developed for a specific situation and are not easily adapted to other settings. Sears and Moustafa,[12] for example, present a conceptual model for simulating the financial viability of an HMO. Illustrations of specific models can be found in Green and Grimes,[13] Thompson,[14] and Hirsch and Miller.[15]

The model developed in this paper extends the work of those who have proposed conceptual models, as well as those who have provided specific models for actual settings. Greater detail of the model is described in a doctoral dissertation.[16]

Overview of the Financial Planning Model (FPM)

The FPM was developed as an aid to decision making in the general process of designing an

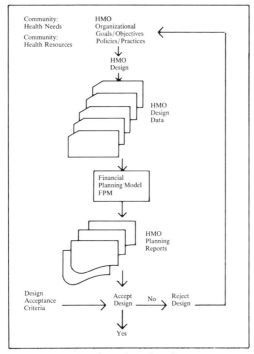

Figure I.   The financial planning model and the HMO planning process

HMO. Use of the model allows planners to determine and evaluate the financial implications of alternative organizational and operational strategies and policies. Figure I illustrates the manner in which the FPM is used in the process of planning an HMO. As shown, input to the planning model consists of several design decisions related to the programs and services to be offered; the method of delivering these services; prices to be charged for services; the cost of health resources, etc.

Operating in a batch-processing mode, the FPM produces a set of reports that provide the planners with informational bases describing the population served, the demand for services, staffing requirements, costs, revenues, and other financial measures which, in turn, are used to evaluate the proposed design. These data are used to prepare outcome measures that can be compared to effectiveness criteria for studying the overall design of the HMO. If the effectiveness criteria are satisfied, the design is accepted. Otherwise, the planning group can modify the design of the HMO and resubmit the new design

for evaluation. This cycle is repeated until the planning group achieves a feasible design—one that would be acceptable to both the providers and consumers affiliated with the HMO.

The FPM was designed to provide planners with the answers to a number of specific design questions, namely:

☐ What will be the expected annual utilization of the plan's medical and health care services?

☐ What effects will various organizational structures and operational policies for delivering services have on the financial security of the plan?

☐ What mix of physicians and allied health and paramedical personnel will be needed to provide directly the services offered by the plan?

☐ What effect will changes in the mix of medical and health care services have on the yearly plan costs and revenues?

☐ What external funding should the plan obtain during its formative years in order to meet its financial obligations?

☐ What are the effects of the plan's size, and the premium and fee-for-service schedules on annual cash flow and financial security?

☐ What copayment and capitation fee schedules and membership levels are needed to break even within the first five years of operation?

☐ What physical resources must be made available each year to provide the services on a direct-service basis?

☐ What will be the effects of changes in the socioeconomic and demographic characteristics of the subscribing population?

☐ What organizational structure and operational policies will result in low initial operation costs, low indebtedness, early break-even?

☐ What are the annual proforma cost and revenue schedules for each HMO configuration evaluated?

The FPM was developed for use by planning groups and sponsor organizations who intend to develop and operate an HMO which satisfies the requirements of the HMO Act of 1973 and other related regulations and guidelines established by the U.S. Department of Health,

Education and Welfare.[17,18,19] Development also was guided by adhering to the following general design criteria:

☐ The model should be sufficiently general to have widespread application in the health industry regardless of the geographic area and type of location of a proposed HMO.

☐ The technical complexity and input data requirements of the FPM should not inhibit its use.

☐ The component models of the FPM should be self-contained, separate entities with their own input-output functions.

☐ The FPM should be constructed so that the user can conduct a number of sensitivity analyses for the major design variables.

☐ The model should be useful to planners who wish to follow the guidelines specified for the HMO Act of 1973 (PL 93-222) and the Social Security Amendments of 1972 (PL 92-603).

☐ The model should provide planners with decision-making data at each of the major stages in the process of designing an HMO and it should provide answers to the many design questions posed by the planner.

The utility of the FPM depends on the degree to which reality can be approximated, whether or not it can answer relevant design questions, and the degree of difficulty encountered in its application. These factors and the major design criteria specified previously led to eleven major assumptions upon which the model is based. In some cases, assumptions were necessary due to the lack of operational data from existing HMOs and similar health insurance plans. In other cases, assumptions were made to reduce the overall technical complexity of the model and minimize the input requirements. Here are the major assumptions:

☐ The proposed HMO involves group practice.

☐ The resource needs of the proposed HMO can be projected by using data from existing HMOs with similar organizational and operational properties.

☐ The HMO will be a direct-service provider of medical services and will either own and operate or lease and operate one or more ambulatory medical facilities.

☐ The HMO will not construct an inpatient care facility of any type during its first five years of operation.

☐ A five-year planning horizon is of sufficient length to make intelligent decisions concerning the financial viability of an HMO.

☐ The HMO can employ fractional physicians and non-physicians.

☐ The HMO will be a non-profit organization exempt from federal and state corporate income tax.

☐ The HMO will not alter the structure of its benefit package, organization, or delivery system within the first five years.

☐ The HMO employs a one-class system of care for its members; that is, the plan will have only one benefit plan for all consumer groups.

☐ The initial monthly premiums and fee structure for plan and fee-for-service patients will be determined by the marketplace.

☐ The HMO's enrollment will not exceed 50,000 plan members at the end of the fifth year of operation.

General Structure of the Model

The FPM consists of eight separate components or "program modules," an EDIT/CONTROL program, and the seven planning models that follow: service population; demand/utilization; staff; space; cost; revenue; financial analysis. These modules, and the input-output relationships between them, are shown in Figure II. The FPM has been written in COBOL to increase the likelihood that more HMO planning groups would have the capability for using the model.

Model Input Requirements

Two data bases are required in the use of the FPM. One is an integral part of the planning model, the other is an external data base. The internal data base is the HMO DATA FILE; the external base, the USER DATA FILE. The former is built into the FPM while the latter is provided by the user.

The HMO DATA FILE consists of two data sets: 1) the Service Population Data Set, and 2) the Service Utilization Data Set. The Service Population Data Set consists of socioeconomic and demographic data for urban and rural areas in the Northeast, North Central,

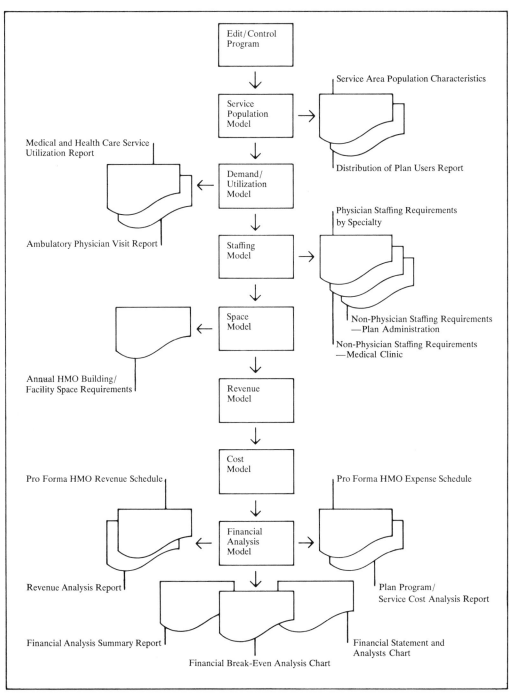

Figure II.   Input-output diagram showing the relationships between the FPM submodels

Table 1. Description of the USER DATA FILE

User Data Set	Contents
1. Geographic, residential and community definition	The census region and types of communities served by the HMO including the fluoridation or non-fluoridation of community water supplies.
2. Annual plan member and fee-for-service patient population levels	The number of Individual, Family, Medicare, Medicaid and Fee-for-Service patients to be served during each of the five years.
3. Annual enrollment levels for supplemental benefit plans	The number of plan members who have elected supplemental benefits during each of the five years.
4. Definition of HMO benefit program service options	The type and scope of service benefits to be provided by the HMO.
5. Definition of HMO services and program delivery options	The delivery system options chosen to provide for the delivery of service benefits selected by the HMO.
6. Definition of HMO facility occupancy options	The medical building and facility occupancy options for the medical and administrative components of the HMO.
7. Planned capacity of medical building and facilities used by the HMO	The service capacity of medical buildings and facilities to be constructed by the HMO during the first five years of plan operation.
8. Plan member utilization rates for inpatient care services	The birth rate, per 1000 women of child-bearing age, length-of-stays in inpatient care facilities, and the hospital days of care per 1000 members.
9. Monthly premium structure for "basic" and "supplemental" benefit plans	The initial monthly premiums for Individual, Family, Medicare, and Medicaid plan members and for all supplemental benefit plans offered by the HMO.
10. Annual percentage price increases in plan premiums	The annual increase in premium prices for "basic" and "supplemental" benefit plans.
11. Co-payment fee schedule for HMO members	The point-of-service charges for services rendered to plan members.
12. Other service fees and annual increases in co-payment fees	Other fees for services rendered to members and the annual increases in co-payment fees.
13. & 14. Service fee schedules for fee-for-service patients	The fees charged non-plan members for services rendered by the HMO.
15. Monthly Medicare cost reimbursement from SSA	The average per-month cost reimbursement from SSA for Medicare members.
16. Revenue from external sources	External income to the HMO from such sources as grants, gifts, endowments, etc.
17. Provider group service cost schedules	The contractual costs to the HMO for contracting with health service groups within the community to provide health services to plan members. These costs are on a capitation and/or unit of service basis.
18. Compensation schedule for HMO physician and non-physician staff members	The annual base salary for physicians and non-physicians employed directly by the HMO including those in administration.

Table 1.   Continued

User Data Set	Contents
19. Fringe benefit, salary increase, and manpower turnover rate for HMO staff members	The annual percentage rates of salary increases for HMO employees. Also included are the percentage rates for fringe benefits, and the annual turnover rates for physicians and non-physicians.
20. Cost inflation rates for hospital and medical care services	Annual rates of cost inflation for hospitalization and medical care services including physician, dental, optical, and pharmaceutical services.
21. HMO loan and investment income data	Annual interest rates and payment periods for capital borrowed from HEW and/or commercial banks to meet operating deficits and for the construction of buildings. Annual interest rates for funds (loans and/or profits) deposited in the bank.

South, and West Census regions of the country. The Service Utilization Data Set contains use rates for the various inpatient and outpatient health services a qualifying HMO may provide. Included in the file are hospital admission rates, physician visit rates, and the distribution of hospital admissions and physician visits by medical specialty and visit site. The utilization rates, which are by sex and age group, were obtained from a sample of operating HMOs located throughout the country. Although the HMO DATA FILE is built into the FPM, the user can modify these data if some of the data do not satisfy local conditions.

The USER DATA FILE is provided by the user and is essentially a data base that defines the HMO under consideration by the planning group. The USER DATA FILE consists of the 21 data sets listed in Table 1. These sets correspond to the major decisions the planning group must make concerning the type and scope of benefits to be offered; how these benefits are to be financed; the method by which these services are delivered; lengths of stay for hospital care; and the price, fee, and compensation schedules and financial policies adopted by the plan. Figure III illustrates the relationships between these data and the seven FPM planning models.

Model Outputs

Using the HMO DATA FILE and the USER DATA FILE, the FPM operates on these data to produce fifteen HMO planning reports.

These reports contain various data describing the dynamic behavior of the HMO over a five-year planning horizon. The reports include the following detailed planning information: age-sex distribution of members and non-members; annual demand for inpatient and outpatient health care services; annual staffing needs of the plan; annual revenue and cost schedules; annual end-of-year financial statements; membership and financial break-even charts. These reports are described in Table 2. Tables 3, 4 and 5 illustrate an annual staffing report, cost report, and financial report for a "sample" HMO configuration.

Sensitivity Analyses

The FPM has been made as general as possible to permit widespread application by health planners and HMO sponsors. It has the flexibility of a simulator, whereby planners can study more fully the economic behavior of the HMO when certain design properties and variables remain fixed while others are allowed to vary (sensitivity analyses). Ten sensitivity analyses have been incorporated into the FPM. Analyses can be performed on the following design variables:

☐ Days of hospital care per 1,000 enrolled members;

☐ Monthly premiums for Individual, Family, Medicare, and Medicaid Plans;

☐ Annual increases in monthly premiums for plan members;

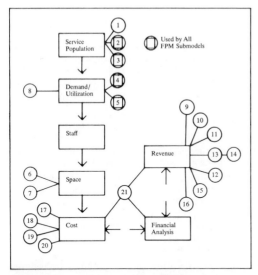

Figure III. USER DATA SETS and FPM planning models

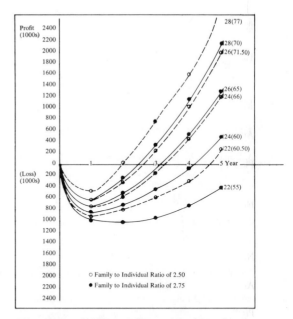

Figure IV. HMO cash flow curves for family to individual plan premium ratios of 2.5 and 2.75

☐ Ratio of Family-to-Individual premium prices;

☐ Annual increases in service fees and charges for Fee-For-Service patients;

☐ Annual salary increases for HMO staff personnel;

☐ Annual staff turnover rates for HMO personnel;

☐ Annual cost inflation rates for hospital care;

☐ Annual cost inflation rates for medical and physician care services;

☐ Annual cost inflation rates for dental care services.

Whenever sensitivity analyses are to be conducted, the FPM will use the "low," "high," and "incremental" values specified by the user. For example, when the user wants to study the economic impact of different premium price increases for the "basic" and "supplemental" benefit plans, a "low" annual increase (say 10%), a "high" annual increase (say 15%), and an "incremental" increase (say 1%) would be supplied. Using these values, the FPM would first operate five years using a 10% annual change in premium prices, then five years with 11%, five years with 12%, and so on up to 15%. In this illustration, the FPM would make six successive "sensitivity runs." Should the plan-

ning group want to study the financial impact of different hospital days per year per 1,000 members, it can vary the hospital days per year per 1,000 from, say, 400 to 600, in 50-day increments.

The sensitivity options listed here are but a few examples of the analyses which can be conducted by the user. Additional analyses and simulations can be performed by repeatedly rerunning the FPM under different values for the input variable to be examined. By using the model as a simulator, a large number of designs can be evaluated by the planning group in a short period of time.

Use of the FPM in a Typical Planning Situation

A typical HMO planning situation requires the planners to examine a number of feasible designs. The purpose of this section is to illustrate how the FPM can be used to choose the "best" HMO configuration once an initial design has been selected for study. Although a large number of design variables can be modified in a real planning situation due to the myriad of decisions involving benefit designs,

Table 2. Description of the HMO Planning Reports Generated by the FPM

Planning Report	Description
Service area population characteristics	Age-sex distribution and socioeconomic data for persons living in the service area of the HMO.
Distribution of plan users report	The age-sex distribution of plan members and Fee-For-Service patients who will use plan services during the year.
Medical and health care service utilization report	The expected utilization of inpatient and outpatient services for the first five years of plan operation.
Ambulatory physician visit report	The expected number of annual ambulatory visits to physicians by medical specialty.
Physician staffing requirements by specialty	Annual staffing patterns for primary and specialty care physicians for each of the first five years of plan operation.
Non-physician staffing requirements—medical clinic	The yearly staffing patterns for the medical clinic including nurses, laboratory technicians, administrative staff, and dental, pharmacy, home care, and mental health services.
Non-physician staffing requirements—plan administration	The yearly staffing pattern for the administrative component of the HMO.
Annual HMO building/facility space requirements	The yearly space needs of fourteen organizational components of the HMO.
Proforma HMO revenue schedule	Estimated yearly income to the HMO from plan operation and external sources including income from borrowed capital and profits if any.
Revenue analysis report	Detailed revenue data by source for the five-year planning period.
Proforma HMO expense schedule	The annual estimated costs of plan operations, including the cost of borrowing capital to meet projected losses during the first five years of plan operation.
Plan program/service cost analysis report	Detailed costs of HMO operations for the year of plan operation. This report is prepared on a yearly basis.
Financial analysis summary report	The financial position of the HMO at the end of each year including when and how much capital must be borrowed and the annual levels of outstanding debt.
Financial statement and analysis chart	The enrollment and financial position of the HMO during each year of plan operation including a graph of revenue vs cost for the first five years.
Financial break-even analysis chart	A graph indicating the time when the HMO's income balances costs and the number of plan members and Fee-For-Service patients using the HMO when this occurs.

delivery systems, and cost and price policies, only a few have been selected to illustrate the model's usefulness and versatility. The design variables modified in the illustrative cases which follow were chosen arbitrarily. These particular variables, however, have the greatest impact on the financial security of an HMO and, therefore, would be likely candidates for modification during the process of designing an HMO.

Sensitivity of Initial Premium Levels

The initial monthly prices for the Individual, Family, Medicare and Medicaid benefit plans will have a significant impact on the financial stability of the HMO. This impact is shown in Figure IV. In this particular case, the Family Premium was assumed to be 2.5 times the Individual Premium. Should the HMO initially

Table 3. HMO prepaid medical plan non-physician staffing requirements—medical clinic

Service Personnel Category	Year 1	Year 2	Year 3	Year 4	Year 5
Primary medical care program:					
Clinical administration	3.00	3.00	3.00	3.00	3.00
Nursing services	10.18	18.83	25.41	30.82	36.11
Laboratory/radiology/PT services	4.20	7.73	10.44	12.65	14.21
Secretarial/receptionist/ clerical services	5.37	7.37	8.90	10.16	11.39
Other ancillary services	.46	.80	1.08	1.32	1.54
Business office	1.75	3.23	4.35	5.28	6.18
Housekeeping-custodial services	1.01	1.88	2.54	3.08	3.61
Dental care program:					
Dentists	.65	1.18	1.65	2.03	2.41
Dental assistants	.97	1.77	2.48	3.04	3.62
Hygienists	.52	.94	1.31	1.63	1.93
Other dental auxiliaries	1.63	2.95	3.00	3.00	3.00
Out-patient drug program:					
Pharmacists	1.75	3.23	4.35	5.28	6.18
Pharmacy support personnel	1.57	2.90	3.91	4.75	5.56
Vision care program:					
Ophthalmologists	.17	.32	.43	.52	.61
Optometrists	.79	1.46	1.98	2.40	2.81
Opticians	..	..	..	..	..
Other vision care personnel	..	..	..	..	..
Out-patient mental health program:					
Psychiatrists	.29	.53	.72	.88	1.03
Psychologists	.43	.80	1.08	1.32	1.54
Psychiatric social workers	.58	1.07	1.45	1.76	2.06
Secretarial/receptionist/ clerical services	1.00	1.00	1.00	1.00	1.00
Home care program:					
Public health nurses	1.00	1.00	1.00	1.00	1.00
Total non-physician personnel	37.32	61.99	80.08	94.92	108.79

charge $22 for an Individual Plan and $55 for a Family Plan, its annual operating cost will always exceed revenue even when the annual premiums are increased annually by 11%. When the premiums are increased to $24 ($60), plan income equals costs during the fifth year. When the initial premiums are $28 to $70, the plan reaches financial equilibrium in the third year of plan operation. When the ratio of Family to Individual is increased to 2.75, the cash flow curves indicate that the HMO will reach financial equilibrium for all Individual premiums from $22 through $28.

Sensitivity of Hospitalization Rates

The impact of hospitalization rates on the annual financial position of an HMO is illustrated by the family of curves given in Figure V. In the first case, the initial monthly premiums were established at $22 for the Individual Plan and $55 for the Family Plan. Here, the HMO did not have favorable annual cash flows until the hospital-days-per-1000 members was kept below 450 days per year. Although the plan finally reached equilibrium in the fifth year for 450, and 400 days-per-1000 members, the cumulative losses for the HMO were extensive. When the monthly premiums were adjusted to $24 and $66 for the Individual and Family Plans respectively, the HMO had a favorable cash flow for the entire range of hospital-days-per-1000 members. Using the premium schedule of $24 and $66, the HMO reached financial equilibrium as early as the third year for all hospitalization rates under 500 days-per-1000 members.

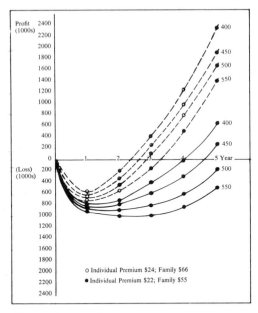

Figure V. HMO cash flow curves for various patient-days-per-1,000-members at two premium levels, $22 (55) and $24 (66)

Sensitivity of Hospital and Medical Cost Inflation

The impact of increasing costs of hospital care and annual inflation rates of hospital and medi-

cal care costs on the financial position of the HMO is shown in Figure VI. As the costs per day decrease for a fixed number of days of care per 1000 members, the time before the HMO reaches financial equilibrium becomes shorter. In our example, the MHO experiences 530 hospital care days per year per 1000 members. Using a premium structure of $22 ($55), the HMO does not reach equilibrium when the annual inflation rate is reduced from 17% down to 13% and the cost per non-maternity day is $130 or $120. When a premium structure of $24 ($60) is instituted, the HMO reaches financial equilibrium for inflation rates ranging from 13% to 17% and the daily cost of hospital cost ranging from $130 down to $120.

As shown in the figure, increases in the cost of a day of hospital care and its annual rate of inflation will cause the HMO to have extended losses unless the premium structure is increased or the number of hospital days of care per 1000 members is reduced to an acceptable level.

Versatility of the FPM

These case examples are just a sample of the many types of analyses which can be performed by members of the HMO planning group. For each design proposed by the planners, the FPM

Table 4. HMO prepaid medical plan proforma HMO expense schedule

Plan expense category	Year of operation				
	Year 1	Year 2	Year 3	Year 4	Year 5
Medical services	$1,181,031.29	$1,867,443.75	$2,467,531.25	$3,133,271.28	$4,318,995.94
Short term inpatient care	468,280.00	997,167.60	1,622,456.81	2,335,862.30	3,241,287.70
Long term inpatient care	0.00	0.00	0.00	0.00	0.00
Psychiatric inpatient care	14,500.00	22,054.50	37,710.44	55,735.68	70,642.26
Dental care program	28,745.57	29,381.95	30,710.44	30,812.82	31,605.34
Vision care program	57,234.62	90,284.97	120,495.38	149,994.27	182,750.56
Home care program	18,288.00	34,003.20	51,609.24	71,264.97	93,299.31
Mental health program	51,306.94	47,878.73	44,827.46	42,110.28	39,690.23
Out-patient drug program	170,923.65	318,941.88	449,296.74	574,673.05	709,711.34
Out-of-area services	26,340.00	48,480.00	65,140.00	79,200.80	92,760.00
Catastrophic illness	11,670.00	23,364.00	35,900.70	48,714.60	63,512.66
Other benefits	0.00	0.00	0.00	0.00	0.00
Community services	0.00	0.00	0.00	0.00	0.00
Plan administration	379,167.05	495,144.34	594,022.90	720,211.52	815,841.60
Carry over losses	0.00	28,251.00	18,025.00	1,905.00	0.00
Debt service	53,719.36	87,994.08	91,617.52	125,549.92	125,549.92
Earnings or admin reserves	18,296.49	37,404.43	50,000.00	50,000.00	50,000.00
Amortization	75,357.82	75,357.82	75,357.82	75,357.82	75,357.82
Other	0.00	0.00	0.00	0.00	0.00
Annual total expenses	**$2,554,860.79**	**$4,203,152.25**	**$5,754,262.70**	**$7,494,633.51**	**$9,881,004.68**
Avg. plan membership (total)	**7,780**	**14,160**	**19,780**	**24,400**	**28,920**
Avg. plan users (total)	**8,780**	**16,160**	**21,780**	**26,400**	**30,920**

Table 5.   HMO prepaid medical plan financial analysis summary report

Plan revenue-expenses-balance	Year of plan operation				
	Year 1	Year 2	Year 3	Year 4	Year 5
Total plan revenue					
Plan operations:	$1,829,649	$3,740,443	$5,705,346	$7,943,848	$10,999,145
Borrowed capital:	671,492	423,434	45,293	00	00
Interest income:	25,468	16,249	1,718	16,691	75,037
Total:	$2,526,609	$4,185,126	$5,752,357	$7,960,539	$11,074,182
Total plan expenses					
Plan operations:	$2,501,141	$4,168,877	$5,750,639	$7,494,663	$9,881,004
New loan principal:	00	00	00	00	00
New loan interest:	53,719	34,274	3,623	00	00
Total:	$2,554,860	$4,203,151	$5,754,262	$7,494,663	$9,881,004
Annual plan balance	($28,251)	($18,025)	($1,905)	$465,876	$1,193,178
Loan interest and principal					
Interest paid—HEW loans:	$58,719	$141,713	$233,330	$324,948	$413,851
Interest paid—other loans:	00	00	00	00	00
Principal paid—HEW loans:	00	00	00	33,932	70,579
Principal paid—other loans:	00	00	00	00	00
Total:	$58,719	$141,713	$233,330	$358,880	$484,430
Capital borrowed to date					
HEW loans:	$671,492	$1,099,926	$1,145,219	$1,145,219	$1,145,219
Bank and other loans:	00	00	00	00	00
Total:	$671,492	$1,099,926	$1,145,219	$1,145,219	$1,145,219

generates substantial information useful in setting policies for enrollment, the service benefits to be covered, how plan and community resources are to be combined together to deliver the services, etc. The FPM is versatile not only in the number and types of analyses which can be conducted, but also gives the planning group latitude in using the model in the design process. The model, for example, can sensitize planners to the dynamic nature of the HMO and the possible ramifications of all of the decisions they might make.

Cost Benefits of the FPM

Performing financial analyses by manual methods is time consuming, tedious, and often leads to computational errors. Once a planning group has formed an initial design of the HMO, it is not uncommon to spend in excess of 500 man hours determining its economic feasibility. In most cases, the HMO needs to be redesigned and, consequently, additional man hours must be consumed. The FPM performs the necessary calculations rapidly and at low cost to the planning group. Experience with the model indicates that the financial position of the HMO

over the first five years can be determined in approximately one minute of computer time at a cost of less than $7 per configuration studied. Furthermore, a feature of the model which allows the user to conduct sensitivity studies provides the planning group with several designs to review at one time.

Summary and Conclusions

Although the planning of both private and public health programs has been exercised for many decades, the state-of-the-art of financial planning in the health industry is still in its embryonic stages. The FPM described in this paper advances the state-of-the-art of health planning in general, and HMO planning in particular. The model and the several research reports prepared during its design bring together the necessary planning data and methodologies to design and evaluate various approaches for a prepaid medical care program. It is general in form and accommodates the most practical choices available to planners designing an HMO for qualification.

The model is capable of assisting HMO planners, sponsor organizations, and HEW officials

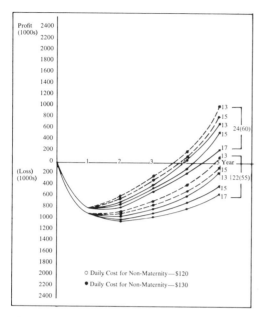

Figure VI.   HMO cash flow curves for various hospital cost inflation rates, premium levels, and daily cost for non-maternity patients

in studying the economic behavior of different HMO design strategies for plan enrollment; the services and benefits offered; the method of delivering these services; the occupancy of medical buildings and facilities; fee and prices for plan services; the cost of plan and community health resources; the borrowing of capital from HEW and other lending institutions.

The FPM is a new tool of analysis for HMO planners. It provides planners with additional inputs to help answer a number of design issues that must be answered inevitably before the HMO can become operational. The information provided by the FPM should not be considered as accurate and foolproof but, instead, should be treated as other "inputs" to the HMO decision-making process.

The simulation features of the FPM allow planners to evaluate a large number of designs at a reasonable cost. In addition, it serves to sensitize and educate those involved in the planning process of the many interactions that must be considered in the planning of a new form of health care delivery.

HMOs currently are being designed and developed at a rapid rate. At the present time, there are approximately 200 HMOs on the drawing board. How many of them will become financially secure HMOs is difficult to project, especially when planning groups have little technology for conducting financial studies. Hopefully, the FPM will help many of these planning organizations to conduct sound financial planning activities.

References

1 U.S. Congress, *The Health Maintenance Organization Act of 1973*, PL 93-222, 93rd Congress, 1973, S. 14.
2 "President Signs Bill for Reform in Medical Care," *New York Times*, December 30, 1973, p. 1.
3 Berman, Howard J. and Weeks, Lewis E. *The Financial Management of Hospitals*, the University of Michigan, 1971.
4 Forsyth, G. C. and Thomas, D. G. "Models for Financially Healthy Hospitals," *Harvard Business Review*, July–August 1971, pp. 107–117.
5 Gent, D. I. "How to Make Cash Forecasting Work for You," *Hospital Financial Management*, July 1972, pp. 27–32.
6 Fayollat, P. D. "Computer Models: Two Ways To Do Financial Forecasts," *Modern Hospital*, April 1973, pp. 103–106.
7 Montague, F. "In This Model, the Question for the Computer Is: What If," *Modern Hospital*, April 1973, pp. 107–109.

8 Serway, G. D. and Rath, G. J. "Computerized Projected Cash Flow Statement to Plan Hospital Expansion," *Inquiry* 9:59–63. (December 1972).
9 U.S. Department of Health, Education and Welfare, *Financial Planning in Ambulatory Health Programs*, Health Services and Mental Health Administration, U.S. Government Printing Office, Washington, D.C., 1973.
10 U.S. Department of Health, Education and Welfare, *Financial Planning Manual for HMOs*, Health Maintenance Organization Service, Health Services and Mental Health Administration, U.S. Government Printing Office, Washington, D.C., 1973.
11 Herbert, M. E. *A Financial Planning Guide for HMO Planners*, Inter-Study, Minneapolis, April 1973.
12 Moustafa, A. T. and Sears, D. W. "Feasibility of Simulation of Health Maintenance Organizations," *Inquiry*, 11:143–150 (June 1974).
13 Greene, L. A. and Grimes, R. M. "A Simulation of

the Financial Requirements of a Pre-Paid Health Care Delivery System," *Examination of Case Studies in Health Facilities Planning*, Proceedings of a Forum held at Washington, D.C., December 3, 4, 1973, National Cooperative Services Center for Hospital Management Engineering, Richmond, VA 1974.

14 Thompson, D. A. "Financial Planning for an HMO," *Health Services Research*, pp. 68–73 (Spring 1974).

15 Hirsch, G. and Miller, S. "Evaluating HMO Policies with a Computer Simulation Model," *Medical Care*, 12, No. 8, pp. 668–681 (August 1974).

16 Coleman, J. R., "A Financial Planning Model for Evaluating the Economic Viability of Health Maintenance Organizations," doctoral dissertation, Department of Industrial Engineering and Operations Research, University of Massachusetts, November 1975.

17 *Health Maintenance Organizations*, Part 110, Sub-Chapter J, Chapter I, Title 42, Code of Federal Regulations, *Federal Register*, Vol. 39, No. 203, Friday, October 18, 1974.

18 *Health Maintenance Organizations; Qualifying Conditions*, Part 405, Chapter III, Title 20, Code of Federal Regulations, *Federal Register*, Vol. 40, No. 128, Wednesday, July 2, 1975.

19 *Principles of Reimbursement for Cost-Basis Health Maintenance Organizations*, Part 405, Chapter III, Title 20, Code of Federal Regulations, *Federal Register*, Vol. 40, No. 146, Tuesday, July 29, 1975.

Myron J. Lefcowitz

Reprinted with permission of the Blue Cross Association, from *Inquiry:* Vol.X, No.1, pp.3-13. Copyright © 1973 by the Blue Cross Association.

Poverty and Health: A Re-examination

Originally Published in March 1973

Current discussions of health policies for the poor typically assume that poverty is a cause of medical deprivation. In these discussions there is much controversy over whether financial or structural barriers are more important in restricting availability and utilization of adequate health services by low-income populations. Whichever side of the argument is taken, two "facts" are accepted as true: 1) Poverty leads to less medical care; and 2) poverty results in diminished health.

In this paper available information that casts doubt on these two statements has been brought together. In addition to making the relationship of income to health problematic, the evidence at times suggests that level of education is a causal factor in individual health status and medical care utilization. When education is taken into account in analyzing the income-health relationship, the correlation is considerably diminished, usually to the point of disappearance. Education, within income levels, however, remains as a factor in health status and behavior. Hence, the observed correlation between income and medical deprivation appears to

Myron J. Lefcowitz, Ph.D. is on the staff of the Institute for Research on Poverty and is Associate Professor, School of Social Work, University of Wisconsin (1180 Observatory Drive, Madison, Wisconsin 53706).
The research reported here was supported by funds granted to the Institute by the Office of Economic Opportunity pursuant to the provisions of the Economic Opportunity Act of 1964. The author wishes to thank Burton Weisbrod, David Elesh, Robinson Hollister, Robert Lampman and Ray Munts for their comments on earlier drafts of this paper. However, the conclusions drawn in this paper are solely the responsibility of the author.

be a consequence of education's relationship with both variables. Unfortunately, the published data provide only a few instances—although they are strategic—having to do with medical care for children and infant mortality.

Some possible implications of this evidence for the current health policy debate are suggested. The major objective of the paper, however, is to clear away some of the myths which have heretofore befogged that debate. Before beginning, two points need to be made. Although some of the material to be presented are recomputations of the available data, the following is primarily a discussion of information as it has been published in various reports of the U.S. National Center for Health Statistics.[1] We do not pretend, therefore, any originality in data analysis. Since the line being pursued is different from the prevailing—or, at least, published—consensus, the use of data well-known to professionals in the field would appear to be particularly appropriate.

Second, we do not want to debate the definition of poverty. Whatever it is, there is agreement that in general economic terms it is at least some minimum access to a bundle of goods and services.[2] One indicator of poverty in that sense is family income. Thus, we shall be using poverty, low income, plus equivalent adjectives synonymously.

Medical Care

There has been almost universal agreement that the poor receive less than the non-poor in the way of actual medical care—both in quantity and quality. The Neigh-

349

borhood Health Center programs sponsored by OEO and then HEW were designed, at least in part, to redress the imbalance. This inequity in medical care, moreover, is apparently observable.[3]

Quantity of Care

The most recent data, however, suggest that there is little correlation between average number of physician visits per person per year and family income. Based on information gathered from household interviews in 1969, the average number of physician visits was 4.8 for persons in families with less than $3,000 income, and 4.3 for persons whose income was over $10,000.[4] But, these averages mask a strong relationship for children under 15 years of age. When family income is under $3,000, the average number of physician visits from July, 1966 to June, 1967 was 4.4 for children under five, and 1.5 for those five to 14 years of age. When income is over $10,000, the averages for the corresponding ages were 7.2 and 3.5[5] Taking education of the head of the family into account, however, the correlation between family income and average annual number of physician visits among children disappears (Table 1). This finding suggests that education of the family head is an important factor in medical care utilization for the young.

However, averages may not reflect the spread of utilization. Perhaps low-income persons visit the physician both less and more often than high-income persons; hence, the similarity in averages. There is little evidence, however, to support that suggestion. Although low-income persons are somewhat more likely than the high-income population *not* to have seen a physician, income is not related to a high frequency (five or more) of visits.[6]

Quality of Care

But what about the quality of that care? Unfortunately, the problem of medical care quality in general has barely been touched. It is an obviously complicated question both in definition and in measure-

Table 1. Number of physician visits per person per year by education of head of family and family income for persons under 15 years of age, July 1966-June 1967

| Family income | Education of head of family | | | |
	Under 5 years	5-8 years	9-12 years	13+ years
Under $5,000	2.1	2.2	3.2	5.4
$5,000 and over	1.4	2.6	4.1	5.0

Source: National Center for Health Statistics. *Volume of Physician Visits, 1966-1967*, Series 10-49 (1968) p. 23.

ment.[7] Hence, we ought to be wary of categorical statements on the relative inferiority of health care received by the poor.

One indicator of quality, however, is use of medical specialists. Specialists relative to other physicians deal more frequently with the diseases which come to their attention and are best-equipped to bring to bear the practices appropriate to management of the disease.[8] The three special services most frequently used, and for which information is available, are pediatrics, obstetrics-gynecology and eye care. In Table 2, the percent of the relevant population using those specialists from July, 1963 to June, 1964 is presented by family income and education of family head. In general, higher income persons had used these services more frequently than the population with incomes less than $4,000. Education also has an impact—one which appears to be sharper than income given the gross categories in Table 2. In almost all instances persons in families where the head had some college education were at least twice as likely to have used the service than when the head had less than nine years of education, regardless of income. These data, then, are consistent with the data reported on physician visits in general; which is, that education seems more strongly related to medical care utilization than income.

Another indicator of quality medical care is the use of private practitioners relative to public clinics. The poor are depicted as relying largely on public clinics and therefore are considered deprived in the quality of their health care compared

Table 2. Percent of population using selected types of medical specialists and practitioners by family income and education of head of family, July 1963-June 1964

Type of visit Income	Education of head of family		
	Under 9 years	9-12 years	13+ years
Pediatric			
Under $4,000	4	15	30
$4,000 and over	10	20	38
Obstetrics-gynecology			
Under $4,000	2	7	11
$4,000 and over	4	10	16
Ophthalmologic			
Under $4,000	4	5	10
$4,000 and over	5	6	11
Optometric			
Under $4,000	7	7	13
$4,000 and over	9	10	9

Source: National Center for Health Statistics. *Characteristics of Patients of Selected Types of Medical Specialists and Practitioners, July 1963-June 1964*, Series 10-28 (1966).

to the non-poor.[9] In fact, low-income persons are more likely to go to a hospital clinic or an emergency room than higher income persons—14 percent of physician visits from July, 1966-June, 1967 when family income is under $3,000 compared with 6 percent when income is over $10,-000. More important, however, 75 percent of the physician visits of low-income persons involved either a home or office visit with a private physician. This proportion, moreover, is the same for persons with higher income.[10] Thus, the image that the poor are at the mercy of public clinics for their medical care is a bit overdrawn.

This is not to argue that quality medicine is indeed distributed equitably across income classes. But, the little evidence available does suggest that an open mind on the issue is in order. Moreover, the data do suggest that when medical care varies by socioeconomic status, it is more across education levels than by family income.

Health of the Poor

But what about the health of the poor? If they are not as healthy as the non-poor, then similarity in medical care utilization would indicate that the poor are relatively deprived given their greater need. Assuming a corresponding demand, equal utilization may be a consequence of a relatively scarce supply of medical care in low-income areas.

Morbidity

Taking age into account, however, there appears to be very little relationship between income and the presence of chronic diseases.[11] This information is based on interviews—and fewer people report ailments than are detected by clinical examination. For example, 6.2 million persons had heart conditions in 1963-1965 according to household interviews.[12] Based on the Health Examination Survey from 1960-1962, however, 14.6 million adults had definite heart disease.[13] This discrepancy might be proportionately larger at lower income levels where people may be less informed about the presence of less obvious chronic conditions. Consequently in an actual clinical examination many more unsuspected ailments could be discovered among low-income persons than among high-income ones. Thus, the correlation between morbidity and income would be increased.

With this possibility in mind, information from the National Health Examination Survey on heart and arthritic conditions, the two leading causes of activity limitation,[14] has been summarized in Table 3. The data presented are the differences between the actual rate per 100 adults, as diagnosed through the Health Examination, and the rate that would have been expected given the age composition of the subgroup. (See the appendixes of the various Health Examination Survey reports for a technical description of the derivation of the expected value.) Thus, a *negative* value indicates *less* actual disease than might be expected for that population and a positive value denotes more. The closer the value is to zero, the closer together are the actual and expected rates.

Looking first at hypertensive heart disease, we can see that there is no apparent

Table 3. Differences between actual and expected* prevalence rates per 100 adults of selected disease conditions by family income, sex and race, 1960-1962

Disease conditions	Family income				
	Under $2,000	$2,000-3,999	$4,000-6,999	$7,000-9,999	$10,000 and over
Definite hypertensive heart disease					
White men	−0.5	−0.8	0.7	−·1.8	1.4
White women	3.8	−0.3	−0.7	−2.1	0.1
Black men	8.2	−6.6	−2.2	−6.9	11.9
Black women	2.7	−1.2	0.8	−6.4	−2.9
Definite hypertension					
White men	−1.6	0.4	1.0	−0.5	−1.6
White women	4.9	−0.7	−1.2	−0.7	−1.6
Black men	7.3	−5.4	−3.4	−13.8	6.5
Black women	4.3	1.9	−6.0	−0.4	−5.6
Definite coronary heart disease					
Men	−0.8	0.2	0.9	0.2	−1.7
Women	0.6	0.3	0.2	0.2	−1.2
Osteoarthritis					
Men	−2.8	0.3	−0.4	1.5	0.5
Women	0.5	0.0	−0.2	−1.0	2.0
Rheumatoid arthritis					
Men	3.0	−0.5	−0.6	−0.2	−0.1
Women	0.0	−0.5	0.7	−0.5	−0.5

*Standardized for age.

Sources: NCHS. *Hypertension and Hypertensive Heart Disease in Adults, 1960-1962*, Series 11-13 (1966) p. 24.
NCHS. *Coronary Heart Disease in Adults, 1960-1962*, Series 11-10 (1965) p. 23.
NCHS. *Osteoarthritis in Adults by Selected Demographic Characteristics, 1960-1962*, Series 11-20 (1966) p. 11.
NCHS. *Rheumatoid Arthritis in Adults, 1960-1962*, Series 11-17 (1966) p. 22.

relationship between family income and the difference between the actual and expected rates per 100 adults. For example, white men with under $4,000 family income have less definite hypertensive heart disease than expected; the next highest income category has more; the next less; those adults with incomes over $10,000 have more. For white women the pattern is quite different—the difference between the actual and expected rates decreases with income from 3.8 to −2.1 in the $7,000-$10,000 category and then increases to 0.1 for the highest income category. Black men exhibit a similar curvilinear pattern as white women—positive in the extreme income categories and negative in the middle categories. Among black women, however, there is no apparent relationship.

For hypertension, the curvilinear pattern appears for both white and black men, but in opposite directions. For women, however, the difference between actual and expected prevalence of hypertension does decrease as income increases (Table 3).

The general relationship is not clear, therefore, between income and hypertension, or income and hypertensive heart disease. Hypertension and hypertensive heart disease can stand for all the disease conditions reported in Table 3—that is, the negative relationship between income and these diseases is problematic. Given the relative importance of heart and arthritic conditions in limiting the activities of people, this conclusion would seem to be significant.

What about other impairments or conditions? The clinical data on diabetes,[15] anemia,[16] vision[17] and hearing[18] are generally consistent with the above conclusion. The available evidence from the Health Examination Survey, then, is consistent with data obtained from household interviews. The only conclusion is that the relationship between health and poverty—as indicated by morbidity—is not proven.

Mortality Rates

Some persons have argued, however, that mortality rates, particularly infant mortality, are a better indicator than morbidity rates of the health status of a population.[19] In general, past research has supported the generalization that these rates decrease with increased socioeconomic status. Nevertheless, the findings have not been unambiguous.[20] Data, however, are now available which permit us to obtain a fix on the variation in infant mortality rates by family income and parents' education. The necessary information was obtained by a follow-back survey of national samples of births and infant deaths for 1964-1966. The data presented suggest that for white births, family income has no consistent relationship with infant mortality when parents' education is taken into account. At all income levels, however, education, whether mother's or father's, is negatively related. For blacks, the patterns are not as clear although both income and education appear to have an impact on infant mortality rates.[21]

This evidence again forces us to be more skeptical about the presumed relationship between poverty and health even when the index of the latter is infant mortality. Rather, as our thesis contends, education appears to be the socioeconomic variable most closely related.

Education and Medical Deprivation

The policy implications of the apparent effect of education on medical deprivation and the concomitant diminution of the income-health correlation when education is taken into account are not readily apparent. In this section a general interpretation of the relationship of education to health will be presented; on the basis of that framework some policy directives are suggested.

Weber[22] pointed out that people are distributed in society along three dimensions —class, status and power. Class refers to economic positions, status to life styles (prestige), and power to control of others. Since persons are distributed with reference to each, policies can be directed to redistributing the values which locate people on each dimension; or, at least by producing enough of the values, we can attempt to move all members of society above some minimum level. Hence, poverty is reduced by increasing family income —and hopefully, the poor's relative share of total income is increased.

In this context, our hypothesis is that health-related and health-oriented behaviors are primarily a function of valued life styles and that education is a primary agent in the development of such tastes. Put some-

what differently, every family—within reasonable limits—has access to any part of the market bundle of goods and services available. How it selects, given its income, from that bundle is the family's life style. Education is a primary determinant in the ordering of those priorities.

What are the dynamics which link education and health? We start with the assumption that reduction of illness and prolongation of life are desired states. Education, in the first instance, is a process that increases the level of information about factors related to those desirable states. It does so directly through what is taught, at least up through the secondary level, but more probably through the acquisition of skills which enable the person to be both more sensitive and more alert to relevant information. Thus, for example, we expect that the more educated a person is, the more likely he is to be aware of the relationship between health and diet or physical exercise, topics much discussed in the mass media. Therefore, we would hypothesize that: The more educated a person is the more likely he is to have the opportunity to be exposed to, to expose himself to, and to be influenced by health information. His opportunities are greater because the mass media to which he is exposed is more likely to provide that information. He is more likely to expose himself because he is more alert to such information. Moreover, he is more influenced because he is more accepting of the claims of science in matters affecting day-to-day life.

Also, through education, the individual develops a life style which may have a greater impact on health status than what he or she may do directly. Diet, for example, may be more a consequence of food preferences or of physical aesthetics than concern about its apparent relationship to health.

This function of education is not explicit in that preferred choices are taught at each level, but rather that the level of education provides the basis for entry into social statuses; and during the distributional process different life styles are acquired—consciously or unconsciously.

More concretely, our educational system is directed toward fitting people into urban society. In that society, for instance, small families are apparently preferred—possibly because the costs for children are larger in cities. Therefore, we should expect that birth rates are related to residential background and education. And, that is indeed the case. Low rates are found for women of nonfarm origin and nonfarm residence. On the other hand, women with a farm background rapidly approach the birth rate for women who have a nonfarm background as farm women's educational level increases.[23] Moreover, family income is unrelated to birth rates in urbanized areas.[24] Whatever the primary social or economic function of small family size, it probably has the additional consequence of affecting the health status of the offspring. Evidence indicates that, in general, infant mortality increases with parity;[25] and moreover, this relationship remains even when socioeconomic status as measured by occupational categories is taken into account.[26] Thus, we can infer that the decreasing number of children per family which flows from increased education has the secondary consequence of reducing infant mortality and, hence, improving the health status of the population concomitantly, albeit indirectly.

One more example of the possible indirect effects of education on health status relates to accidents. The accident rate for a population is in some degree a consequence of the potentiality for injury inherent in that population's physical location and movement within a social environment. Presumably, this location and movement is a function of life style. Therefore, it is interesting to note that although income, controlling for age, is only slightly related to the current injury rate, education, again taking age into account, is strongly and negatively related in general. Thus, for persons 25-44 years of age, the current injury rate per 100 persons per year drops from 35.2 for persons with only some high school to 20.5 for persons with a college degree.[27]

One explanation is that education is also negatively related to the accident potential in occupations. Some evidence for this hypothesis is that men have higher injury rates than women at all age levels up to 65. This difference is largely attributable to the much greater incidence of work injuries among men. Following the same reasoning, we would also expect that nonwhites would have a higher accident rate than whites; that is, they are more likely to be in accident-risking situations—particularly at work. On the contrary, the nonwhite accident rate is two-thirds the white one for persons under 45 and about the same for persons over 45. These data at least bring into question occupation as an explanation for the relationship between education and injury rate. We would suggest that differential life styles may be the explanation.

Consumption Patterns and Permanent Income

An alternative explanation for the analytic importance of education relative to income for health status and health care is that consumption patterns are more directly tied to permanent income, for which level of education is a proxy. There is no way using available data, however, to test directly the permanent income hypothesis. Presumably, the relationship of education to family consumption of medical care and to infant mortality rates might be explained in part by the permanent income hypothesis. However, since most physician visits are a direct response to an illness and injury—only about 20 percent of the visits by children under 15 are for a general check-up or immunization and vaccination[28]—permanent income might be less important in the consumption of medical care than in expenditures for durable consumer goods.

Unfortunately, the above is only supposition. Efforts to find published data which could provide a more direct test was, with one exception, largely unavailing. The exception relates to cigarette smoking. We would expect in that case that average number of cigarettes smoked per day by men would increase with income—and indeed it does among present smokers. What we also find is that income is positively related to the age-adjusted percentage of men who have *never* smoked and who are former smokers. The same relationship holds for education.[29] It would be difficult to predict the fact that higher income is positively associated with not smoking cigarettes from a permanent income hypothesis. Actually, we would be more likely to predict the opposite in keeping with the generally positive relationship between income and the consumption of other goods and services.

Given the current state of our knowledge, however, the permanent income hypothesis is not so easily disproven. The above data do bring it into question, while leaving the life-style hypothesis untouched. Probably both mechanisms are in operation so that the main issue is their relative importance.

If our contention is correct that preferences (life styles) are of more moment in health behavior than access to a market basket of goods and services, what does this hypothesis have to say about whether to emphasize a financial or structural approach in our health policy? If the hypothesized lower preferences for health care among the less educated is correct, the price elasticity with respect to health care is small. Moreover, our data suggest that the income elasticity is also small (see Table 1). Although reduction in cost would clearly increase utilization (we assume, of course, that supply increases correspondingly or is already sufficient to handle the increased demand), the change would be small if the elasticities are as predicted. Whether the magnitude of that effect is optimum from society's viewpoint —that is, whether the consumption of medical services by the lower educated will move up to some level of adequacy—is problematic given the hypothesis.

The problem, then, is to increase the preference for health care and other health-inducing behaviors among the lower educated. This guideline suggests that alterations in the structure of the delivery system, as it relates to the less well-educated, be considered the appropriate policy direction. Most discussions of structural reform focus on increased supply and/or proximity of services, none of which addresses the heart of the problem as here stated. What is needed are changes that will decrease the psychic distance and that will enhance the significance of modern health practices for the medically deprived. Such programs as outreach workers sensitive to the life styles of the low-educated, medical translators to facilitate communication between the practitioner and client, reinforcement of preferred behaviors which are causally linked to health (e.g., making available at low cost preferred food which provides an adequate diet) appear to be mechanisms which in the short-range policy horizon would be more conducive to improving the health and medical care of the population concerned. An examination of the social-anthropological literature on the introduction of modern health technology among underdeveloped groups might be most instructive for our own society. If programs of this type were directed toward the low-income population, they would, by their nature, scoop in a large part of that subset which is deprived as a result of their life patterns.

Health and Poverty Restated

But what about the consequences of illness? It is our contention that illness and medical care have more serious consequences for lower income populations than for the affluent. In economic terms, the costs of illness are inequitably distributed among the income categories and hence may cause or increase impoverishment. We claim no originality for this idea for which the supportive data are generally known. What we do assert is that incorrect policy implications have been drawn.

First, even though the prevalence of persons with one or more chronic ailments

Table 4. Percent of adults with family incomes under $3,000 by their chronic condition and activity limitation status, 1965-1966

| | Percent under $3,000 income | | | | |
| | | Persons with 1+ chronic conditions | | | |
Age	Persons with no chronic conditions	No limitation of activity	Limitation, but not in major activity	Limitation in amount or kind of major activity*	Unable to carry on major activity
17-44	12	11	16	24	41
45-64	12	13	21	36	51
65+	43	47	54	55	57

*Major activity refers to ability to work, keep house, or engage in school or preschool activities.
Source: NCHS. *Limitation of Activity and Mobility Due to Chronic Conditions, 1965-1966*, Series 10-45 (1968) p. 26.

is unrelated to income, persons whose chronic conditions limit their major activity are much more likely to have incomes under $3,000 than where the ailment is less restrictive (Table 4). This relationship is particularly true for non-aged adults. In the 17-44 age group, among those who have no chronic conditions, one out of every eight or nine has a family income under $3,000; in the same group among those unable to carry on their major activity two out of every five have family incomes under $3,000 (Table 4). The pattern is similar for 45-64 year olds. Among the aged, where advanced years restrict activity in any case, low income is much less related to the limitations imposed by chronic conditions.

This finding is not surprising. Income and the physical demands of occupational activity are, in general, negatively related. Among persons with similar ailments, moreover, we would expect those engaged in physical labor to be more restricted in their work activity than persons in nonmanual occupations.

Some evidence for this hypothesis is presented in Table 5. Among currently employed persons over 44 years of age who report one or more chronic conditions, those in farm and nonfarm labor occupations are most likely to say that their condition limited their major activity. Alternatively, professional, technical, and clerical workers are least likely to report such restrictions (see Table 5).

Haber[30] presents corroborating data from the Social Security Disability Survey. The occupations in which the workers are most limited are also somewhat more likely to include workers having one or more chronic conditions (Table 5). Thus, it is possible that the chronic condition may be a consequence of work, particularly farm work, itself. That possibility aside, however, the data are consistent with, but do not confirm our thesis that the economic consequences of poor health are more serious for persons in more physically demanding occupations.

Income and Work Days Lost

Unfortunately, these data are not available by employment status and income. However, we do have, by income, the average number of days lost from work during 1968-1969 for currently employed persons. What is instructive to note is that income is correlated with work days lost for men between 25 and 64 years of age. Moreover, the relationship is quite strong. Men 25-44 years old lose twice as much time from work if their income is less than $3,000 than if it is over $10,000. Among men 45-64 years old, those with less than $3,000 income lose more than twice as many days as men with more than $10,000 family income. Thus, precisely among primary wage earners, the differential cost of illness is greatest.[31]

Lower income families, then, lose a greater proportion of their income as a result of illness than do more affluent per-

Table 5. Chronic conditions and limitation of major activity by occupation of currently employed persons over 44 years of age, 1965-1966

Occupation	Of all in occupation, percent with chronic conditions	Of all with 1+ chronic conditions, percent with limitation of major activity
Professional, technical	68	7
Managers, officials proprietors (nonfarm)	69	15
Clerical	68	9
Sales	72	15
Craftsmen and foremen	67	14
Operative	66	13
Service, except private household	69	15
Private household	77	24
Laborers, except farm and mine	69	24
Farm laborers and foremen	72	33
Farmers and farm managers	77	33

Source: NCHS. *Limitation of Activity and Mobility Due to Chronic Conditions, 1965-1966,* Series 10-45 (1968) pp. 48-49.

sons. This conclusion assumes that days lost from work means wages lost for everyone. But, it is plausible that persons in higher paying jobs are more likely to have sick leave benefits, formal or informal, and therefore, are less likely to lose any income as a result of illness. In fact, that is the case. The higher the family income, the more likely are currently employed persons to report that they are reimbursed for work time lost through illness.[32] Thus, the impact on income for wage earners in the lower income categories is even greater relative to high-income persons than just missing more days at work.

Costs of illness, obviously, can also mean direct out-of-pocket expenses for the necessary treatment and care. Such out-of-pocket costs are proportionately greater for lower income families.[33] In 1961, families with less than $4,000 money income after taxes spent between 7.5 and 10 percent of it on medical care compared to 6 to 7 percent

for higher income families.[34] Family income was negatively and sharply related to coverage by hospital and surgical insurance.[35] Since the proportion of persons hospitalized in a given year does not vary by income,[36] we can assume that lower income persons are more likely to be confronted with a large medical bill than are persons with higher incomes. For example, of those persons hospitalized for surgical treatment, where family income was under $2,000, about one-third of the discharges had some part of the surgeon's bill paid for by insurance compared with four-fifths when the income was over $7,000.[37] The threat of a catastrophic medical bill is underlined by the fact that hospitalized lower income persons tend to be in the hospital somewhat longer than their higher income counterparts.[38]

The conclusion that illness has a greater financial impact on the poor than the more affluent is hardly surprising. After all, Medicare and Medicaid are attempts to correct this inequity—at least insofar as direct out-of-pocket costs are concerned—as are the various health bills currently in the Congressional hopper. What the data point to, however, is that vocational rehabilitation and cash transfer programs may be more productive in ameliorating the consequences of poor health than are health programs.

Conclusion

This paper has attempted to focus the available, mostly published data about income and health on the public debate over whether financial barriers or structural barriers are more important in restricting availability and utilization of adequate health services to lower income populations. This debate has assumed in part that medical deprivation is caused by poverty. Through reviewing the data, however, that assumption has been questioned. Hence, insofar as the policy controversy has been based on poverty as a causal factor in poor health and inadequate medical care, the demarcation of alternative approaches to improving health standards and increasing medical care utilization has rested on an unstable assumption. Instead, the evidence presented indicates that education is negatively related to health and health care.

Policy Directions

The policy directions for intervention between education and health status and care are not immediately apparent. We have suggested that education functions to distribute the population by valued life styles (preferences, in economic terms) and that these styles include elements which directly or indirectly affect health and utilization of health services. Presumably, as the educational level increases, the health status of the population will improve in response to the hypothesized change in life styles. At the same time, effective demand for health care will also increase. It is very difficult, of course, to demonstrate both trends as well as their causal relationship to education. If the general hypothesis is correct, however, it does suggest that policies designed to reduce medical deprivation on the basis of poverty as a cause are misguided. In this framework the current policy issue may be reformulated: What changes in health policy—financial and/or structural—will increase utilization among the less educated given their relatively lower preference for health care?

A policy explicitly for the less educated does not appear reasonable. We would hardly want to add a taste test as an analog to the means test. Since education and income are highly correlated, a health policy directed toward the poor would cover a large portion of the low-educated population. But, which type of remedy—financial or structural—should be emphasized?

The argument is presented that the effect of a financial policy would lead to only a small increase in health care utilization and/or health-improving behavior among the low-educated. The basis for that hypothesis is that both income elasticity and price elasticity with respect to such behavior are small. Thus, if we are interested in the medically deprived, policies directed to changing the preferences and/or to reinforcing existing health-inducing preference patterns are required. This conclusion suggests, then, that structural changes be given central consideration over financial changes in the health arena.

But, can we then ignore the poor as such in our development of policy? The evidence presented in the paper does support the notion that a loss of health and the use of medical care are more costly to the poor than non-poor. This cost is twofold. First, the share of income required for medical care is greater for the poor. Any policy which picks up the tab for services can to that extent redress the inequity. Clearly, however, this objective is more income-distributional than health-improving. Second, poor health can drastically affect earnings, making poor out of previously non-poor and creating a barrier to movement out of poverty for those persons already there. Policies designed to reduce the income consequences of ill health would focus on transfer payments during an illness or disability period (e.g., broader disability insurance both in coverage of working population and to other than work-related disabilities) and/or an expansion of our vocational rehabilitation programs.

To a large extent, then, a serious attempt to deal with the health and poverty issue would involve only in part what is typically considered a health program and would address itself to the relative cost inequities between poor and non-poor.

References and Notes

1 See the following National Center for Health Statistics (NCHS) publications for a more detailed description of their surveys: *Origin, Program, and Operation of the U.S. National Health Survey*, Series 1-1 (1963); *Cycle I of the Health Examination Survey: Sample and Response*, Series 11-1 (1963); and *Plan and Initial Program of the Health Examination Survey*, Series 1-4 (Washington, D.C.: GPO, 1964).

Since the Government Printing Office is the publisher for all NCHS publications, that information will not be repeated.

2 Watts, Harold. "An Economic Definition of Poverty." In: Moynihan, D.P. (ed.) *On Understanding Poverty* (New York: Basic Books, 1969) pp. 316-329.

3 White, Elijah L. "A Graphic Presentation on Age and Income Differentials in Selected Aspects of Morbidity, Disability and Utilization of Health Services," *Inquiry* 5:18-30 (March 1968).

4 NCHS. *Age Patterns in Medical Care, Illness, and Disability, 1968-1969*, Series 10-70 (1972) p. 10.

5 NCHS. *Volume of Physician Visits, 1966-1967*, Series 10-49 (1968) p. 19.

6 *Ibid.*, p. 39.

7 Roth, Julius. "The Treatment of the Sick." In: Kosa, John, *et al.* (eds.) *Poverty and Health* (Cambridge: Harvard University Press, 1969) pp. 222-226.

8 Mechanic, David. *Medical Sociology* (New York: The Free Press, 1968) p. 354.

9 Roth, *op. cit.*, pp. 217-218.

10 NCHS. Series 10-49, *op. cit.*, p. 30.

11 NCHS. *Limitation of Activity and Mobility Due to Chronic Conditions, 1965-1966*, Series 10-45 (1968).

12 NCHS. *Age Patterns in Medical Care, Illness, and Disability, 1963-1965*, Series 10-32 (1966) p. 55.

13 NCHS. *Heart Disease in Adults, 1960-1962*, Series 11-6 (1964) p. 7.

14 NCHS. Series 10-45, *op. cit.*, p. 6.

15 NCHS. *Blood Glucose Levels in Adults, 1960-1962*, Series 11-18 (1966).

16 NCHS. *Mean Blood Hematocrit of Adults, 1960-1962*, Series 11-24 (1967).

17 NCHS. *Binocular Visual Acuity of Adults, by Region and Selected Demographic Characteristics, 1960-1962*, Series 11-25 (1967).

18 NCHS. *Hearing Level of Adults by Education, Income, and Occupation, 1960-1962*, Series 11-31 (1968).

19 Lerner, Monroe. "Social Differences in Physical Health." In: Kosa, *et al.* (eds.) *Poverty and Health, op. cit.* p. 91.

20 Mechanic, *op. cit.*, pp. 244-257.

21 NCHS. *Infant Mortality Rates: Socioeconomic Factors*, Series 22-14 (1972) pp. 13-14.

22 Weber, Max. "Class, Status, Party." In: Gerth, H. H., and Mills, C. Wright. (trs.) *From Max Weber: Essays in Sociology* (New York: Oxford University Press, 1946) pp. 180-195.

23 Duncan, Otis Dudley. "Farm Background and Differential Fertility," *Demography* 2:240-249 (1965).

24 Sweet, James. "Some Demographic Aspects of Income Maintenance Policy." In: Orr, Larry L.; Hollister, Robinson G.; and Lefcowitz, Myron J. (eds.) *Income Maintenance: Interdisciplinary Approaches to Research* (Chicago: Markham Press, 1971).

25 Illsley, Raymond. "The Sociological Study of Reproduction and Its Outcome." In: Richardson, Stephen A., and Guttmacher, Alan F. (eds.) *Childbearing: Its Social and Psychological Aspects* (Baltimore: Williams and Wilkins, 1967) pp. 96-98.

26 Chase, Helen C. "Infant Mortality and Weight at Birth: 1960 United States Birth Cohort," *American Journal of Public Health* 59:1618-1628 (September 1969).

27 NCHS. *Types of Injuries: Incidence and Associated Disability, 1965-1967*, Series 10-57 (1969) p. 7.

28 NCHS. *Volume of Physician Visits by Place of Visit and Type of Service, 1963-1964*, Series 10-18 (1965) p. 26.

29 Hedrick, James L. *Facts on Smoking, Tobacco, and Health* (National Clearinghouse for Smoking and Health, 1968) pp. 10-11.

30 Haber, Lawrence D. "Disability and Social Planning: Implications of The Social Security Disability Survey." Paper presented at the annual meeting of the National Conference on Social Welfare, June 3, 1970, Chicago, Illinois.

31 NCHS. *Time Lost From Work Among the Currently Employed Population, 1968*, Series 10-71 (1972) p. 15.

32 *Ibid.*, p. 23.

33 Tucker, Murray A. "Effect of Heavy Medical Expenditures on Low Income Families," *Public Health Reports* 85:419-425 (May 1970).

34 U.S. Bureau of Labor Statistics. *Consumer Expenditure Survey Report, 1960-61*, Report 237-93 (Washington, D.C.: GPO, 1965) p. 16.

35 NCHS. *Family Hospital and Surgical Insurance Coverage, 1962-1963*. Series 10-42 (1967) pp. 13-17.

36 NCHS. *Persons Hospitalized by Numbers of Hospital Episodes and Days in a Year, 1965-1966*. Series 10-50 (1969).

37 NCHS. *Proportion of Surgical Bill Paid by Insurance, 1963-1964*. Series 10-31 (1966) p. 8.

38 NCHS. Series 10-50, *op. cit.*, p. 14.

Part VI

Applications

Among the tools of economic analysis, cost-benefit analysis or a variation of it is most often used as a practical way to assess the desirability of public projects. This involves drawing on a variety of traditional sections of economic study—welfare economics, public finance, resource economics—and trying to weld these components into a coherent whole. Most of the papers in this section deal with applying the cost-benefit technique to problems in the health field.

The first paper by Crystal and Brewster serves as an introduction to acquaint people in the health field with cost-benefit analysis and how it may be used for dealing with the problems at hand. The following three papers cite examples of actual applications of cost-benefit analysis as used in assessing the desirability of a phenylketonuria screening program, alcoholism rehabilitation program, and infectious kidney disease prevention program respectively.

Whatever program one chooses, the decision will have to rest on some form of quantification of benefits and costs. These papers provide insight into some of the theoretical and procedural problems that are likely to be encountered in carrying out the task of evaluating costs and benefits. Readers will realize from these examples the importance of taking a long view (in the sense of looking at repercussions in the future) and a wide view (in the sense of allowing for side effects of many kinds of many persons, industries, regions, etc.).

The Martin Feldstein and James Schuttinga paper develops a sophisticated statistical method for assessing the effect of case-mix on hospital cost. Evaluations of interhospital differences in hospital cost usually encounter the problem of how to hold the effect of case-mix on cost constant so that more meaningful cost comparisons may be made. This paper offers a method that goes a long way toward solving this classic dilemma. The problem addressed here is similar to that dealt with by Thompson, et al. and Berry, albeit their respective approaches differ.

361

Royal A. Crystal
Agnes W. Brewster

Reprinted with permission of the Blue Cross Association, from *Inquiry*: Vol.III, No.4, pp.3-13. Copyright © 1966 by the Blue Cross Association.

Cost Benefit and Cost Effectiveness Analyses in the Health Field: An Introduction

Originally Published in December 1966

This study presents a discussion of the related analytical techniques of cost effectiveness and cost benefit analyses. The utilization of these techniques in the health field makes it possible to examine problems and estimate yield or return for given investments. The cost benefit approach measures the magnitude of a disease, problem, or group of these, while the cost effectiveness analysis is employed to estimate the anticipated return for the various alternatives. The methods of constructing cost benefit and cost effectiveness models are explained, and some ways they can be used in the health field are pointed out.

The purpose of this discussion of cost benefit and cost effectiveness analyses is to present an introduction to these techniques in a clear and concise manner for the use of those responsible for planning and policy making in the health field. Cost benefit and cost effectiveness analyses are primarily analytical techniques which are used by the manager in making his choice. By their use it is possible to select what is considered to be an optimal approach from a group of feasible alternatives. The cost benefit approach has been used in industry in various forms. It is not a

Royal A. Crystal is Associate Director, Health Services and Resources Data Center, Division of Medical Care Administration, Public Health Service, Department of Health, Education, and Welfare, and **Agnes W. Brewster** is Chief, Health Economics Branch, Division of Medical Care Administration, Public Health Service, Department of Health, Education, and Welfare.

new tool; it is only new to many health program planners.

For some time the Department of Defense has been using these analytical techniques to review some of its programs and problems, in determining which weapons systems to select or how best to deploy forces for a given mission. This is probably where the phrase "more bang for the buck" originated. The results of these types of analyses in defense planning have interested the Bureau of the Budget to the extent that it is working to have all other federal agencies evaluate their programs in this manner, using what is referred to as "Program Planning Budgeting."

The results and efficiency of these techniques, as used in government, have rapidly become of interest to planners and decision makers outside of government. In the health field especially, they open the door to a wide range of decision possibilities, both administrative and technical, which heretofore have not been taken advantage of. In the not too distant future as these tools are refined for use in what is essentially a service industry, it will be possible to rank diseases and health problems according to the economic burden they place on our communities, and to select and develop our programs along lines which will assure the greatest return for our investment in health services. Through the application of cost effectiveness analysis particularly, it will be possible to maximize the efficiency of both the programs which serve people and the administrative procedures which these programs dictate.

COST BENEFIT ANALYSIS

Briefly stated, a cost benefit analysis is a series of mathematical calculations which provide an estimate of the potential value of following a given course of action, such as undertaking or instituting a new program or procedure or revising an old one. In the health field, cost benefit calculations frequently relate to the gain or benefit which will accrue to society as a result of following a stipulated course. An excellent definition of the conceptual framework for cost benefit analysis has been developed by Klarman in his book, *The Economics of Health*,[1] and is abstracted below.

1. "The total costs of a disease per case serve as the measure of benefits derived from preventing that case. In a cost benefit calculation the comparison is between contemplated additional expenditures for health and medical services, on the one hand, and the anticipated reduction in costs (direct plus indirect), on the other hand . . . In practice, difficulties may arise as decisions are made on the methods of handling the several elements of the calculation and, as compromises are struck, by measuring the elements for which data are available rather than those which are indicated by the conceptual framework or theoretical model.

2. "One difficulty is that few (if any) health services are pure investment goods or pure consumption goods. It is customary to recognize the consumption benefit of most health and medical care expenditures, to comment on the difficulty of measuring it, and then to dismiss it. What is measurable may not be necessarily important, but it is recorded and, therefore, cited. The measurable part (the investment component) is not likely, however, to bear a uni-

form relationship to the consumption component in all health and medical care programs. Attaching a value to the consumption part of the benefit, lest it be totally neglected (or treated as zero), is a challenging task."

In discussing cost benefit analysis, it is necessary to recognize that we are dealing primarily with concepts. The first concept is that of the total or gross cost of a disease. We define gross cost as the measure of the total benefit which will accrue to society as a result of total control or eradication; *i.e.*, of not having the disease. The gross cost consists of two elements: actual dollar expenditures for care and services, and theoretical dollar losses as a result of lost productivity. It is necessary to grasp this concept if cost benefit analysis is to be used as a tool in assigning program priorities, since it provides a measure not only of the direct cost of a disease, but also of the total economic cost of the disease. The second concept is that of the net benefit to society, which is defined as the gross cost of the disease less the cost of control or eradication. This concept is most useful since it provides us with a working measure of the value of control.

There are two types of cost associated with any given disease: the direct or "real cost," and the indirect or theoretical cost. The components of these costs are shown in Figure I.

The direct cost area is concerned with actual medical care expenditures which are associated with the disease or condition and which are made by people in a given time period; people are defined as individuals, government, other third parties, or any combination of these. Direct costs include both personal and nonpersonal service costs. Expenditures for personal services include the costs for hospital care, nursing homes, physicians' services, drugs, and nursing care, to list a few of the items. Nonpersonal services include the cost of research and training, a portion of the annual expenditures for health insurance, and expenditures for other non-

[1] Herbert E. Klarman, *The Economics of Health* (New York: Columbia University Press, 1965), pp. 163-4.

FIGURE I
Components of Economic Cost of Disease

I. DIRECT COSTS—

Personal Services
Hospital Care
Nursing Home Care
Physiciar.s' Service
Drugs
Nursing Service
Other Services

Nonpersonal Services
Research Costs
Training Costs
Other Health Services Costs
Cost of Facilities Construction
Net Cost of Insurance

II. INDIRECT COSTS—

Dollar Losses Due to Mortality
Current Years
Previous Years

Dollar Losses Due to Morbidity
Institutionalized Patients
Noninstitutionalized Patients

personal services. The direct cost component concept may be easily understood and requires less complex computation procedures than those used for indirect costs.

In a study entitled *Estimating the Cost of Illness* (1963),[2] Dorothy P. Rice estimated the cost of various disease groups based on total health care expenditures in the United States in 1963 and on projections of the value of lost productivity for 1963 and all future years for the affected populations. The cost components varied slightly from the model shown in Figure I, in that direct costs were allocated entirely to personal services, rather than to personal and nonpersonal services. This study found that the total cost of the grouping *Diseases of the Circulatory System* was $20.9 billion, as shown in Figure II.

Of the $20.9 billion total, the direct cost was $2.2 billion. Therefore, the bulk of the cost, approximately $18.7 billion, is not yet explained. This $18.7

[2] Dorothy P. Rice, *Estimating the Cost of Illness* (U.S. Department of Health, Education, and Welfare, Public Health Service Publication No. 947-6 [Washington, D.C.: U.S. Government Printing Office, May, 1966]), pp. 7-8.

billion is the indirect, or theoretical cost. In analyzing this amount, one begins to mix theoretical losses with real costs (expenditures).

The concept of indirect cost, as indicated here, is that the present value of current and future productivity losses for those with circulatory diseases is $18.7 billion when computed for 1963. If the group of patients with circulatory diseases had not been so affected, the value of their output would have accounted for this additional amount being added to the gross national product in 1963 and later years.

In *Estimating the Cost of Illness*,[3] Rice states the underlying economics of indirect cost and its relationship to the present value of future earnings in the following manner:

"From the economist's point of view, however, single year cost estimates represent only a portion of the estimated losses in output resulting from illness, disability and death, thereby seriously under-estimating the economic costs to society. If an individual had not died in this year, he would have continued to be productive for a number of years. If he is ill and disabled this year and his disability continues into future years, his future productivity will be affected. It is the present value of these future losses that constitutes the appropriate measure of the costs of a disease.

"For mortality, the estimated cost or value to society of all deaths is the product of the number of deaths and the expected value of an individual's future earnings with sex and age taken into account. This method of derivation must consider life expectancy for different age and sex groups, changing patterns of earning at successive ages, varying labor force participation rates, imputed value for housewives' services, and the appropriate discount rate to convert a stream of costs or benefits into its present worth."

As described, the economic cost of a disease is a combination of the direct (or actual) cost and the indirect cost

[3] *Ibid.*, p. 85.

FIGURE II

Estimated Economic Cost for Diseases of the Circulatory System, 1963*

Type of Cost	Amount (millions)	Percent
Total	$20,948.3	100.0
Direct costs	2,267.3	10.8
Hospital care	1,272.7	
Nursing home care	207.1	
Physicians' services	714.2	
Nursing care†	73.3	
Indirect costs	18,681.0	89.2
Morbidity losses—1963		
institutional population	328.9	
noninstitutional population	2,590.7	
Mortality losses—1963 and		
future years, discounted at 4 percent	15,761.4	

* Abstracted from Dorothy P. Rice, *Estimating the Cost of Illness*, Public Health Service Publication No. 947-6, May, 1966, Tables 2, 4, 8, 10, 26.
† Includes the services of private duty professional nurses in the hospital and home, private duty practical nurses, and visiting nurses.

(the value of lost productivity). However, in cost benefit analysis, because some diseases cannot be eradicated, but rather can only be controlled (as may be true for most diseases), an additional cost is computed and labeled as a "control or eradication factor."

For instance, Figure II indicates that circulatory diseases carry an annual cost of approximately $20.9 billion for 1963. With this $20.9 billion in mind, we then ask how much more it would cost to reduce circulatory diseases' morbidity and mortality rates by a given percent, because while these conditions cannot be eradicated their incidence can be reduced. The additional expenditures for research, training, and services, and for new construction if required for morbidity and mortality reduction is defined as the control factor. By assuming some level of morbidity and mortality reduction, we also imply a reduction in the economic cost of the disease.

In those conditions where eradication or total control is possible, for example polio through the use of new vaccines, the direct plus the indirect economic cost less the cost of control or eradication is considered to be the net benefit to society. In those programs that only

lend themselves to partial control, such as heart disease, the proportion of cost saved is described as an interim benefit; therefore, the net benefit to society is defined as the proportional saving which accrues as a result of stipulated control activities. Figure III presents models of highly simplified cost benefit formulae to illustrate the general application of these concepts.

COST EFFECTIVENESS ANALYSIS

A second major area in which interest has developed over the last several years is that of cost effectiveness analysis. Cost effectiveness analysis is best defined as a series of analytical and mathematical procedures which aid in the selection of a course of action from among various alternative approaches. The cost effectiveness approach has evolved into an effective tool for management decision making, planning, and resource allocation. The Division of Indian Health Services of the Public Health Service was one of the first service organizations to utilize this technique, and has proven that it can be applied successfully in the health field.

In cost effectiveness analysis, as in

cost benefit analysis, there are several basic concepts which must be considered. Among these concepts, the following three are most important:

1. There are alternative ways to accomplish an objective and we must select the optimal alternative, which may not be the least costly one.
2. There must be at least two alternative ways to accomplish a task in order to undertake cost effectiveness analysis.
3. Cost effectiveness analysis is not cost reduction; it is optimization of an approach to a specific goal or set of goals.

From a managerial standpoint cost effectiveness analysis is directed by two basic economic considerations: (1) A minimum expectation that in either social or economic terms, for the program being undertaken, there will be a dollar of return for each dollar of investment. (2) An optimal expectation that one dollar plus some additional increment of economic or social return will accrue for each dollar of investment.

A cost effectiveness analysis is ultimately reduced to a series of models. These models, which are frequently but not always complex, set out alternatives and indicate the anticipated return of each alternative relative to a given level of investment. Operationally, the procedure requires a separate set of models for each available alternative.

In undertaking cost effectiveness analysis we must consider the inputs which go into the development of the analytic models. Essentially, the same inputs are used that have always been used in decision making and planning. For example: (1) Capital—What dollars are available to do the job? (2) Labor—How many people are available to accomplish the goal? (3) Tools— What techniques, facilities, etc., are available? (4) Data—What sources of information are available?

FIGURE III

Illustrative Cost Benefit Models

DEFINITION OF SYMBOLS

DC = Direct cost (the expenditure for care and services)

IC = Indirect cost (the value of lost productivity)

TC = Total cost of the disease $(DC + IC)$

F = Control or eradication factor (expenditures for additional research, services, training, and construction necessary to achieve a given level of control or eradication)

NB = Interim or net benefit to society (proportion of benefit derived from partial control or eradication)

G = Gross benefit to society

COST BENEFIT MODELS

Cost Benefit Concept—$TC = G$

Where the total cost of a disease $(TC = DC + IC)$ is defined as the benefit in dollars which would accrue to society if the disease was eradicated, i.e., without the disease there would be no direct expenditures for care and services and no loss in productivity.

Eradication Program—$NB = DC + IC — F$

Where the net or actual benefit to society (NB) is defined as the cost of the disease $(DC + IC)$ less the added or incremental cost (F) required to bring about total control or eradication.

Control Program—

$$NB = (DC)(B) + (IC)(B) — F$$

Where the net or actual benefit to society (NB) is defined as a proportion of the cost of the disease less the added or incremental cost (F) required to bring about a stipulated level of control or eradication.

It is important to recognize that in many respects cost effectiveness analysis uses procedures which are similar to those currently used in program evaluation. However, a more disciplined look is being taken in order to fully analyze information, alternatives, and problems and, where possible, take advantage of various new technological developments which are available. In this disciplined process, the initial step is to delineate clear and specific objectives, which ask why it is necessary to do a given task and what is expected in return for the undertaking. We do not merely say we want to reduce condition X by 20 per-cent or build 500 new hospital beds in community Y. Rather, we ask why we should be doing this and what our real short and long range objectives are. After the objectives have been deter-mined, the cost effectiveness approach evaluates the alternatives, asking the questions, "To attain this objective, how many alternatives and what types of alternatives are available? Do we only have one way to do the job? Are there two alternatives open to us? Are there more than two alternatives? If there are several alternatives, what specifically are they?"

In determining available alternatives the procedure requires looking beyond the obvious. For example, is there the possibility of a time-cost trade-off? It may be that if a community continues to add hospital beds at the current rate over a period of 15 years, its needs will be met. However, if expenditures are increased for years one through five, it may be possible to reach necessary ca-pacity within five years and thereby satisfy demand much sooner. In another approach, it might be decided that while one could spend $4 billion adding hospi-tal beds over the next 15 years and thus spread expenditures, it would be more advantageous if part of the expenditure was for increased research to provide a major breakthrough for a specific disease which would then reduce the need for many additional hospital beds.

For another example of the possible use of cost effectiveness analysis, it is of interest to review the program which was implemented after the development of the polio vaccine. In the United States, vaccination programs for chil-dren were initiated through the private sector of the economy. Our sister coun-try, Canada, did this through a public program. If the techniques of cost effec-tiveness were applied prior to reaching a program decision, information would have been provided on the cost to the government as well as the cost that did enter into the formula, the cost to the family of paying the physician. The ul-timate objective of universal vaccina-tion probably was not considered in the original proposal. Cost effectiveness analysis would have forced an evalua-tion of this consideration. Estimates of the possible extra cost of a completely public program, or some other combina-tion, might have been in terms of its effectiveness if in fact the goal was to have every child protected against polio.

After setting objectives and deter-mining possible alternative ways to at-tain these objectives, it is necessary to specify what resources are required for each alternative—resources in terms of people, money, equipment, and facilities. Having thus developed objectives, al-ternatives, and resource needs, the analyst then prepares cost effectiveness models for each alternative and also de-termines the criteria to be used for the selection of the preferred alternative or alternatives.

As the cost effectiveness models are built, we are concerned with several pertinent measurements which will be used in making a decision and which form parts of the model. These include:

1. Measures of effectiveness — the criteria which indicate how well the alternative satisfies the objec-tives.
2. Measures of operational use—the criteria for consideration of alter-natives in light of the other re-sponsibilities which must be un-dertaken.
3. Measures of personnel and equip-ment needed—the determination for each alternative of the num-ber and kinds of people and equip-ment required.
4. Cost factors.
5. Measures of cost—the determina-tion of cost for each alternative way of doing the job and the manner in which cost will be measured.

FIGURE IV

Illustration of Interacting Cost Effectiveness Models

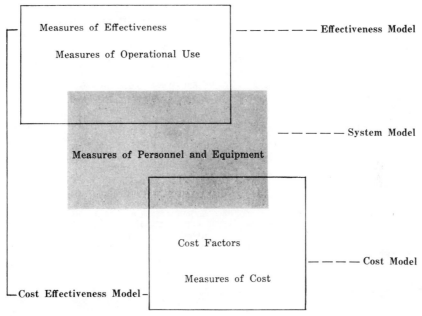

There are therefore five types of measurement which must be considered. These measurements are combined into what is called the cost effectiveness model. In practice there is not one, but three interacting models which form the cost effectiveness analysis, as shown in Figure IV.

The three models in Figure IV are built around the five measurements, since the individual measurements are generally meaningless by themselves. Measurements of effectiveness and operational use are related to the personnel and equipment needed, and these in turn are related to the various cost factors involved. When taken together, these three models form the overall cost effectiveness model for any given alternative.

Figure V presents a group of simplified models which were developed for demonstration purposes in the Public Health Service.

The objective, which had been thought through in a clear and precise manner, is stated "to increase research grant applications in health economics by 10 percent in the next 12 months." Given this specific objective, it was possible to look at the number of alternative ways in which it could be accomplished. It was found that there were five alternatives.

Having delineated these alternatives, the assumption was made that data were available, since it is known what university departments of economics exist in the United States, what level of degrees they offer, and the size and qualification of the faculties. At this point, consideration was given to the personnel required for each alternative. The type of non-branch staff required was also considered; for instance, regional office staff that would be required. After estimating what staff was needed for each alternative, a dollar cost for each alternative was developed. This cost included staff costs, additional costs of printing, additional travel, and other elements which could be foreseen. In summary, these costs represent both current costs

FIGURE V

Theoretical Cost Effectiveness Model

Objective—To increase research grant applications in health economics by 10 percent in the next 12 months

Assumption—All necessary information is available

MEASUREMENT EFFECTIVENESS MODEL	ALTERNATIVES				
	1	**2**	**3**	**4**	**5**
Effectiveness—Yield (percent)	6.0	9.0	10.5	2.0	0.5
Operational Use—Man Days					
Central Office					
a. Preparation	300	300	250	50	—
b. Contact	200	200	150	350	125
c. Follow-up	300	400	400	150	—
d. Meetings	200	400	300	—	—
e. Travel	250	200	100	—	—
Regional Office					
a. Preparation	150	50	50	—	—
b. Contact	70	50	50	150	—
c. Follow-up	125	100	200	50	—
d. Meetings	75	100	50	—	—
e. Travel	30	100	100	—	—
Total Man Days	1,700	1,900	1,650	750	125
SYSTEM MODEL					
Equipment Required					
Central Office					
a. Current	yes	yes	yes	yes	yes
b. Additional	yes	yes	yes	yes	no
Regional Office					
a. Current	no	no	no	no	no
b. Additional	yes	yes	yes	yes	no
Personnel Required					
Central Office					
a. Current Staff					
(1) Professional	2	2	2	1	—
(2) Clerical	1	1	1	1	1
b. Additional Staff					
(1) Professional	1	2	1	—	—
(2) Clerical	1	1	1	1	—
Regional Office					
a. Current Staff					
(1) Professional	—	—	—	—	—
(2) Clerical	—	—	—	—	—
b. Additional Staff					
(1) Professional	1	2	1	—	—
(2) Clerical	1	—	1	1	—
Total Staff Required	7	8	7	4	1
COST MODEL					
Cost Factors					
(thousands)					
Salaries					
a. Central Office	$50	$60	$56	$14	$2
b. Regional Office	18	28	75	18	—
Travel					
a. Central Office	10	44	32	—	—
b. Regional Office	8	22	12	—	—
Equipment—Total	2	3	2	1	1
Supplies and Printing	2	2	2	3	1
Miscellaneous	1	1	1	—	—
Total Cost	$91	$160	$180	$36	$4

COST MEASUREMENT
   Salaries—cost based on annual rate by personnel category
   Travel—cost per trip and miscellaneous expense
   Equipment—cost per unit of equipment
   Supplies—cost based on estimated use
   Printing—cost based on estimate of volume and number of jobs
   Miscellaneous—cost based on appropriate items involved

DESCRIPTION OF ALTERNATIVES
   1. Hold nine regional meetings and have individual follow-up.
   2. Make contact with selected faculty members at colleges and universities with graduate programs in economics.
   3. Address departments of economics, business and public administration at selected universities with graduate programs and have appropriate follow-up.
   4. Send informational material to departments of economics, business and public administration.
   5. Do nothing until specifically asked for information.

CHOICE: Alternative 3, with an estimated yield of 10.5 percent.

which would be incurred in any case, and also additional or incremental costs.

Once all of the above factors were determined, an estimate was made of the potential additional yield in research grants over a 12-month period for each alternative: alternative one, 6 percent; alternative two, 9 percent; alternative three, 10.5 percent; alternative four, 2 percent; and alternative five (where nothing would be done until asked) where there would be only a natural increase of 0.5 percent. Alternative three was selected in this case (to address departments of economics at universities to get the message across to a large number of people in a short period of time) which would increase our yield by almost 11 percent.

There are advantages and disadvantages to all five alternatives. Combinations of alternatives could have been chosen, but for simplicity of illustration only a single alternative was selected. This alternative appears reasonable when all of the pertinent factors are considered. The cost would be $180,000 which, while not the least expensive, is not too expensive in view of the return. In terms of staff, only four persons would have to be added, as opposed to alternative two which required adding five persons. On a yield basis, a 10.5 percent return was estimated, which was above our 10 percent goal.

CONCLUSION

As the foregoing discussion indicates, cost effectiveness and cost benefit analyses are related analytical techniques. In order to measure the magnitude of a disease, problem, or group of these, the cost benefit approach (and especially the economic cost aspect) is used. Cost effectiveness analysis is then undertaken to estimate the anticipated return for the various alternatives which are open to solve the problem at hand. Both processes, but especially cost benefit analysis, represent a mixture of real and theoretical costs. When these costs are developed and analyzed, a new method is available to look at problems and to estimate yield or return for given investments.

From the standpoint of Blue Cross, other third-party payers and health agencies of all kinds, the use of these tools can help to maximize the value of the services which are provided. For instance, using this method, a third-party payer could explore the possibility that exists for the development of new benefits programs based on the analysis of the specific effect of various conditions or on the cost of specific modalities of care. In the area of health service planning these analytical methods could lead to a sound determination of the correct mix of inpatient and outpatient services and other community resources. For the administrator, the techniques could lead to a high level of systems and budget allocation efficiency.

Having presented this discussion of cost benefit and cost effectiveness analyses in a highly positive vein and having pointed out the many uses, it is, perhaps, necessary to end on a note of caution. These techniques will not make decisions for us. They are tools which help in the decision-making process and not scientific procedures which stand up under rigid tests of objectivity. Their proper use hopefully will bring a degree of orderliness to a system which too often has been characterized as being irrationally organized to meet irrational demand.

Kenneth C. Steiner
Harry A. Smith

Application of Cost-Benefit Analysis to a PKU Screening Program

Reprinted with permission of the Blue Cross Association, from *Inquiry:* Vol.X, No.4, pp.34-40. Copyright © 1973 by the Blue Cross Association.

Originally Published in December 1973

Although the cost-benefit model had its primary origin and application in this country in the Department of Defense, its theoretical base, which combines welfare economics, public finance, and resource economics, has been used indirectly for centuries.[1,2] It was one means of evaluating a proposed project; therefore, the approaches used were alternately called "investment planning" or "project appraisal." The cost-effectiveness model is a variation of the original cost-benefit model.

Both cost-benefit and cost-effectiveness models are pragmatic approaches to very real problems and have little abstract theory underlying their development and application. Certain assumptions are necessarily somewhat theoretical in nature, but this need not detract from the use of the models. The decisions based on the data resulting from these analyses are far better than the intuitive decisions that otherwise would be made. The purpose, then, of cost-benefit and cost-effectiveness analyses is to improve the decision-making process in very real situations.

Cost-benefit analysis is based on the assumption that the problem can be identified; the cost of its consequence can be measured within a permissible range of accuracy; the problem can be eradicated or controlled at some predetermined level by

a new program; and the cost of the new program also can be measured. Thus, the costs associated with the old problem become the benefits against which the costs of the new program are compared. Conceptually, this is sound when the assumptions made are reasonably true, the calculations are accurate, and the methodology is reasonably acceptable. Cost-benefit analysis requires more definitive assumptions than cost-effectiveness, but it is an easier model to use where its application is valid.

Cost-effectiveness, on the other hand, is based on a more fluid conceptual framework. In fact, Quade[3] defines cost-effectiveness analysis as "any analytical study designed to assist a decision-maker identify a preferred choice from among possible alternatives." Even Quade, however, states that this definition is too broad. A more precise definition would be that cost-effectiveness analysis is a methodical approach of identifying alternative solutions to a problem (or courses of action) in terms of costs and their effectiveness in attaining some specific objective. While the costs of the alternatives are always measured in terms of dollars, the effectiveness may be measured in any of a number of terms as long as the term selected is applicable to the alternative under study. One can readily see the wider scope of factors and measurements opened to the investigator in a cost-effectiveness study; for example, comparable rates of incidence of diseases, mortality rates, fewer physician visits, etc., just to mention a few in the health field. One may compare the relative rates of effectiveness against a standard or budgeted cost, or even against variable costs as

Kenneth C. Steiner, M.S. is a graduate student in the Department of Health Care Administration, University of Mississippi School of Pharmacy (University, Mississippi 38677).
Harry A. Smith, Ph.D. is Professor of Pharmacy Administration, University of Kentucky College of Pharmacy.
The research reported in this paper was supported by the Research Institute of Pharmaceutical Sciences, University of Mississippi.

long as the ratios remain comparable and the results aid in the decision to be made.

Solutions to certain public health problems are more amenable to one model, while solutions to other problems require the other approach. Equally sound decisions may be reached by either method, while some problems will not yield to either. The choice of the best model or analysis is not always clear-cut; however, one of the models usually is best suited for a particular problem.

Usually the cost-benefit model is the best approach for screening programs for diseases. Use of this model in screening programs assumes first of all a valid test; that is, a relatively high rate of success in detection of the disease and a reliable statistical estimate of the success of the test. Second, the model assumes there is a cure for the disease or that it can be controlled to the extent that the patient may live a productive life, or at least a measurable percent of cases can be cured or controlled. Third, it assumes that estimates of the cost of the various parameters can be measured.

Cost-Benefit Analysis of a PKU Screening Program

The cost-benefit approach was used successfully to measure the cost-benefit parameters of a phenylketonuria (PKU) screening program for Mississippi and relating the costs to the benefits.

Phenylketonuria is a hereditary condition in which the patient possesses a simple Mendelian autosomal, recessive gene. It is caused by a rare, inborn error of metabolism and usually results in mental retardation. This disease is somewhat unique in the area of mental deficiency as it is readily detected, and when diagnosed early in life, the deficiency can be modified or prevented with dietary treatment. PKU develops because of the patient's inability to metabolize phenylalanine properly. The result is a deficiency in the amount of phenylalanine that is converted to tyrosine, and large amounts of phenylalanine are found in the blood and spinal fluid. There are no physical standards for comparison

in the diagnosis of children with suspected PKU at birth. The child will be apparently normal, but at three or four months of age signs of retardation will appear. The first noticeable change will be the infant's loss of interest in his surroundings, followed by a decrease in mental development, which finally ceases at the age of 10 to 14.

Costs of PKU

The costs associated with PKU were categorized into two areas: direct costs and indirect costs. Direct costs were defined as the actual expenditures for medical and other services attributable to the disease, reflecting the use of resources. These include both personal and non-personal costs. Personal service expenditures included the cost of hospital care, professional medical care, and pharmaceutical services, to list the major items. Non-personal service expenditures included medical supplies, drugs, medical research cost, government grants, charges for depreciation of facilities, and any other non-personal cost associated with the disease.[4,5]

Indirect costs were defined as a loss of economic productivity attributable to the disease, resulting from either death or disability. These indirect costs were calculated on the basis of the annual loss of production as measured by the loss of wages for the work years or months attributable to disease. It was presumed that the patients would have been gainfully employed in a full employment period.[6] The median incomes of the population segmented by age and sex were used in this study. Future earnings were discounted at the rate of 4 percent to ascertain their current value.[7]

The total cost per case, direct and indirect, served as the measure of benefits derived from preventing that case. Three types of benefits are identifiable: 1) reduction in the use of health resources; 2) gains in economic output; and 3) satisfaction from better health. Much too little attention has been given to the latter benefit, according to some economists.[8, 9] But this benefit, the satisfaction or feeling of well-being of the patient, is very difficult to measure, especially in economic terms. Thus this factor is normally treated as a bonus or windfall to society after all the other calculations are made.

There are two basic approaches in the application of the cost-benefit analysis— the retrospective and the prospective approaches. Both approaches were used in this study. The retrospective approach measures the direct and indirect costs of the current population with a disease entity, PKU in this instance. After these calculations are made, an estimate of the costs of screening, detecting, and treating these patients from among the entire population encompassing the life spans of the patient population is calculated.

The other technique, utilizing the prospective approach, calculates the cost of screening, detecting, and treating all of the live-births in a given year. The future savings (cost to society) of preventing the direct medical cost of the people who are successfully detected and treated plus the indirect costs of future economic productivity of these patients are compared to the cost of screening and detection.

Results of the Retrospective Method

Information from the three mental institutions in Mississippi provided the data for computing the direct and indirect costs associated with PKU patients. Demographic characteristics of the patients provided the base line data as shown in Table 1. The direct costs for all mentally retarded patients in the three institutions are summarized in Table 2.

Since PKU patients were not identified among the retarded patients in the three Mississippi institutions, the direct cost of maintaining PKU patients had to be estimated by the most reliable means available. First, the personal service costs for all patients in the institutions were calculated on a per patient per year basis. These figures were multipled by the known number of mentally retarded patients in all the three institutions. This gave an overall annual cost of $3,762,398 for personal services for all mentally retarded patients in

Table 1. Age and sex distribution of mentally retarded patients in Mississippi mental institutions in 1967

Age	Male	Female	Total
Under 5	3	0	3
5-9	32	36	68
10-14	83	49	132
15-19	158	74	232
20-24	176	74	250
25-34	260	148	408
35-44	234	175	409
45-54	201	210	411
55-64	148	234	382
65+	84	109	193
Total	1,379	1,109	2,488

the three institutions. The total non-personal service cost per year for the three institutions was $367,748. In addition, $73,346 in research grants was awarded to other institutions to study mental retardation during the baseline year. The total annual direct cost was $4,203,492. Based on the reported statistic that 1 percent of all mentally retarded patients are PKU patients,[10] the best estimate of the direct cost per year per PKU patient was 1 percent of $4,203,492 or $42,035. PKU patients have been reported to be institutionalized 30 years on the average;[11] therefore, the the estimated total direct cost for PKU patients was $1,261,050.

Indirect costs are measured by the loss of income. It was assumed that once a mentally retarded patient was institutionalized, he remained incapacitated for life and was a complete loss to the work force. The indirect costs for all the institutionalized mental retardates were computed and reported in Tables 3 and 4.

The total estimated indirect cost for the mentally retarded population was $105,354,-512. One percent of this amount, $1,053,-545, was allocated to the PKU patient population. The sum of the direct and indirect costs was summarized in Table 5.

The total cost (the sum of direct and indirect costs) to society to care for the 25 PKU patients (1 percent of the 2,488 institutionalized mentally retarded patients) was $2,314,595.

Table 2. Summary of direct costs for institutionalized mentally retarded patients

	Whitfield	Ellisville	Meridian	Total
Personal services				
Cost/patient/year	$ 1,847	$ 1,241	$ 1,322	$ 1,512[a]
Number of patients[b]	1,094	1,248	146	2,488
Total	$2,020,618	$1,548,768	$193,012	$3,762,398
Non-personal services				
Depreciation	$ 83,510	$ 78,215	$ 13,041	$ 174,766
Imputed interest	113,991	66,951	12,040	192,982
Research grants	....	....	....	73,346
Total	$ 197,501	$ 145,166	$ 25,081	$ 441,094
Total direct cost	$2,218,119	$1,693,934	$218,093	$4,203,492

[a]Rounded average for the three institutions.
[b]The numbers represent the mentally retarded patient population; there were other patients with various mental disorders in these institutions.

Table 3. Adjusted present value of lifetime earnings for males: amount discounted at 4 percent, adjusted to 1967 dollars and for Mississippi, by age

(1)	(2)	(3)	(4)	(5)	(6)	(7)
Age	Earnings[a]	Inflator factor[b]	Inflated lifetime earnings[c]	Lifetime earnings deflated[d]	Number of mentally retarded[e]	Adjusted lifetime earnings for mentally retarded[f]
0-4	$ 62,026	1.090	$ 67,608	$34,480	3	$ 103,440
5-9	79,333	1.090	86,473	44,101	32	1,411,232
10-14	96,736	1.090	105,442	53,775	83	4,463,325
15-19	114,613	1.090	124,928	63,713	158	10,066,654
20-24	126,688	1.192	151,012	77,016	176	13,554,816
25-34	125,801	1.141	143,539	73,205	260	19,033,300
35-44	104,629	1.158	121,160	61,792	234	14,459,328
45-54	71,676	1.178	84,434	43,061	201	8,655,261
55-64	37,168	1.143	42,483	21,666	148	3,206,568
65+	6,560	1.155	7,577	3,864	84	324,576
Total						$75,278,500

[a]From: Rice, D. P. *Estimating the Cost of Illness*, Health Economics Series No. 6, Publication #947-6 (Washington, D.C.: GPO, May 1966) Table 24, p. 93.
[b]Ratio of 1966 median income to 1963 median income.
[c]Column 2 times column 3.
[d]Column 4 times ratio of 1967 median income for Mississippi to 1967 median income for U.S.
[e]Obtained from Table 1.
[f]Column 5 times column 6.
Source: Column 3 derived from: U.S. Bureau of the Census. *Current Population Reports*, Series P-60, No. 43, "Income of Families and Persons in the United States: 1963" (Washington, D.C.: GPO, September 29, 1964) Table 20, p. 36; and *ibid.*, No. 53, "Income in 1966 of Families and Persons in the United States" (Washington, D.C.: GPO, December 28, 1967) Table 20, p. 38.

Estimated Detection Cost

This cost was compared to the estimated program cost to have detected this number of PKU patients and maintained them at a self-supporting status in society. This estimated cost was computed retrospectively as follows. The incidence rate of PKU among a white population is 1:15,000,[12] while the incidence rate among the non-white population is 1:100,000.[13] The 1967 ratios of live-births among white and non-white populations in Mississippi were 49 percent and 51 percent, respectively. Based on 46,714 live-births in 1967, 1.76 PKU cases would have been detected if all 46,714 newborns had been tested, or 1 case of PKU could be found in 26,542 newborns. Therefore, testing approximately 660,000 newborns over a period of 14 years would have been required to have detected the 25 institutionalized PKU patients. The cost of screening the newborns and treating this number of patients has been outlined in Table 6.

Table 4. Adjusted present value of lifetime earnings for females: amount discounted at 4 percent, adjusted to 1967 dollars and for Mississippi, by age

(1) Age	(2) Earnings[a]	(3) Inflator factor[b]	(4) Inflated lifetime earnings[c]	(5) Lifetime earnings deflated[d]	(6) Number of mentally retarded[e]	(7) Adjusted life- time earnings for mentally retarded[f]
0-4	$36,280	0.964	$34,974	$17,837	0	$ 000,000
5-9	46,289	0.964	44,623	22,758	36	819,288
10-14	56,422	0.964	54,391	27,739	49	1,359,211
15-19	64,936	0.964	62,598	31,925	74	2,362,450
20-24	67,960	1.150	78,154	39,859	74	2,949,566
25-34	65,608	1.110	72,825	37,141	148	5,496,868
35-44	58,801	1.119	65,798	33,557	175	5,872,475
45-54	47,634	1.130	53,826	27,451	210	5,764,710
55-64	33,816	1.116	37,739	19,247	234	4,503,798
65+	12,525	1.361	17,047	8,694	109	947,646
Total						$30,076,012

[a]From: Rice, D. P. *Estimating the Cost of Illness, op. cit.*, Table 24, p. 93.
[b]Ratio of 1966 median income to 1963 median income.
[c]Column 2 times column 3.
[d]Column 4 times ratio of 1967 median income for Mississippi to 1967 median income for U.S.
[e]Obtained from Table 1.
[f]Column 5 times column 6.
Source for Column 3: Same as in Table 3.

Table 5. Total costs for institutionalized PKU patients in 1967[a]

Direct costs	
30-year extended direct costs	$1,261,050
Indirect costs	
Present value of lifetime earnings lost	1,053,545
Total direct and indirect costs	$2,314,595

[a]Determined by taking 1 percent of the respective costs for mentally retarded patients.

Table 6. Retrospective analysis of program costs

Number of screening tests required	660,000[a]
Cost of initial screening	$561,000[b]
Cost of retesting within six weeks	$561,000[b]
Number of confirmation tests required	3,300[c]
Cost of confirmation tests	$ 12,375[d]
Cost of retesting while on special diet	$ 3,937[e]
Cost of special diet for seven years	$127,750[f]
Administrative cost (10% of other costs)	$126,606
Total program cost	$1,392,668

[a]Figure rounded to the nearest 1,000.
[b]Based on mean cost of $.85 per test from a survey of 42 health departments.
[c]Based on national statistic of 0.5 percent cases requiring confirmation test.
[d]Based on mean cost of $3.75 from survey of the health departments.
[e]Based on average cost of $3.75 per test once every two months for 7 years.
[f]Based on national statistics of an average cost of $2.00 per day per patient.

This total, $1,392,668, is the estimated cost to detect and treat the 25 suspected PKU patients in the Mississippi mental institutions. This figure can then be compared to the total cost of institutionalization and earnings lost of $2,314,595. The resulting cost-benefit ratio was calculated to be 1 to 1.66. Stated positively, each dollar spent in the detection and control of the disease would have yielded a net gain of $0.66 above the cost of the detection and control program.

Results of the Prospective Method

The prospective method based on 1967 live-births in Mississippi was thought to yield more valid results than the retrospective method. As previously noted, testing the 46,714 live-births in 1967 would have detected an average of 1.76 PKU cases. The total costs to conduct such a screening program were tabulated in Table 7.

It was assumed that the total number of live-births would be tested initially and again within six weeks. Also, it was assumed that an average number of confirmation tests would be made, and a test monitoring the PKU urine level would be performed every two months. A diet cost of

Table 7. Program costs for live-birth data

Number of live-births in Mississippi in 1967	46,714
Average cost per screening test	$0.85
Number of confirmation cases	233.6
Number of cases of whites	1.52
Number of cases of nonwhites	.24
(A) Cost of initial screen test	$39,707
(B) Cost of retest at six weeks	$39,707
(C) Cost of confirmation at $3.75 per test	$ 876
(D) Diet cost of 1.76 cases for seven years	$ 8,994
(E) Cost of retest while on diet	$ 278
(F) Administration cost	$ 8,956
Total cost of program	$98,518

$2.00 per patient per day was used in the computations, which is the highest cost reported in the literature.[14] The statistics used in Table 7 maximized the cost of the detection and treatment program.

Based on the data used in the retrospective method, the direct cost of institutionalized care was estimated at $1,690 per case per year. If the 1.76 cases had been detected in 1967, it would have cost $89,232 for institutional care for 30 years, the minimum expected length of time of institutionalization, or $210,588 for the 70.8 years of normal life expectancy of a one-year-old child born in 1967. The indirect cost for loss of future earnings, discounted at 4 percent per annum,[7] totaled $45,830. The total direct and indirect costs were $135,062 for 30 years of institutional care and $256,418 for 70.8 years of institutional care. These data yielded cost-benefit ratios of 1 to 1.37 and 1 to 2.60, respectively.

Again, the gain to society using live-birth data and the prospective method was substantial, even if we use the minimum of 30 years of institutionalization. In all of the calculations, costs of the detection and control programs were maximized, while direct and indirect costs (benefits) were minimized.

Conclusion

The conclusion to be drawn from this study is that a PKU screening program is beneficial not only to the person who has the disease but also to society. The retrospective approach yielded a cost-benefit ratio of 1:1.66. Using the more valid prospective approach, the cost-benefit ratio was 1:1.37 when the direct costs were minimized to correspond to the 30 year average time a patient is institutionalized. A ratio of 1:2.60 resulted when the full life expectancy was used. Neither the time and money spent for a PKU preventive program nor the economic benefits derived from such a program reveal the additional financial burden and amount of personal care required by the families of the undiagnosed patients. In addition, the emotional stress which is inflicted upon the families cannot be measured in economic terms.

Cost-benefit analysis proved to be a satisfactory technique in evaluating a PKU screening program as it has in several other diseases. It provides the model to determine the social validity of such programs as family planning, day care centers, preventive dental care, fluoridation of water supply, and vaccination against communicable diseases. Cost-benefit estimates have been made of cancer and other major diseases. Both models have been applied to various aspects of maternal and child health. This enumeration is not exhaustive, but does represent some of the more obvious applications of the models.

The cost-effectiveness model could also be used to determine the desirability of using non-physicians in limited areas of primary health care; this category could include the pediatric nurse, physician's assistant, the clinical pharmacist, and the emergency paramedic. Cost-effectiveness analysis might also be applied to cardiac emergency ambulance service.

One area in which cost-effectiveness analysis can and should be applied is to new health care delivery systems such as the health maintenance organization concept. One of the weaknesses in these emerging government-sponsored experimental health care models is the internal evaluation included in the grant. The evaluation, using the cost-effectiveness model, should be performed by an outside agency.

Special education for the various categories of mentally deficient children is another field in which cost-benefit analysis would provide proof of the social value of these programs. It is the opinion of the authors that the programs in special education could have one of the highest benefit-to-cost ratios of all the various social programs.

The application of cost-benefit and cost-effectiveness models is far-reaching. It seems axiomatic that more money should be funded for this type of research before appropriating huge sums of money for the many supposedly worthwhile social projects.

References

1 Prest, A. R. and Turvey, R. "Cost-Benefit Analysis: A Survey," *The Economic Journal* 75:683-735 (1965).

2 Marshall, A. W. "Cost-Benefit Analysis in Health." Paper presented in Monterey, California, November 10, 1965, and reproduced by the Rand Corporation.

3 Quade, E. S. "Cost-Effectiveness: An Introduction and Overview." Paper presented at a Symposium on Cost Effectiveness Analysis, June 14-16, 1965, sponsored by the Washington Operations Research Council and reproduced by the Rand Corporation.

4 Rice, D. P. "Estimating the Cost of Illness," *American Journal of Public Health* 57:424-440 (1967).

5 Rice, D. P. *Estimating the Cost of Illness*, Health Economics Series No. 6, PHS Publication #947-6 (Washington, D.C.: GPO, May 1966) p. 3.

6 Fein, R. *Economics of Mental Health*, (New York: Basic Books, 1958).

7 Rice, *Estimating the Cost of Illness, op. cit.*, Parts II & III, Appendix B.

8 Marshall, *op. cit.*, p. 3.

9 Klarman, H. E. *The Economics of Health* (New York: Columbia University Press, 1965).

10 Hsia, D. Y. Y. "Recent Developments in Inborn Errors of Metabolism," *American Journal of Public Health* 50:1653-1661 (1960).

11 Cunningham, G. C. "Two Years of PKU Testing in California," *California Medicine* 111:11-16 (1969).

12 Hormuth, R. P., specialist in services for mentally retarded children, Children's Bureau, Department of Health, Education and Welfare, personal communication.

13 Katz, H. P. and Menkes, J. H. "Phenylketonuria Occurring in an American Negro," *Journal of Pediatrics* 65:71-74 (1964).

14 Centerwall, W. R.; Centerwall, S. A.; Acosta, P. B.; and Chinnock, R. F. "Phenylketonuria. I. Dietary Management of Infants and Young Children," *Journal of Pediatrics* 59:93-101 (1961).

J. Michael Swint
William B. Nelson

The Application of Economic Analysis to Evaluation of Alcoholism Rehabilitation Programs

Reprinted with permission of the Blue Cross Association, from *Inquiry:* Vol.XIV, No.1, pp.63-72. Copyright © 1977 by the Blue Cross Association.

Originally Published in March 1977

The extensive nature of the alcoholism problem in the United States has naturally resulted in a variety of efforts to control it. And given an excess of "desirable" rehabilitation programs over the number allowable by the scarcity of resources, there is a need for objective program evaluation; i.e., for the calculation of a program's expected benefits for comparison with its costs. As such, our primary objective is to illustrate the potential value of cost-benefit analysis (CBA) in the objective evaluation of an individual alcoholism rehabilitation program. After a brief discussion of the nature, value and limitations of CBA, we develop an algorithm to make the necessary calculations and a case study to illustrate the potential utility of the analysis in this regard.

Cost-Benefit Analysis

Generally CBA may be thought of as a technique for allocating the public sector's resources efficiently among competing uses. Prest and Turvey offer the following broad definition for CBA.[1]

Cost-benefit analysis is a practical way of assessing the desirability of projects where it is important to take a long view (in the sense of looking at repercussions in the further, as well as the nearer, future) and

J. Michael Swint, Ph.D. is Assistant Professor of Economics, School of Public Health, University of Texas Health Science Center (Houston, TX 77025).

William B. Nelson, Ph.D. is Assistant Professor of Finance, Cleveland State University (Cleveland, OH 44115).

Financial support for this research was provided by the Department of Health, Education and Welfare.

a wide view (in the sense of allowing for side-effects of many kinds on many persons, industries, regions, etc.), i.e., it implies the enumeration and evaluation of all the relevant costs and benefits.

The use of cost-benefit analysis forces the analyst to make a complete enumeration of expected costs and benefits as well as an explicit consideration of the assumptions underlying the quantitative evaluation of costs and benefits. Essentially, it provides the decision-maker with information designed to improve his ability to make rational decisions. It is only meant to function as one source of information, along with other relevant information, to be evaluated by the decision-maker. Thus, CBA is not intended to provide the sole decision-making criterion; that has only been incorrectly imputed to it by non-practitioners. It merely provides economic information that must be combined with distributional, socio-political, humanitarian and other information by the decision-maker (vis-à-vis the analyst) for his net evaluation. It should be noted that whenever program evaluation decisions are made without the benefit of net economic impact data, a value for the net economic impact has nevertheless been implicitly assumed, perhaps without decision-makers realizing it themselves. We see no value in forcing decision-makers to assume, either implicitly or explicitly, the magnitude of the economic impact of a program rather than having it provided as the result of an objective analytical exercise.

As CBA normally represents an attempt to quantify outputs as well as costs in monetary terms, it is most easily applied to areas where a project's outputs are of a measurable tangible

Table 1.   Alcoholism prevalence

Industry type	Employees	Average age	Percent males	Percent who are alcoholics	Number of alcoholics
Heavy	11,074,000	40 years or over	90 or more	10.0	1,107,400
Medium	29,142,000	38 to 40 years	60–89	5.9	1,719,378
Light	18,069,000	37 years or less	59 or less	1.5	271,035
Total	58,285,000				3,097,813

nature. Naturally, this is not always the case in the health field as not all benefits are readily monetized. Many attempts have been made to impute monetary values to intangibles,[2] but none with much success. In health program areas where there are few *economic* benefits to be derived—nursing home programs, for example—CBA is of relatively little use.[3] This does not imply that those programs are not of high priority, but rather that the benefits flowing from them are primarily intangible (in the form of consumption rather than investment) and beyond the purview of the analyst to evaluate. In many other areas of the health field, such as alcoholism rehabilitation programs, the losses of productivity due to death, absenteeism and debility on the job are great and the programs are amenable to CBA.

Economic Costs of Alcoholism

Prevalence of Alcoholism

Although the experts do not agree on precise figures, there appears to be a general consensus that approximately 5 percent of the nation's work force suffers from alcoholism. A report from the National Commission on Alcoholism estimated that as of January, 1968, there were 3.1 million alcoholics employed in business and government combined.[4] A breakdown of their findings, according to type of industry, is shown in Table 1.

These data of course do not include alcoholics that are either unemployed or not in the labor force. A study by Efron and Keller[5] in 1970 estimated the number of alcoholics to be in excess of 5 million, while DeLint and Schmidt[6] put it at 6 million in 1971. Despite the lack of precision in these prevalence data, the number of alcoholics is quite substantial.

Costs of Alcoholism

Alcoholism imposes both immeasurable costs, in terms of human suffering, and economic costs. The latter include at least the following:

1 Increased mortality due to cirrhosis of the liver and other diseases.
2 The output loss due to the higher unemployment rate of alcoholics.
3 Work loss, due to increased absenteeism from work and lower productivity on the job.
4 Hospitalization costs, due to the mental health problems of alcoholics.
5 Traffic accident costs, including death, disability, property loss and hospitalization; and also the costs of the higher rate of imprisonment of alcoholics.

While the estimates are very rough, the economic costs of alcoholism in the United States have been put as high as $15-billion per year;[7] i.e., $10-billion in the cost of work loss, $2-billion in health and welfare service costs, and $3-billion for property damage, medical expenses, etc. Additionally, about 30,000 alcohol-related traffic fatalities occur per year; and the costs of alcoholism-related crime has been placed near $100-million per year, with about 2 million arrests.[8,9]

Also, Holtman has estimated that the discounted present value of the costs of alcoholism among U.S. males in 1959 was approximately $41.7-billion.[10] This figure was composed of: 1) decreased life expectancy, $9.93-billion (23.8 percent of the costs); 2) unemployment, $23.86-billion (57.2 percent); 3) absenteeism, $7.74-billion (18.6 percent); 4) imprisonment, $.029-billion (0.07 percent); 5) hospitalization, $.052-billion (0.12 percent); and 6) auto accidents, $.388-billion (0.93 percent).

Treatment Alternatives

There is a wide variety of programs attempting to deal with alcoholism. They are normally curative in approach and take the form of either individual or group therapy, or some combina-·tion of the two.[11] Currently there exists no systematic manner of detecting alcoholics and channeling them into an appropriate form of treatment. Instead there is a patchwork of programs in industry, various levels of government, and various types of "independent" treatment centers, funded by either private or public sources. The variety of approaches is manifested in alcoholism clinics, detoxification centers, transitional facilities (or half-way houses), mental hospital inpatient care for alcoholics and, of course, Alcoholics Anonymous.

Unfortunately, the objective evaluation of treatment programs remains very inadequate.[12] There has not been rigorous development in standardized program design, outcome definition or outcome measurement, leaving decision-makers relatively little to work with.

For evaluative purposes it is at a minimum important to know:

1 What the assumptions are regarding the parameter magnitudes of a proposed program so the reviewing group can judge them.
2 The sensitivity of the evaluated outcome to modest changes in the assumptions. Where there exists uncertainty as to the appropriate value of certain parameters (e.g., the rate of successful rehabilitation), and the evaluated outcome is quite sensitive to a change in an assumption, the review agency would have to take this into account. The reviewers' preference or distaste for uncertainty would help determine their decision.
3 Where there are weak links in terms of empirical evidence so that the values assigned them can be closely scrutinized by reviewers.

Fortunately, there is sufficient evidence to establish a range of values for relevant parameters and to allow sensitivity analysis with each. At a minimum this would force an explicit presentation of assumptions. While it would of course be preferable to have complete data, allocation decisions in the funding of alcoholism programs must nevertheless be made in their absence. As these decisions are currently often based on implicit unreviewed assumptions regarding outcome parameters, an improvement in information of this sort would certainly contribute to the objective evaluation of these programs. Thus, in the next section we develop and illustrate an algorithm for the use of CBA in an individual rehabilitation program.

Case Study

Let us assume that a health planning agency is given a proposal for the funding of an alcoholism rehabilitation program. Specifically, the proposal calls for a clinic serving outpatients only. As is traditional with outpatient alcoholism facilities, "Patients at these clinics are generally from middle-class backgrounds and because of the selection policies governing admission, skid row alcoholics are virtually excluded. For instance, considerable emphasis is placed on the patient's family situation, verbal ability, and motivation—all of which tend to be reflections of social class, education, occupation, and family's financial standing."[13] Thus, we shall assume that the target population is composed of middle-income working males.[14]

The rehabilitation approach used will be multifaceted, recognizing that individual clients will have diverse psychological backgrounds and will presumably require a variety of therapies. As such, a combination of group therapy and individual therapy will be utilized. Hence, it is stated by the sponsors of the proposal that there will be:

☐ Two psychiatric social workers (PSW) to conduct group therapy daytime sessions. Each PSW would have one group of six patients per day for each of the week days, or five groups per week. Each group thus meets once per week such that one PSW has 30 different patients per week.
☐ Two PSWs to conduct group nighttime therapy sessions. They would accommodate the same patient load as the day PSWs.
☐ One full-time-equivalent psychiatrist who would engage in individual therapy with patients as needed to complete the rehabilitation effort.
☐ One program administrator, 2,000 square

Table 2.   Direct costs

	Annual costs
Labor	
Psychiatric social workers $14,000 p.a. × 4	$56,000
Psychiatrist (one full-time-equivalent)	20,000
Administrator	14,000
Voluntary workers (one full-time-equivalent)	....
Total labor costs	$90,000
Rental, utilities and materials	
One facility, 2,000 sq. feet (rental)	$14,400
Utilities	1,000
Materials and office supplies	2,600
Total facility costs	$18,000
Total annual costs	$108,000
Capital purchases	
Medical equipment and office equipment, in year 1 only	$50,000
Scrap value of equipment at end of year 7	$10,000

feet of office space and various equipment and materials.

Furthermore, it is estimated by the program's sponsors that the average successful rehabilitation effort will require approximately 50 weeks (one work year). Upon successful rehabilitation a patient would be replaced in the group by a new patient. Also as patients who are not successfully treated by the program drop out, they are replaced by new patients such that at any one time there are 120 patients enrolled.[15] For example, if we assume the probability of success of rehabilitation is 25 percent, then 30 patients will be rehabilitated in any given year; in the following year those 30 will be replaced, in addition to replacements for any of the remaining 90 (unsuccessful patients) that decide not to continue in the program.[16]

The assumption of the one-year probability of success of 25 percent refers to the average length of successful treatment. Some may require six months and others 18 months, but during any given 12 month period 30 patients will be rehabilitated (.25 × 120). Additionally, of the unsuccessful patients that decide to remain in the program, it may be said that they clearly have strong motivation which in effect serves as an offset to their deeper problem

(which itself is manifested by its persistence). Thus it can be assumed that their probability of successful rehabilitation will continue at 25 percent—although the analysis could readily incorporate different probabilities for different years.

In addition, while the sponsor believes the program will be successful and continue indefinitely, the proposal is for an initial program life of seven years. As we cannot operate under the sponsor's "belief" that the program will continue indefinitely, it must be evaluated on the basis of its initial request for a seven-year life.

Direct Costs

The sponsor's estimated program costs are shown in Table 2. Given these figures, the annual total costs (needed for the CBA discounting process) are: year 1, $158,000 ($108,000 + $50,000 in capital equipment); years 2–6, $108,000 per year; and year 7, $98,000 ($108,000–$10,000 capital equipment scrap value).

Indirect Costs

In addition to these direct costs, we must include any indirect costs that will accrue to the program. Let us assume that each of the patients attending the day sessions is forced to miss work to do so, and that each of the patients attending evening sessions is not forced to miss work. Of the 60 day patients enrolled at any one time there are 12 full-time-equivalent day patients (one day per week per patient for an average of 50 weeks, ⅕ of a working year, × 60 patients). Thus, the social cost of work loss due to attendance at the rehabilitation program, or indirect cost, is 12 × the annual patient salary level. For our base case this is $10,039 × 12 = $120,468 per year of the program (this will of course vary when alternative salary levels are used).[17]

Thus, total annual social costs levels are (direct and indirect):[18]

☐ Year 1—$278,468
☐ Years 2–6—$228,468
☐ Year 7—$218,468.

Later in the analysis adjustments will be made in these cost levels for cases where the relevant level of patient income is assumed to be $7,500 and then $11,000.

Benefits

The next question is what benefits of alcoholism rehabilitation can we define, isolate and measure? That is, what costs to society (in addition to the humanitarian costs to the alcoholic's friends, family and himself) would have occurred that are now averted due to the rehabilitation of the 30 alcoholics per year?[19] These costs constitute the program's *economic benefits.*

As indicated in the introduction to the case study, there are several categories of benefits from reduced alcohol abuse, the first of which is decreased mortality due to alcoholism. There is a longer life expectancy for non-alcoholics, and hence the working years that would have been lost for this reason, after the alcoholic's death, are avoided upon his rehabilitation. The economic value of these working years will be evaluated at the median annual income of working males in 1973 ($10,039). As the alcoholic has a higher probability of dying, his expected income must be lower than a non-alcoholic.

The difference in life expectancy of alcoholics versus non-alcoholics is available from Raymond Pearl's *Alcohol and Longevity.*[20] Pearl computed the probabilities of future life expectancy for abstainers and heavy drinkers, based on a cohort of 5,000 individuals. The difference in probabilities will be multiplied by the median annual income for each potential work year remaining in the successfully rehabilitated patient's life to reflect the loss in income to an alcoholic attributable to his lower life expectancy.[21]

Next, there exist the social costs due to the higher expected future unemployment rate of currently employed alcoholics as versus currently employed non-alcoholics. That is, all of the proposed program's target patients are now employed, but some of these lose their jobs due solely to their alcoholism problem. This higher probability that rehabilitated alcoholics would have otherwise become unemployed must be evaluated at their annual income level to yield the value of the eliminated costs (benefits to society).

Estimates of aggregate unemployment among alcoholics normally reveal very high percentages (15–25 percent); however, we are not concerned with national averages, but rather, the expected rate for alcoholics and non-alcoholics that are currently employed in occupations paying in the vicinity of $10,000 per year. While we lack precise data on this score, indications are that the difference between these groups is at least 4 percentage points. As such, we will use a 6 percent rate of unemployment for alcoholics and a 2 percent rate for non-alcoholics. Again, the expected rate of unemployment among alcoholics will be varied in the sensitivity analysis and can be utilized in this manner by planners in accordance with the nature of any given program.

Then, the alcoholic employee has a higher rate of absenteeism on the job and, often, a lower productivity on the job than the non-alcoholic employee. Estimates combining these indicators of inefficiency have been made by a variety of investigators. Generally, estimates of inefficiency of the working alcoholic, in terms of lower productivity due to absenteeism *and* lowered work output while on the job, range from 20 percent to 30 percent of his potential output (of that achievable by the otherwise equivalent non-alcoholic).[22] In our base case we shall assume a rate of (combined) inefficiency of 20 percent for the average alcoholic employee. This indicates that an alcoholic employee, in our definition, includes only those with serious drinking problems (but one can easily adjust the nature of target populations to that of his choosing). The method of this adjustment will be delineated in the discussion on the method of computation.

As was mentioned earlier, there are also social costs of alcoholism due to 1) increased hospitalization costs for mental health problems, 2) traffic accident costs, and 3) imprisonment and the other costs associated with the higher crime rate of alcoholics. While these costs, in humanitarian terms, can be quite substantial, they represent only a very small percentage of the total *economic* costs. For example, Holtman[23] found that the present value of expected future total social costs, as estimated for all male alcoholics in 1959, attributed about 1 percent of that total to the combined effects of hospitalization, traffic accidents, and imprisonment. As such, these social costs will not be included in the total of benefits to be computed from the program; i.e., the costs of information in this case are too high as the data necessary to compute these costs are very difficult to obtain (and of dubious quality). And clearly the benefits of this information would be minimal as they provide only about 1 percent of the total benefits of rehabilitated alcoholics.

Analysis

With this background material and the information presented us by the program sponsors, we can proceed to analyze the economic merits of the proposal utilizing cost-benefit analysis.

Benefits

In our initial case (as many of the values of the basic parameters were developed over the preceding pages) we assume that:

y = median annual income of non-alcoholics and the successfully rehabilitated patients, or $10,039.

U_A = the expected future unemployment rate of our currently employed patients, or .06.

U_{NA} = the expected future unemployment rate for employed non-alcoholics, or .02.

I_A = the percent of job efficiency lost, from both absenteeism and lower on-the-job productivity, due to an employee's alcoholism, or 20 percent.

d = the expected annual percent increase in worker productivity, or 3 percent.

r = the discount rate, .10. Naturally, as a decrease in costs or an increase in benefits is of more value today than, say, 10 years from now, it is necessary to adjust for this by a discounting process wherein future values are converted into current values for common denominator comparison purposes. The current value of benefits to be received t years hence is simply

$$PV = B_t/(1 + r)^t$$

where, PV = the present value of the benefits.

B_t = the value of benefits in year t (measured in year t terms).

r = the rate of discount.

a = the age of the successfully rehabilitated patient. As the majority of alcoholics fall in the 35–54 year age range, the program sponsor has decided, in an effort to achieve maximum early impact on the alcoholic, to concentrate on alcoholics of the ages 35 through 44. In other words, at any one time there are 12 patients of each of these ages in the program—or 120 total. And in absence of any evidence to the contrary there is assumed to be equal probability of cure for any given age group among the patients.

P_t = the probability of a male non-alcoholic surviving through year t.[24]

Given these we can develop the framework for the analysis.

First, to arrive at the present discounted value of the future income of non-alcoholics, we must sum their annual earnings, y (adjusted for expected future productivity increases, d) from their current age, a, to the assumed retirement age, 65. Thus we have,

$$\sum_{t=a}^{65} \left[y(1 + d)^{t-a} \right]$$

Adding in the appropriate discount factor for each of the years between a and retirement, we arrive at,

$$(1) \quad PV = \sum_{t=a}^{65} \left[\frac{y(1 + d)^{t-a}}{(1 + r)^{t-a}} \right].$$

For example, for a worker of age 42, the formula sums and discounts the next 23 years of his income (adjusted for his annual increasing productivity, d).

Next, to arrive at the expected present discounted value of future income of non-alcoholics, i.e., adjusted for the probability of survival (PV above assumes all workers will live to age 65), we must include P_t to reduce the gross discounted value of future income in (1) to that mathematically expected. Thus,

$$(2) \quad PV_{NA} = \sum_{t=a}^{65} \left[\frac{y(1 + d)^{t-a}}{(1 + r)^{t-a}} \right] \cdot P_t$$

= present value of expected future income of non-alcoholics.

Repeating this adjustment for alcoholics,

$$(3) \quad PV_A = \sum_{t=a}^{65} \left[\frac{y(1+d)^{t-a}}{(1+r)^{t-a}} \right] \cdot P_t{}^A$$

= present value of expected future income of alcoholics

where, $P_t{}^A$ is the probability of an average male alcoholic surviving through year t.[25]

Given this, the cost of alcoholism due to lower life expectancy is C_1,

(4) $C_1 = PV_{NA} - PV_A$; i.e., the present value of the future earnings of non-alcoholics less the same for alcoholics. This figure is not adjusted for expected unemployment rates. Thus, the cost of alcoholism due to the higher expected rate of unemployment of alcoholics is C_2,

(5) $C_2 = PV_A \cdot U_A - PV_{NA} \cdot U_{NA}$. Neither of these figures is adjusted for expected rates of inefficiency among alcoholic workers. As such, the cost of alcoholism due to lower rates of efficiency on the job and higher rates of absenteeism is C_3,

(6) $C_3 = PV_A (1 - U_A) I_A$, where $1 - U_A$ is the expected future rate of employment of alcoholics who are currently employed.

Thus, we can simply sum the three types of costs as computed,

(7) $C = C_1 + C_2 + C_3$, or the total economic costs of alcoholism. As we are interested in age groups 35 through 44, we must restrict the computations to them,

$$(8) \quad n \cdot \sum_{a=35}^{44} \cdot C_a = B_k,$$ or the total economic

benefits from the program's k^{th} year of operation, e.g. year 1 for $k = 1$; where $n =$ the number of alcoholics in each age group who are successfully rehabilitated during year t. To recall, the initial assertion made by the program's sponsor was that 25 percent would be rehabilitated. This is three of the 12 per age group and thus $n = 3$ for our base case. The proposal called for an initial period of funding of seven years and, as such, we must add the benefits of the remaining six years of its operation to B_k in (8). Thus,

$$(9) \quad \sum_{t=1}^{7} \left[\frac{B_k(1+d)^t}{(1+r)^t} \right] = B^*$$

= the total discounted

present value of expected economic benefits of the entire seven-year operation of the alcoholism program.

The results for these and other computations will be presented after the development of the cost calculations.

Costs

To recall, the cost figures as presented by the program sponsor were as follows (base case):

☐ Year 1—$278,468.
☐ Years 2–6—$228,468 each year.
☐ Year 7—$218,468.

The present discounted value of these costs is C^*,

$$(10) \quad C^* = \sum_{t=1}^{7} \left[\frac{C_t}{(1+r)^t} \right] = C^*.$$

The decision parameters we are interested in are straightforward comparisons of B^* and C^*; B^*/C^*, the benefit-cost ratio; and $B^* - C^*$, the net present value of the program. When the former exceeds 1.0 and the latter exceeds 0 the program qualifies under the CBA criterion as being "socially profitable."

Base Case Results

Given the parameters as assumed in the base case, the calculations were performed as indicated in equations (1) through (10). The results are seen in Table 3. Clearly, both easily pass the economic criteria (i.e., $B^*/C^* > 1$ and $B^* - C^* > 0$) and hence the program, to the extent we believe in the base case parameters, is clearly to be recommended on an economic basis.

Additionally, as the other major category of benefit (accruing to society) from the program is humanitarian in nature, and is obviously positive in an alcoholism rehabilitation program, there is no reason not to recommend the program as represented by the base case. If $B^*/C^* < 1$ and $B^* - C^* < 0$, such that the program failed to pass the economic criteria, then the decision-making body would have to assign a value to the humanitarian benefits to determine the program's net desirability. The

Table 3. Base case results

Total benefits: $6,457,002 = B*
1 Attributable to the increased life expectancy of the successfully rehabilitated patients: $3,045,398.
2 Attributable to the lower unemployment rate of the successfully rehabilitated patients: $548,305.
3 Attributable to the higher work efficiency of the successfully rehabilitated patients: $2,863,299.

Total costs: $1,157,146 = C*
Benefit-cost ratio $(B*/C*) = 5.6$
Net present value $(B* - C*) = $5,299,856$

Table 4. Pessimistic case results

Total benefits: $1,183,188
1 Attributable to the increased life expectancy of the successfully rehabilitated patients: $758,392.
2 Attributable to the lower unemployment rate of the successfully rehabilitated patients: $2,863,299.
3 Attributable to the higher work efficiency of the successfully rehabilitated patients: $2,863,299.

Total costs: $1,008,815
Benefit-cost ratio = 1.2
Net present value = $174,373

point here is that when the economic criteria are satisfied, it is unnecessary to evaluate the humanitarian benefits as they are positive and will merely agree with the economic criteria.

If the reviewing body is not confident in the validity of the parameters as presented by the program sponsor, it may wish to see the results of computations with a different set of parameters. As the case as presented is strongly positive, let us examine a somewhat more pessimistic case.

Assume that y (income) = $7,500 (as versus $10,039); I_A (inefficiency) = .10 (as versus .20); U_A (unemployment) = .04 (as versus .06); n (rehabilitations per age group); and that the remainder of the parameters are unchanged. The results using these parameters are shown in Table 4. As can be seen, the results are indeed rather sensitive to changes in the parameters, they remain quite robust such that even with this pessimistic set of assumptions the economic criteria are satisfied. This should serve to allay many misgivings that reviewers may have had.[26] To allow various combinations of parameters and allow an examination of the next impact of changing a given parameter we use sensitivity analysis.

Sensitivity Analysis

Calculations were made for a series of possibilities at discount rates of 10 percent and 5 percent (Table 5). Setting $I_A = .20$, $U_A = .06$, and $d = .03$, we see the effects of varying n (the number of successfully rehabilitated patients per group per year), y (income) and r (the discount rate).

The results are quite sensitive to changes in n and r, but nevertheless they $(B*/C*)$ remain substantially greater than 1.0 throughout.

example, in Table 5, when $r = .10$, at $y = $7,500, a change from $n = 1$ to $n = 3$ results in an increase in the benefit-cost ratio from 1.6 to 4.8. Similarly, that ratio of 1.6 increases to 2.9 in Table 5, when $r = .05$, with no changes other than the decline in r from .10 to .05. The results do not, however, vary nearly as much with the range of levels in y (income) tested for the program at hand. In Table 5, when $r = .10$, note that increasing y from $7,500 to $10,039 (at $n = 1$) increases the benefit-cost ratio from 1.6 to 1.9. While this is not an impact to be ignored, it is certainly less important than the changes in r and n.

This sensitivity analysis will allow program reviewers to make their own assumptions and observe the final result in that light. In the present case, the results clearly indicate "recommendation" on economic grounds, regardless of the parameter values chosen from the tables. However, this is not always the case and the availability of sensitivity impacts of changes in the various critical parameters would, for many sponsored proposals, be of yet more substantial value.

Table 5. Benefit-cost ratio, $B*/C*$

Successful rehabilitations (n)[1]	Income (y)		
	$7,500	$10,039	$11,000
r = .10			
1	1.6	1.9	1.9
3	4.8	5.6	5.8
5	8.0	9.3	9.7
r = .05			
1	2.9	3.4	3.5
3	8.7	10.1	10.6
5	14.5	16.9	•17.7

[1] Number of successful rehabilitations per age group per year.

Summary

We have presented an algorithm designed to facilitate the application of economic analysis to the evaluation of individual alcoholism rehabilitation programs. In doing so we have attempted to delineate the limitations of such analyses as well as the type and value of information they provide. After a brief review of the basic principles of cost-benefit analysis and a listing of the economic costs of alcoholism, a case study was developed as an heuristic device to illustrate the algorithm and the potential utility of cost-benefit analysis, particularly when used in conjunction with sensitivity analysis, as a logical framework for the evaluation effort.

References and Notes

1 Prest, A. R. and Turvey, R. "Cost-Benefit Analysis: A Survey," *The Economic Journal* 75:683–735 (December 1965).

2 As Klarman states, "Among the approaches that have been proposed and attempted are those of insurance or game theory, expenditures for an analogous disease at old age, jury verdicts, the implications of past decisions on public expenditures, and the sheer listing of known consequences without quantification of valuation." In: Klarman, H. E. "Present Status of Cost-Benefit Analysis in the Health Field," *American Journal of Public Health* 57:1948 (November 1967).

3 In instances such as this, an alternative technique, cost-effectiveness analysis, may be utilized. The primary difference between cost-benefit analysis and cost-effectiveness analysis (CEA) is that in the former a social value in monetary terms is estimated for a program's achieved health objectives for comparison with its costs, whereas in the latter costs are merely compared to various levels of health objectives obtained (or health service inputs delivered), measured in physical terms, without a social valuation placed on the attainment of these objectives. As such, while CBA may be instrumental in determining the social desirability of a proposed project, CEA can only help determine the most efficient manner of achieving a given health objective—the social desirability of which is taken as predetermined. It is most useful when many of the benefits of a given health program are intangible or difficult to isolate. The comparative roles of CBA and CEA will be analyzed in a forthcoming paper in the *Journal of Studies on Alcohol*.

4 National Council on Alcoholism. *Prevalence of Alcoholism Among Employees in Business, Industry, and Civilian Government* (New York: NCA, March 1968).

5 Efron, V. and Keller, M. *Selected Statistics on Consumption of Alcohol, 1950–1968, and on Alcoholism, 1930–1968* (New Brunswick, N.J.: Rutgers Center of Alcohol Studies, 1970).

6 DeLint, J. and Schmidt, W. "Consumption Averages and Alcoholism Prevalence: A Brief Review of Epidemiological Investigations," *British Journal of Addiction* 66:97–107 (September 1971).

7 Chafetz, M. and Demone, H., Jr. "Program to Control Alcoholism," in: Caplan, G. (ed.) *American Handbook of Psychiatry*, Vol. II, *Child and Adolescent Psychiatry, Socio-cultural and Community Psychiatry* (New York: Basic Books, 1974) pp. 712–722.

8 *Alcoholism and Highway Safety Report* (Washington, D.C.: GPO, August 1968).

9 *Substantial Cost Savings from Establishment of Alcoholism Program for Federal Civilian Employees*, Report to the Special Subcommittee on Alcoholism and Narcotics, Committee on Labor and Public Welfare, U.S. Senate, October 1970.

10 Holtman, A. G. "Estimating the Demand for Public Health Services: The Alcoholism Case," *Public Finance* 19:351–360 (1964).

11 See: Trice, H. M. *Alcoholism in America* (New York: McGraw-Hill, 1966).

12 See: Blum, E. M. and Blum, R. H. *Alcoholism* (San Francisco: Jossey-Bass, 1967).

13 Commission of Inquiry into the Non-Medical Use of Drugs. "The Treatment of Alcoholism," in: Whitehead, P.; Grindstaff, C.; and Boydell, C. (eds.) *Alcohol and Other Drugs: Perspectives on Use, Abuse, Treatment, and Prevention* (Toronto: Holt, Rinehart and Winston of Canada, Ltd., 1973) p. 79.

14 The analysis could easily be generalized to include employed women and non-workers of either sex.

15 With 120 patients enrolled in the program at any one time, the cost calculations, as will be seen, turn out to be quite straightforward.

16 "Successful rehabilitation," as used here, excludes those patients just temporarily or partially rehabilitated. In this sense the calculated benefits will represent a lower bound as they will exclude the short-term benefits (if any) of those who have relapses.

17 The median annual income of working males in 1973. Source: Bureau of Labor Statistics. *Employment and Earnings.*

18 Note that this excludes any fees that patients may be required to pay as these would be purely distributional in nature and would not involve the reallocation of any real resources. As such, while fees may impact on the financial feasibility of a program, they do not affect its "social profitability."

19 The assumption of a probability of success of 25 percent, and hence 30 successfully rehabilitated alcoholics per year, will be altered higher and lower during the sensitivity analysis. Evidence from a wide variety of sources suggests that documented alcoholism treatment programs have had success rates of anywhere from 10 percent to 75 percent (see, for example, Blum and Blum, *op. cit.*, pp. 86–87).

20 Pearl, R. *Alcohol and Longevity* (New York: Alfred Knopf, 1926).

21 This approach was used by, Holtman, A. *The Value of Human Resources and Alcoholism,* unpublished Ph.D. dissertation, Washington University, 1963.

22 *Substantial Cost Saving from Establishment of Alcoholism Program for Federal Civilian Employees, op. cit.*

23 Holtman, *op. cit.*

24 This is obtained by defining $P_t = N_{t+1}/N_t$ where, N_t = the number of surviving males out of the 100,000 that begin in the cohort at age 0. N_{t+1} is thus the number surviving to the year following N_t.

25 The data for these probabilities (P_t^A) are available from Pearl, *op. cit.*

26 Clearly, the very positive nature of the results is due to the construction of the program. That is, only currently employed individuals of moderate levels of income and of relatively low ages (i.e., long-life expectancies) are allowed to participate. Indeed, if the sponsor would have structured the program toward a mix of people, many of whom were not in the labor force, the results would be less robust. For example, a set of calculations was made assuming: average y (income) = \$3,000 (many patients are not in the labor force); r = .10; U_A = .04; I_A = .10; n = 1. The results were B^*/C^* = 0.63 and $B^* - C^*$ = −\$272,646 (the age of the target population remained 35 to 44) and, hence, the program failed to satisfy the economic criteria.

Fredric C. Menz

Economics of Disease Prevention: Infectious Kidney Disease

Reprinted with permission of the Blue Cross Association, from *Inquiry:* Vol.VIII, No.4, pp.3-18. Copyright © 1971 by the Blue Cross Association.

Originally Published in December 1971

Dramatic advances in the treatment of diseases are for the most part universally welcomed. However, because of economic constraints, differences in philosophical or ethical judgments, and conflicting medical viewpoints concerning the efficacy of alternative methods of disease control, proposals to guarantee unlimited access to such treatments, by whatever means, are usually met with some dissent.

Often, the disagreements are based upon differences in the sources of the arguments rather than on simple differences of view. Three viewpoints may be contrasted. First, there is the uninformed humanitarian who wishes to provide immediate response to urgent problems, and who on that account would always put first the need to keep the dying alive. Second, there is the view of the medical professional whose interest is in the prevention of disease, where possible, and in control and mitigation of its effects. Third, there is the view of the policy-maker who is attracted to competing alternatives, constrained by budget, and devoted to achieving optimal results

Fredric C. Menz, Ph.D. is Assistant Professor of Economics, Temple University, Philadelphia. This paper is adapted from the author's unpublished dissertation for the James Wilson Department of Economics, University of Virginia, "An Economic Analysis of Disease Control Programs," August, 1970.

Support for this research was provided by the National Institute of Allergy and Infectious Diseases (PHS), Training Grant A1-00266, and the Temple University Computer Activities Center.

The author would like to thank Harold M. Hochman, Calvin M. Kunin, Roland N. McKean, and Azriel A. Teller for their advice on the dissertation; and Arnold H. Raphaelson for his comments on this paper. All responsibilities are assumed by the author.

from a combination of choices. This paper presents and illustrates a model which permits accommodation of the analysis of the medical and economic professionals with that of social preference by combining consideration of medical and economic data in a way that permits explicit recognition of social preferences.

Variation of opinion within the medical community concerning the most effective means of controlling the morbidity and mortality associated with kidney diseases provides a case in point. There have been advances in artificial kidney therapy (and in other forms of dialysis), and in kidney transplantation; and recent proposals have suggested an expansion of governmental financing of "kidney centers" in order to eventually insure treatment for all persons with otherwise terminal chronic kidney failure.

A lack of consensus on such proposals can be ascribed to differing viewpoints concerning:

1 The feasibility as well as the ethical implications of employing costly procedures involving artificial and borrowed organs to prolong for an uncertain period of time the lives of a limited number of selected individuals with terminal chronic kidney failure; and

2 The effectiveness of medical treatment administered earlier in the kidney disease process in terms of its ability to prevent chronic kidney disease and thereby reduce the need for treatment facilities in the future.

One view contends that the "prevention" of chronic kidney disease is not a viable alternative to providing facilities for treating persons with kidney failure; and that kidney disease control programs should, therefore, emphasize the "treatment" rather than the "prevention" of kidney disease. The contrary view holds that the costs of a large-scale dialysis and kidney transplantation program would be "excessive" because its success—measured in terms not only of patient survival but also of their medical and vocational rehabilitation—is not assured, especially if treatment is offered to "unselected" patients; and because its drain on both human and non-human medical resources is severe at a time when such resources appear to be in critically short supply. The implication, of course, is that expenditures by the Federal government for dialysis and transplantation would be more wisely invested in a broadly based medical program for "preventing" kidney disease by detecting and treating it in the early stages of its natural history.

This paper will attempt to clarify discussion of this issue by presenting a framework for determining the effectiveness of medical programs designed to "prevent" infectious kidney disease. This particular type of kidney disease was chosen because it is one of the major types, causing about one-fourth of the morbidity and mortality associated with kidney diseases; and is considered to be more susceptible to "prevention," based on its prevalence, natural history, and other factors, than the other major types. It should be stressed at the outset that the effectiveness of disease control programs should not be considered in terms of an all-or-nothing "prevention" as opposed to "treatment" framework. It is conceivable that prevention is so costly and its effect on reducing the flow of patients requiring dialysis and/or transplantation so insignificant as to render it an unreasonable alternative under certain conditions. But it is more likely that the choice confronting decision-makers is one between incremental changes in the allocations among alternatives for disease control, with some being spent for dialysis and transplantation and some for preven-

tion—and the question is how much more for one or the other. After presenting an analysis of infectious kidney disease prevention programs, we will consider how the analysis could be extended to assist the development of an optimal strategy for allocating the infectious kidney disease budget among the various alternatives for controlling the morbidity, mortality, and treatment costs associated with this disease.

Methodology

One criterion for evaluating the effectiveness of a proposed medical program is to compare its costs with its expected benefits. The costs would be based on the costs of detecting the disease and the costs of administering medical treatment. The benefits would be related to the sequence of events—the morbidity, mortality, and treatment costs—that would be prevented as a result of the program. The benefits can be stated either in physical magnitudes, such as the number of deaths or bed-days of sickness that have been avoided, or in terms of a specified *numeraire,* such as dollars. The program's benefits can then be compared with its costs to facilitate policy choice.

Several methodological and analytical problems accompany the use of benefit and cost analysis. Some relate to the implications as well as the applicability of cost-benefit analyses; some to determining the quantitative magnitudes of certain costs and benefits ("measurement" problems); and others to assigning a dollar measure to the quantitative estimates of costs and benefits ("valuation" problems). Discussion of these problems is warranted since they have received substantial attention and affect the merits of the present study.

One commonly voiced objection is that selecting among different types of health programs by comparing their costs and benefits is contrary to physicians' attitudes in the care of individual patients. Nevertheless, such decisions are constantly made. Prior decisions concerning the allocation of health resources affect the current mix of health programs; and, given the scarcity of health resources, it seems desirable to base such decisions on an explicitly enumerated set of criteria.

Specification of Criteria

This leads to a fundamental set of methodological issues: those related to the specification of criteria for program selection. Not only must the relevant criteria be identified, but weights must be assigned to a given level of achievement for each criterion. Criteria frequently suggested for selecting among health programs include:

1 The relative magnitudes of the various disease problems;
2 The effectiveness of the budgetary allotments among different types of health problems;
3 The differences between the costs and benefits of the proposed programs;
4 The impact of the costs and benefits of the various alternatives upon the income distribution of the population.

In the absence of a "social objective" function, which would essentially identify the goals of society and weight the criteria appropriately—so as to make likely the choice of the "best" mix of health programs—choices are made within a certain political decision-making process with legislative actions presumably revealing social preferences. It must be concluded, therefore, that a cost-benefit comparison provides pertinent and valuable information to facilitate choice; and there is a presumption that projects "passing" a benefit-cost test should be preferred to those that "fail." However, such a test need not provide fully correct evaluations of costs and benefits in the view of decision-makers voting for their actual preferences.

Even under circumstances where cost and benefit calculations seem particularly applicable, the actual calculation of costs and benefits introduces many complex problems. "Measurement" problems arise because it is difficult or impossible (and therefore costly) to attempt to measure the quantitative significance of certain costs and benefits due to uncertainty, lack of knowledge about future events, and spillovers of benefits and costs to third parties. For example, it is difficult to predict with certainty the number of deaths that an infectious kidney disease program will prevent; it is impossible to measure the contributions of kidney transplantation and hemodialysis to the general stock of medical knowledge. Failure to include explicit estimates of such benefits and costs results in a decision reflecting implicit judgments as to their quantitative significance.

"Valuation" problems result from difficulties in expressing certain disparate costs and benefits in terms of a common measure of value. For example, the detection, treatment, and permanent cure of infectious kidney disease in an early stage will eliminate the costs associated with morbidity, mortality, and treatment—including the pain, discomfort, and fear of incapacitating illness—that would have accompanied subsequent stages of the disease process. While analysts can readily measure and assign dollar values to the avoided medical costs (assuming knowledge of the disease's natural history), they may be unwilling or unable to express the reductions in morbidity, mortality and pain costs in terms of dollar values. This difficulty arises not because societies and individuals do not, at least implicitly, place valuations on human lives, but because of diverse opinions concerning the specific value to be assigned. Under these circumstances the customary procedure in a cost-benefit analysis is to either assign an "appropriate" value to the benefits or costs,[1] or to present the full array of expected results without expressing them in the form of a single index of value.

Problems associated with the measurement and valuation of costs and benefits can be circumvented to some extent so as to make policy assessment more conscious and systematic and more nearly in accord with a society's range of preferences. This can be done by incorporating within the analysis a range of alternative estimates for the magnitude of certain "immeasurable" benefits and costs, or for the value of certain expected results, and showing how the costs, benefits, and conclusions of the analysis would thereby be affected. For example, if the mortality rate associated with a certain disease is not known precisely, alternative estimates can be used to demonstrate how the costs and benefits would be affected. If certain "immeasurable" external benefits are expected to result from a proposed course of action, it might be worthwhile (as a way to make them explicit) to show how the benefits would vary with alternative estimates of their quantitative magnitude. The costs of a proposed medical program could be estimated using alternative assumptions about costs of medicine, laboratory fees, incidence of the disease, or other key variables, with some indication as to how policy conclusions would be altered with different assumptions. If the "correct" discount rate for converting future costs and benefits to their present values is not known, alternative rates yielding different results should be provided. If there are diverse opinions regarding the specific "value" of certain expected results, such as preventing illness or prolonging an individual's life, the analysis should include an evaluation of the policy implications using alternative valuations of the expected results. Such a procedure would tend to forestall criticism concerning the "correctness" of particular assumptions that have been employed, enhance the applicability and conclusions of the analysis, and make explicit any judgments as to the quantitative significance of certain "immeasurable" costs and benefits as well as the relative valuations of expected outcomes.

Infectious Kidney Disease Prevention Program

Based on medical data presented elsewhere,[2] the following assumptions pertaining to the infectious kidney disease process underlie the basic model:

1 The natural history of infectious kidney disease is comprised of four basic stages: uncomplicated urinary tract infection (UTI); urinary tract infection involving the kidneys (KI); chronic kidney disease (CKD); and chronic irreversible kidney failure (CKF).

2 Especially in the first two stages, but also in the third, the disease is frequently asymptomatic so that individuals must be screened for the disease if it is to be detected.

3 Unless administered early in the first stage, medical treatment is ineffective in permanently halting the progression of the disease process although it may result in short-term eradication of the infection.

4 The disease becomes symptomatic in the fourth stage and unless some form of long-term palliative treatment (either dialysis or transplantation) is used to relieve the symptoms that accompany this stage of the disease, the patient will die.

5 There is, therefore, a certain probability that unless the disease process is halted in either the first or second stage it will progress over a certain time span to the stage of chronic irreversible kidney failure.

Costs of a Disease "Prevention" Program

Infectious kidney disease is frequently asymptomatic in its first two stages (UTI and KI), so its presence can only be determined by detection programs in certain population cohorts. Once detected, the infection is usually treated with various antibiotics until eradicated. However, since urinary infections are difficult to cure or eradicate permanently—especially if longstanding, and if the kidneys are involved—there is a certain probability of recurrence in subsequent time periods. An infectious kidney disease prevention program would involve, therefore: 1) selecting a target population, 2) screening it for stages 1 and/or 2 of the disease, 3) administering treatment to individuals with infections, and 4) conducting follow-up tests on those with infections—even if "successfully" treated—for a certain time period.

The total costs of a medical program to prevent urinary infections from progressing through subsequent stages of the disease would depend, therefore, on four principal elements. First, an important factor is the number of tests needed to detect the urinary infections in the population cohort. The number of tests would be determined by: the size of the target population; the number of tests required to confirm the presence of the disease (individuals who are positive on the initial test are usually re-tested twice subsequently); the number of persons followed and re-tested for either persistence or a recurrence of the disease each year; and the number of times the entire cohort is to be screened in its lifetime. Second, the cost per test would enter the calculation. Third, the average costs of medical treatment, including laboratory fees, urologic examinations, drugs, and doctors' fees would be considered. Fourth, the number of persons treated would be involved. This figure depends on the number of persons initially detected with the disease, the short-term success in eradicating the infection, the probability of recurrences in successfully treated patients, and the success in treating recurrences. The number of persons treated and the number of treatments required per person would thus be related to total treatment costs. Program costs would then include total costs of screening and treatment.[3]

Benefits of a Disease "Prevention" Program

The benefits of a medical program serve as a measure of the observed or simulated willingness of consumers to pay for the services rendered, and thus represent an estimate of the value placed on the reductions in morbidity, mortality, treatment costs and pain costs that result from the program. The benefits are related not only to the sequence of events that would have occurred in the absence of medical treatment, but also to the effectiveness of the treatment in preventing the progression of the disease through its various stages. There are two sets of primary beneficiaries

from an infectious kidney disease prevention program: 1) those in whom the infection has been eliminated and the progression of the disease thereby halted; and 2) those in whom the entire disease process is pushed into the future though the infection is never completely or successfully eradicated as a result of the prevention program.[4] The second group of direct beneficiaries will be ignored and, to this extent, the benefits will be understated.

To estimate the benefits of an infectious kidney disease prevention program, individuals who have been detected with the disease, treated, and permanently cured, will be followed through subsequent stages of the disease process to determine the sequence of events if the "prevention program" had not been administered. It is assumed that the infectious kidney disease process is comprised of four stages—UTI, KI, CKD, and CKF—and that, after an individual develops CKF, either dialysis or transplantation is required to prevent death. It is also assumed that individuals must progress through the infectious kidney disease process sequentially (i.e., stage 1 to 2 to 3 to 4 to dialysis or transplantation). The probabilities of an individual being sick, of his dying or developing the next stage of the disease, or of his being spontaneously cured (and thereby "leaving" the process) are assumed to depend on the particular stage of the disease, the length of time the individual has been in that stage, and his clinical status in previous time periods.

Persons who are cured as a result of the prevention program are classified as having been in either stage 1 (UTI) or stage 2 (KI) at the time of cure. There are certain probabilities that those who were in stage 1 when cured would have been sick or well, developed an infection of the kidneys (stage 2), spontaneously "lost" their UTI, or died during time period 1. Similarly, there are certain probabilities that individuals who were in stage 2 when cured would have been sick or well, developed chronic kidney disease (stage 3), or died during the first time period. During a second time period, some who were initially in stage 1 will remain there (and either be sick, well, die or spontaneously cured); some will develop stage 2; some will remain in stage 2 (having either been classified initially in this stage or developed it during time period 1); and some will develop stage 3 (CKD). By the fourth time period, some of the cohort detected with UTI and cured would have required medical treatment—dialysis and/or transplantation—for CKF. There are certain probabilities of survival and clinical rehabilitation for persons receiving this treatment.

Assuming certain probabilities — or ranges of probabilities—for these events, the number of persons in each stage of the disease and the number sick, well, dead, and receiving treatment for the final stage of the disease can be estimated for each year the cohort is followed. Additional data are needed to estimate the costs of morbidity and mortality associated with the various stages of the disease. For example, the morbidity losses for persons in stage 2 in the second time period are calculated by: 1) multiplying the number of persons in stage 2 in time period 2 by the probability of sickness to determine the number of sick persons; 2) multiplying the number of sick persons by the average number of bed-days or restricted days per episode of morbidity; and 3) multiplying the total number of bed-days by a dollar value for each bed-day. Then, to express the dollar costs for stage 2 in time period 2 in terms of their present value, the costs must be discounted. Algebraically

$$\binom{\text{Present value}}{\text{of morbidity}} = \binom{\text{Total persons}}{\text{in stage 2}} \times$$

$$\binom{\text{Probability}}{\text{of sickness}} \times \binom{\text{Average bed-days}}{\text{sick person}} \times$$

$$\binom{\text{Dollar value}}{\text{per bed-day}} \times \binom{\text{Discount}}{\text{rate}}$$

Similarly, the present value of mortality is the result of applying the probability of death, an arbitrary current value for each death, and a discount rate to the number of persons in stage 2. The present values

of morbidity and mortality are then in common terms and can be combined. The dollar figure that results is the present value of the costs of morbidity and mortality during time period 2 for persons from the original target cohort who would have been in the second stage of the infectious kidney disease process if their infections had not been detected, treated, and cured in the prevention program. To determine the total benefits of the prevention program, similar calculations for each stage of the disease, as well as for the costs associated with the treatment required for stage 4, would be aggregated over a certain time span.

Since the models for estimating costs and benefits explicitly allow the inclusion of alternative arrays of values for certain variables, there are many opportunities for analysis. Alternative assumptions about discount rates, prevention costs, morbidity and mortality rates, treatment costs, and other variables, might be used to determine their effects on cost and benefit estimates. If a given program were not worthwhile (in a cost-benefit sense) under a particular set of assumptions, the analysis could show what changes in assumptions would be necessary to make the program worthwhile. The analysis could also show how new, more effective ways to "prevent" infectious kidney disease or new methods to treat CKF would affect cost and benefit estimates, and how such changes would alter the optimal strategy for controlling the costs associated with this disease.

Hypothetical Kidney Disease Medical Program

In this section, the techniques for estimating the costs and benefits of infectious kidney disease control programs will be more fully elaborated and applied to a hypothetical medical program for detecting and treating "kidney infections" in a certain population cohort. This is a purely hypothetical example, and the specific probabilities and dollar values for the various events have been chosen primarily to simplify the exposition of the models.

Table 1. Costs of a hypothetical kidney disease prevention program for a single population cohort

Year	Number screened[a]	Present value of screen costs[b]	Number treated[c]	Number of successes[d]	Present value treatment costs[e]	Present value total costs[f]
1	1,300,000	$13,000,000	50,000	25,000	$5,000,000	$18,000,000
2	50,000	462,950	25,000	12,500	2,314,800	2,777,750
3	50,000	428,650	12,500	6,250	1,071,620	1,500,270
4	50,000	396,900	6,250	3,125	496,120	893,020
5	50,000	367,500	3,125	1,563	229,690	597,190
6	50,000	340,300	1,563	781	106,380	446,680
7	50,000	315,100	781	390	49,220	364,320
8	50,000	291,750	390	195	22,760	314,510
9	50,000	270,150	195	97	10,540	280,690
10	50,000	250,100	98	49	4,900	255,000
11	50,000	231,600	49	25	2,270	233,870
12	50,000	214,450	24	12	1,030	215,480
13	50,000	198,850	12	6	480	119,330
14	50,000	183,800	6	3	220	184,020
15	50,000	170,250	3	1	100	170,350
	Total program cost					$26,432,480

[a]Year 1: $(1 + .15 + .15) \times (1,000,000)$; Year 2 (*et seq.*): $.05 (1,000,000)$.
[b]$10 (discounted at 8 percent to present value) $\times$ column 2.
[c]Year 1: $.05 (1,000,000)$; Year 2 (*seq.*): .5 of preceding year.
[d]50 percent of column 4.
[e]$100 (discounted at 8 percent to present value) $\times$ column 4.
[f]Column 6 + column 3.

Costs of Early Detection and Treatment Program

The costs of a medical program to prevent kidney infections from progressing beyond the first two stages of the disease process are based on the costs of detecting and the costs of treating the disease in its early stages. Since infectious kidney disease is usually asymptomatic in its earliest stages (UTI and KI), the target population must be screened to determine the presence of disease. Assume the following: 1) 1,000,000 individuals are to be screened for "kidney infections"; 2) three consecutive positive urine specimens are needed to verify the diagnosis; 3) 15 percent of the group are found to be positive on the first test, two-thirds of whom are positive on the second test, and the overall prevalence after the third test (i.e., the actual UTI prevalence rate as determined by three consecutive positive tests) is 5 percent; 4) all persons in whom a "kidney infection" has been detected are rescreened once per year for 15 years; 5) the cost per test is $10; and 6) the discount rate for converting future costs to their present

value is 8 percent.[5] The number of persons screened per year and the present value of screening costs are shown in Table 1, columns 2 and 3.

Once the infection is detected, the cost of treatment varies depending on the specific medical procedures employed. Some patients are merely given antibacterial therapy and, if the infection is not eradicated within a certain time period, a different drug is prescribed. Others are given an extensive urologic workup in order to determine the extent to which the kidneys are also infected. The cost of treatment also varies with the degree of difficulty in eradicating the infection, with some patients requiring several years of continuous treatment to eradicate the UTI. In other cases, however, the UTI is eradicated with the first round of treatment, though there is still a certain probability of relapse thereafter. Because there is a relatively high frequency of recurrence in persons who are apparently treated "successfully" for UTI, "successful" treatment is assumed to mean short-term eradication of the infection rather than permanent cure of the infectious kidney disease process. Therefore, there is a certain probability that persons treated "successfully" will have a recurrence of their infection in subsequent time periods; and this, too, will affect the costs of treating "kidney infections" in their early stages.

Assume that 50 percent of the persons entering the treatment program are treated "successfully" initially and that 50 percent of the remainder are treated "successfully" each time period thereafter. Assume also in this example that success means zero probability of future recurrence (i.e., permanent cure). Assuming treatment costs of $100 per episode and a discount rate of 8 percent, the number of patients treated, the number of "successes," and the present value of the treatment costs each year are shown in columns 4, 5 and 6, respectively, of Table 1. Column 7 shows the present value of the treatment and detection costs for each year of this prevention program. The total costs—$26,-432,480—represent the present value of the total costs for an infectious kidney disease control program based on the above assumptions.

Benefits of the Program

It is assumed that unless infectious kidney disease is detected, treated and permanently cured at an early stage, there is a certain probability that the disease will progress from an uncomplicated UTI (stage 1) to chronic irreversible kidney failure (stage 4).[6] Therefore, the benefits of an infectious kidney disease prevention program can be estimated by measuring the morbidity, mortality, and treatment costs that will be avoided as a result of the program.

It was assumed in the prevention program illustrated above that 50 percent of those with UTI were treated successfully the first year and 50 percent of the remainder were successfully treated each year thereafter until all the UTI's were eradicated. It was also assumed that the probability of the infection recurring after

being successfully treated was zero. Thus successful treatment in this example is assumed to result in permanent cure of the UTI and permanent cessation of the disease process. The number of persons successfully treated (permanently cured) per year is shown in column 6, of Table 1. Each year's "successes" must be followed through the infectious kidney disease process to determine what would have occurred if their UTI had not been successfully treated.

Persons who have been permanently cured are initially classified as having been in either stage 1 (UTI) or stage 2 (KI) at the time of cure. Each group is then followed through the remainder of the disease process. During the first time period, a certain number of those permanently cured would have been sick; some would have remained well;[7] in some the UTI may have spontaneously cured; some would have developed a kidney infection; and a certain number would have died. In time period 2, persons remaining in stage 1 (i.e., those who were either sick or well during period 1) must be followed for morbidity, mortality, spontaneous cure, or a worsening of the disease. Since the probability of these events is assumed to be related to medical status in previous time periods, those who were sick in the first time period are more likely to be sick, die, or develop stage 2, and less likely to be spontaneously cured or well, than those who had remained well. Similarly, the probability of morbidity differs in time period 3 and subsequent periods, with totals for these periods calculated over the entire cohort.

Since it has been assumed that some, but not all, persons being treated for "kidney infections" (UTI or KI) are cured in the first year of treatment, new "permanently cured" persons enter the benefit flow over an extended time span.[8] Therefore the total number of UTI's who would have been sick, well, cured, dead, or developed KI in a certain time period would be an aggregate based on the UTI's from previous time periods' cohorts who are still

Table 2. The first stage of the kidney disease process: number of persons morbid, dead, well, spontaneously cured, and developing stage 2 each year

Year	Enter stage 1 (UTI)[a]	Enter stage 2 (KI)[b]	UTI Morbidity[c]	UTI Okay[d]	UTI Cured[e]	UTI Mortality[f]
1	12,500	17,500	2,500	1,250	2,500	1,250
2	6,250	9,688	2,000	1,187	1,875	1,500
3	3,125	5,172	1,244	809	1,181	1,031
4	1,563	2,701	704	483	680	610
5	782	1,391	381	269	372	338
6	391	709	200	144	197	180
7	195	359	104	76	102	94
8	98	181	53	39	53	48
9	49	91	27	20	27	25
10	25	46	14	10	14	13
11	13	23	7	5	7	6
12	6	11	3	3	3	3
13	3	6	2	1	2	2
14	2	3	1	1	1	1
15	1	1	....	....	....	....

[a]50 percent of "successes" (Table 1, column 5).
[b]Year 1: 50 percent of successes + 40 percent of column 2; Year 2 (*et seq.*): 50 percent of successes + certain percentages of previous years' UTI cohorts (see text).
[c]Year 1: 20 percent of column 2; Year 2 (*et seq.*): 20 percent of column 2 + certain percentages of previous years' UTI's in columns 4 and 5.
[d]Same as column 4, with different probabilities (see text). Persons who remain well still have the disease, but suffer no morbidity or mortality, are not cured, and do not worsen in that time period.
[e]Same as column 4, with different probabilities (see text). Persons who are "cured" have spontaneously cured themselves of the disease.
[f]Same as column 4, with different probabilities (see text).

being followed plus the UTI cohort that entered the benefit flow in that particular time period. For example, by the fourth time period, four separate cohorts would have entered the benefit flow: the initial cohort, comprised of those whose "kidney infections" were permanently cured the first year of the prevention program, would be in their fourth year in the UTI stage; the cohort which was cured in the second year of the prevention program would be in its third year; the third year's "permanent cures" would be in their second year in the benefit flow; and those who were treated successfully (in this example, permanently cured) in time period 4 would be in their first year.

Table 2 shows the number of UTI's sick, well, spontaneously cured, dead and developing KI each year, and is based on the following assumptions:

1 Fifty percent of the persons cured each year are initially found to have a kidney infection (stage 2 of the disease process);

2 During the first year, 20, 10, 20, 40, and 10 percent of each entering UTI group are sick, well, spontaneously cured, moved to stage 2, and dead, respectively;

3 Each year thereafter there are probabilities of 25, 10, 10, 25 and 30 percent that a person who was sick in the previous period will be sick, well, spontaneously cured, develop stage 2 and dead, respectively; and probabilities of 10, 25, 30, 25, and 10 percent that one who was well in the previous period will be sick, well, cured, develop KI, and dead, respectively.[9]

Each year's figures are an aggregate comprised of each of the UTI groups being followed in that year. For example, the morbidity for year 3 is comprised of the number of UTI's morbid in each of the three groups being followed in that year, including the third year's morbidity for the 12,500 UTI's from year 1 (representing 50 percent of those permanently cured the first year of the program), plus the second year's morbidity for the 6,250 UTI's

Table 3. Total morbidity and mortality losses associated with stage 1 (UTI) of the infectious kidney disease process for the original population cohort

Year	Bed-days[a]	Morbidity losses[b]	Mortality losses[c]	Total indirect losses, stage 1[d]	Present value total indirect losses[e]
1	2,500	$25,000	$1,250,000	$1,275,000	$1,275,000
2	2,000	20,000	1,500,000	1,520,000	1,407,368
3	1,244	12,440	1,031,000	1,043,000	894,541
4	704	7,040	610,040	617,000	489,806
5	381	3,810	338,000	341,810	251,230
6	200	2,000	180,000	182,000	123,869
7	104	1,040	94,000	95,040	59,894
8	53	530	48,000	48,530	28,317
9	27	270	25,000	25,270	13,653
10	14	140	13,000	13,140	6,573
11	7	70	6,000	6,070	2,812
12	3	30	3,000	3,030	1,300
13	2	20	2,000	2,020	802
14	1	10	1,000	1,010	371
Total benefits if stage 1 were prevented					$4,555,536

[a]UTI morbidity (Table 2, column 4) × 1 day (representing average length of illness for each episode of morbidity).
[b]Column 1 × $10 (representing average "value" per bed-day of illness).
[c]UTI mortality (Table 2, column 7) × $1000 (representing average "value" of each death).
[d]Column 3 + column 4.
[e]Column 5 discounted at 8 percent to present value.

who were successfully treated in year 2, plus the first year's morbidity for the 3,125 UTI's who entered the benefit flow in year 3.

In Table 3, a certain number of bed-days are assigned each episode of morbidity, certain values are attributed to each death and to each bed-day of morbidity, and the present value of the total morbidity and mortality losses associated with stage 1 of infectious kidney disease are estimated, based on the foregoing assumptions.[10] The present values of each year's total losses are calculated using an 8 percent discount rate. The present value of the total morbidity and mortality losses—$4,555,536—represents the benefits if stage 1 were prevented from occurring as a result of an infectious kidney disease prevention program.

The same procedure can be used to estimate the benefits expected to result from the prevention of the second and third stages of infectious kidney disease in a certain cohort. Over a certain time duration, persons are in stage 2 (KI) either because they had a kidney infection when permanently cured or had advanced to stage 2 from the first stage of the disease. For any particular year the total number of KI's sick, well, dead, and advancing to stage 3 (CKD) would be based on the number of persons entering and remaining in stage 2 as of that year. The same is true for individuals in the third stage of the disease. The primary difference between the different stages of the disease process would be in the probabilities of the various events, which would be directly related to the severity (stage) of the disease. The total indirect losses associated with the second and third stages of the disease process — representing the benefits expected to result if these stages were prevented from occurring — are presented below.[11]

Chronic Irreversible Kidney Failure

The fourth stage of the infectious kidney disease process is chronic irreversible kidney failure (CKF). After progressing to this stage of the disease, persons either die within a short time period or are selected to receive some form of long-term treatment—either dialysis or transplantation. The number of persons entering CKF

Table 4. Results for patients requiring long-term treatment for CKF

Year	Enter long-term treatment[a]	Total on HD[b]	HD patients fully rehabilitated[c]	HD mortality[d]	Total receiving transplants[e]
4	4,288	2,144	1,286	429	2,573
5	4,868	3,720	2,232	742	3,178
6	3,452	3,959	2,375	792	2,519
7	2,053	3,402	2,041	680	1,707
8	1,128	2,569	1,563	521	1,085
9	597	1,862	1,117	372	671
10	309	1,272	763	254	409
11	158	842	505	168	247
12	80	545	327	109	149
13	40	347	208	69	89
14	21	219	132	44	55
15	10	137	82	27	32
16	4	84	51	17	19
17	....	51	31	10	10
18	....	31	18	6	6
19	....	18	11	4	4
20	....	11	7	2	2

[a]Certain percentage of persons with CKF (see footnote 12).
[b]Year 4: 50 percent of column 2; Year 5 (*et seq.*): 50 percent of column 2 + 60 percent of the previous year's column 3.
[c]60 percent of column 3. Additional columns to account for partial rehabilitation and inactive cases should be added where information permits or assumptions require them.
[d]20 percent of column 3.
[e]50 percent of column 2 + 20 percent of column 3.

in any time period is related to the number of persons sick or well with CKD in the previous time period.[12] The total benefits if stage 4 were prevented from occurring are presented below.

Persons who have progressed through the four stages of the infectious kidney disease process and have been selected to receive long-term treatment for CKF must also be followed to determine the treatment costs and indirect losses associated with treatment for CKF, since these could have been avoided if the disease had been prevented in the original population cohort. Each year a certain number of persons are selected from those with chronic kidney failure and are either put on dialysis therapy or given a kidney transplant. Thereafter, dialysis patients will either remain alive on dialysis, be given a transplant, or die; and patients who are alive on dialysis will be either fully or partially rehabilitated or totally inactive. The probabilities of full and partial rehabilitation, inactivity, death, and receiving a transplant are assumed to depend on the patient's clinical status in the preceding

period.[13, 14] Table 4 presents data on the flow of patients from the original population cohort, showing the number selected each year to receive treatment, the total on dialysis, and the numbers fully rehabilitated, dying, and given transplants. Table 5 shows the direct and indirect costs associated with dialysis treatment, based on the above assumptions, and discounted at 8 percent. The total annual direct costs of dialysis are a function of the number of persons being maintained on home dialysis (HD) and the cost per patient per year. The column entitled "rehabilitation losses" would include an estimate of the losses associated with incomplete rehabilitation. The present value of the direct and indirect losses represent an approximation of the "costs" associated with dialysis therapy which could have been avoided with a disease prevention program for the original population cohort.

The direct and indirect costs associated with kidney transplants must also be determined. Since survival rates depend on whether the graft is from a related living donor, unrelated living donor, or cadaver, transplant recipients are initially classified according to the source of their graft and then followed to determine the subsequent course of events. During their first year with a transplant, recipients will either remain alive with the transplant, die, or be given dialysis therapy after transplant failure. During the second year, recipients of transplants are classified into one of the following groups: 1) alive with the same transplant; 2) alive with a second transplant; 3) alive, but due to transplant failure, given dialysis therapy; or 4) dead due to transplant failure. Patients transferred back to dialysis must also be followed. To simplify this illustration, it is assumed that patients whose transplants fail simply die rather than receive another transplant or dialysis therapy. The mortality rate is assumed to be 50 percent per year; each transplant is assumed to cost $1,000; each death "costs" $1,000; and costs are discounted using an 8 percent discount rate. The total costs associated with kidney transplantation, representing the benefits if the disease process were

prevented in the original population cohort, are shown in Table 6.

Table 6. Present values of costs and benefits of a hypothetical disease control program for a single population cohort

	Total	
Stage 1 (UTI)	$ 4,555,536	
Stage 2 (KI)	10,231,673	
Stage 3 (CKD)	18,437,808	
Stage 4 (CKF)	3,961,684	
Dialysis	16,035,607	
Transplantation	16,662,042	
Program benefits		$69,884,350
Program costs		$26,432,480

Table 6 totals the indirect losses expected to be incurred in each stage of the disease process and the indirect losses and direct costs of treatment for CKF to arrive at the present in Table 1. Obviously the costs and benefits of the program depend on the particular assumptions that have been made; but, based on this illustrative comparison of costs and benefits, the program would be worthwhile.

Table 5. Present value of the direct and indirect losses associated with dialysis treatment for CKF (stage 4)

Year	Total costs of HD[a] (in 000's)	Mortality losses, HD[b] (in 000's)	Rehabilitation losses[c]	Total losses[d] (in 000's)	Present value total dialysis losses[e]
4	$2,144	$429	....	$2,573	$2,042,447
5	3,720	742	....	4,462	3,279,570
6	3,959	792	....	4,751	3,233,530
7	3 402	680	....	4,082	2,572,478
8	2,569	521	....	3,090	1,803,015
9	1,862	372	....	2,234	1,207,030
10	1,272	254	....	1,526	763,305
11	842	168	....	1,010	467,832
12	545	109	....	654	280,501
13	347	69	....	416	165,194
14	219	44	....	263	96,705
15	137	27	....	164	55,842
16	84	17	....	101	31,835
17	51	10	....	61	17,806
18	31	6	....	37	10,001
19	18	4	....	22	5,504
20	11	2	....	13	3,012
Total benefits if HD were avoided					$16,035,607

[a]Total on HD (Table 4, column 3) × $1,000.
[b]HD mortality (Table 4, column 5) × $1,000.
[c]In this illustration, all dialysis patients are assumed to be fully rehabilitated.
[d]Column 2 + column 3.
[e]Column 5 discounted at 8 percent to present value.

Conclusions

The preceding section illustrated the application of various models for estimating the costs and benefits of infectious kidney disease prevention programs. In this section, the implications as well as limitations of the models will be discussed.

The most important limitation of the preceding analysis, and of the cost-benefit technique per se, is the assumption that what consumers should be willing to pay for a service (because of its expected benefits) represents its "value." In this study, the benefits are assumed to be based on the morbidity, mortality, and treatment costs that would have been necessary had the prevention program not been administered. As was stressed earlier, difficult problems arise not only with respect to the criterion itself (i.e., the use of attributed "willingness to pay" as a proxy for a service's value), but also in determining the specific dollar amount that consumers would be willing to offer for the provision of a certain service. There will, after all, be very little information on the probabilities of a *particular* person going on to the next stage of the disease (or becoming ill) even if he is aware of its presence. Further, the choice of treatment alternatives is limited to what may be prescribed. Therefore, a model must substitute assumption for information on cost parameters as well as value.

The model could be extended to determine the costs and benefits of preventing infectious kidney disease in successive cohorts over an extended time span. For example, it might be proposed that all females be screened for "kidney infections" on their fifth birthday, and thereafter as necessitated by the initial findings. The annual costs of such a program would be based on the number of persons screened in each of the cohorts that have entered and are being followed as of that year. The costs and benefits that are estimated for a single entering cohort could not, however, be merely multiplied by the number of entering cohorts to determine the aggregate costs and benefits because the cohorts would be entering the program in different time periods.[15]

As a means of by-passing the important problems associated with the estimation of benefits and costs, the model has treated many of the relevant parameters as variables rather than as certain specified values. While space limitations preclude further illustration, different dollar estimates could be assumed for each episode of morbidity and mortality, alternative discount rates could be utilized, different dollar "values" could be used to estimate the costs associated with the partial rehabilitation of dialysis patients, and different probabilities could be associated with stages of the disease. For example, if it is thought that a certain society "prefers" to direct the bulk of its medical care resources to caring for the aged, weights that appropriately reflect such preferences could be used in estimating a medical program's benefits for different age groups. Thus social preferences could be reflected in the assessment of candidate programs for government support. Or, if each bedday of morbidity is thought to be "worth" $100, the indirect losses associated with morbidity could be estimated using $100 as the value that consumers would have placed on preventing a bed-day of morbidity from occurring. Better clinical and economic data could make the assumptions more realistic, and uniform application to different medical programs of comparable data would permit comparison among programs.

Applicability to Other Disease Control Programs

The specific models that have been presented pertain to infectious kidney disease. With simple modifications these models could be used to analyze the effectiveness of other kidney disease control programs as well. More important, however, the basic analysis—not necessarily "cost-benefit," but simply the method of viewing a disease as a process which begins at some point in time and "progresses" to more advanced stages—can be applied to the analysis of medical programs for any disease if the disease can be thought of in analogous terms. For example, concern has been voiced recently about the procedure of routinely vaccinating children against smallpox in view of the frequency of the complications (including death) associated with the administration of the smallpox vaccine.[16] One way of analyzing whether routine smallpox vaccinations are worthwhile would be to utilize a cost-benefit framework and to weigh the expected costs of routine vaccination against the expected benefits. The "costs" would include: 1) the cost of administering the vaccination, which would depend on the size of the population cohort and the cost per vaccination; 2) the effectiveness of the vaccination in preventing smallpox from occurring; and 3) the estimated total indirect losses due to the morbidity and mortality that result from the vaccination.[17] Various estimates of morbidity, mortality, discount rates, and other key variables could be postulated to determine how the costs of smallpox control programs would be affected.

The "benefits" of a smallpox vaccination program would be the decrease in morbidity, mortality, and treatment costs that would be expected to result from the program.[18] Assuming that vaccinations permanently halt the smallpox disease process, individuals who are given the vaccination could be followed through the natural history of the disease in order to determine the number of persons who would have been sick or died if the vaccination program had not been administered. If the expected benefits of the smallpox vaccination program exceed its costs, the program would—using the cost-benefit criterion—be judged worthwhile. If not, the recommendation would be to discontinue the routine vaccination of children against smallpox.

Allocation of Resources

To conclude that a medical program is worthwhile does not necessarily mean, however, that it should be undertaken. For one thing, the cost-benefit basis for evaluating the effectiveness of alternate medical programs is only one of many criteria that are used by decision-makers in choosing between various policy proposals. Even if a program were worthwhile by the cost-benefit criterion, this does not necessarily lead to the conclusion that the program should be adopted. First, "health" is only one of many competitors for scarce resources. Second, "disease control" is only one method for utilizing funds that have been allotted for purposes of "health." Funds might also be used for research to find new methods for treating chronic renal failure, additional ways to detect urinary tract infections, or more effective treatment for UTI.

Finally, if the "disease control" budget is to be effectively allocated among various diseases, the medical programs for these diseases must be evaluated in terms of their *relative* effectiveness in reducing the morbidity, mortality, and treatment costs associated with each of the diseases. This is most simply illustrated in a two-disease case. For example, assume 1) that smallpox and infectious kidney diseases are the only diseases that exist; 2) that programs to prevent each would be worthwhile according to the cost-benefit criterion; and 3) that resource limitations require a choice between the two programs. The choice as to the appropriate expenditure levels for each program should depend on a comparison of their relative effectiveness in reducing the direct and indirect losses that result from the advanced stages of the two diseases.

It is interesting that the Federal government—as well as several state governments—are providing funds for establishing artificial kidney centers to treat individuals with chronic kidney failure. In terms of the framework discussed above, this implies, first, that they put a higher priority on reducing the morbidity and mortality resulting from kidney disease than for certain other diseases; and, second, that the "kidney disease budget" is more effectively used to prevent the morbidity and mortality caused by CKF than to prevent the morbidity and mortality caused by other stages of the kidney disease process (and thereby to avoid CKF). There remains the question of whether the present budgetary allotment is the most effective way to distribute the kidney disease budget among the various stages of the disease. An analysis of this question would include a comparison of the marginal costs and benefits associated with the expenditure of funds in each of the stages. Maximum benefits will occur when such costs and benefits are equated at the margin. Since the benefits are reflections of the reduction of the morbidity, mortality, and treatment costs caused by kidney disease, the budget should be distributed among the stages of the disease in a way that will maximize the total benefits expected from the overall expenditure.

If the problem were reduced to that of determining the most effective allocation of the kidney disease budget between the "prevention" of the disease, on the one hand, and its "treatment," on the other, the marginal costs and benefits associated with expenditures for "preventing" the disease in a certain cohort would have to be compared with the marginal costs and benefits associated with "treating" the disease in that cohort. In this study a model was developed and applied to estimate the costs and benefits of "prevention" programs. Using the same framework, the marginal costs and benefits of various "treatment" programs could also be determined if treatment for chronic renal failure is viewed as a means by which life is prolonged in certain individuals. The costs would be comprised of the expenditures for dialysis and transplantation facilities, and the benefits would be the reductions in morbidity and mortality expected to result from the provision of such facilities. Integrating such data with that in this study would give an indication of how the kidney disease budget should be allocated if total benefits are to be maximized.

These elements involved in achieving maximum efficiency and approaching optimal use of certain budget are well established in economic literature. They have been explored in recent discussions of planning-programming-budgeting systems (PPBS), for example.[19] It is time for the integration of such economic analysis with the knowledge of disease management and control. Application of models that relate them can lead to informed choices for government's health agenda, choices that give proper weight to urgent needs, such as treatment of CKF, and that give proper (discounted) weight to the values of disease prevention.

References and Notes

1 For example, the present value of expected lifetime earnings is frequently used as a proxy for an individual's "value" to society. This procedure tends to weight programs in favor of wealthy, young, able-bodied Caucasian males.

2 See Chapter 2, pages 33-75, of the author's dissertation, *An Economic Analysis of Disease Control Programs*, unpublished, University of Virginia, 1970.

3 Treatment-caused complications, such as drug reactions, will be ignored in cost estimates since they occur infrequently, and when they do are easily controlled by either reducing the dosage or by changing drugs.

4 There are secondary beneficiaries as well. Preventive programs may lead to the discovery of other previously undetected diseases and may also prevent certain other kidney-disease-caused disorders from occurring.

5 It should be emphasized that it is assumed here that the entire population is screened only once and only those found to have UTI's initially will be rescreened yearly thereafter. This is for purposes of simplification only. Those who were initially negative might also be rescreened over a certain time span, or a new target population might be screened each year. If so, the costs as well as the benefits would differ, but the logical framework of these models would still apply.

6 Based on the following: 1) until the third and fourth stages, infectious kidney disease is asymptomatic and will, therefore, not be detected until the kidneys have suffered permanent and irreversible damage, and 2) as the disease worsens, medical treatment becomes progressively less effective in eliminating the infection and halting damage to the kidneys (see footnote 2).

7 Persons who remain well are still in the UTI stage of the disease process but are not sick in that particular time period; persons who are "spon-

taneously cured" leave the disease process entirely.

8 In this example, 15 years (Table 1, column 5).

9 The probabilities are hypothetical but were chosen to illustrate that in this study it is *not* assumed that the probability of the various events is a constant geometric rate; that is, the probabilities of each of the various events occurring is assumed to depend on the patient's status in the preceding period(s). The method utilized is similar to a period analysis in the sense that a flow of persons is followed over a certain time span.

10 The measure for morbidity as well as the assumed values per bed-day and death are hypothetical (and treated as variables) in this illustration. The particular values were chosen so to simplify actual calculations. Alternative estimates could be assumed to show their affect on the benefit estimates.

11 The following assumptions apply to stage 2 (KI): 1) 10, 20, 50, and 20 percent of each group that enters stage 2 (or is in that stage at the time of cure) are sick, well, moved to CKD, and dead, respectively, that first year; 2) after the initial year, there are probabilities of 20, 0, 60, and 20 percent that a KI who was sick in the previous period will be sick, well, moved to CKD, and dead, respectively, and probabilities of 20, 0, 60, and 20 percent that a person who was well in the previous period will be well, sick, moved to CKD, and dead, respectively.

For stage 3, the following assumptions apply: 1) during the first year 10, 5, 70, and 15 percent of each entering CKD cohort are sick, well, develop CKF, and dead, respectively; and 2) each year thereafter there are probabilities of 10, 5, 60, and 25 percent that a person who was sick in the previous period will be sick, well, develop CKF, and dead, respectively, and the same probabilities that a CKD who was well in the previous period will be well, sick, develop CKF, and dead, respectively.

For both stages, each episode of morbidity is assumed to result in 10 days of restricted activity "costing" $10 per day; each death is valued at $1000; and future costs are discounted using an 8 percent discount rate.

12 The following assumptions apply to the fourth stage: 1) in their initial year with CKF 10, 0, 70, and 20 percent of each group are sick, well, selected to receive long-term treatment, and dead, respectively; 2) thereafter there are probabilities of 5, 0, 65, and 30 percent that a CKF who was sick in the previous period will be sick, well, accepted for treatment, and dead, respectively; and 3) each episode of morbidity results in 10 days of restricted activity "costing" $10 per day; each death "costs" $1000; and present values are computed using an 8 percent discount rate.

13 For simplification, it is assumed in this illustration that all patients on dialysis therapy are fully rehabilitated. Partial rehabilitation would entail additional economic losses and could be estimated in a manner similar to that for estimating morbidity losses in the various stages of the disease.

14 The following assumptions are used to estimate the costs associated with dialysis therapy: 1) 50 percent of the CKF's selected to receive treatment each year are initially given dialysis therapy; 2) during that year, and subsequently, 60, 20, and 20 percent of the patients remaining on dialysis are fully rehabilitated, given a kidney transplant, and die, respectively; 3) the cost per patient per year for dialysis is $1000; and 4) deaths are assumed to "cost" $1000.

15 For example, if a prevention program were initiated in 1970, then the fifth year of the prevention program for the 1970 cohort would be 1975, and the fifth year's costs would be discounted using 1970 as the base year. But the cohort that is followed beginning in 1971 would not be in the fifth year of the prevention program until 1976, and the costs of the prevention program in its fifth year (which would be the same undiscounted amount for two identical cohorts) should be discounted using 1971 as the base year. Thus the present value of the costs incurred in the fifth year of the disease prevention program will differ, and simple aggregation (over otherwise identical cohorts) will not yield the correct present value of the prevention program's cost. A meaningful aggregated cost figure would result only if the appropriate time factors for each cohort were taken into account. Analogous considerations apply to aggregation of benefits in the situation described here, so that extension to other cohorts and years present the need for further calculation but add few conceptual problems.

16 Lane, J. M. and Millar, J. D. "Routine Vaccination against Smallpox Re-Considered," *New England Journal of Medicine* 281:1220-1224 (1969).

17 It was assumed for infectious kidney disease that no complications resulted from the medical treatment that was administered to eradicate the urinary infection and thereby halt the disease process. Screening was used, without side effects, to detect the disease, and only positives were treated. This is clearly not true with smallpox vaccinations. Instead, disease prevention requires a treatment (vaccination) of the healthy population. Another difference between the two prevention programs results because the smallpox vaccination is usually more effective in preventing smallpox from occurring than antibiotic treatment is in preventing the advanced stages of kidney disease from occurring. Both are important factors that determine the costs (and relative effectiveness) of various disease "prevention" programs.

18 Since smallpox is a contagious disease, the benefits to persons other than those receiving the vaccine must also be estimated. Also, benefits resulting from the prevention of smallpox-caused disorders must be accounted for.

19 See: Joint Economic Committee of the U.S. Congress, *The Analysis and Evaluation of Public Expenditures: The PPB System*, three volumes (1969).

Martin S. Feldstein
James Schuttinga

Hospital Costs in Massachusetts: A Methodological Study

Originally Published in March 1977

Reprinted with permission of the Blue Cross Association, from *Inquiry:* Vol.XIV, No.1, pp.22-31. Copyright © 1977 by the Blue Cross Association.

The rapid increase in hospital costs and the dominant financial role of private and public insurance programs have made the variations in hospital costs a subject of careful public scrutiny. Unfortunately, the ability to compare costs in different hospitals in a meaningful way is substantially limited by differences among institutions in the mix of cases treated. Without further analysis, it is not clear how much of the variation in hospital costs is simply a reflection of these differences in case-mix. Similarly, it is not clear whether any particular hospital has a relatively high average cost per case because it treats a case-mix that is inherently expensive or because it treats a more ordinary case-mix in a costly way.

The purpose of the current study is to develop a method of adjusting hospital costs for interhospital differences in case-mix. This case-mix adjusted measure of hospital costliness is intended as a management aid for understanding and perhaps guiding hospital costs. The statistical analysis provides:

1 A measure of the general impact of case-mix on hospital costs, i.e., an estimate of the fraction of the variation in hospital case costs that is a reflection of case-mix;

2 A costliness rating for each individual hospital, i.e., a measure of each hospital's cost after purging the effect of case-mix.

We find that about one-half of interhospital cost variation among Massachusetts short-term hospitals can be explained by our measure of case-mix variation. About 40 percent of the variation in average cost per day is also explained in this way.

Several alternative costliness measures are developed. These are quite highly correlated with each other but have a lower correlation with average cost per case, implying that the choice among these costliness measures is less important than the use of costliness rather than cost. In presenting these costliness measures, we wish to stress that they should be regarded as a managerial guide and not as a mechanical tool. It would be unwise to tie any cost control formula to these individual costliness values. If they are used in the cost regulation process, it should be as a method of identifying hospitals that *may* have costs that are inappropriately high or low and that therefore warrant further analysis.

This paper provides a brief analysis of the methods and a description of the quantitative conclusions. The first section discusses the basic regression analysis method by which costliness is defined and calculated. The second section describes the data that we have analyzed. The next section deals with the technique of principal component analysis that has been used to summarize case-mix information. The results for average cost per case are pre-

Martin S. Feldstein, D. Phil. is Professor of Economics, Harvard University (1737 Cambridge Street, Cambridge, MA 02138).

James Schuttinga, Ph.D. is Assistant Professor of Economics, Gordon College (Wenham, MA 01984).

This work was supported by the Department of Human Services of the Commonwealth of Massachusetts. The authors would like to express their gratitude to William Brady, Thomas Gagnon, Carolyn Lipsett and Joseph Steinberg of the Massachusetts Rate Setting Commission; to Maureen Steinbrunner and Charles Stover of the Department of Human Services, and to the Massachusetts Hospital Association.

sented in the fourth section, and the corresponding results for average cost per patient day are presented in the fifth section.

Hospital Costliness

The basic idea of the hospital costliness measure is to compare the actual cost per case[1] in each hospital with the cost per case that would be expected for that hospital because of its case-mix.[2] To make this idea more precise, assume for the moment that we know a "standard cost" for each diagnostic type of case, i.e., the average cost for that type of case for all hospitals in the state taken together. For each individual hospital, we do know the average cost per case and the proportion of cases of each diagnostic type. This information on proportional case-mix and "standard cost" for each type of case can be used to calculate the average cost per case that the hospital would have if its cost for each case type were the same as the standard cost for that case type. More formally,

$$(1) \quad \begin{array}{l}\text{Expected average} \\ \text{cost per case in} \\ \text{hospital } i\end{array} = \sum_{j=1}^{J} p_{ij} c_j^s$$

where p_{ij} is the proportion of cases of type j in hospital i and c_j^s is the standard cost per case of type j.

The costliness of a hospital can then be defined as the ratio of its actual average cost per case to the average cost per case that would be expected on the basis of its case-mix:

$$(2) \quad \begin{array}{l}\text{Costliness of} \\ \text{hospital } i\end{array} = \dfrac{\text{Actual average cost per case in hospital } i}{\text{Expected cost per case in hospital } i}$$

or

$$(3) \quad (\text{Costliness})_i = C_i / \sum_{j=1}^{J} p_{ji} c_j^s$$

where C_i is average cost per case in hospital i. Costliness is thus a measure of cost per case that has "purged" the effect of the hospital's particular case-mix.

This measure of hospital costliness cannot be applied directly because no measure of the "standard cost" for each type of case is available. The basic idea of comparing actual cost to the cost predicted on the basis of the hos-

pital's case-mix can be implemented by using multiple regression analysis. Instead of using the theoretical "standard costs," the multiple regression method calculates the expected cost per case in each hospital as the fitted value of a least squares regression. Costliness is then defined as the ratio of the hospital's actual cost per case to the cost per case predicted by the regression equation.

Since this is the approach that we have actually used, it is worthwhile to present the method in more detail. Assume that the average cost per case and the proportion of cases of J different types is known for N hospitals. We estimate the following equation by the ordinary least squares method of multiple regression:

$$(4) \quad C_i = \sum_{j=1}^{J} \beta_j p_{ij} + U_i$$

where U_i is a random disturbance and β_j is a regression coefficient. The least squares regression estimates, which will be denoted by $\hat{\beta}_j$'s, define the predicted value of the hospital's cost:

$$(5) \quad \hat{C}_i = \sum_{j=1}^{J} \hat{\beta}_j p_{ij} .$$

The costliness value for hospital i is then defined by:

$$(6) \quad \text{Costliness}_i = C_i / \hat{C}_i .$$

The use of least squares multiple regression assures that the $\hat{\beta}_j$'s are chosen to make the predicted $\hat{C}_i$'s correlate as highly with the observed C_i's as possible. This implies that the least squares values of the $\hat{\beta}_j$'s explain as much of the observed variance in the C_i's as possible. Finally, the $\hat{C}_i$'s have the same average value as the observed C_i's.[3]

If the J types of cases are mutually exclusive, the $\hat{\beta}_j$'s can be interpreted as estimates of the standard cost for each case type. More generally, cases may be classified according to several criteria, e.g., diagnosis, age, and surgical procedures. One of the p_{ji}'s may refer to the proportion of patients in a particular age group (regardless of their diagnosis), while another p_{ji} refers to the proportion of patients with a particular diagnosis (regardless of age).[4] This allows the costliness measure to purge the effects of these other factors in a way that assumes no interaction.

In practice, we have modified the multiple regression method by using principal component analysis. This technique will be discussed in the third section. First, however, the data will be described.

The Data

Our analysis brings together two bodies of data on short-term nonteaching hospitals in Massachusetts for 1972. First, all hospitals are required to prepare a detailed statement of hospital costs for use by the Massachusetts Rate Setting Commission in setting official reimbursement rates for Blue Cross, Medicaid and workmen's compensation.[5] The report also indicates the number of inpatient days, discharges and beds in each hospital.

We used these reports to derive total inpatient expenses. Inpatient expenses exclude depreciation and capital expenditures, and expenses for outpatient services, research, education, and other non-patient activities. Newborn infant expenses are excluded for days coinciding with the mother's stay. Although any such allocation of total costs involves arbitrary choices, we believe that the resulting estimates represent a careful, consistent and uniform calculation.

During the 12 months ending on September 30, 1972, the Massachusetts Hospital Association collected information about all of the discharges in 55 short-term nonteaching hospitals. These hospitals represent about half of all the cases in the 119 Massachusetts short-term general hospitals during that year. Cases were classified by primary diagnosis according to the three- or four-digit International Classification of Diseases, Adapted, Eighth Re-

vision.[6] For surgical procedures, cases were classified according to 99 two-digit ICDA8 codes. Finally, information on the age and sex of the patient was recorded.

For the purpose of our analysis, this detailed information was summarized by 152 diagnostic groups, 51 surgical groups and 10 age-sex categories. These aggregations were guided by the logical structure of the ICD code, by information on the number of cases in each detailed category in the entire sample, and by earlier work of Robert Evans on the appropriate classification of case types by relative cost.[7] The age categories for each sex were: 0–14 years, 15–29 years, 30–49 years, 50–64 years, and over 64 years old.

Some basic characteristics of the sample of 55 short-term hospitals used in this sample are described in Table 1. The hospitals ranged in size from 55 beds to 449 with an average of 188. The number of cases discharged in the year varied from less than 1,000 to more than 16,000 with a mean of 6,652. There was very substantial variation in average cost per case. The range from $442 to $1,039 had a mean of $752 and a standard deviation of $152. Similarly, average cost per day varied from $62 to $126, with a mean of $92 and a standard deviation of $13.

Principal Component Analysis

Because we have only 55 observations and more than 200 case-mix variables, it is not possible to include all of the case-mix information directly in a regression equation. We have used the method of principal component analysis to aggregate the detailed case-mix information into a more manageable number of indices that can represent the case-mix of each hospital

Table 1. Characteristics of the sample of 55 short-term hospitals

Variable	Mean	Standard deviation	Minimum	Maximum
Beds	188	102	55	449
Cases	6,652	3,770	756	16,513
Inpatient days	53,768	31,708	8,261	140,800
Average cost per case	$751.91	$151.50	$442.22	$1,039.3
Average cost per day	$99.32	$13.33	$62.37	$125.53
Average length of stay	8.15	1.20	6.09	10.93

Table 2.   Cumulative proportion of total variance accounted for by principal components of diagnostic proportions

Principal component	For cases	For days
1	.11	.09
2	.20	.17
3	.26	.23
4	.31	.29
5	.36	.33
6	.41	.37
7	.45	.41
8	.48	.45
9	.51	.48
10	.54	.51
20	.75	.73
30	.87	.87
40	.95	.94
50	.99	.99

Table 3.   Cumulative proportion of total variance accounted for by principal components of surgical proportions

Principal component	For cases	For days
1	.18	.18
2	.29	.27
3	.36	.34
4	.43	.40
5	.49	.46
6	.54	.51
7	.58	.55
8	.62	.59
9	.65	.63
10	.68	.66
20	.88	.87
30	.96	.96
40	.99	.99
50	1.00	1.00

Since principal component analysis is less familiar than other standard statistical techniques, a brief and nontechnical description is worthwhile.[8] In the current analysis, a principal component index variable is a weighted sum of the individual case-mix proportions. If p_{ji} is the proportion of cases of type j in hospital i, the first principal component variable for hospital i is defined by

$$(7) \quad X_{1j} = \sum_{j=1}^{K} W_{1j} p_{ji}$$

where the weights (W_{1j}'s) are chosen to make X_{1i} the "best possible single representative of all K case-mix proportions." More specifically, X_{1j} is the "best possible" representation of the p_{ji}'s in the sense that X_{1i} accounts for as much of the variance of the p_{ji}'s as possible. Equivalently, if V_j is the variance of the p_{ji}'s and r_{j1} is the correlation of X_1 and p_j, the W_{1j}'s are chosen to maximize $\sum_j r^2_{j1} V_j$.

The first principal component variable will be able to account for much of the variance in the case-mix proportions if the p_{ji}'s are themselves highly intercorrelated. For example, if a hospital with a high fraction of cases of one type is likely to have a high fraction of some other type, the principal component analysis can well summarize the two types with a single variable. More generally, the success of principal component analysis depends on the existence of common characteristics of the hos-

pitals. Fortunately, our analysis shows that this condition prevails.[9]

Table 2 shows the proportion of the variance of the diagnostic case-mix proportions accounted for by different numbers of principal component variables. Thus, the first principal component variable accounts for 11 percent of the variance of all 152 diagnostic categories. Similarly, the first 10 component variables account for 54 percent of the variance. Adding an additional 10 variables only increases this to 75 percent. If the diagnostic mix is recalculated as the proportions of patient days instead of cases, the principal component variables again explain a very large proportion of the variance in the raw proportions. For example, 10 principal component variables account for 51 percent of the original variance.

Principal component variables can also be used to represent the mix of patients according to surgical procedures. Table 3 shows that 10 principal component variables account for 68 percent of the case-mix variance and 66 percent of the patient-day mix.

Finally, Table 4 shows that just two principal component variables can account for two-thirds of the variance in age-sex proportions.

In short, the structure of the hospitals' case-mix is such that a small number of principal component variables can effectively represent the much more detailed data that cannot otherwise be used in the regression.

Table 4. Cumulative proportion of total variance accounted for by principal components of age-sex proportions

Principal component	For cases	For days
1	.48	.39
2	.68	.62
3	.83	.75
4	.90	.84
5	.95	.93
6	.97	.96
7	.98	.98
8	1.00	1.00

Costliness per Case

The principal component variables have been used to derive costliness per case measures based on the method described in the first section. The basic step in this modified procedure is to relate cost per case to the case-mix principal component variables:

$$(8) \quad C_i = \sum_{k=1}^{K} \beta_k X_{ki} + U_i .$$

Least squares regression is used to estimate the β_k's and a fitted or predicted cost per case is calculated as:

$$(9) \quad \hat{C}_i = \sum_{k=1}^{K} \hat{\beta}_k X_{ki}$$

where the $\hat{\beta}_k$'s are the least squares estimates of the β_k's. Costliness is then defined as

$$(10) \quad \text{Costliness}_i = C_i / \hat{C}_i .$$

A variety of different specifications of the X_{ki}'s have been used: diagnostic mix, diagnostic and surgical mix, hospital size, etc. The results are fortunately quite similar. After presenting summary information about each equation, the costliness values will be compared.[10]

Our simplest specification relates average cost per case to the first 10 diagnostic case-mix principal component variables. This specification explains 64 percent of the observed variation in average cost per case; i.e., $R^2 = 0.64$. Even after correcting for the 10 degrees of freedom that are used up in this way, the corrected $\bar{R}^2 = 0.56$. *In short, more than half of the interhospital variation in cost per case can be explained by differences in their case-mix.*[11]

We also experimented with adding to this specification variables that represent hospital size,[12] an indication of whether the hospital is in Boston, and a further case-mix variable that measures the expected average duration per case.[13] Because the estimated coefficients of the hospital size variables have large standard errors despite the substantial variation in observed sizes, it is reasonable to conclude that hospital size *as such* does not affect cost per case.[14]

A hospital's location in Boston raises average cost per case by an estimated $139 after adjusting for case-mix, but this coefficient is also not significantly different from zero; the standard error is $124. Since the number of Boston hospitals in the sample is small (only four), judgment must be reserved on this issue.

Finally, the expected duration variable does add to the explanatory ability of the other case-mix variables. This variable was constructed by finding the average duration for each of the 152 diagnostic types in each of the 10 age-sex groups. These 1,520 average durations were then applied to the corresponding composition of each hospital to get that hospital's average duration. An extra one day's average expected duration, after adjusting for case-mix, adds $109 to average cost per case.

The third specification summarized in Table 5 adds the first five surgical principal component variables to the 10 diagnostic principal component variables. This information on surgical composition adds almost no additional explanatory power. The adjusted $\bar{R}^2$ increases from 0.56 without the surgical variables to 0.57 in the current specification. When the diagnostic mix is given, there appears to be no additional information relevant to hospital costs in the surgical principal component variables.

The fourth equation adds the surgical variables to the expanded specification of equation 2. Hospital size, a Boston location and the surgical variables are again statistically insignificant.

Some evidence that knowledge of the surgical procedures may be important even when the diagnostic variables are given is provided by the fifth equation. Here the number of surgical principal component variables is extended to 10. While equation 4 explained 59 percent of

Table 5. Specifications of cost per case regression equation

Specification	Diagnostic principal components	Surgical principal components	Other variables	$\bar{R}^2$
1	1–10	....	......	0.56
2	1–10	....	Beds, (Beds)² Boston, Expected duration	0.61
3	1–10	1–5	......	0.57
4	1–10	1–5	Beds, (Beds)² Boston, Expected duration	0.59
5	1–10	1–10	Beds, (Beds)² Boston, Expected duration	0.68

the cost per case variation ($\bar{R}^2 = 0.59$), the current specification explains 68 percent ($\bar{R}^2 = 0.68$). Although the difference is not large, it suggests that this more detailed information on case-mix may be relevant.

In this specification, the coefficient of the Boston variable becomes much larger and statistically significant. The coefficient implies that a Boston location raises cost per case by $402 (standard error, $172) after adjustment for diagnostic and surgical procedure differences. Since average cost per case was $760, this represents a very substantial differential. Again, the very small number of Boston hospitals must caution against drawing any strong conclusions from this estimate.

Comparison of Costliness Values

Before comparing the costliness values based on these five specifications, it is worthwhile to point out that our analysis shows that at least two-thirds of the variation in cost per case can be explained by differences in case-mix and location. Only the residual variation can reflect differences in efficiency or quality that are not correlated with case-mix. Recall from Table 1 that average cost per case had a mean of $752 and a standard deviation of $152. With two-thirds of the variance accounted for, the standard deviation of adjusted costs is reduced to only $87. Thus about two-thirds of hospitals (i.e., the range from one standard deviation below the average to one standard deviation above) have an adjusted cost that is within

about 12 percent of the mean instead of the 20 percent if case-mix adjustments are not made. Although there remain some hospitals with unwarrantedly high or low costs, the great majority of hospitals have costs that are very close to the average once case-mix differences are taken into account.[15]

Figure I illustrates how adjusting for case-mix substantially reduces the dispersion of cost per case. The first graph shows the frequency distribution of relative cost per case without any adjustment for case-mix. The relative cost of a hospital is defined here as its cost per case divided by the mean cost per case of $752. The second graph shows the much less disperse distribution of costliness per case using specification 5.

Table 6 shows the intercorrelation of the five costliness variables based on these five specifications. In addition, the correlation of each case-mix variable with observed average cost per case is presented. The costliness values are all more highly correlated with each other than any of them is with cost per case. The low correlation of costliness and cost per case implies that there is a very substantial difference between hospitals' average cost per case and these costs adjusted for differences in case-mix. The observed cost per case is a very poor proxy for the more relevant costliness values. In contrast, the high correlations among the costliness values indicate that each of these alternative measures tells approximately the same story about the costliness of different hospitals.

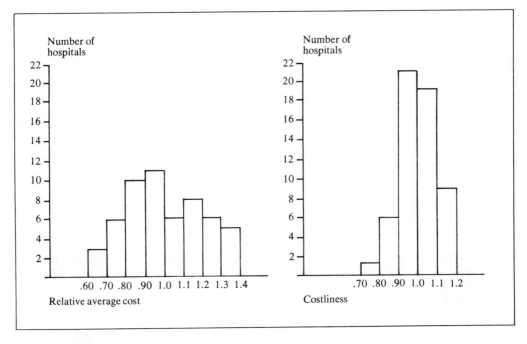

Figure I. **Frequency of hospitals by relative cost and costliness**

The one exception is costliness specification 5 in which 10 surgical case-mix principal component variables are included. The correlation of about 0.75 with the other costliness variables suggests that costliness 5 provides some additional information. Since specification 5 has the highest explanatory power, this costliness measure may be regarded as the most appropriate. There is, however, the danger that the significance of the second five surgical principal components in equation 5 (recall that the first five components were insignificant) is a statistical artifact and that costliness 5 is therefore misleading. A verification with a future set of data is required to resolve this ambiguity.

Costliness per Patient Day

Cost per patient day provides an alternative to cost per case as a crude measure of a hospital's performance. When no adjustment for case-mix has been made, cost per case will vary among hospitals because different case types have different mean durations of stay. The use of cost per patient day is thus a way of eliminating one source of the effect of case-mix on cost. Of course, the effect of case-mix on cost per day is not eliminated by this procedure. Moreover, a new source of distortion is introduced. Hospitals that have longer durations of stay will, other things (including case-mix) equal, have lower cost per day. In general, this reduc-

Table 6. Correlations of cost and costliness values per case

| | Cost per case | Costliness per case | | | | |
		1	2	3	4	5
Cost per case	1.00	0.59	0.51	0.53	0.49	0.38
Costliness 1	...	1.00	0.88	0.91	0.84	0.69
Costliness 2	...	...	1.00	0.87	0.95	0.77
Costliness 3	...	...	...	1.00	0.92	0.73
Costliness 4	...	...	...	...	1.00	0.80
Costliness 5	...	...	...	...	...	1.00

Table 7. Costliness per patient day specifications

Specification	Diagnostic principal components	Surgical principal components	Other variables	$\bar{R}^2$
1	1–10	. . .	. . . .	0.38
2	1–10	. . .	Beds	0.39
3	1–10	1–5	. . . .	0.36
4	1–10	1–5	Beds	0.44
5	1–10	1–10	Beds	0.45

tion in cost per day will be accompanied by a higher cost per case, i.e., an increase in duration of stay causes a less than proportionate reduction in cost per day. For this reason, cost per day, even if adjusted for case-mix, can be a misleading indicator of hospital performance.

We nevertheless estimated costliness measures based on the proportions of patient days in different diagnostic and surgical categories. Table 7 analyzes the results of these specifications which parallel those of Table 5 for cost per case.

The first 10 diagnostic categories account for only 38 percent of the variation in cost per patient day ($\bar{R}^2 = 0.38$).[16] This lower explanatory power in comparison with cost per case is to be expected since part of the cost per case variation reflects case-mix differences in durations of stay. But the remaining explanatory power of case-mix indicates that the use of cost per day is a very inadequate adjustment for case-mix differences.

The Boston location variable never had a significant effect on cost per patient day in our sample. Not surprisingly, the expected duration of stay of the hospital's case-mix was also insignificant in all specifications that we examined. Although the number of beds had a significant negative influence in several specifications, the square of beds was always insig-

nificant. The specifications reported in Table 7 therefore contain the number of beds as the only non-case-mix variable.

Adding beds alone to the 10 diagnostic principal components does not increase the explanatory power of the equation (see equation 2 of Table 7). Similarly, the first five surgical principal components are insignificant in specification 3. But when both the number of beds and the five surgical principal components are combined (specification 4), the coefficients of the number of beds and of the five surgical principal component variables are significant. The specific coefficient of the number of beds implies that an additional 100 beds reduces cost per patient day by $6.86 (standard error, $2.73). Including the first 10 surgical components (specification 5) does not increase the explanatory power of the equation and leaves the effect of size essentially unchanged at $7.36 per 100 beds (standard error, $3.11).

The correlations among cost per patient day and the five costliness values shown in Table 8 generally resemble the pattern shown for cost per case in Table 6. First, cost per patient day has lower correlations with the costliness values than they have among themselves. Second, the individual costliness values are themselves highly intercorrelated. In short, cost per patient day is not a good measure of costliness per

Table 8. Correlations of cost and costliness values per patient day

	Cost per patient day	Costliness per patient day				
		1	2	3	4	5
Cost per patient day	1.00	0.70	0.69	0.67	0.63	0.56
Costliness 1	. . .	1.00	0.98	0.95	0.89	0.80
Costliness 2	. . .	. . .	1.00	0.91	0.90	0.82
Costliness 3	. . .	. . .	. . .	1.00	0.93	0.85
Costliness 4	. . .	. . .	. . .	. . .	1.00	0.92
Costliness 5	. . .	. . . .	. . .	. . .	. . .	1.00

patient day but there is great similarity among the costliness measures.

In concluding this discussion of cost per patient day, it is worthwhile to note that the correlation between cost per patient day and cost per case is only 0.69. More important, the correlations among the costliness values are also low. For example, the specification with 10 diagnostic principal components produces costliness indices with correlation 0.59. The correlations associated with the other specifications are between 0.46 and 0.68. Thus even after eliminating the effects of case-mix, the cost per patient day is a poor measure of cost per case.

Conclusion

We conclude from our analysis that case-mix adjusted costliness is a potentially useful tool of health service management. More than half of the observed variation in cost per case can be explained by a basic principal components measure of case-mix. With the addition of information on location and size and of further information on case-mix, more than two-thirds of the variation in cost per case can be explained. The costliness measure that results from this specification has only a very low correlation with observed cost per case (0.38). Similar results were obtained for cost per patient day. Moreover, even after adjusting for case-mix differences the costliness per patient day had a low correlation with costliness per case.

In short, neither cost per case nor cost per patient day is an adequate measure of a hospital's performance. The case-mix adjusted measure of costliness provides a way of elim-inating a substantial amount of extraneous variation in cost. Because of the limited sample size and the need to use principal component variables, the current specifications are likely to understate the amount of variation that can be explained by a correct case-mix specification. There is, of course, the possibility that differences in efficiency or quality are correlated with case-mix so that these regressions "overcorrect" for the pure effect of case-mix differences.

The costliness per case measure nevertheless provides a basis for dividing hospitals into those with costs that do not depart substantially from their predicted level (e.g., a costliness between 0.90 and 1.10), those with costs that *may* be unduly high (e.g., costliness above 1.10) and those with costs that *may* be unduly low. Administrative attention may then be focused more fruitfully on those hospitals in the high and low categories.

A useful extension of this work would be an analysis of costliness indices for individual components of cost per case, e.g., nursing cost or laboratory fees. It would also be worthwhile to enlarge the sample so that a greater number of variables could be examined.

It is appropriate in conclusion to emphasize that this analysis deals only with *relative* costs. While the dispersion of relative costs is substantial, the rate of increase in all hospital costs is a potentially much more serious problem. The greater challenge to public policy is to develop a mechanism for guiding this increase in average costs so that the scope of hospital services corresponds to the preferences of the people and to their willingness to pay for those services.

References and Notes

1 A similar measure of costliness per patient day can also be constructed. This will be discussed in the fifth section of this paper. To avoid repetition, all of the description will be in terms of costliness per case.

2 The idea of a case-mix adjusted measure of costliness was first developed in: Feldstein, M. *Economic Analysis for Health Service Efficiency* (Amsterdam: North Holland Publishing Co., 1967).

3 The method of least squares regression is a very standard statistical technique. For a more detailed description, see, for example: Johnston, J. *Econometric Methods* (New York: McGraw-Hill, 1963).

4 For a technical reason, one subcategory of each classification beyond the first is not explicitly accounted for.

5 This is the HCF-400 Form, "Hospital Statement for Reimbursement," Commonwealth of Massachusetts, Rate Setting Commission.

6 These classifications are commonly referred to as ICDA8 codes.

7 The final lists of diagnostic categories and of surgical procedures are available from the authors. Evans developed his classification with the assistance of physicians who advised on the likely differences among diagnoses in clinical costliness. See: Evans, Robert G. "Behavioral Cost Functions for Hospitals," *Canadian Journal of Economics* 4:198–215 (May 1971); and Evans, Robert G. and Walker, H. D., "Information Theory and the Analysis of Hospital Cost Structure," *Canadian Journal of Economics* 5: 398–418 (August 1972).

8 For a technical discussion of principal component analysis, see, for example: Kendall, M. G. *A Course in Multivariate Analysis* (New York: Hafner, 1957).

9 The second principal component variable is also constructed as a weighted sum of the individual case-mix proportions. The weights are chosen to account for as much of the variance of the p_{ji}'s not already accounted for by X_1. Further principal component variables are constructed in the same way.

10 The principal component variables for the age and sex mix were never significant; these results are therefore not reported.

11 The basic regression used to derive the costliness measures is as follows: Consider first the regression of cost per case on 10 case-mix principal component variables. Each such variable is a weighted average of the proportions of cases in different diagnostic categories. A weighted average with most of the weight given to predominantly expensive cases will have a positive coefficient, while if the most weight is given to cases of less than average expensiveness its coefficient will be negative.

The principal component variables are constructed to have mean zero, constant standard deviation and statistical independence from each other. The constant term is therefore equal to the mean cost per case and all of the regression coefficients therefore have the same standard deviation, 13.78. We present the t-statistics which show that six of the coefficients are significantly different from zero by standard statistical criteria.

Cost
per $= 752 + 60.1 \times 1 - 9.5 \times 2$
case   (4.4)   (0.7)

$$21.4 \times 3 + 51.0 \times 4 + 24.9 \times 5 + 54.6 \times 6$$
$$(1.6) \qquad (3.7) \qquad (1.8) \qquad (4.0)$$

$$53.9 \times 7 + 22.1 \times 8 - 7.4 \times 9$$
$$(3.9) \qquad (1.6) \qquad (0.5)$$

$$+ 34.8 \times 10$$
$$(2.5)$$

$$\bar{R}^2 = 0.56$$

The corresponding equation for average cost per day is:

Average cost
per day $= 92.3 + 3.1 \times 1 + 5.5 \times 2$
                (2.2)   (3.8)

$$+ 0.3 \times 3 + 2.8 \times 4 - 0.10 \times 5$$
$$(0.2) \qquad (2.0) \qquad (0.1)$$

$$+ 3.1 \times 6 - 1.46 \times 7 + 2.5 \times 8$$
$$(2.1) \qquad (1.6) \qquad (1.7)$$

$$+ 4.3 \times 9 - 2.3 \times 10$$
$$(2.9) \qquad (1.6)$$

$$\bar{R}^2 = 0.38$$

12 Actually, the number of hospital beds and the square of that number.

13 The specifications and their ability to explain the variation in cost per case are summarized in Table 5.

14 Neither coefficient would be significant at the 30 percent level. The point estimates imply a maximum cost per case in hospitals of about 300 beds. But a 500-bed hospital has costs that are only $40 lower, and a 100-bed hospital has costs that are only $80 lower. These estimates are subject to large error and are not statistically significantly different from zero.

15 This represents a much greater explanation of inter-hospital variation in cost per case than Feldstein found for British hospitals. (Feldstein, *Economic Analysis for Health Service Efficiency, op. cit.*) This occurs despite the similar coefficients of variation in Massachusetts (a coefficient of variation of 0.20) and Britain to 0.25. It may reflect the cruder quality of the case-mix data in England. But it may actually say that more of the interhospital cost variation in Massachusetts is justified by case-mix differences.

16 See note 11 for this equation.